GANTZ'S MANUAL OF CLINICAL PROBLEMS IN INFECTIOUS DISEASE

Sixth Edition

James W. Myers, MD

Professor of Internal Medicine, Infectious Diseases
Quillen College of Medicine
East Tennessee State University
Johnson City, Tennessee

Jonathan P. Moorman, MD, PhD, FACP

Professor
Department of Internal Medicine
Division Chief, Infectious Diseases
Quillen College of Medicine
East Tennessee State University
Johnson City, Tennessee

Cassandra D. Salgado, MD, MS

Associate Professor of Medicine
Hospital Epidemiologist
Division of Infectious Diseases
Medical University of South Carolina
Charleston, South Carolina

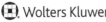
. Wolters Kluwer | Lippincott Williams & Wilkins
Health
Philadelphia · Baltimore · New York · London
Buenos Aires · Hong Kong · Sydney · Tokyo

Acquisitions Editor: Julie Goolsby
Product Manager: Leanne Vandetty
Vendor Manager: Bridgett Dougherty
Senior Manufacturing Manager: Benjamin Rivera
Marketing Manager: Kimberly Schonberger
Design Coordinator: Teresa Mallon
Production Service: SPi Global

Library of Congress Cataloging-in-Publication Data
Gantz's manual of clinical problems in infectious disease / [edited by] James W. Myers, Jonathan P. Moorman, Cassandra D. Salgado. — 6th ed.
    p. ; cm.
    Manual of clinical problems in infectious disease
    Rev. ed. of: Manual of clinical problems in infectious disease / Nelson M. Gantz ... [et al.]. 5th ed. c2006.
    Includes bibliographical references and index.
    ISBN 978-1-4511-1697-7 — ISBN 1-4511-1697-7
I. Myers, James W. (Internist) II. Moorman, Jonathan P. III. Salgado, Cassandra. IV. Gantz, Nelson Murray, 1941- V. Manual of clinical problems in infectious disease. VI. Title: Manual of clinical problems in infectious disease.
    [DNLM: 1. Communicable Diseases–Handbooks. WC 39]
    616.9—dc23

                                                                          2012026643

Care has been taken to confirm the accuracy of the information presented and to describe generally accepted practices. However, the authors, editors, and publisher are not responsible for errors or omissions or for any consequences from application of the information in this book and make no warranty, expressed or implied, with respect to the currency, completeness, or accuracy of the contents of the publication. Application of the information in a particular situation remains the professional responsibility of the practitioner.

The authors, editors, and publisher have exerted every effort to ensure that drug selection and dosage set forth in this text are in accordance with current recommendations and practice at the time of publication. However, in view of ongoing research, changes in government regulations, and the constant flow of information relating to drug therapy and drug reactions, the reader is urged to check the package insert for each drug for any change in indications and dosage and for added warnings and precautions. This is particularly important when the recommended agent is a new or infrequently employed drug.

Some drugs and medical devices presented in the publication have Food and Drug Administration (FDA) clearance for limited use in restricted research settings. It is the responsibility of the health care provider to ascertain the FDA status of each drug or device planned for use in their clinical practice.

To purchase additional copies of this book, call our customer service department at (800) 638-3030 or fax orders to (301) 223-2320. International customers should call (301) 223-2300.

Visit Lippincott Williams & Wilkins on the Internet: at LWW.com. Lippincott Williams & Wilkins customer service representatives are available from 8:30 am to 6 pm, EST.

10 9 8 7 6 5 4 3 2 1

This 6th edition is dedicated to the original authors of *Manual of Clinical Problems in Infectious Disease*—Dr. Richard Gleckman and Dr. Nelson Gantz. They will be remembered by a generation of infectious disease fellows and medical residents as outstanding teachers, clinicians, and scholars.

To my wife Donna who stands by me faithfully as I pursue my career. I would like to thank Dr. Berk for his investment in my career. He has served as my mentor and friend for many years. From my internship through my junior attending years, Dr. Berk has been instrumental in furthering my career. I thank him for inviting me as an editor on the previous edition of this book and hope that we have lived up to his high standards.

— *James W. Myers*

To the many mentors who have steered me throughout the years, and to Susan, my most important guide.

— *Jonathan P. Moorman*

To each student, resident, and fellow I have had the privilege of working with; you all inspire me.

— *Cassandra D. Salgado*

Contributors

Waseem Ahmad, MD
Assistant Professor
Department of Internal Medicine
Division of Infectious Diseases
Quillen College of Medicine
East Tennessee State University
Johnson City, Tennessee

Yasir Ahmed, MD
Department of Internal Medicine
Division of Infectious Diseases
University of South Carolina
Columbia, South Carolina

Helmut Albrecht, MD
Heyward Gibbes Distinguished Professor of
* Internal Medicine*
Division Chief, Division of Infectious
* Diseases*
Department of Internal Medicine
University of South Carolina
Vice Chief of Staff
Palmetto Health Richland
Columbia, South Carolina

Stephan Albrecht
University of South Carolina
Aiken, South Carolina

David B. Banach, MD, MPH
Fellow
Department of Medicine
Mount Sinai School of Medicine
Mount Sinai Hospital
New York, New York

Michael S. Boger, MD, PharmD
Assistant Professor
Division of Infectious Diseases
Attending Physician
Department of Medicine
Medical University of South Carolina
Charleston, South Carolina

Kelsey Burr, MD
Resident Physician
Department of Internal Medicine
University of Tennessee
Nashville, Tennessee

David P. Calfee, MD, MS
Associate Professor
Departments of Medicine and Public Health
Weill Cornell Medical College
Chief Hospital Epidemiologist
Department of Infection Prevention and
* Control*
New York-Presbyterian Hospital/Weill Cornell
New York, New York

Mark B. Carr, MD
Assistant Professor
Department of Internal Medicine
University of Tennessee
Medical Director
Department of Infection Prevention
Baptist Hospital
Nashville, Tennessee

Ioana Chirca, MD
Fellow
Department of Infectious Diseases
Medical University of South Carolina
Charleston, South Carolina

L.W. Preston Church, MD
Hospital Epidemiologist
Ralph H. Johnson VA Medical Center
Charleston, South Carolina

Curtis J. Coley II, MD
Division of Pulmonary and Critical Care
* Medicine*
University of Michigan
Ann Arbor, Michigan

Paul Cook, MD
Professor
Department of Infectious Diseases
East Carolina University
Chief
Department of Infectious Diseases
Vidant Medical Center
Greenville, North Carolina

Sean Cook, MD
Department of Internal Medicine
Division of Infectious Diseases
University of South Carolina
Columbia, South Carolina

Michael Davis, MD
Fellow
Department of Medicine
Division of Infectious Diseases
Quillen College of Medicine
Eastern Tennessee State University
Johnson City, Tennessee

Santosh Dhungana, MD
Medical Resident
University of Tennessee Health Science
Center
Memphis, Tennessee
Baptist Hospital
Nashville, Tennessee

Ivar L. Frithsen, MD
Assistant Professor
Department of Family Medicine
Medical Director
Employee Health Services
Medical University of South Carolina
Charleston, South Carolina

Melanie Gerrior, MD
Division of Infectious Diseases
Medical University of South Carolina
Charleston, South Carolina

Amanda Guedes de Morais, MD
Fellow
Department of Internal Medicine
Division of Infectious Diseases
Quillen College of Medicine
East Tennessee State University
Johnson City, Tennessee

Keith W. Hamilton, MD
Instructor
Infectious Diseases Division, Department of
Medicine
University of Pennsylvania
Associate Director of Healthcare
Epidemiology, Infection Prevention and
Control
Infectious Diseases Division, Department of
Medicine
Hospital of the University of Pennsylvania
Philadelphia, Pennsylvania

Susan Harwell, MD
Resident Physician
Department of Medicine
University of Tennessee Health Sciences
Center
Memphis, Tennessee
Consultant
Department of Internal Medicine
Baptist Hospital
Nashville, Tennessee

Lamis Ibrahim, MD
Assistant Professor
Department of Internal Medicine
Division of Infectious Diseases
Quillen College of Medicine
East Tennessee State University
Johnson City, Tennessee

Michael G. Ison, MD, MS
Associate Professor
Division of Infectious Diseases and Organ
Transplantation
Northwestern University Feinberg School of
Medicine
Medical Director
Transplant and Immunocompromised Host
Infectious Diseases
Northwestern Memorial Hospital
Chicago, Illinois

Oluwatosin Jaiyeoba, MD
Fellow
Department of Obstetrics and Gynecology
Division of Infectious Diseases, Department
of Medicine
Medical University of South Carolina
Charleston, South Carolina

Joseph F. John, Jr, MD
Associate Chief of Staff for Education
Ralph H. Johnson Department of Veterans
Affairs Medical Center
Division of Infectious Diseases
Medical University of South Carolina
Charleston, South Carolina

Evgenia Kagan, MD
Assistant Professor of Medicine
Department of Medicine, Infectious Disease
  Division
Medical University of South Carolina
Charleston, South Carolina

Amit Kalra, MD
Internal Medicine Resident PGY III
Department of Internal Medicine
East Tennessee State University
Johnson City, Tennessee

Abdel Kareem Abu Malouh, MD
Fellow
Department of Internal Medicine
Division of Infectious Diseases
Quillen College of Medicine
East Tennessee State University
Johnson City, Tennessee

J. Michael Kilby, MD
Professor
Department of Medicine
Medical University of South Carolina
Charleston, South Carolina

Jayalakshmi Kuseladass, MD
Resident Physician
Department of Medicine
University of Tennessee Health Sciences
  Center
Memphis, Tennessee
Resident Physician
Department of Internal Medicine
Baptist Hospital
Nashville, Tennessee

Ebbing Lautenbach, MD, MPH, MSCE
Associate Professor of Medicine
Department of Medicine
University of Medicine
Director of Research
Hospital Epidemiology
Hospital of the University of
  Pennsylvania
Philadelphia, Pennsylvania

Paul Lewis, PharmD, BCPS
Clinical Pharmacist Specialist – Infectious
  Diseases
Johnson City Medical Center
Johnson City, Tennessee
Adjunct Faculty, Clinical Preceptor
Gatton College of Pharmacy
East Tennessee State University
Johnson City, Tennessee

Claire E. Magauran, MD
Department of Internal Medicine
Tufts University School of Medicine
Boston, Massachusetts
Infectious Disease Attending
Division of Infectious Diseases
Baystate Medical Center
Springfield Massachusetts

Sunanda Mangraj, MD
Fellow
Department of Medicine
Division of Infectious Diseases
Quillen College of Medicine
Eastern Tennessee State University
Johnson City, Tennessee

Camelia E. Marculescu, MD, MSCR
Assistant Professor of Medicine
Department of Medicine, Infectious Disease
  Division
Medical University of South Carolina
Charleston, South Carolina

Anil Mathew, MD
Fellow
Department of Medicine
Division of Infectious Diseases
Quillen College of Medicine
Eastern Tennessee State University
Johnson City, Tennessee

Paul C. McNabb, MD
Professor, Medicine-Infectious Disease
The University of Tennessee Health Science
  Center
Memphis, Tennessee

Holly B. Meadows, PharmD
Clinical Assistant Professor
Department of Clinical Pharmacy and
  Outcome Sciences
South Carolina College of Pharmacy
Clinical Pharmacy Specialist—Solid Organ
  Transplant
Department of Pharmacy Services
Medical University of South Carolina
Charleston, South Carolina

Melissa A. Miller, MD, MS
Clinical Lecturer
Department of Internal Medicine, Division
  of Pulmonary and Critical Care Medicine
University of Michigan
University of Michigan Hospital and Health
  Systems
Ann Arbor, Michigan

Jonathan P. Moorman, MD, PhD, FACP
Professor
Department of Internal Medicine
Division Chief, Infectious Diseases
Quillen College of Medicine
East Tennessee State University
Johnson City, Tennessee

Carlene A. Muto, MD, MS
Associate Professor of Medicine and
  Epidemiology
Division of Hospital Epidemiology and
  Infection Control
University of Pittsburgh Medical Center
Presbyterian Campus
Pittsburgh, Pennsylvania

James W. Myers, MD
Professor of Internal Medicine, Infectious
  Diseases
Quillen College of Medicine
East Tennessee State University
Johnson City, Tennessee

Tue H. Ngo, MD, MPH
Assistant Professor of Medicine
Department of Medicine
Medical University of South Carolina
Charleston, South Carolina

Emmanuel Okon, MD
Fellow
Department of Medicine
Division of Infectious Diseases
James H. Quillen College of Medicine
East Tennessee State University
Johnson City, Tennessee
Infectious Diseases Consultant
Virtua Voorhees Hospital
Voorhees, New Jersey

Christopher H. Parsons, MD
Assistant Professor
Department of Medicine
Medical University of South Carolina
Charleston, South Carolina

Paras Patel, MD
Assistant Professor
Department of Internal Medicine
Division of Infectious Diseases
Quillen College of Medicine
East Tennessee State University
Johnson City, Tennessee

Sabena Ramsetty, MD
Hospitalist
Hudson Valley Hospital Physicians
Orange Regional Medical Center
Middletown, New York

Ramzy H. Rimawi, MD
Fellow
Department of Infectious Diseases
East Carolina University
Vidant Medical Center
Greenville, North Carolina

Hana Saleh, MD
Internal Medicine Resident
Department of Internal Medicine
East Tennessee State University,
  James H. Quillen College of Medicine
Johnson City, Tennessee

Cassandra D. Salgado, MD, MS
Associate Professor of Medicine
Hospital Epidemiologist
Division of Infectious Diseases
Medical University of South Carolina
Charleston, South Carolina

Michael J. Satlin, MD
Instructor in Medicine
Department of Internal Medicine
Weill Cornell Medical College
Assistant Attending Physician
Department of Internal Medicine
New York-Presbyterian Hospital
New York, New York

Wael E. Shams, MD
Assistant Professor
Department of Internal Medicine
Division of Infectious Diseases
East Tennessee State University
Johnson City, Tennessee

Christopher Trabue, MD
Assistant Professor
Department of Internal Medicine
University of Tennessee Health Sciences
  Center
Memphis, Tennessee
Consultant
Department of Infectious Diseases
Baptist Hospital
Nashville, Tennessee

Ashley Tyler, PharmD, BCPS
Clinical Assistant Professor
College of Pharmacy
University of Tennessee Health Sciences
  Center
Memphis, Tennessee
Clinical Pharmacy Specialist
Department of Pharmacy
Baptist Hospital
Nashville, Tennessee

Ellie S. Walker, MD
Resident Physician
Department of Internal Medicine
Northwestern University Feinberg School of
  Medicine
Northwestern Memorial Hospital
Chicago, Illinois

Zhi Q. Yao, MD, PhD
Associate Professor
Department of Internal Medicine
Division of Infectious Disease
Quillen College of Medicine
East Tennessee State University
Johnson City, Tennessee

Dima Youssef, MD
Assistant Professor
Department of Internal Medicine
Division of Infectious Disease
Quillen College of Medicine
East Tennessee State University
Johnson City, Tennessee

Preface

In 1979, at the request of their students and house officers, Drs. Richard Gleckman and Nelson Gantz prepared the first edition of *Manual of Clinical Problems in Infectious Disease*. At the time, their aim was to provide medical students, house officers, and practitioners with a contemporary approach to selected problems in infectious disease: key annotated references supported the text. Since that time, numerous infectious agents have been recognized, new concepts have evolved, and new treatments have emerged. Nevertheless, our target audience and objective are the same as our predecessors'.

The sixth edition of *Manual of Clinical Problems in Infectious Disease* is not simply an updated version of the five earlier books but a new approach: it focuses on key problems in infectious disease in a terse, organized, user-friendly fashion that capitalizes on the wealth of Internet information currently available to clinicians. Advances in many areas of infectious disease, including HIV, HCV, and transplantation infection, are presented. We have added additional topics for which there are limited resources, including interpreting antimicrobial sensitivity reports, therapeutic drug monitoring, and antibiotic dosing in obesity and pregnancy. For this edition, we are pleased to add Drs. Cassie Salgado and Jonathan Moorman to the team. Every effort has been made to add contemporary references and links to the text to enhance the accuracy of the manual and to provide a springboard for further reading; many references are annotated.

Like all previous editions, this manual is not meant to be all-inclusive. Numerous major texts that fulfill this mission have already been published. The sixth edition of *Manual of Clinical Problems in Infectious Disease* represents an attempt to provide contemporary, scientifically accurate, and readable material on selected topics of concern to the practicing physician, house officer, and medical student. All of the editors are clinicians who see patients on a regular basis and have written chapters based on a "real world" approach to patient care while keeping with a scientific basis of management. Chapters have been added, removed, or revised in keeping with changes in infectious disease over the past several years. We are proud of our effort and feel that this book will prove valuable to the clinician in the day-to-day management of patients with infectious disease.

Since the fifth edition was published, we have mourned the loss of Nelson Gantz and Richard Gleckman. They were both superb clinicians, scholars, mentors, and educators whose vision brought this manual to fruition over 30 years ago. We dedicate this current edition to their memory.

James W. Myers, MD
Cassandra D. Salgado, MD, MS
Jonathan P. Moorman, MD, PhD, FACP

Contents

AIDS

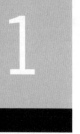

1

Role of HIV Resistance Testing in the Treatment of HIV Infection

Melanie Gerrior and Christopher Parsons

INTRODUCTION

- Acquired resistance of HIV to available antiretroviral agents (ARVs) remains a worldwide concern. Soon after zidovudine (AZT, ZDV) received approval by the FDA in 1987 for the treatment of HIV infection, patients began experiencing treatment failure related to HIV resistance to this agent.[13]
- Early-generation resistance tests, developed in 1989, identified the dose for individual ARVs necessary to inhibit 50% of HIV growth.[7] Technology ultimately advanced with the use of polymerase chain reaction (PCR) to identify mutations within the HIV genome responsible for resistance to specific ARVs.
- HIV genome sequencing uncovered additional complexities related to HIV resistance. For example, although HIV encodes only nine genes, mutations were identified that confer resistance to one drug or an entire class of drugs or that actually *increase* HIV sensitivity to ARVs.
- HIV-1 subtype B predominates in the developed world and is the focus of the majority of susceptibility studies, though it accounts for only 12% of all HIV subtypes worldwide.[12]
- Results of HIV resistance testing are best interpreted by experienced HIV providers in the context of many factors that may influence drug resistance, including compliance and the results of laboratory determinants of successful therapy.

ACQUISITION OF RESISTANCE

- The genome sequence of HIV recovered prior to initiation of highly active antiretroviral therapy (HAART) is referred to as the "wild-type" (WT) sequence. This "WT virus" does not reflect the genetic code of a single viral "clone," but rather the most replication-competent viral clones (or "species") within the patient's circulation. In other words, it reflects many species (referred to as "quasispecies"), all of which replicate billions of times per day. WT virus exhibits drug resistance in 15% to 20% of patients.[9]
- Intrinsic drug resistance may occur due to errors in viral transcription in the absence of exposure to HAART.[6]
- Fully suppressive HAART was not available to patients until the mid-1990s (with the advent of protease inhibitors [PIs]). Therefore, many patients diagnosed with HIV early in the epidemic were receiving ARVs that did not fully suppress HIV replication, facilitating the development of drug resistance mutations.[8]
- Suboptimal medication adherence, AVR interactions with other medications that increase or decrease effective blood levels (i.e., P450 inducers), and transmission of

drug resistance from person to person (intravenous drug abuse and mother-to-child transmission) also contribute to the prevalence of HIV drug resistance.

- Resistant quasispecies are often not identified until the predominant WT virus is suppressed during HAART therapy. Drug-resistant quasispecies are typically present in insufficient quantities (>10% of all circulating species in the presence of the more replication-competent WT virus) to permit their detection. Therefore, for treatment-experienced patients, HIV resistance testing should be performed in the presence of HAART therapy.

HIV GENOTYPE TESTING

- Commercial assays, referred to as "genotypes," sequence the HIV genome to identify mutations associated with drug resistance for HIV.
- An individual patient's collective HIV species, isolated from whole blood following venipuncture, is typically labeled as "susceptible," "possibly resistant," or "resistant" to each ARV tested based on the presence or absence of well-characterized mutations in the HIV genome.
- Reports include mutations that confer resistance of HIV to ARVs *in vitro* (cell culture) and that have been associated with treatment failure for HIV patients.
- Mutations are reported as a letter-number-letter sequence. The first letter represents the wild-type amino acid; the number represents the position of the mutation within the genome, and the second letter represents the amino acid substituted that confers resistance. Some mutations have not exhibited significant individual or synergistic contributions to HIV drug resistance, and we will not discuss these further.
- Some drug classes exhibit a high barrier to resistance (e.g., HIV PIs), requiring the presence of several mutations before partial or complete drug resistance occurs.[4,5] Other classes exhibiting a low barrier to resistance (e.g., nucleoside and nonnucleoside reverse transcriptase inhibitors) may require only one mutation to render drugs in these classes inactive.[10]
- Some mutations occur in a predictable pattern when HIV is only partially suppressed, as with thymidine analogue-associated mutations (TAMs) arising with inadequate treatment using nucleoside/nucleotide reverse transcriptase inhibitors (NRTIs).
- Several genotype assays are available involving allele-specific PCR, multiplex primer extension, and so-called deep sequencing. Frequently utilized assays employ some variation of these protocols to identify specific mutations within the most prevalent quasispecies (comprising >10% of all species).
- Indications for performing the genotype assay include the following scenarios: (i) after HIV diagnosis and before HAART administration, (ii) during HAART therapy with repeatedly detectable HIV viral load (typically >1,000 copies/mL to allow for optimal genome sequencing), (iii) pregnancy, and (iv) postexposure prophylaxis (we recommend genotype testing for the source individual in cases of high-risk exposure if possible in order to help guide therapy in the event of eventual HIV infection of the exposed patient).[7]
- Genotypes are less costly, and their results are available in a more timely manner, relative to other resistance assays. However, genotypes do not account for the impact of combinations of different mutations, nor do they account for mechanisms of resistance unrelated to well-characterized mutations (including potential impact of novel mutations).[11]
- More information regarding resistance mutations can be obtained from a number of resources, including The Stanford University HIV Drug Resistance Database (http://hivdb.stanford.edu/) and the DHHS HIV Treatment Guidelines.

- The following are lists of well-characterized mutations for each class of currently available ARVs, including specific mutations conferring resistance to individual ARVs (with most common and clinically relevant mutations in bold):

Nucleoside/Nucleotide Reverse Transcriptase Inhibitors

- See Table 1-1 for further characterization
- 69 insertion complex: renders all NRTIs ineffective via impairment of drug incorporation
- Q151M: renders all NRTIs except tenofovir ineffective via impairment of drug incorporation
- TAMs: (M41L[1], D67N[2], K70R[2], L210W[1], T215Y/F[1], K219Q/E[2]) render all NRTIs ineffective via an increased rate of excision of drug from the DNA terminus. Two TAM resistance patterns are noted (superscripts 1 and 2). Type 2 resistance mutations may increase susceptibility to nonnucleoside reverse transcriptase inhibitors (NNRTIs) in NNRTI-naïve patients.
- L74V and M184V: increase susceptibility to AZT, TDF, and d4T
- M184V: confers resistance to other NRTIs through impairment of drug incorporation, although ddI, FTC, and 3TC retain some activity (Table 1-1)
- Abacavir (ABC)—**K65R**
- Didanosine (ddI)—K65R
- Emtricitabine (FTC)—**K65R, M184V**
- Lamuvidine (3TC)—**K65R, M184V**
- Tenofovir (TDF)—**K65R**, K30E
- Stavudine (d4T)—M41L, K65R, D67N, K70R, L210W, T215Y/F, K219Q/E
- Zidovudine (AZT, ZDV)—M41L, D67N, K70R, L210W, T215Y/F, K219Q/E

Nonnucleoside Reverse Transcriptase Inhibitors

- K103N/S is the most common mutation identified following initiation of NNRTI therapy. It confers resistance to first-generation NNRTIs efavirenz and nevirapine but not to second-generation NNRTIs etravirine or rilpivirine
- Efavirenz (EFV)—**K103N**, Y181C/I, Y188I
- Nevirapine (NVP)—**K103N**, Y181C/I, Y188C/L/H
- Etravirine (ETR)—**Y181C/I/V**, **G190S/A**, L100I, K101E/H/P, E138KA/G/K[2], Y181C/I/V, M230L; no single mutation conferring high-level resistance has been identified, and two weighted scoring systems (Monogram and Tibotec) are used to

Table 1-1	Nucleoside Analogue	
Nucleoside, Nucleotide	**HAART Analogue**
Adenosine	Didanosine (ddI)
	Tenofovir (TDF)
Cytosine	Zalcitabine (ddC)
	Lamivudine (3TC)
	Emtricitabine (FTC)
Thymidine	Zidovudine (AZT, ZDV)
	Stavudine (d4T)
Guanosine	Abacavir (ABC)

predict Etravirine resistance: Tibotec scoring ≥4 = resistant, 2.5–3.5 = intermediate, 0–2 = susceptible; Monogram scoring ≥4 = reduced susceptibility; Y181C/I/V is the most common mutation and is assigned a score of 4 per Monogram system; G190S/A is the second most common mutation and is assigned a score of 4 per Tibotec system

• Rilpivirine (RPV)—**E138K**, **M184I**, Y181I/V, K101E/P; E138K increases resistance by 2.8 fold; E138K + M184I combination increases resistance by 6.7 fold

Protease Inhibitors

• Atazanavir (ATV)—**I50L**, **I84V**, **N88S**, V82 A/T/F/I, L10I/F/V/C, I90M; I50L does not produce cross-resistance with other PIs
• Darunavir (DRV)—**I50V**, **I54M/L**, **I47V**, **I84V**, L76V, T74P, V32I
• Fosamprenavir (FPV)—**I50V**, **I84V**, L10F/I/R/V, V82 A/F/S/T, I90M
• Indinavir (IDV)—**I84V**, **M46I/L**, **V82A/F/T**, L10I/R/V, M36I, L90M
• Lopinavir (LPV)—**V32I**, **I47V/A**, **L76V**, **V82A/F/T/S**, L10F/I/R/V, I84V, L90M
• Nelfinavir (NFV)—**L90M**, **D30N**, L10F/I, V82A/F/T/S, I84V
• Saquinavir (SQV)—**L90M**, **G48V**, L10I/R/V, V82A/F/T/S, I84V
• Tipranavir (TPV)—**I47V**, **Q58E**, **T74P**, **N83D**, **I84V**, **V82L/T**, L10V

Integrase Inhibitors

• Raltegravir (RAL)—**N155H**, **Q148H/K/R**, Y143R/H/C, E92Q; most common is N155H that increases resistance 10-fold; Q148H/K/R, increases resistance 25-fold

PHENOTYPE TESTING

• Two commercial phenotypic resistance assays (or "phenotypes") are currently available: the Antivirogram (Virco NV, Belgium) and PhenoSense (LabCorp, Burlington, North Carolina). These assays involve creation of recombinant viruses incorporating HIV-encoded genes from a patient's circulating HIV isolate, followed by assessment of their replication capacity in the presence of individual ARVs over a range of drug concentrations. Both assays compare the concentration of drug required to inhibit 50% of baseline replication (IC50) of the recombinant virus to the IC50 for a reference strain.
• Results are displayed as a fold change in IC50 (relative to the reference strain).
• One advantage of phenotypes is that they evaluate drug activity in the presence of all mutations found in the patient's viral genome (thereby accounting for the potential importance of all mutations collectively rather than only well-characterized individual mutations).[3] In addition, they can be used to assess drug activity against non–B subtype viruses for which only limited data are available regarding the relative importance of individual mutations.
• Phenotypes are more expensive than genotypes, and phenotype results are available in a less timely fashion relative to genotypes.

TROPISM TESTING

• HIV proteins bind to chemokine receptors during initial viral entry to host cells. The two best characterized of these receptors are CCR5 and CXCR4.
• New agents, referred to as "entry inhibitors," inhibit HIV interactions with these receptors.

- Only one of these agents, maraviroc, is currently available for clinical use and is approved only for treatment-experienced patients in whom it may further suppress HIV replication. It must be used with other ARVs to which a patient's HIV isolate is fully susceptible.
- The utility of this agent can be reasonably predicted with either of two commercially available tests: the Trofile assay (LabCorp, Burlington, North Carolina) and the Phenoscript assay (VIRalliance, Paris, France).
- These assays involve creation of recombinant viruses incorporating genes expressing patient-derived HIV envelope proteins that are then used to infect cell lines expressing either CCR5 or CXCR4.
- Results of these infectivity assays define tropism for the patient's isolate and are reported as CCR5 ("R5") tropic, CXCR4 ("X4") tropic, or dual/mixed ("D/M," meaning that the virus utilizes both X4 and R5 receptors).
- Optimal clinical results with maraviroc are anticipated when R5 tropic virus is identified using this assay.

REFERENCES

1. Adams J, Patel N, Mankaryous N, et al. Nonnucleoside reverse transcriptase inhibitor resistance and the role of the second-generation agents. *Ann Pharmacother* 2010;44:157.
2. Asahchop EL, Oliveira M, Wainberg MA, et al. Characterization of the E138K resistance mutation in HIV-1 reverse transcriptase conferring susceptibility to etravirine in B and non-B HIV-1 subtypes. *Antimicrob Agents Chemother* 2011;55:600–607.
3. Barbour JD, et al. Evolution of phenotypic drug susceptibility and viral replication capacity during long-term virologic failure of protease inhibitor therapy in human immunodeficiency virus-infected adults. *J Virol* 2002;76:11104–11112.
4. Delaugerre C, Buyck JF, Peytavin G, et al. Factors predictive of successful darunavir/ritonavir-based therapy in highly antiretroviral-experienced HIV-1-infected patients (the DARWEST study). *J Clin Virol* 2010;47:248–252.
5. De Meyer S, Lathouwers E, Dierynck I, et al. Characterization of virologic failure patients on darunavir/ritonavir in treatment-experienced patients. *AIDS* 2009;23:1829–1840.
6. Gianella S, Richman DD. Minority variants of drug-resistant HIV. *J Infect Dis* 2010;202(5):657–666.
7. Hirsch MS, Günthard HF, Schapiro JM, et al. Antiretroviral drug resistance testing in adult HIV-1 infection: 2008 recommendations of an International AIDS Society-USA panel. *Clin Infect Dis* 2008;47:266–285.
8. Larder BA, Kemp SD. Multiple mutations in HIV-1 reverse transcriptase confer high-level resistance to zidovudine (AZT). *Science* 1989;246(4934):1155–1158.
9. Little SJ, Holte S, Routy J-P et al. Antiretroviral-drug resistance among patients recently infected with HIV. *N Engl J Med* 20;347(6):385–394.
10. Li J, et al. Low-frequency HIV-1 drug resistance mutations and risk of NNRTI-based antiretroviral treatment failure. *JAMA* 2011;305(13):1327–1335.
11. Llibre JM, Schapiro JM, Clotet B. Clinical implications of genotypic resistance to the newer antiretroviral drugs in HIV-1-infected patients with virological failure. *Clin Infect Dis* 2010;50:872–881.
12. Osmanov S, et al. Estimated global distribution and regional spread of HIV-1 genetic subtypes in the year 2000. *J Acquir Immune Defic Syndr* 2002;29(2):184–190.
13. Richman DD. Susceptibility to nucleoside analogues of zidovudine-resistant isolates of human immunodeficiency virus. *Am J Med* 1990;88(5B):8S–10S.

Opportunistic Infections in AIDS

Yasir Ahmed, Sean Cook, and Helmut Albrecht

An opportunistic infection (OI) is an infection caused by pathogens that usually do not cause disease in a host with a healthy immune response but may have an "opportunity" to do so in patients with a compromised immune system. In patients with HIV infection, OIs are defined as infections that are either more frequent or more severe due to advancing immunosuppression.

In the early 1990s, the introduction of prophylactic medications and better treatment strategies for the management of acute OIs led to improved survival in patients with HIV. In the mid-1990s, the introduction and widespread use of potent antiretroviral therapy (ART) regimens led to a profound reduction of OI-related mortality.[1] Despite the availability of potent ART, however, OIs continue to be a leading cause of both morbidity and mortality in patients with HIV and AIDS.[2]

The degree of immunosuppression, as measured by CD4 cell counts, in most instances correlates with the risk of specific OIs (Table 2-1).

While the list can be used for risk stratification, it should be noted that CD4 cell counts are unreliable in acutely ill patients or in patients with other immunocompromising conditions (such as end-stage renal disease or postsplenectomy). The following lists pertinent features of common or important OIs. Additional information is available elsewhere[2] and treatment options are summarized in Table 2-2.

PNEUMOCYSTIS JIROVECII PNEUMONIA

Pulmonary infection with the fungal pathogen *Pneumocystis jirovecii* causes *Pneumocystis jirovecii* pneumonia (PJP or PCP). PCP clinically presents as a subacute process with progressive dyspnea, fever, and nonproductive cough that has been worsening over several weeks prior to presentation.

Initial radiography may not show disease, but patients with severe illness typically present with bilateral interstitial infiltrates with perihilar distribution. A significant elevation of the serum lactate dehydrogenase (LDH) is often present, but this finding is nonspecific. Hypoxemia may be present and may become severe. HIV-infected adults should receive primary PCP prophylaxis if they have a CD4+ count of <200 cells/μL, a CD4+ cell percentage of <14%, or a history of an AIDS-defining illness or oropharyngeal candidiasis. Trimethoprim-sulfamethoxazole one double-strength tablet daily is the preferred agent, but dapsone, atovaquone, and aerosolized pentamidine constitute alternative options.[2]

TOXOPLASMOSIS ENCEPHALITIS

Toxoplasmosis encephalitis (TE) caused by *Toxoplasma gondii* is almost exclusively due to reactivation of preexisting disease. Initial presentation typically involves

Table 2-1	Risk Stratification for Specific Opportunistic Infections by CD4 Cell Count

CD4 Count	Opportunistic Infection(s)
>200	Tuberculosis, KS
<200	Tuberculosis, KS, PCP, disseminated histoplasmosis
<100	*Toxoplasma gondii* encephalitis, cryptococcal meningitis, cryptosporidiosis, microsporidiosis
<50	DMAC, CMV infection, PML

Table 2-2	Drug Therapy for Treatment and Chronic Maintenance Therapy of AIDS-Associated OIs in Adults and Adolescents

OI	Preferred Therapy, Duration of Therapy, Chronic Maintenance	Alternative Therapy
PCP	*Preferred treatment for moderate to severe PCP* • Trimethoprim-sulfamethoxazole (TMP-SMX) (15–20-mg TMP and 75–100-mg SMX)/kg/day IV administered q6h or q8h **(AI)**, may switch to PO after clinical improvement **(AI)** *Indications for corticosteroids **(AI)*** $PaO_2 < 70$ mm Hg at room air or alveolar-arterial O_2 gradient >35 mm Hg Dose of prednisone: Days 1–5: 40 mg PO b.i.d. Days 6–10 40 mg PO q.d. Days 11–21: 20 mg PO q.d. *Preferred treatment for mild to moderate PCP* •Trimethoprim-sulfamethoxazole (TMP-SMX) DS 2 tablets PO t.i.d. **(AI)** • Duration of therapy for PCP is 21 days **(AII)**.	*Alternative therapy for moderate to severe PCP* • Pentamidine 4 mg/kg IV daily infused over ≥60 minutes **(AI)**, certain specialists reduce dose to 3 mg/kg IV daily because of toxicities **(BI)**; or • Primaquine 15–30 mg (base) PO daily plus clindamycin 600–900 mg IV q6h to q8h or clindamycin 300–450 mg PO q6h to q8h **(AI)** *Alternative therapy for mild to moderate PCP* • Dapsone 100 mg PO daily and TMP 15 mg/kg/day PO (three divided doses) **(BI)**; or • Primaquine 15–30 mg (base) PO daily plus clindamycin 300–450 mg q6–8h **(BI)**; or • Atovaquone 750 mg b.i.d. PO **(BI)**

Table 2-2	Drug Therapy for Treatment and Chronic Maintenance Therapy of AIDS-Associated OIs in Adults and Adolescents *(Continued)*

OI	Preferred Therapy, Duration of Therapy, Chronic Maintenance	Alternative Therapy
Toxoplasma gondii encephalitis	*Preferred therapy* • Pyrimethamine 200 mg PO × 1, then 50–75 mg PO daily plus sulfadiazine 1,000–1,500 mg PO q6h plus leucovorin 10–25 mg PO daily **(AI)** Duration for acute therapy • At least 6 weeks **(BII)**; longer duration if clinical or radiologic disease is extensive or response is incomplete at 6 weeks • Adjunctive corticosteroids (e.g., dexamethasone) should be administered when clinically indicated.	*Alternative therapy regimens* • Pyrimethamine (leucovorin)* plus clindamycin 600 mg IV or PO **(AI)**; or • TMP-SMX (5 mg/kg TMP and 25 mg/kg SMX) IV or PO b.i.d. **(BI)**; or • Atovaquone 1,500 mg PO b.i.d. with food (or nutritional supplement) plus pyrimethamine (leucovorin)***(BII)**; or • Atovaquone 1,500 mg PO b.i.d. plus sulfadiazine 1,000–1,500 mg PO q6h **(BII)**; or • Atovaquone 1,500 mg b.i.d. PO **(BII)**; or • Pyrimethamine (leucovorin)* plus azithromycin 900–1,200 mg PO daily **(BII)**
Cryptosporidiosis	*Preferred therapy* • Initiate or optimize ART for immune restoration **(AII)** • Symptomatic treatment of diarrhea **(AII)** • Aggressive oral or IV rehydration and replacement of electrolyte loss **(AIII)**	*Alternative therapy for cryptosporidiosis* • A trial of nitazoxanide 500–1,000 mg PO b.i.d. with food for 14 days **(CIII)** + optimized ART, symptomatic treatment and rehydration and electrolyte replacement
Microsporidiosis	Initiate or optimize ART; immune restoration to CD4+ count >100 cells/μL is associated with resolution of symptoms of enteric microsporidiosis **(AII)**.	
M. tuberculosis (TB)	Empiric treatment should be initiated and continued in HIV-infected persons in whom TB is suspected until all diagnostic workup is complete **(AII)**.	

(Continued)

Table 2-2	Drug Therapy for Treatment and Chronic Maintenance Therapy of AIDS-Associated OIs in Adults and Adolescents *(Continued)*

OI	Preferred Therapy, Duration of Therapy, Chronic Maintenance	Alternative Therapy
	Treatment of drug-suscepti-ble active TB disease Initial phase (2 months) **(AI)** • Isoniazid (INH)† + [rifampin (RIF) or rifabu-tin (RFB)] + pyrazinamide (PZA) + ethambutol (EMB); if drug suscepti-bility report shows sen-sitivity to INH and RIF and PZA, then EMB may be discontinued before 2 months of treatment is completed **(AI)** Continuation phase • INH + (RIF or RFB) daily or t.i.w. **(AIII)** or biw (if CD4+ count >100/μL) **(CIII)** Duration of therapy: Pulmo-nary TB—6 months **(AI)** Pulmonary TB with cavitary lung lesions and (+) cul-ture after 2 months of TB treatment **(AII)**—9 months Extrapulmonary TB with CNS, bone, or joint infec-tions—9 to 12 months **(AII)** • Directly observed therapy (DOT) is recommended for all HIV patients under-going treatment for active TB **(AII)**.	*Treatment for drug-resistant active TB* Resistant to INH • Discontinue INH (and streptomycin, if used) • (RIF or RFB) + EMB + PZA for 6 months **(BII)**; or • (RIF or RFB) + EMB for 12 months (preferably with PZA during at least the first 2 months) **(BII)** • A fluoroquinolone may strengthen the regimen for patients with extensive disease **(CIII)**. • Therapy should be individ-ualized based on resis-tance pattern and with close consultation with experienced specialist **(AIII)**.
DMAC disease	*Preferred therapy for DMAC* At least two drugs as initial therapy with • Clarithromycin 500 mg PO b.i.d. **(AI)** + ethambutol 15 mg/kg PO daily **(AI)**	*Alternative therapy for DMAC* • Azithromycin 500–600 mg + ethambutol 15 mg/kg PO daily **(AII)**

Table 2-2	Drug Therapy for Treatment and Chronic Maintenance Therapy of AIDS-Associated OIs in Adults and Adolescents *(Continued)*

OI	Preferred Therapy, Duration of Therapy, Chronic Maintenance	Alternative Therapy
	Addition of rifabutin may also be considered: • Rifabutin 300 mg PO daily (dosage adjustment may be necessary based on drug-drug interactions) **(CI)**	Addition of a third or fourth drug should be considered for patients with advanced immunosuppression (CD4+ count <50 cells/μL), high mycobacterial loads (>2 log CFU/mL of blood), or in the absence of effective ART **(CIII)**. • Other drugs used are amikacin, streptomycin, ciprofloxacin, levofloxacin, and moxifloxacin.
Cryptococcal meningitis	*Preferred induction therapy* • Amphotericin B deoxycholate 0.7 mg/kg IV daily plus flucytosine 100 mg/kg PO daily in four divided doses for at least 2 weeks **(AI)**; or • Lipid formulation amphotericin B 4–6 mg/kg IV daily (consider for persons who have renal dysfunction on therapy or have high likelihood of renal failure) plus flucytosine 100 mg/kg PO daily in four divided doses for at least 2 weeks **(AII)**	*Alternative induction therapy* • Amphotericin B (deoxycholate or lipid formulation, dose as preferred therapy) plus fluconazole 400 mg PO or IV daily **(BII)** • Amphotericin B (deoxycholate or lipid formulation, dose as preferred therapy) alone **(BII)** • Fluconazole 400–800 mg/day (PO or IV) plus flucytosine 100 mg/kg PO daily in four divided doses for 4–6 weeks **(CII)**—for persons unable to tolerate or unresponsive to amphotericin B
	Preferred consolidation therapy • Fluconazole 400 mg PO daily for 8 weeks **(AI)**	*Alternative consolidation therapy* • Itraconazole 200 mg PO b.i.d. for 8 weeks **(BI)**, or until CD4+ count ≥200 cells/μL for >6 months as a result of ART **(BII)**

(Continued)

Table 2-2	Drug Therapy for Treatment and Chronic Maintenance Therapy of AIDS-Associated OIs in Adults and Adolescents *(Continued)*

OI	Preferred Therapy, Duration of Therapy, Chronic Maintenance	Alternative Therapy
	Preferred maintenance therapy	*Alternative maintenance therapy*
	• Fluconazole 200 mg PO daily **(AI)** lifelong or until CD4+ count ≥200 cells/ μL for >6 months as a result of ART **(BII)**	• Itraconazole 200 mg PO daily.
Histoplasma capsulatum infections	*Preferred therapy for moderately severe to severe disseminated disease*	*Alternative therapy for moderately severe to severe disseminated disease*
	Induction therapy (for 2 weeks or until clinically improved)	*Induction therapy* (for 2 weeks or until clinically improved)
	• Liposomal amphotericin B at 3 mg/kg IV daily **(AI)**	• Amphotericin B deoxycholate 0.7 mg/kg IV daily **(BI)**
		• Amphotericin B lipid complex 5 mg/kg IV daily **(CIII)**
		Maintenance therapy same as "preferred therapy"
	Maintenance therapy	
	• Itraconazole 200 mg PO t.i.d. for 3 days, then b.i.d. **(AII)**	
	• Itraconazole levels should be obtained in all patients to ensure adequate absorption (AIII)	
	Preferred therapy for less severe disseminated disease	
	Induction and maintenance therapy	
	• Itraconazole 200 mg PO t.i.d. for 3 days, then 200 mg PO b.i.d. **(AII)**	
	Duration of therapy: at least 12 months	
CMV disease	*Preferred therapy for CMV retinitis*	*Alternative therapy for CMV retinitis*
	For immediate sight-threatening lesions	• Ganciclovir 5 mg/kg IV q12h for 14–21 days, then 5 mg/kg IV daily **(AI)**; or
	• Ganciclovir intraocular implant + valganciclovir 900 mg PO (b.i.d. for 14–21 days, then once daily) **(AI)**	• Ganciclovir 5 mg/kg IV q12h for 14–21 days, then valganciclovir 900 mg PO daily **(AI)**; or

Table 2-2	Drug Therapy for Treatment and Chronic Maintenance Therapy of AIDS-Associated OIs in Adults and Adolescents *(Continued)*

OI	Preferred Therapy, Duration of Therapy, Chronic Maintenance	Alternative Therapy
	• One dose of intravitreal ganciclovir may be administered immediately after diagnosis until ganciclovir implant can be placed **(CIII)** For small peripheral lesions • Valganciclovir PO daily **(BII)** *Preferred therapy for CMV esophagitis or colitis* • Ganciclovir IV or foscarnet IV for 21–28 days or until resolution of signs and symptoms **(BII)** • Oral valganciclovir may be used if symptoms are not severe enough to interfere with oral absorption **(BII)**. • Maintenance therapy is usually not necessary, but should be considered after relapses **(BII)**. *Preferred therapy for CMV pneumonitis* • Treatment should be considered in patients with histologic evidence of CMV pneumonitis and who do not respond to treatment of other pathogens **(AIII)**	• Foscarnet 60 mg/kg IV q8h or 90 mg/kg IV q12h for 14–21 days, then 90–120 mg/kg IV q24h **(AI)**; or • Cidofovir 5 mg/kg/week IV for 2 weeks, then 5 mg/kg every other week with saline hydration before and after therapy and probenecid 2 g PO 3 hours before the dose followed by 1 g PO 2 hours after the dose, and 1 g PO 8 hours after the dose (total of 4 g) **(AI)** Note: This regimen should be avoided in patients with sulfa allergy because of cross hypersensitivity with probenecid
VZV disease	*Varicella (chickenpox) Uncomplicated cases* • Acyclovir (20 mg/kg body weight up to a maximum of 800 mg PO 5 × daily), valacyclovir 1,000 mg PO t.i.d., or famciclovir 500 mg PO t.i.d. × 5–7 days **(AII)**	*Infection caused by acyclovir-resistant VZV* • Foscarnet 90 mg/kg IV q12h **(AII)**

(Continued)

Table 2-2	Drug Therapy for Treatment and Chronic Maintenance Therapy of AIDS-Associated OIs in Adults and Adolescents *(Continued)*

OI	Preferred Therapy, Duration of Therapy, Chronic Maintenance	Alternative Therapy
	Severe or complicated cases • Acyclovir 10–15 mg/kg IV q8h × 7–10 days **(AIII)** • May switch to oral acyclovir, famciclovir, or valacyclovir after defervescence if no evidence of visceral involvement is evident **(AIII)** *PORN* • Ganciclovir 5 mg/kg IV q12h, plus foscarnet 90 mg/kg IV q12h, plus ganciclovir 2 mg/0.05 mL intravitreal twice weekly, and/or foscarnet 1.2 mg/0.05 mL intravitreal twice weekly **(AIII)** • Optimization of ART **(AIII)** *ARN* • Acyclovir 10 mg/kg IV q8h × 10–14 days, followed by valacyclovir 1,000 mg PO t.i.d. × 6 weeks **(AIII)**	
HHV-8 diseases (KS, PEL, MCD)	Initiation or optimization of ART should be done for all patients with KS, PEL, or MCD **(BII)**. *Preferred therapy for visceral KS (BII), disseminated cutaneous KS (CIII), and PEL (BIII)* • Chemotherapy + ART **(BII)** • Oral valganciclovir or IV ganciclovir might be useful as adjunctive therapy in PEL **(BII)** *Preferred therapy for MCD* • Valganciclovir 900 mg PO b.i.d. **(BII)**; or • Ganciclovir 5 mg/kg IV q12h **(BII)**	*Alternative therapy for MCD* Rituximab 375 mg/m² given weekly × 4–8 weeks, may be an alternative to antiviral therapy **(BII)**

Table 2-2	Drug Therapy for Treatment and Chronic Maintenance Therapy of AIDS-Associated OIs in Adults and Adolescents *(Continued)*	
OI	**Preferred Therapy, Duration of Therapy, Chronic Maintenance**	**Alternative Therapy**
HHV-6 infection	If HHV-6 has been identified as cause of disease in HIV-infected patients, use same drugs and doses as treatment for CMV disease **(CIII)** • Ganciclovir (or valganciclovir) • Foscarnet	
HPV disease	Treatment of condylomata acuminata (genital warts) *Patient-applied therapy* • Podofilox 0.5% solution or 0.5% gel—apply to all lesions b.i.d. × 3 consecutive days, followed by 4 days of no therapy, repeat weekly for up to four cycles **(BIII)**; or • Imiquimod 5% cream—apply to lesion at bedtime and remove in the morning on three nonconsecutive nights weekly for up to 16 weeks. Each treatment should be washed with soap and water 6–10 hours after application **(BII)**	*Provider-applied therapy* • Cryotherapy (liquid nitrogen or cryoprobe)—apply until each lesion is thoroughly frozen; repeat every 1–2 weeks. Some providers allow the lesion to thaw, then freeze a second time in each session **(BIII)** • Trichloroacetic acid or bichloroacetic acid cauterization—80%–90% aqueous solution, apply to each lesion, repeat weekly for 3–6 weeks **(BIII)** • Surgical excision (BIII) or laser surgery **(CIII)** 100% efficacy.

Ratings Scheme for Prevention and Treatment Recommendations—Category Definition: A, Both strong evidence for efficacy and substantial clinical benefit support recommendation for use. Should always be offered. B, Moderate evidence for efficacy—or strong evidence for efficacy but only limited clinical benefit—supports recommendation for use. Should generally be offered. C, Evidence for efficacy is insufficient to support a recommendation for or against use. Or evidence for efficacy might not outweigh adverse consequences Optional. D, Moderate evidence for lack of efficacy or for adverse outcome supports a recommendation against use. Should generally not be offered. Quality of the Evidence Supporting the Recommendation: I, Evidence from at least one properly designed randomized, controlled trial. II, Evidence from at least one well-designed clinical trial without randomization, from cohort or case-controlled analytic studies (preferably from more than one center), or from multiple time-series studies, or dramatic results from uncontrolled experiments. III, Evidence from opinion of respected. ART, antiretroviral therapy; b.i.d., twice a day; b.i.w., twice weekly, t.i.d., three times a day; t.i.w., three times weekly; g, gram; IM, intramuscular; IV, intravenous; μL, microliter; mg, milligram; PO, oral. Based on Guidelines for prevention and treatment of opportunistic infections in HIV-infected adults and adolescents: Recommendations from CDC, the National Institutes of Health, and the HIV Medicine Association of the Infectious Diseases Society of America. *MMWR Morb Mortal Wkly Rep* 2009;58:1–198.

headache, confusion, and focal neurologic findings. Contrast computed tomography (CT) imaging of the brain usually shows a single or multiple ring-enhancing lesions. The empiric diagnosis is confirmed through clinical and radiographic improvement following treatment initiation.

MICROSPORIDIOSIS/CRYPTOSPORIDIOSIS/ENTERIC BACTERIAL INFECTIONS

In patients with AIDS, microsporidiosis and cryptosporidiosis usually present at CD4+ levels below 100 cells/μL. Acute or subacute onset of potentially significant watery, nonbloody diarrhea with and without fever is the most common presenting symptom. Diagnosis of cryptosporidiosis can be achieved through stool antigen tests or partial acid-fast staining of oocysts. Microsporidiosis can be visualized using fluorescent or modified trichrome staining. Some cases require intestinal biopsy for diagnosis.[2] Enteric bacterial infections, predominantly with *Salmonella*, *Shigella*, and *Campylobacter* are 20 to 100 times more common in HIV-infected individuals. Clinical presentation ranges from acute self-limiting diarrhea to overt septicemia. Recurrent salmonella bacteremia is considered an AIDS defining illness. For all three enteric pathogens, fluoroquinolones are the recommended treatment even though some physicians recommend empiric macrolide therapy, especially in certain geographic locations.[2] In salmonella bacteremia, the addition of a third-generation cephalosporin may also be warranted pending antibiotic susceptibilities.

MYCOBACTERIUM TUBERCULOSIS INFECTION (TB)

Mycobacterium tuberculosis infection (TB) disease can develop immediately after exposure (primary disease) or after reactivation of latent TB infection (LTBI) disease (reactivation disease). Primary disease accounts for one-third or more of cases of TB disease in HIV-infected populations. Unlike other AIDS-defining OIs, CD4+ count is not a reliable predictor of TB. Persons with LTBI are, by definition, asymptomatic. Diagnosis can be accomplished by tuberculin skin test (TST) or interferon gamma release assay (IGRA) based–testing. Both, however, are less reliable in patients with advanced immunodeficiency. In HIV-infected patients without pronounced immunosuppression, TB clinically resembles TB among HIV-uninfected persons. The evaluation of suspected TB should include a chest radiograph regardless of the possible anatomic site of disease. Sputum samples for acid-fast bacilli (AFB) smear and culture should be obtained from patients with pulmonary symptoms. For patients with signs of extrapulmonary TB (more common in HIV-infected patients), needle aspiration or tissue biopsy of skin lesions, lymph nodes, or pleural or pericardial fluid should be performed.[2]

DISSEMINATED *MYCOBACTERIUM AVIUM* COMPLEX DISEASE

M. avium is the etiologic agent in >95% of patients with AIDS who present with disseminated *Mycobacterium avium* complex (DMAC) disease. The mode of transmission is thought to be through inhalation, ingestion, or inoculation via the respiratory or gastrointestinal tract. DMAC infection usually presents with fever, night sweats, weight loss, fatigue, diarrhea, abdominal pain, visceromegaly, and lymphadenopathy. A confirmed diagnosis of DMAC disease is based on compatible clinical features coupled with the isolation of *Mycobacterium avium* complex (MAC) from cultures of blood, bone marrow, or other normally sterile tissue or body fluids. HIV-infected adults with a CD4+ cell count of <50 cells/μL should receive chemoprophylaxis with azithromycin (1,200 mg weekly or 250 mg daily). In patients with symptoms compatible with DMAC, active disease should be ruled out with negative AFB blood or tissue culture before azithromycin is initiated in order to avoid macrolide monotherapy which could result in resistant development.

CRYPTOCOCCAL MENINGITIS

Cryptococcal meningitis is caused by several species of the fungal pathogen *Cryptococcus* and presents with signs of increased intracranial pressure (headache, altered mental status, visual problems) and fever. True meningeal signs are rare, especially in patients with advanced immunosuppression. Disseminated disease with skin lesions or pulmonary disease can be present. Infection can be caused by multiple types of *Cryptococcus* species, most notably *C. neoformans*. Meningitis is often subacute with common presenting complaints of generalized headache and malaise with low-grade fever. Brain imaging is often unrevealing or shows nonspecific findings. India ink staining of cerebrospinal fluid (CSF) is positive in 50% of infections but is more rapid than culture. Cryptococcal antigen can be detected in the CSF or serum of most patients with cryptococcal infections, and this may be helpful to monitor response to treatment.

HISTOPLASMOSIS

Histoplasmosis is endemic to certain regions of the continental United States, Puerto Rico, and South America, and the most common etiologic species is the fungus *Histoplasma capsulatum*. Organisms are inhaled and usually cause a self-limited disease of the respiratory tract in patients without immunodeficiency. Systemic spread, most notably to organs of the reticuloendothelial system (spleen, liver, bone marrow), is the hallmark of disseminated disease usually seen in patients with low CD4+ cell counts. Symptoms include fever, fatigue, lymphadenopathy, and dyspnea. Gastrointestinal symptoms include dysphasia or odynophagia. A travel history to an endemic region and compatible symptoms in a patient with a CD4+ cell count of ≤150 cells/μL should result in specific diagnostic testing. Urine histoplasma antigen testing is highly sensitive (85% to 98%) and specific. In advanced cases, the fungus can be isolated in tissue or blood samples.

CYTOMEGALOVIRUS DISEASE

Disease caused by reactivation of cytomegalovirus (CMV) disease is usually found in persons with advanced immunosuppression (CD4+ counts <50 cells/μL). Retinitis is the most common clinical manifestation of CMV end-organ disease. It presents as a unilateral retinal vasculitis in two-thirds of patients at initial diagnosis but in the absence of therapy or immune recovery spreads to involve both eyes in the majority of patients. Depending on the location, retinal CMV disease may be asymptomatic or present with floaters, scotoma, or visual field defects. The characteristic ophthalmologic appearance is fluffy yellow-white retinal lesions tracking with vasculature structures. Intraretinal hemorrhage or retinal detachment may be present. Other presentations of CMV include esophagitis, colitis, pneumonitis, and CMV neurologic disease like dementia, ventriculoencephalitis, or ascending polyradiculomyelopathy.

CMV viremia can be detected by polymerase chain reaction (PCR) or antigen assays but is not specific for end-organ disease. Detection of CMV in endothelial cells of affected tissue is diagnostic.

VARICELLA-ZOSTER VIRUS DISEASE

Shingles or zoster results from reactivation of latent varicella-zoster virus (VZV). The incidence of shingles is >15-fold higher in HIV-infected adults than in the general population, especially if their CD4+ count is <200 cell/μL. It manifests as an eruption of painful cutaneous vesicles in a dermatomal distribution, often preceded by prodromal pain. VZV can cause other neurologic syndromes including CNS vasculitis, multifocal leukoencephalitis, ventriculitis, myelitis, cranial nerve palsies, focal brain-stem lesions, and aseptic meningitis. Acute retinal necrosis (ARN) and progressive outer retinal necrosis (PORN) are variants of necrotizing retinopathy caused by VZV and associated with high rates of visual loss. When lesions are atypical or the diagnosis is uncertain, swabs from a fresh lesion or tissue biopsies can be submitted for viral culture, direct fluorescent antigen testing, or PCR. Prompt antiviral therapy should be instituted in all immunosuppressed patients within 1 week of rash onset or start of symptoms.

PROGRESSIVE MULTIFOCAL LEUKOENCEPHALOPATHY/JC VIRUS INFECTION

Progressive multifocal leukoencephalopathy (PML) is an OI of the CNS, caused by polyoma JC virus and characterized by focal demyelination. PML manifests as focal neurologic deficits, usually with insidious onset and steady progression. The magnetic resonance imaging (MRI) typically shows distinct white matter lesions in areas of the brain corresponding to the clinical deficits that are usually hyperintense (white) on T2-weighted image. In most cases, clinical picture and imaging findings support a confident presumptive diagnosis of PML. JC virus by PCR is positive in CSF in 70% to 90% cases. The treatment involves ART to reverse the immunosuppression that interferes with the normal host response to this virus and approximately half of patients experience a remission with ART.[1]

HUMAN HERPESVIRUS 8 DISEASE

Human herpesvirus 8 (HHV-8) is associated with all forms of Kaposi sarcomas (KS) and certain rare neoplastic disorders, for example, primary effusion lymphoma (PEL) and multicentric Castleman disease (MCD). MCD manifests with generalized adenopathy and fever and can progress to multiorgan failure. Detection of HHV-8 in the peripheral blood or in tissue biopsy via PCR is a helpful adjunct in the diagnosis. Highly active ART should be administered to all HIV-infected persons with KS, PEL, or MCD, but many patients require chemotherapy.

HUMAN PAPILLOMAVIRUS DISEASE

Human papillomavirus (HPV), a common sexually transmitted DNA virus, is the most frequent cause of cervical and anal cancer in patients with HIV. HPV serotype 16 accounts for 50% of cervical cancers, and serotypes 6 and 11 cause 90% of genital warts. HPV 16 is also present in the majority of noncervical cancers including anus, vulva, vagina, penis, and oropharynx. Diagnosis of genital and oral warts is made by visual inspection and can be confirmed by biopsy.

IMMUNE RECONSTITUTION INFLAMMATORY SYNDROME

Most studies suggest that unless other individual compelling contraindications are present, early initiation of ART near the time of initiating OI treatment should be considered for most patients with an acute OI.[2] Antiretroviral therapy, however, improves immune function and CD4+ cell count in HIV-infected patients within the first few months after starting treatment, and some patients develop a paradoxical inflammatory response by their reconstituted immune system to infectious or noninfectious antigens, resulting in apparent clinical worsening. In the case of OIs, this can be severe and has been referred to as immune reconstitution inflammatory syndrome (IRIS). IRIS has been observed most commonly for mycobacterial infections (TB and DMAC disease), but also for other OIs, including PCP, cryptococcal infection, TE, and PML. Antiretroviral therapy should generally be continued through this phase. One randomized trial has shown some benefit of adding steroids in patients with paradoxical worsening of TB following initiation of ART.[3]

REFERENCES

1. Walensky RP, Paltiel AD, Losina E, et al. The survival benefits of AIDS treatment in the United States. *J Infect Dis* 2006;194:11–19.
2. Kaplan JE, et al. Guidelines for prevention and treatment of opportunistic infections in HIV-infected adults and adolescents: recommendations from CDC, the National Institutes of Health, and the HIV Medicine Association of the Infectious Diseases Society of America. *MMWR Morb Mort Wkly Rep* 2009;58:1–198.
3. Meintjes G, Wilkinson RJ, Morroni C, et al. Randomized placebo-controlled trial of prednisone for paradoxical tuberculosis-associated immune reconstitution inflammatory syndrome. *AIDS* 2010;24:2381–2389.

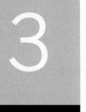

3

Drug Interactions in Patients with HIV Infection

Christopher H. Parsons and Michael S. Boger

INTRODUCTION

- The number of antiretroviral agents (ARVs) approved for treatment of HIV continues to expand, offering patients more effective, tolerable, and convenient options. As a result of this and other advances in HIV management, the life span of patients living with HIV has increased, approaching an age comparable to patients afflicted with other chronic diseases.[1]
- Interactions between ARVs and other drugs used to treat comorbid illnesses have become increasingly important for patients and health care providers.
- Psychiatric illness, diabetes, hypertension, hyperlipidemia, and bacterial and other infections are frequently encountered among HIV patients. Drugs used to treat these conditions may interact with ARVs by utilizing the same hepatic metabolism pathway.
- Other drugs may influence ARV pharmacokinetics through their effects on gastrointestinal absorption, protein binding, and renal filtration or excretion.
- ARVs share toxicities with many other drugs, a portion of which are listed in Table 3-1.
- Drug interactions are often complex and should be considered carefully when choosing an ARV regimen for HIV patients. Potential interactions should be discussed with an experienced HIV provider in consultation with a pharmacist. However, the growing number of HIV patients with comorbid chronic conditions who interact with primary care physicians necessitates that all providers achieve some level of familiarity with drug interactions.

NUCLEOSIDE REVERSE TRANSCRIPTASE INHIBITORS

- Table 3-2 summarizes clinically significant drug-drug interactions for nucleoside reverse transcriptase inhibitors (NRTIs). These agents have minimal drug interactions because they are not metabolized by the hepatic cytochrome P450 (CYP450) enzyme system, and are eliminated via renal excretion.
- Tenofovir reduces atazanavir levels through induction of CYP3A4; therefore, these drugs should only be coadministered in the presence of ritonavir "boosting" (see section on Protease Inhibitors below for more details).
- The combination of zidovudine and stavudine is contraindicated due to their mutual antagonism and competitive inhibition of intracellular stavudine phosphorylation, resulting in reduced stavudine levels.
- Because the chewable tablet and solution forms of didanosine are manufactured as a buffer, administration with agents dependent on gastric acid for absorption,

Table 3-1	Major Toxicities of Common Drugs Used to Manage HIV Infection	

Bone Marrow Suppression	Renal Toxicity	Liver Toxicity
Zidovudine	Tenofovir	NRTI
Co-trimoxazole	Indinavir	NNRTI
Dapsone	Acyclovir	Protease inhibitors
Ganciclovir	Amphotericin	Macrolides
Pyrimethamine	Aminoglycosides	Fluconazole
Sulfadiazine		Itraconazole
Flucytosine		Ketaconazole
Amphotericin		Voriconazole
Interferon alpha		Rifampin
Ribavirin		Rifabutin
Linezolid		Valproic acid
β-lactam agents		
Valproic acid		

HIV, human immunodeficiency virus; NRTI, nucleoside reverse transcriptase inhibitor; NNRTI, nonnucleoside reverse transcriptase inhibitor.

including atazanavir and azole antifungals, may reduce their bioavailability. Administration of tenofovir with enteric-coated didanosine may also lead to significant elevations in didanosine levels.
• The combination of didanosine and allopurinol is not recommended due to potential for didanosine toxicity.[2]

NONNUCLEOSIDE REVERSE TRANSCRIPTASE INHIBITORS

• Nonnucleoside reverse transcriptase inhibitors (NNRTIs) interact with a number of ARVs and other drugs, as illustrated in Table 3-3, due largely to their influence on hepatic metabolism. All five agents are substrates of CYP3A4, with efavirenz, etravirine, nevirapine, and rilpivirine inducing CYP3A4 activity, and delavirdine inhibiting CYP3A4 activity. Etravirine also inhibits activity of CYP2C19.[3]
• Rosuvastatin, atorvastatin, and pravastatin are the preferred HMG-CoA reductase inhibitors for use with NNRTIs because they incur fewer drug interactions, although myopathies and rhabdomyolysis may be more likely when these medications are used with NNRTIs.
• Anticonvulsants, including carbamazepine, phenobarbital, and phenytoin, induce CYP450 and reduce NNRTI levels, particularly for etravirine.[4]
• Clarithromycin should not be used with NNRTIs.[5]
• Rifabutin (in lieu of rifampin) is preferred for the treatment of mycobacterial infections arising in patients receiving NNRTIs.
• Proton pump inhibitors (PPIs) significantly reduce rilpivirine concentrations and should be avoided. H_2 blockers and antacids may be coadministered with rilpivirine if taken at sufficient intervals before or after rilpivirine dosing.[3,6]
• Etravirine has demonstrated utility in ARV-experienced patients, but providers should be aware of significant drug interactions, several of which are noted above.

Table 3-2	Clinically Significant Interactions with NRTIs[a]	
Agent	**Interacting Drug**[a]	**Result**
Tenofovir (TDF)[20]	Atazanavir	↓ atazanavir levels, ↑ tenofovir levels—atazanavir should be boosted with ritonavir
	Didanosine	↑ didanosine levels—reduce didanosine dose to 250 mg a day
	Probenecid	inhibits tubular secretion of tenofovir—**contraindicated**
Abacavir (ABC)	Methadone	↓ methadone levels—monitor for signs of withdrawal
Zidovudine (ZDV)[20]	Stavudine	antagonistic—**contraindicated**
	Ganciclovir	↑ zidovudine levels—avoid combination if possible
	Ribavirin	*In vitro* antagonism of zidovudine—**contraindicated**
Emtricitabine (FTC)	No significant interactions reported	
Lamivudine (3TC)	Chlorpropamide	↓ chlorpropamide levels—consider alternative agents
Didanosine (ddI)[20]	Atazanavir	↓ atazanavir absorption (with buffered didanosine formulations)—administer at different times
	Tenofovir	↑ didanosine levels—reduce didanosine dose to 250 mg
	Ganciclovir, indinavir, itraconazole (capsule), ketoconazole, fluoroquinolones	↓ levels of these agents Indinavir may ↓ bioavailability of didanosine
	Lopinavir/ritonavir	↓ lopinavir/ritonavir absorption—administer at different times
	Ribavirin	↑ risk of mitochondrial toxicity—**contraindicated**

[a]Clinically significant interactions with commonly used agents are included—additional interactions are reported in the literature.
NRTI, nonnucleoside reverse transcriptase inhibitor; TDF, tenofovir; ABC, abacavir; ZDV, zidovudine; FTC, emtricitabine; 3TC, lamivudine; ddI, didanosine

Table 3-3 Clinically Significant Interactions with NNRTIs[a]

Agent	Interacting Drug[a]	Result
Etravirine[4,5,7,20,21]	**Other ARVs**	
	Fosamprenavir	↑ amprenavir levels—**contraindicated**
	Tipranavir	↓ etravirine levels—**contraindicated**
	Atazanavir	↓ atazanavir levels, ↑ etravirine levels—**contraindicated**
	Maraviroc	↑ maraviroc levels—increase maraviroc to 600 mg b.i.d. unless etravirine given with maraviroc + ritonavir-boosted PI comparable to darunavir, where maraviroc dose should be reduced to 150 mg b.i.d.
	Antibiotics	
	Rifampin, rifapentine	↓ etravirine levels—**contraindicated**
	Rifabutin	↓ etravirine levels, ↓ rifabutin levels—dose rifabutin at 300 mg daily if administered with unboosted PI, but avoid combination if used with ritonavir boosted PI
	Antifungals	
	Ketoconazole, itraconazole	Use with caution: ↓etravirine and antifungal levels
	Voriconazole	↑ etravirine and voriconazole levels—monitor voriconazole levels
	Fluconazole	↑ etravirine levels—use with caution
	Others	
	Immunosuppressants[3]	↓ immunosuppressant levels—monitor closely
	Warfarin	↑ ↓ INR—monitor INR closely
	Antiarrhythmics[4]	May ↓ antiarrhythmic levels—monitor closely
	Digoxin	↑ digoxin levels—monitor digoxin levels and for signs of digoxin toxicity
	Anticonvulsants: phenytoin, carbamazepine, phenobarbital	↓ etravirine levels—**contraindicated**
Rilpivirine[5,6,20,22]	Dexamethasone	↓ rilpivirine levels—**contraindicated**
	Phenytoin	↓ rilpivirine levels—**contraindicated**
	Carbamazepine	↓ rilpivirine levels—**contraindicated**

(Continued)

Table 3-3	Clinically Significant Interactions with NNRTIs[a] (Continued)	
Agent	**Interacting Drug**[a]	**Result**
	PPIs: omeprazole, lansoprazole, esomeprazole, pantoprazole, rabeprazole	→ rilpivirine levels—**contraindicated**
	Rifamycins: rifampin, rifabutin, rifapentine	→ rilpivirine levels—**contraindicated**
	St. John's wort	→ rilpivirine levels—**contraindicated**
	H₂-receptor antagonists: famotidine, ranitidine, cimetidine, nizatidine	→ rilpivirine levels—administer 12 hours before or 4 hours after rilpivirine dose
	Antacids	→ rilpivirine levels—administer 2 hours before or 4 hours after rilpivirine dose
	Methadone	→ methadone levels—monitor for opiate withdrawal
	Azoles: voriconazole, ketoconazole, itraconazole, posaconazole, fluconazole	↑ rilpivirine levels, ↓ azole levels—monitor closely
Efavirenz[8,20,23]	**Other ARVs**	
	NNRTI: etravirine, nevirapine, rilpivirine	→ efavirenz/NNRTI levels and ↑ NNRTI toxicity—**contraindicated**
	Atazanavir/ritonavir	→ atazanavir levels—increase atazanavir to 400 mg with 100 mg ritonavir
	Lopinavir/ritonavir	→ lopinavir levels—consider increase lopinavir/ritonavir to 600/150 mg twice daily
	Fosamprenavir/ritonavir	→ amprenavir levels—total of 300 mg of ritonavir recommended per day
	Antibiotics	
	Rifampicin, rifampin	→ efavirenz levels—**avoid combination** if possible. In patients ≥50 kg, increase efavirenz dose to 800 mg once daily
	Rifabutin	→ rifabutin levels—increase rifabutin dose by 50%
	Voriconazole	→ voriconazole levels, ↑ efavirenz levels—increase voriconazole to 400 mg every 12 hours and decrease efavirenz to 300 mg once a day
	Posaconazole	→ posaconazole levels—**contraindicated**
	Itraconazole, ketoconazole	↓ azole levels—**avoid combination** if possible
	Clarithromycin	↓ clarithromycin levels—**avoid combination** if possible

Nevirapine[20,24]

Others

St. John's wort — ↓ efavirenz levels—**contraindicated**

Ergot derivatives — ↑ ergot toxicity—**contraindicated**

Benzodiazepines: triazolam, midazolam — ↑ benzodiazepine toxicity—**contraindicated**

Immunosuppressives: sirolimus, tacrolimus, cyclosporin — ↓ levels of immunosuppressive agents—**avoid combination** if possible

Methadone — ↓ methadone levels—monitor for opiate withdrawal

HMG-CoA reductase inhibitors: atorvastatin, simvastatin, pravastatin — ↓ HMG-CoA reductase inhibitors levels—monitor cholesterol levels

Oral contraceptives — ↓ ethinyl estradiol levels—use alternative method of contraception

Carbamazepine — ↓ efavirenz/carbamazepine levels—use with caution

Atazanavir/ritonavir — ↓ atazanavir, ↑ nevirapine—**contraindicated**

Oral contraceptives — ↓ ethinyl estradiol levels—use alternative method of contraception

Fluconazole — ↑ nevirapine levels—monitor for side effects, use with caution

Fosamprenavir — ↓ amprenavir levels, ↑ nevirapine levels—do not coadminister unless fosamprenavir is used with ritonavir at 700/100 mg b.i.d.

Lopinavir/ritonavir — ↓ lopinavir levels—increase lopinavir/ritonavir to 600/150 mg twice daily

Methadone — ↓ methadone levels—monitor for opiate withdrawal

Rifabutin — ↑ rifabutin levels—monitor for signs of toxicity and use with caution

Rifampin — ↓ nevirapine levels—consider alternative agent for HIV

Delavirdine[20,25]

Certain benzodiazepines,[2] ergot derivatives, pimozide — ↑ levels of these agents with possible toxicity—**contraindicated**

Rifampin, rifabutin — ↓ delavirdine levels—**contraindicated**

Antacids — ↓ delavirdine levels—separate by at least 1 hour

Trazodone, certain antiarrhythmics,[2] warfarin, clarithromycin, certain HMG-CoA reductase inhibitors,[4] methadone — ↑ levels of all of these—use cautiously

[a]Clinically significant interactions are included—other interactions have been studied and reported in the literature.
ARVs, antiretroviral agents; PI, protease inhibitor; INR, international normalized ratio; NNRTI, nonnucleoside reverse transcriptase inhibitor; HMG-CoA, hydroxymethylglutaryl-CoA.

Some protease inhibitors (PIs) can be coadministered with etravirine in the presence of ritonavir to minimize CYP3A4-induced reductions in PI levels.[5,7]

- Use of nevirapine or efavirenz may lead to failure of oral contraceptives, and alternative methods of contraception should be offered to women of childbearing age receiving these agents. Of note, efavirenz is contraindicated during pregnancy due to its demonstrated teratogenicity in animal studies.

- The dose of lopinavir/ritonavir should be increased in the presence of nevirapine or efavirenz, and we do not recommend using these agents together given increased toxicities.

- Atazanavir should be administered at a higher dose (400 mg) and boosted with ritonavir when coadministered with efavirenz for treatment-naïve patients, and we recommend avoiding this combination in ARV-experienced patients.[8]

- The combination of atazanavir and nevirapine is contraindicated, and fosamprenavir requires dose adjustment when used with nevirapine.[9]

PROTEASE INHIBITORS

- Table 3-4 summarizes clinically significant drug-drug interactions for the four PIs recommended for use by most published HIV treatment guidelines: atazanavir, darunavir, lopinavir, and fosamprenavir (the latter is the pro-form of the bioactive amprenavir).[10]

- Although other PIs (saquinavir and indinavir) may be used in specific situations for treatment-experienced patients whose HIV exhibits multiclass resistance to ARVs, these agents incur significant toxicities and drug interactions, and their unfavorable pharmacokinetics require more frequent daily dosing. Therefore, they should only be used in consultation with an experienced HIV provider, and we do not elaborate further on drug interactions involving these agents.

- Ritonavir, a first-generation PI, is no longer recommended for HIV treatment due to excessive toxicity (gastrointestinal intolerance) observed with standard doses of this agent.

- All PIs are substrates of the cytochrome P450 enzyme CYP3A4, and, therefore, interact with a large number of other drugs.

- Of particular importance is the concept of PI "boosting": PIs are coadministered (and in some cases coformulated) with ritonavir in order to increase drug levels for PIs by virtue of ritonavir inhibition of CYP3A4 activity.[11,12] A dose of 100 mg daily of ritonavir is sufficient to inhibit CYP3A4 activity while minimizing inherent toxicities. Darunavir and lopinavir should always be coadministered with ritonavir. Atazanavir and fosamprenavir should also be coadministered with ritonavir in most situations, although these agents may not require boosting when administered with certain ARVs from other classes. Unfortunately, ritonavir boosting has the undesirable effect of increasing clinically significant drug interactions for PIs.[12]

- Concurrent use of PIs and NNRTIs is generally discouraged since NNRTIs reduce PI levels and since their concurrent use potentiates NNRTI toxicity (see prior section). An exception to this is coadministration of etravirine and darunavir—a combination demonstrating safety and efficacy for treatment-experienced patients.[13]

- Use of multiple PIs in the same patient (with the exception of low-dose ritonavir) is also discouraged since their concurrent use incurs significant drug interactions, and since multiple PI regimens have not exhibited durable suppression of HIV replication in clinical trials.

- Caution should be exercised when using PIs with drugs from the following classes: antibiotics (antibacterial and antifungal agents), psychotropic and neuroleptic

Table 3-4   Clinically Significant Interactions with PIs

Agent	Interacting Drug[a]	Result
Atazanavir/ritonavir[26]	**Other ARVs**	
	NNRTIs: efavirenz, etravirine, nevirapine, rilpivirine	↓ atazanavir/NNRTI levels and NNRTI toxicity—**avoid combination**
	Saquinavir	↑ saquinavir levels and PR prolongation—**avoid combination**
	Fosamprenavir	↓→ atazanavir levels—**avoid combination**
	Tipranavir	↓→ atazanavir levels—**avoid combination**
	Lopinavir	↑ PR prolongation—**avoid combination**
	Indinavir	↑ risk of hyperbilirubinemia
	Maraviroc	↑ maraviroc levels
	Tenofovir	↓ atazanavir levels—approved for concurrent use with ritonavir-boosted atazanavir
	Antibiotics	
	Rifampin	↓ atazanavir levels—**avoid combination**
	Rifabutin	↑ rifabutin levels—avoid combination if possible
	Minocycline	↓→ atazanavir levels—avoid combination if possible
	Clarithromycin	↑ clarithromycin levels, may increase cardiotoxicity (QT prolongation)—**avoid combination if possible**
	Azole antifungals: voriconazole, posaconazole	↑ atazanavir levels and ↓ voriconazole levels (ritonavir)
	Ketoconazole[b]	↑ ketoconazole/ritonavir levels and risk for hepatotoxicity
	Others	
	HMG-CoA reductase inhibitors[b]: lovastatin, simvastatin	↑ HMG-CoA reductase inhibitors levels and likely increase risk for myopathy and rhabdomyolysis—**contraindicated**
	HMG-CoA reductase inhibitors: rosuvastatin, atorvastatin	↑ HMG-CoA reductase inhibitors levels, may increase risk for myopathy and rhabdomyolysis—**use with caution and monitor for HMG-CoA reductase inhibitor toxicity**
	Benzodiazepines[b]: triazolam, midazolam	↑ benzodiazepine toxicity—**contraindicated**

(Continued)

Table 3-4   Clinically Significant Interactions with PIs *(Continued)*

Agent	Interacting Drug[a]	Result
	St. John's wort	↓ atazanavir levels—**contraindicated**
	Sildenafil[b]	↑ sildenafil levels and may increase risk for hypotension and priapism—**contraindicated**
	Ergot derivatives[b]	↑ ergot toxicity—**contraindicated**
	Colchicine[b]	↑ colchicine levels, may increase colchicine toxicity—**contraindicated**
	Amiodarone[b]	↑ amiodarone toxicity—**contraindicated**
	Fluticasone[b]	↑ plasma fluticasone levels and decreased cortisol, increased risk of Cushing syndrome—**contraindicated**
	Antihypertensives: diltiazem, esmolol, metoprolol, sotalol, labetalol, timolol, amlodipine	↑ risk of cardiotoxicity and PR prolongation—use with caution
	digoxin[b]	↓ digoxin levels—use with caution
	PPIs: omeprazole, lansoprazole, esomeprazole, pantoprazole, rabeprazole	↓ atazanavir levels—use only with ritonavir—boosted atazanavir
	H₂-receptor antagonists: famotidine, ranitidine, cimetidine, nizatidine	↓ atazanavir levels—use only with ritonavir-boosted atazanavir
	Antacids	↓ atazanavir levels—use only with ritonavir-boosted atazanavir
	Class Ia antiarrhythmics	↑ levels of Ia antiarrhythmics—use with caution
	Phenytoin	↓ atazanavir levels
	Garlic extracts	↓ atazanavir levels—use with caution
	Immunosuppressives: temsirolimus, tacrolimus	↑ levels of immunosuppressives—use with caution
	Methadone[b]	↓ methadone levels—monitor for opiate withdrawal
	Fentanyl	↑ fentanyl toxicity—avoid combination if possible
	Tamoxifen[b]	↓ tamoxifen levels—recommend avoiding during tamoxifen treatment for breast cancer

Darunavir/ritonavir[27]	
Narcotic analgesics[b]	↑ narcotic analgesic levels and sedation—use with caution
Tricyclic antidepressants[b]	may ↑ QT prolongation—avoid combination if possible
Oral contraceptives	↓ ethinyl estradiol levels; **use alternative method of contraception**
Levothyroxine[b]	↓ levothyroxine efficacy
Other ARVs	
Efavirenz	↓ darunavir, ↑ efavirenz levels
Protease inhibitors: saquinavir, lopinavir	↓ darunavir levels—avoid combination if possible
Indinavir	↑ darunavir/indinavir levels
Maraviroc	↑ maraviroc levels
Others	
HMG-CoA reductase inhibitors[a]: lovastatin, simvastatin	↑ HMG-CoA reductase inhibitors levels, likely increase risk for myopathy and rhabdomyolysis—**contraindicated**
Amiodarone[b]	↑ amiodarone toxicity—**contraindicated**
Colchicine[b]	↑ colchicine levels, may increase colchicine toxicity—**contraindicated**
Sildenafil[b]	↑ sildenafil levels, may increase risk for hypotension and priapism—**contraindicated**
Ergot derivatives[b]	↑ ergot toxicity—**contraindicated**
Benzodiazepines[b]: triazolam, midazolam	↑ benzodiazepine toxicity—**contraindicated**
Rifabutin	↑ rifabutin/darunavir levels—avoid combination if possible
Carbamazepine	↑ carbamazepine toxicity—**contraindicated**
Voriconazole	↓ voriconazole levels—**contraindicated**
Itraconazole	↑ itraconazole and ↓ darunavir levels
Posaconazole	↑ posaconazole levels—avoid combination if possible
Ketoconazole[b]	↑ ketoconazole/ritonavir levels and risk for hepatotoxicity
Fluticasone[b]	↑ plasma fluticasone levels and decreased cortisol, increased risk of Cushing syndrome—**contraindicated**
Immunosuppressives: sirolimus, cyclosporine	↑ levels of immunosuppressives—use with caution
Antihypertensives: metoprolol, timolol, nifedipine	↑ levels of antihypertensives

(Continued)

Table 3-4   Clinically Significant Interactions with PIs *(Continued)*

Agent	Interacting Drug[a]	Result
	vardenafil	↑ vardenafil levels
	digoxin[b]	↑ digoxin levels—use with caution
	Anticonvulsants: phenytoin; phenobarbital	↓ anticonvulsant levels
	Oral contraceptives	↓ ethinyl estradiol levels; **use alternative method of contraception**
	Warfarin	Alters warfarin levels, monitor INR
	Methadone[b]	→ methadone levels—monitor for opiate withdrawal
	Fentanyl	↑ fentanyl toxicity—avoid combination if possible
	Garlic extracts	↓ atazanavir levels—use with caution
	Tamoxifen[b]	↓ tamoxifen levels—recommend avoiding during tamoxifen treatment for breast cancer
	Narcotic analgesics[b]	↑ narcotic analgesic levels and sedation—use with caution
	Tricyclic antidepressants[b]	may ↑ QT prolongation—avoid combination if possible
	SSRIs: paroxetine, sertraline	↓ SSRI levels
	Levothyroxine[b]	↓ levothyroxine efficacy
	Other ARVs	
	Saquinavir	↑ saquinavir levels and PR/QT prolongation—**avoid combination**
	Fosamprenavir	↓ lopinavir levels
	Atazanavir	may ↑ PR prolongation
	NNRTIs: efavirenz, nevirapine	↓ lopinavir levels, ↑ NNRTI toxicity
	Maraviroc	↑ maraviroc levels
	Others	
	Colchicine[b]	↑ colchicine levels, may increase colchicine toxicity—**contraindicated**
	Sildenafil[b]	↑ sildenafil levels, may increase risk for hypotension and priapism—**contraindicated**
	Rifampin	↓ lopinavir levels—**contraindicated**
	Ergot derivatives[b]	↑ ergot toxicity—**contraindicated**

Lopinavir/ritonavir[28]

Benzodiazepines[b]: triazolam, midazolam	↑ benzodiazepine toxicity—**contraindicated**
Amiodarone[b]	↑ amiodarone toxicity—**contraindicated**
HMG-CoA reductase inhibitors[a]: lovastatin, simvastatin	↑ HMG-CoA reductase inhibitors levels, likely increase risk for myopathy and rhabdomyolysis—**contraindicated**
Voriconazole[b]	→ voriconazole levels—use with caution
Ketoconazole[b]	↑ ketoconazole/ritonavir levels and risk for hepatotoxicity
Posaconazole	↑ lopinavir levels and QT prolongation—avoid combination if possible
St. John's wort	→ lopinavir/ritonavir levels—**contraindicated**
Fluticasone[b]	↑ plasma fluticasone levels and decreased cortisol, increased risk of Cushing syndrome—**contraindicated**
HMG-CoA reductase inhibitors: rosuvastatin, atorvastatin	↑ HMG-CoA reductase inhibitors levels, may increase risk for myopathy and rhabdomyolysis—**use with caution and monitor for HMG-CoA reductase inhibitor toxicity**
Rifabutin[b]	↑ rifabutin levels—avoid combination if possible
Fentanyl[b]	↑ fentanyl toxicity—avoid combination if possible
Garlic extracts	→ lopinavir levels—use with caution
Phenytoin	→ lopinavir levels
Carbamazepine	↑ carbamazepine toxicity—**contraindicated**
Tamoxifen[b]	→ tamoxifen levels—recommend avoiding during tamoxifen treatment for breast cancer
Azithromycin	may ↑ QT prolongation—avoid combination if possible
Fluoroquinolones: moxifloxacin, ciprofloxacin, levofloxacin, norfloxacin	may ↑ QT prolongation—avoid combination if possible
Chlorpromazine	may ↑ QT prolongation—avoid combination if possible
Erythromycin	may ↑ QT prolongation—avoid combination if possible
Trazodone	may ↑ QT prolongation—avoid combination if possible
Fluconazole	may ↑ QT prolongation—avoid combination if possible
Immunosuppressives: sirolimus, tacrolimus	↑ levels of immunosuppressives—use with caution

(Continued)

Table 3-4   Clinically Significant Interactions with PIs (Continued)

Agent	Interacting Drug[a]	Result
	Tricyclic antidepressants[b]	may ↑ QT prolongation—avoid combination if possible
	Narcotic analgesics[b]	↑ narcotic analgesic levels and sedation—use with caution
	Oral contraceptives	↓ ethinyl estradiol levels; **use alternative method of contraception**
	Warfarin	Alters warfarin levels, monitor INR
	Levothyroxine[b]	↓ levothyroxine efficacy
	Methadone[b]	↓ methadone levels—monitor for opiate withdrawal
	Benzodiazepines[b]: triazolam, midazolam	↑ benzodiazepine toxicity—**contraindicated**
	SSRIs: paroxetine	↑ paroxetine levels
Fosamprenavir/ ritonavir[29]	**Other ARVs**	
	NNRTIs: nevirapine, efavirenz	↓ amprenavir levels and ↑ NNRTI toxicity—**avoid combination**
	Etravirine	↑ amprenavir levels
	Raltegravir	↓ raltegravir/amprenavir levels—**avoid combination**
	Atazanavir	↓ atazanavir levels—**avoid combination**
	Saquinavir	↓ amprenavir levels—**avoid combination**
	Maraviroc	↑ maraviroc levels
	Others	
	Colchicine[b]	↑ colchicine levels and may increase colchicine toxicity— **avoid combination**
	Sildenafil[b]	↑ sildenafil levels, may increase risk for hypotension and priapism—**contraindicated**
	Rifampin	↓ amprenavir levels—**contraindicated**
	Ergot derivatives[b]	↑ ergot toxicity—**contraindicated**
	Benzodiazepines[b]: triazolam, midazolam	↑ benzodiazepine toxicity—**contraindicated**
	Amiodarone[b]	↑ amiodarone toxicity—**avoid combination**
	digoxin[b]	↑ digoxin levels—use with caution

HMG-CoA reductase inhibitors[b]: lovastatin, simvastatin	↑ HMG-CoA reductase inhibitors levels and likely increase risk for myopathy and rhabdomyolysis—**contraindicated**
HMG-CoA reductase inhibitors: rosuvastatin, atorvastatin	↑ HMG-CoA reductase inhibitors levels, may increase risk for myopathy and rhabdomyolysis—**use with caution and monitor for HMG-CoA reductase inhibitor toxicity**
Fluticasone[b]	↑ plasma fluticasone levels and decreased cortisol, with increased risk of Cushing syndrome—**contraindicated**
Fentanyl[b]	↑ fentanyl toxicity—avoid combination if possible
Rifabutin[b]	↑ rifabutin levels—avoid combination if possible
Garlic extracts	→ amprenavir levels—use with caution
Tamoxifen[b]	→ tamoxifen levels—recommend avoiding during tamoxifen treatment for breast cancer
Tricyclic antidepressants[b]	may ↑ QT prolongation—avoid combination if possible
SSRIs: paroxetine	↑ paroxetine levels
Narcotic analgesics[b]	↑ narcotic analgesic levels and sedation—use with caution
Oral contraceptives[b]	→ ethinyl estradiol levels; **use alternative method of contraception**
Methadone[b]	→ methadone levels—monitor for opiate withdrawal
Levothyroxine[b]	→ levothyroxine efficacy
Benzodiazepines[b]: triazolam, midazolam	↑ benzodiazepine toxicity—**contraindicated**
Azole antifungals: voriconazole, ketoconazole	↑ azole/amprenavir/ritonavir levels and risk for hepatotoxicity
St. John's wort	→ amprenavir levels—**contraindicated**
Phenytoin	→ phenytoin/amprenavir levels
Immunosuppressives: cyclosporine, tacrolimus	↑ levels of immunosuppressives—use with caution
Voriconazole	↑ voriconazole/amprenavir levels—use with caution
Warfarin	↑ warfarin levels, monitor INR
H$_2$-receptor antagonists: ranitidine, cimetidine	→ amprenavir levels—use only with ritonavir-boosted amprenavir

[a] clinically significant interactions are included-additional interactions are reported in the literature

[b] denotes interactions primarily with ritonavir.

AVRs, Antiretroviral agents; PI, protease inhibitor; NNRTI, nonnucleoside reverse transcriptase inhibitor; HMG-CoA, hydroxymethylglutaryl-CoA; SSRI, selective serotonin reuptake inhibitor.

medications (benzodiazepines, serotonin reuptake inhibitors (SSRIs), tricyclic anti-depressants, narcotic analgesics, and antiepileptics), HMG-CoA reductase inhibitors (simvastatin and lovastatin should be avoided), antihypertensives (particularly beta-blockers), antiarrhythmic agents, acid-reducing agents (drugs from all classes in this category reduce PI bioavailability), and immunosuppressive medications (PIs increase levels of these medications).

- Care should be exercised with coadministration of PIs and warfarin, as warfarin levels are less predictable in this setting.[14] We recommend more frequent monitoring of the international normalized ratio (INR) or avoidance of PIs if warfarin is used.
- Estrogen-based oral contraceptives should not be used as the principal method of contraception in patients taking PIs, which reduce estrogen levels.[15] In addition, garlic extract and St. John's wort reduce PI levels and should be avoided.[16]

OTHER ANTIRETROVIRAL AGENTS

- A selective inhibitor of the HIV-encoded integrase, raltegravir, was recently approved for use in HIV-infected patients. Raltegravir is metabolized through uridine diphosphate glucuronosyltransferase-mediated glucuronidation in the liver, thereby exhibiting fewer drug interactions than other ARVs.
- Coadministration of raltegravir with rifampin, etravirine, or PPIs (particularly omeprazole) reduces raltegravir bioavailability.
- Fosamprenavir should not be coadministered with raltegravir due to reductions in levels of both agents when used together.[5,17]
- Two other drugs approved more recently for treatment of HIV include an antagonist of the chemokine receptor CCR5 (maraviroc) and an inhibitor of HIV fusion with the target cell membrane (enfuvirtide). Maraviroc is only approved for use in treatment-experienced patients in the presence of other more potent ARVs and is metabolized in the liver as a substrate of CYP3A.[18]
- Concurrent use of PIs and maraviroc may result in increased levels of maraviroc, whereas coadministration of rifampin, NNRTIs, antiepileptics (carbamazepine and phenytoin), and St. John's wort may reduce plasma maraviroc levels.[5] Interestingly, concurrent use of maraviroc and the yellow fever vaccine may incur an increased risk of yellow fever vaccine-associated viscerotropic disease in HIV-infected patients.[19] Significant interactions between commonly used drugs and enfuvirtide have not been reported.

REFERENCES

1. Losina E, Freedberg KA. Life expectancy in HIV. *BMJ* 2011;343:d6015.
2. Moreno S, Hernandez B, Dronda F. Didanosine enteric-coated capsule: current role in patients with HIV-1 infection. *Drugs* 2007;67(10):1441–1462.
3. Fulco PP, McNicholl IR. Etravirine and rilpivirine: nonnucleoside reverse transcriptase inhibitors with activity against human immunodeficiency virus type 1 strains resistant to previous nonnucleoside agents. *Pharmacotherapy* 2009;29(3):281–294.
4. Kakuda TN, Scholler-Gyure M, Hoetelmans RM. Pharmacokinetic interactions between etravirine and non-antiretroviral drugs. *Clin Pharmacokinet* 2011;50(1):25–39.
5. Brown KC, Paul S, Kashuba AD. Drug interactions with new and investigational antiretrovirals. *Clin Pharmacokinet* 2009;48(4):211–241.
6. Ford N, Lee J, Andrieux-Meyer I, et al. Safety, efficacy, and pharmacokinetics of rilpivirine: systematic review with an emphasis on resource-limited settings. *HIV AIDS* 2011;3:35–44.

7. Scholler-Gyure M, Kakuda TN, Raoof A, et al. Clinical pharmacokinetics and pharmaco-dynamics of etravirine. *Clin Pharmacokinet* 2009;48(9):561–574.

8. Rakhmanina NY, van den Anker JN. Efavirenz in the therapy of HIV infection. *Expert Opin Drug Metab Toxicol* 2010;6(1):95–103.

9. Barry M, Mulcahy F, Merry C, et al. Pharmacokinetics and potential interactions amongst antiretroviral agents used to treat patients with HIV infection. *Clin Pharmacokinet* 1999;36(4):289–304.

10. Thompson MA, Aberg JA, Cahn P, et al. Antiretroviral treatment of adult HIV infection: 2010 recommendations of the International AIDS Society-USA panel. *JAMA* 2010;304(3):321–333.

11. Hull MW, Montaner JS. Ritonavir-boosted protease inhibitors in HIV therapy. *Ann Med* 2011;43(5):375–388.

12. Josephson F. Drug-drug interactions in the treatment of HIV infection: focus on pharma-cokinetic enhancement through CYP3A inhibition. *J Intern Med* 2010;268(6):530–539.

13. Katlama C, Clotet B, Mills A, et al. Efficacy and safety of etravirine at week 96 in treatment-experienced HIV type-1-infected patients in the DUET-1 and DUET-2 trials. *Antivir Ther* 2010;15(7):1045–1052.

14. Liedtke MD, Rathbun RC. Warfarin-antiretroviral interactions. *Ann Pharmacother* 2009;43(2):322–328.

15. El-Ibiary SY, Cocohoba JM. Effects of HIV antiretrovirals on the pharmacokinetics of hormonal contraceptives. *Eur J Contracept Reprod Health Care* 2008;13(2):123–132.

16. Dasgupta A. Herbal supplements and therapeutic drug monitoring: focus on digoxin immunoassays and interactions with St. John's wort. *Ther Drug Monit* 2008;30(2):212–217.

17. Burger DM. Raltegravir: a review of its pharmacokinetics, pharmacology and clinical stud-ies. *Expert Opin Drug Metab Toxicol* 2010;6(9):1151–1160.

18. Yost R, Pasquale TR, Sahloff EG. Maraviroc: a coreceptor CCR5 antagonist for manage-ment of HIV infection. *Am J Health Syst Pharm* 2009;66(8):715–726.

19. Roukens AH, Visser LG, Kroon FP. A note of caution on yellow fever vaccination during maraviroc treatment: a hypothesis on a potential dangerous interaction. *AIDS* 2009;23(4):542–543.

20. HIV InSite: hivinsite.ucsf.edu

21. *Intelence (etravirine) full prescribing information*. Raritan, NJ: Tibotec Therapeutics; 2008.

22. *Endurant (rilpivirine) full prescribing information*. Raritan, NJ: Tibotec Therapeutics; 2011.

23. *Sustiva (efavirenz) full prescribing information*. Princeton, NJ: Bristol-Myers Squibb; 2011.

24. Viramune (nevirapine) full prescribing information. Ridgefield, CT: Boehringer Ingelheim; 2011.

25. Recriptor (delavirdine) full prescribing information. New York, NY: Pfizer; 2008.

26. Reyataz (atazanvir) full prescribing information. Princeton, NJ: Bristol-Myers Squibb; 2003.

27. Prezista (darunavir) full prescribing information. Raritan, NJ: Tibotec; 2006.

28. Kaletra (lopinavir/ritonavir) full prescribing information. Chicago, IL: Abbott Laborato-ries; 2012.

29. Lexiva (fosamprenavir) full prescribing information. Cambridge, MA: GlaxoSmithKline; 2009.

4 Primary Care in HIV

Sabena Ramsetty

With earlier initiation of highly active antiretroviral therapy (HAART) and increased longevity of HIV patients, practitioners are providing more comprehensive primary care. HIV increases the risk of heart disease, particularly at CD4 cell counts <500 cells/mm[14] as well as certain malignancies including cervical cancer, non-Hodgkin lymphoma, and anal cancer; however, since the advent of HAART, the majority of cancers affecting HIV patients are non–AIDS defining (i.e., lung and liver cancer, Hodgkin lymphoma).[9] Thus, it is imperative to address cardiovascular risk factors such as hyperlipidemia, diabetes, and tobacco abuse, and perform appropriate cancer screening.

HYPERLIPIDEMIA

HIV patients should have cholesterol goals guided by the National Cholesterol Education Program (see Table 4-1).[10] Diet alone at 24 weeks can lower low density lipoprotein (LDL) by 5.5%. Advise patients to increase intake of whole grains, fruits, and vegetables and decrease saturated fats and refined sugars.[16] Baseline fasting lipids should be checked prior to initiating HAART and at 3 to 6 months after starting any new antiretroviral regimen.[7] One multicenter prospective study found increased rates of hyperlipidemia in HIV patients on protease inhibitor based regimens compared to patients not receiving protease inhibitors(11). Also, certain antiretrovirals are associated with hyperlipidemia including efavirenz, stavudine, ritonavir, and lopinavir/ritonavir (see Table 4-2).

Check a fasting lipid profile and liver function tests (LFTs) prior to starting lipid therapy, and consider discontinuing therapy if patients have persistent transaminitis greater than three times the upper limit of normal, or creatine phosphokinase greater than five to ten times the upper limit of normal. Drug interactions with ritonavir and other protease inhibitors (PIs) are common as they are potent inhibitors of the cytochrome P450. Pravastatin and atorvastatin are first-line agents for patients with hyperlipidemia on PI-based regimens. Lovastatin and simvastatin are contraindicated for patients on PI regimens. Choose cholesterol drugs with respect to type of dyslipidemia. For example, in patients with isolated hypertriglyceridemia (>500), consider fibrates; for patients with isolated low high density lipoprotein (HDL), consider niacin; if LDL is above goal, triglycerides are 200 to 500 mg/dL, and non-HDL cholesterol is elevated, consider an HMG-CoA reductase inhibitor (statin).[7] Monitor LDL cholesterol levels 4 to 6 weeks after starting lipid therapy and monitor LFTs closely when initiating statins in patients who are concurrently receiving potentially hepatotoxic medications (i.e., ritonavir, saquinavir, amprenavir, efavirenz, and nevirapine).

If patients are at high cardiovascular risk (>20% risk of heart disease within 10 years using the Framingham score) and their lipids are not sufficiently controlled by medications, consider adjusting HAART to include more lipid friendly drugs.[7,10] Amprenavir and nelfinavir have intermediate effects, indinavir and saquinavir have little effect on lipids, and atazanavir has minimal effect.

Table 4-1	Cholesterol Goals and Indications for Therapy	
Risk Factors	**LDL Goal**	**Indications for Therapy**
Established CHD or risk equivalent (i.e., diabetes) >2 risk factors[a] +10 year risk of CHD >20%	<100 mg/dL	If LDL 100–129, can give trial of dietary therapy alone. If LDL >130mg/dL, begin lipid-lowering medication + diet.
2+ risk factors[a] and 10 year risk for CHD ≤20%	<130 mg/dL	If LDL 130–160, and 10-year risk of CHD <10%, can give trial of dietary therapy alone. If LDL 130–160, and 10-year risk of CHD >10%, give lipid-lowering medication +diet. If LDL >160, give lipid-lowering medication +diet.
0–1 risk factor[a]	<160 mg/dL	If LDL >160, can give trial of dietary therapy alone. If LDL >190, consider lipid-lowering medication.

[a]Risk factors include cigarette smoking, hypertension (sbp >140, family history of premature CHD, age (men >45 and women >55), and low HDL (HDL < 40).

HYPERTENSION

There is no significant difference between the incidence of hypertension in HIV-positive individuals compared to seronegative patients, and treatment of hypertension in HIV patients should be guided by the American Heart Association recommendations: target BP is <140/90 for patients with no cardiovascular risk factors, <130/80 for patients at high cardiovascular risk, and <120/80 for patients with left ventricular dysfunction (decreased ejection fraction, diastolic dysfunction, or history of congestive heart failure).[12,17]

Table 4-2	Percentage Increase in Total Cholesterol/Triglycerides in Common Regimen				
Regimens	**TDF/FTC/ Efavirenz**	**TDF/FTC r/Atazanavir**	**TDF/FTC r/Darunavir**	**TDF/FTC/ Raltegravir**	**AZT/3TC/ Efavirenz**
Total Cholesterol >240 mg/dL	22%	11%	23%	Rare reports	24%
Triglycerides >750 mg/dL	4%	—	2%	Rare reports	2%

TDF (tenofovir), FTC (emtricitabine), AZT (Zidovudine), 3TC (lamivudine).

HYPERGLYCEMIA

Compared to HIV-negative men, those infected with HIV on HAART have a four times greater incidence of diabetes.[4] Thus, HIV patients should be screened for hyperglycemia prior to starting HAART and periodically after initiation.[18] Diabetes is diagnosed with any two of the following values: a fasting blood glucose >126 mg/dL, HbA1C >6.5, or an abnormal glucose tolerance test (2). Several antiretrovirals may cause hyperglycemia including indinavir, ritonavir, nelfinavir, lopinavir, and saquinavir.[18] Nevirapine, efavirenz, and atazanavir do not have adverse effects on glucose.

Oral hypoglycemic agents should be offered to diabetic HIV patients. Thiazolidinediones (TZDs) increase insulin sensitivity in peripheral tissues and reduces insulin resistance.[18] LFTs should be checked prior to starting TZDs. Metformin improves insulin resistance but side effects include lactic acidosis which may be increased in combination with certain nucleoside reverse transcriptase inhibitors (NRTIs) such as stavudine, zidovudine, and didanosine.[18] Consider endocrine consultation in patients who may require insulin therapy for better diabetes control.

TOBACCO ABUSE

All HIV patients should be screened for tobacco abuse and counseled on cessation. HIV patients who smoke cigarettes are at higher risk for cardiovascular disease, bacterial pneumonia, non–AIDS-related malignancies, and AIDS-related events.[15] There are several options to aid in tobacco cessation. Buproprion improves success by approximately 10% at 1 year[13,20]; however, it is contraindicated in patients with severe cirrhosis, a history of seizures, or bipolar disorder. Nicotine replacement therapy (patch, gum, spray, inhaler) improves success by 1.5- to 2-fold when coupled with brief counseling from the provider.[13]. There is no good evidence to suggest one method over another, but combined therapy may be better than single therapy.

Varencycline (Chantix), a nonnicotine medication that blocks nicotine receptors in the brain, increases smoking cessation success by 26%, and has been found to be more effective than nicotine replacement therapy.[3,8] Neuropsychiatric side effects may occur and include hostility, agitation, depression, and suicidal ideation. Thus, this medication should be avoided in patients with psychiatric conditions and used with caution in patients on efavirenz.[8]

DEPRESSION

Major depression among HIV patients occurs twice as often compared to HIV-negative patients.[5] Depression can affect medication compliance and contribute to physiologic stress. The Beck Depression Scale can be used as a screening tool. Men with symptoms of depression should also be screened for low testosterone as this is potentially treated with replacement therapy.[5] Medical treatment should be offered in conjunction with counseling to depressed patients; however, it is important to note that certain antiretrovirals interact with antidepressant drugs. PIs can increase concentrations of buproprion and fluoxetine to toxic levels.[6] Also, consider avoiding efavirenz use in patients with depression or anxiety as it may intensify these symptoms. Psychiatric consultation is strongly recommended for depressed HIV patients with active substance abuse or symptoms of mania.

OBESITY

Obesity (body mass index > 30 kg/m^2) increases the risk of many comorbidities including hypertension, diabetes, and respiratory problems. After initiation of HAART, many HIV patients experience weight gain. This can be excessive and patients must be counseled on appropriate dietary habits and exercise. The American Heart Association currently recommends at least 150 minutes of moderate exercise or 75 minutes of vigorous exercise per week.[19]

INITIAL SEROLOGIC TESTING

Several serologies should be obtained upon diagnosis of HIV. Toxoplasma IgG results will affect the use and choice of prophylaxis if CD4 < 100.[1] Serum cryptococcal antigen, if positive, could suggest disseminated disease and prompt more thorough evaluation with a lumbar puncture. Hepatitis A, B, and C serologies should also be obtained at baseline to help guide immunization as well as to consider treatment strategies. Coccidiomycoses serologies should be considered for patients with residence or travel to the southwest, and histoplasma serologies for patients with residence or travel to the Ohio/Mississippi River Valley.

HLAB5701 should be checked at baseline as a positive test predicts a hypersensitivity reaction to abacavir, and tropism testing should be considered if using a CCR5 inhibitor such as maraviroc. G6PD should be checked before starting patients on dapsone, primaquine, or sulfonamides.[1]

Baseline and annual rapid plasma reagin (RPR) for syphilis screening should also be obtained. If RPR is positive and the patient has late latent syphilis, neurologic symptoms, or active tertiary syphilis, then a lumbar puncture should be performed.[1]

OTHER TESTING

A baseline chest x-ray should be obtained regardless of tobacco use. Urinalysis and creatinine clearance (CrCl) should also be assessed as this can help identify patients with HIV associated nephropathy. Patients with ≥1+ proteinuria or glomerular filtration rate (GFR) <60 should have further renal workup.

Patients on tenofovir and indinavir should have urinalysis and CrCl checked every 6 months.

A funduscopic exam should be performed for patients with CD4 counts <50.[1] Additionally, age-appropriate screening for colon cancer should begin at age 50 with annual fecal occult blood testing, flex sigmoidoscopy at 5-year intervals, or colonoscopy at 10-year intervals.

GENDER-SPECIFIC ISSUES

Men: HIV-positive men are at risk for hypogonadism.[1] A morning serum total cholesterol should be obtained in patients reporting fatigue, erectile dysfunction/poor libido, and symptoms of depression. While there are no formal national guidelines for the screening of anal cancer, the New York State Department of Health recommends performing baseline and annual anal pap smears on HIV-positive men who have sex with men, as well as any patient with a history of anal or genital warts.

Women: HIV-positive women have a higher risk of cervical cancer and should be screened at baseline and annually with Pap smears.[1] All women should be referred for screening mammograms from age 40.

ADULT IMMUNIZATIONS

All HIV patients should receive the following vaccines: pneumococcal vaccine every 5 years regardless of age, tetanus toxoid, diphtheria toxoid, hepatitis A and B vaccines if not immunized, and an annual influenza vaccine.[1] Live viruses are generally contraindicated in immunosuppressed individuals, but the varicella vaccine is proven to be safe in HIV patients with a CD4 count greater than 200cells/mm^3 and is recommended for those who are not already immunized.[1] Lastly, the human papillomavirus vaccine is currently approved for women aged 13 to 26 for prevention of cervical cancer, but data regarding efficacy and safety in HIV patients remain under investigation.[1]

REFERENCES

1. Aberg J, Kaplan J, Libman H, et al. Primary care guidelines for the management of persons infected with human immunodeficiency virus: 2009 update by the HIV medicine Association of the Infectious Diseases Society of America. *Clin Infect Dis* 2009;49(5): 651–681.
2. American Diabetes Association. Standards of medical care in diabetes—2010. *Diabetes Care* 2010;33:S11–S61.
3. Aubin HJ, Bobak A, Britton JR, et al. Varenicline versus transdermal nicotine patch for smoking cessation: results from a randomised open-label trial. *Thorax* 2008;63(8): 717–724.
4. Brown TT, Cole SR, Li X, et al. Antiretroviral therapy and the prevalence and incidence of diabetes mellitus in the multicenter AIDS cohort study. *Arch Intern Med* 2005;165: 1179–1184.
5. Ciesla JA, Roberts JE. Meta-analysis of relationship between HIV infection and risk for depressive disorders. *Am J Psychiatry* 2001;158:725–730.
6. DeSilva KE, Le Flore DB, Marston BJ, et al. Serotonin syndrome in HIV-infected individuals receiving antiretroviral therapy and fluoxetine. *AIDS* 2001;15:1281–1285.
7. Dube MP, Stein JH, Aberg JA, et al. Guidelines for the evaluation and management of dyslipidemia in human immunodeficiency virus (HIV)-infected adults receiving antiretroviral therapy: recommendations of the HIV Medical Association of the Infectious Disease Society of America and the Adult AIDS Clinical Trials Group. *Clin Infect Dis* 2003;37: 613–627.
8. Ebbert JO, Wyatt K, Hays JT, et al. Varenicline for smoking cessation efficacy, safety, and treatment recommendations. *Patient Prefer Adherence* 2010;4:355–362.
9. Engels EA, Biggar RJ, Hall HI, et al. Cancer risk in people infected with human immunodeficiency virus in the United States. *Int J Cancer* 2008;123(1):187–194.
10. Expert Panel on Detection, Evaluation, and Treatment of High Blood Cholesterol in Adults. Executive Summary of the Third Report of the National Cholesterol Education Program (NCEP) Expert Panel on Detection, Evaluation, and Treatment of High Blood Cholesterol in Adults (Adult Treatment Panel III). *JAMA* 2001;285(19):2486–2497.
11. Fellay J, Boubaker K, Ledergerber B, et al. Prevalence of adverse events associated with potent antiretroviral treatment: Swiss HIV Cohort Study. *Lancet* 2001;358:1322–1327.
12. Jerico C, Knobel H, Montero M, et al. Hypertension in HIV-infected patients: prevalence and related factors. *Am J Hypertens* 2005;18:1396–1401.
13. Lancaster T, Stead L, Silagy C, et al. Effectiveness of interventions to help people stop smoking: findings from the Cochrane Library. *BMJ* 2000;321(7257):355–358.

14. Lichtenstein KA, Armon C, Buchacz K, et al. Low CD4+ T cell count is a risk factor for cardiovascular disease events in the HIV outpatient study. *Clin Infect Dis* 2010;51(4): 435–447.

15. Lifson AR, Neuhaus J, Arribas JR, et al. Smoking-related health risks among persons with HIV in the Strategies for Management of Antiretroviral Therapy clinical trial. *Am J Public Health* 2010;100:1896–1903.

16. Moyle GJ, Lloyd M, Reynolds B, et al. Dietary advice with or without pravastatin for the management of hypercholesterolaemia associated with protease inhibitor therapy. *AIDS* 2001;15(12):1503.

17. Rosendorff C, Black H, Cannon C, et al. Treatment of hypertension in the prevention and management of ischemic heart disease. A scientific statement from the American Heart Association Council for High Blood Pressure Research and the Councils on Clinical Cardiology and Epidemiology and Prevention. *Circulation* 2007;115:2761–2788.

18. Spollet GR. Hyperglycemia in HIV/AIDS. *Diabetes Spectrum* 2006;19(3):163–166.

19. Roger VL, Go AS, Lloyd-Jones DM, et al. Heart disease and stroke statistics—2011 update: a report from the American Heart Association. *Circulation* 2011;123:e18–e209.

20. West R. Bupropion SR for smoking cessation. *Expert Opin Pharmacother* 2003;4(4): 533–540.

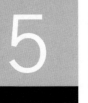

5

HIV Infection and Pregnancy

Oluwatosin Jaiyeoba and J. Michael Kilby

INTRODUCTION

Significant advances have been made in the prevention of mother-to-child HIV transmission (MTCT) to the extent that in countries with access to modest health care resources, it is a reasonable goal that no child should be born with HIV. With the implementation of recommendations for universal prenatal HIV counseling and testing, antiretroviral prophylaxis (including multidrug highly active antiretroviral regimens, rather than monotherapy, for infected mothers), scheduled cesarean delivery, and avoidance of breast-feeding, the rate of perinatal transmission of HIV has dramatically diminished to <2% in the United States and Europe.

EPIDEMIOLOGY

- Men and women are equally affected by HIV infection worldwide. However, the United States has consistently experienced a relative increase in the number of HIV-infected women in recent years. In 2009, women accounted for 24% of new US HIV infections.
  - Fifty-seven percent occurred in African American women, 21 % in Caucasian women, and 16% in Hispanic/Latinas.

ANTIRETROVIRAL THERAPY

Importance of Antiretroviral Therapy

- Decreases maternal viral load (VL) in blood and genital secretions, reduces perinatal transmission, and functions as infant preexposure prophylaxis.
- Three-part strategy: antepartum, intrapartum, infant prophylaxis.
- Three-drug combination therapy is recommended, generally:
  2 nucleoside/nucleotide reverse transcriptase inhibitors (NRTI)

  PLUS

  1 nonnucleoside reverse transcriptase inhibitor (NNRTI)

  OR

  1 protease inhibitor (PI) boosted with 100 mg oral ritonavir

Consideration Should Be Given to Drug Distribution in Pregnancy

- Altered drug pharmacokinetics (PK) during pregnancy
  - Placental transport of the drug, compartmentalization of the drug in the embryo/ fetus and placenta, biotransformation of the drug by the fetus and placenta, and elimination of the drug by the fetus

- Altered drug dosing requirements and susceptibility to toxicity
- NRTI and NNRTI have similar PK properties in pregnant and nonpregnant women.
- PI show variable PK properties in pregnant women particularly in the second and third trimesters. See Table 5-1.

When to Initiate Antiretroviral Therapy

- Always counsel about antiretroviral therapy (ART) use during pregnancy and prevention of perinatal transmission, regardless of plasma HIV RNA levels.
- Perform genotypic resistance testing before initiating ART if HIV RNA levels are above the threshold for resistance testing.
- Begin ART
  - Immediately in women requiring treatment for their own health.
  - After the first trimester in women not requiring immediate therapy.
  - See Table 5-1 for commonly used preferred and alternative regimens.
- Continue ART unchanged in women who become pregnant during therapy
  - ART-experienced patients should continue medication unless regimen includes efavirenz, which is not recommended for use in the first trimester and should only be used in the second and third trimesters if there are no alternatives.

Importance of Viral Load and Immune Status on Risk of HIV Transmission

- Plasma HIV RNA VL correlates predictably with transmission risk. However, there is no absolute VL threshold below which there is no known risk of transmission.

ANTEPARTUM MANAGEMENT

- Management to include the recommendations in Table 5-2 and routine obstetric care following American College of Obstetricians and Gynecologists (ACOG) guidelines.
- Monitor CD4 cell count at initial antenatal visit and at least every 3 months.
- HIV RNA VL monitoring:
  - Initial visit or before initiation of therapy
  - Two to four weeks after initiating or changing therapy
  - Every 4 to 8 weeks until plasma HIV RNA levels are undetectable
  - Every 2 months for the remainder of the pregnancy
- One log decline in plasma viremia expected 1 month after initiation of therapy.
- Complete viral suppression achieved within 12 to 24 weeks after initiation of therapy
- Plasma HIV RNA viral level assessment at 36 weeks of gestation to decide mode of delivery
  - Plasma HIV RNA VL >1,000 copies/mL = cesarean delivery
  - Plasma HIV RNA VL <1,000 copies/mL = may have vaginal delivery if no obstetric contraindication
- Repeat genotypic resistance testing in patients who report adherence but experience suboptimal viral suppression or viral rebound to detectable levels.
- Monitor for common complications of ART during pregnancy (renal dysfunction when receiving tenofovir, or anemia due to zidovudine).
- Ultrasound

Table 5-1   List of Anti-retrovirals Commonly Used in Pregnancy. (List includes individual medications and co-formulations)

Drug (Abbreviated Name) Trade Name	Dosage Recommendation	Co-Formulations	PKs	Recommendations for Use in Pregnancy
NRTI				
Lamivudine (3TC) Epivir	150 mg b.i.d. or 300 mg once daily	Combivir (AZT+3TC) 3TC 150 mg + ZDV 300 mg	PK not significantly altered. High placental transfer	Recommended dual-NRTI backbone in ART-naïve patients
Zidovudine (AZT, ZDV) Retrovir	300 mg b.i.d. or 200 mg t.i.d.	Combivir 1 tablet b.i.d.	PK not significantly altered. High placental transfer	Recommended dual-NRTI backbone in ART-naïve patients. Monitor for anemia
Abacavir (ABC) Ziagen	Ziagen 300 mg b.i.d. or 600 mg once daily	Epzicom (ABC+3TC) ABC 600 mg + 3TC 300 mg	PK not significantly altered. High placental transfer	Alternative NRTI for dual-NRTI backbone
Emtricitabine (FTC) Emtriva	Emtriva 200-mg capsule once daily or 240 mg (24 mL) oral solution once daily	Truvada (FTC+TDF) FTC 200 mg + TDF 300 mg. Atripla[a] (EFV+FTC+TDF) 1 tablet at or before bedtime. Take on an empty stomach to reduce side effects.	PK slightly lower levels in third trimester. No clear need to increase dose. High placental transfer	Alternative NRTI for dual-NRTI backbone
Tenofovir Disoproxil Fumarate (TDF) Viread	Viread 300-mg tablet once daily	Truvada 1 tablet once daily. Atripla[a] 1 tablet at or before bedtime	High placental transfer to fetus	Preferred NRTI in combination with 3TC or FTC in women with chronic HBV infection. Because of potential for renal toxicity, renal function should be monitored.

NNRTIs

Drug	Dosing	Combination	PK/Placental transfer	Comments
Nevirapine (NVP) Viramune	200-mg tablets or 50-mg/5-mL oral suspension		PK not significantly altered. High placental transfer	Initiate in pregnant women with CD4 counts >250 cells/mm³ only if benefit clearly outweighs risk because of the increased risk of potentially life-threatening hepatotoxicity in women with high CD4 cell counts
Efavirenz[a] (EFV) Sustiva	600 mg once daily at or before bedtime Take on an empty stomach to reduce side effects.	Atripla[a] 1 tablet once daily at or before bedtime	No change in dose indicated. Moderate placental transfer to fetus	EFV should be avoided in the first trimester. Use after the first trimester can be considered if, after consideration of other alternatives, this is the only choice for a specific woman.
Etravirine (ETR) Intelence	200 mg b.i.d. Take following a meal		No PK studies in human pregnancy, placental transfer rate unknown	No experience in human pregnancy
Rilpivirine (RPV) Endurant	25 mg once daily with a meal.	Complera (RPV+TDF+FTC) RPV 25 mg + TDF 300 mg + FTC 200 mg	No PK studies in human pregnancy, placental transfer rate unknown	No experience in human pregnancy

PIs

Drug	Dosing	Combination	PK/Placental transfer	Comments
Lopinavir + Ritonavir (LPV/r) Kaletra	Tablets: (LPV 200mg + RTV 50mg) or (LPV 100mg + RTV 25mg) standard dose is LPV/r 400mg/100mg b.i.d	Increase dose to LPV/r 600mg/150mg b.i.d. in second and third trimester	PK suggests dose should be increased to 600mg/150mg b.i.d. in second and third trimester. Low placental transfer	Recommended PI in ART-naïve patients. There is extensive experience with use in pregnancy.

(Continued)

Table 5-1 List of Anti-retrovirals Commonly Used in Pregnancy. (List includes individual medications and co-formulations) *(Continued)*

Drug (Abbreviated Name) Trade Name	Dosage Recommendation	Co-Formulations	PKs	Recommendations for Use in Pregnancy
Atazanavir (ATV) Reyataz (combined with low-dose ritonavir [RTV] boosting)	ATV 300 mg + RTV 100 mg once daily		PK suggests that standard dosing results in decreased plasma concentration compared with non-pregnant adults. However, for most pregnant women, dose adjustment of ATV is not needed. Low placental transfer to fetus	Alternative PI. ART-experienced pregnant women on either tenofovir or H2-receptor blocker (not both) should increase ATV dose to 400 mg (with ritonavir 100 mg).
Darunavir (DRV) Prezista (combined with low-dose RTV boosting)	(DRV 800 mg + RTV 100 mg) once daily. (DRV 600 mg + RTV 100 mg) b.i.d. if any DRV resistance mutations		No PK studies in human pregnancy. Minimal to low placental transfer to fetus	No data about the use of DRV in pregnancy but clinically there has been an increase in its use in pregnancy.
Integrase Inhibitors				
Raltegravir (RAL) Isentress	400-mg tablets b.i.d.	With rifampin: 800 mg b.i.d.	Standard dose appears appropriate during pregnancy. Variable but high placental transfer to fetus	No experience in human pregnancy

[a]Avoided in first trimester, and may be considered by some clinicians as a last resort later in pregnancy. But generally to be avoided.

Table 5-2	Initial Evaluation of the HIV-Infected Pregnant Woman

- Degree of immunodeficiency (defined by past and current CD4 cell counts)
- Plasma HIV RNA VL and antiretroviral resistance testing if VL detectable
- Need for opportunistic infection prophylaxis (*Toxoplasma gondii*, *Pneumocystis jiroveci* pneumonia, *Mycobacterium avium* complex)
- Presence of coinfections that may require curative or maintenance therapy (tuberculosis, syphilis, gonorrhea, chlamydia, genital herpes simplex, hepatitis B, and hepatitis C)
- Evaluation of immunization status (tetanus-pertussis-diphtheria, hepatitis A, hepatitis B, influenza, and pneumococcus)
- Baseline hematologic, renal and hepatic parameters
- HLA-B*5701 testing, if abacavir use is anticipated
- Assessments of adequate housing, nutrition, and supportive care needs

- First trimester: confirms gestational age and guides time of cesarean delivery if indicated
- Second trimester (18 to 21 weeks): assessment of fetal anatomy
- Follow with nonstress testing (NST)/fetal well-being assessment if appropriate.
- Amniocentesis and other invasive procedures are not contraindicated in virologically suppressed patients but typically avoided unless necessary.

INTRAPARTUM MANAGEMENT

- Continue ART during labor or before cesarean delivery. Administer IV zidovudine (initial loading dose of 2 mg/kg intravenously over 1 hour, followed by continuous infusion of 1 mg/kg/h until delivery) beginning 3 hours before scheduled cesarean delivery.

Management of Women Who Present with Ruptured Membranes

- HIV-infected patients with plasma RNA levels of <1,000 copies who present with ruptured membranes (ROM) near term or at term may have a vaginal delivery.
- When ROM occurs before 34 weeks of gestation, decisions about delivery should be based on gestational age, HIV RNA level, current ART regimen, and evidence of acute infection such as chorioamnionitis.
- Administration of steroids to accelerate fetal lung maturity is not contraindicated and should follow ACOG guidelines.
- Clinicians may consider administration of oxytocin, if clinically appropriate, to expedite delivery.

POSTPARTUM MANAGEMENT

- HIV-infected women in the United States should not breast-feed their infants. Lack of breast-feeding is associated with earlier return of ovulation; thus, counsel regarding contraception is warranted. Screen for postpartum depression and offer appropriate therapy.

Care of Exposed Neonate

- HIV DNA polymerase chain reaction (PCR) is required to diagnose HIV infection in infants <18 months of age. Consultation with an expert in the diagnosis and management of the infant born to an HIV-positive mother is encouraged.
- AZT is recommended for all HIV-exposed infants. Dosage should be weight based.

Breast-feeding Infants of Mothers Diagnosed with HIV Infection Postpartum

- Breast-feeding should be stopped until infection is confirmed. Pumping and temporarily discarding breast milk is recommended until infection is ruled out.
- Infants of women who develop acute HIV infection while breast-feeding are at greater risk of becoming infected than are those of women with chronic HIV infection.

SUMMARY

- All pregnant HIV-infected women should be strongly encouraged to take ART regardless of their CD4 cell count for MTCT prevention.
- ART should be initiated as soon as possible in women requiring it for their health and after the first trimester for MTCT prevention.
- Pregnant women should receive AZT infusion prior to cesarean delivery or during labor.
- Patients with plasma HIV RNA VL>1,000 copies/mL should have a scheduled cesarean delivery at 38 weeks of gestation.
- Avoid breast-feeding, and provide newborns with prophylactic zidovudine for 6 weeks or longer depending on their virologic status.
- Considerations regarding continuation of ART for maternal therapeutic indications after delivery are the same as for nonpregnant women.

SUGGESTED READINGS

ACOG Practice Bulletin No. 99. Management of abnormal cervical cytology and histology. *Obstet Gynecol* 2008:112(6):1419–1444, (Reaffirmed 2010).
    Provides guidance on how to triage and manage abnormal Pap smears. This is especially important in HIV-infected women.
ACOG Practice Bulletin No. 80. Premature rupture of membranes. *Obstet Gynecol* 2007;109(4):1007–1019, (Reaffirmed 2009).
    Provides evidence-based guidance on how to manage women who present with ROM. Management is discussed based on gestational age.
Best BM, Stek AM, Mirochnick M, et al. Lopinavir tablet pharmacokinetics with an increased dose during pregnancy. *J Acquir Immune Defic Syndr* 2010;54(4):381–388.
    Higher dose of lopinavir should be used in the second and third trimesters.
Cooper ER, Charurat M, Mofenson L, et al. Combination antiretroviral strategies for the treatment of pregnant HIV-1-infected women and prevention of perinatal HIV-1 transmission. *J Acquir Immune Defic Syndr* 2002;29(5):484–494.
    Levels of HIV-1 RNA at delivery and prenatal antiretroviral therapy were independently associated with transmission. The protective effect of therapy increased with the complexity and duration of the regimen.

Hart CE, Lennox JL, Pratt-Palmore M, et al. Correlation of human immunodeficiency virus type 1 RNA levels in blood and the female genital tract. *J Infect Dis* 1999;179(4):871–882. *Initiation of antiretroviral therapy significantly reduced the amount of HIV-1 RNA in vaginal secretions. These findings suggest that factors that lower blood plasma virus load may also reduce the risk of perinatal and female-to-male heterosexual transmission by lowering vaginal virus load.*

Morrison CS, Demers K, Kwok C, et al. Plasma and cervical viral loads among Ugandan and Zimbabwean women during acute and early HIV-1 infection. *AIDS* 2010;24(4):573–582. *Cervical VLs were strongly correlated with plasma VLs during the first 6 months of HIV-1 infection (p < 0.0001) and were significantly higher (0.7 to 1.1 $\log_{10}$ copies/ mL higher) during acute infection than subsequently during the early infection period. Subtype D infection, pregnancy, and breast-feeding at the time of HIV infection were associated with a higher plasma viral setpoint, while young age was associated with a decreased plasma setpoint.*

Recommendations for Use of Antiretroviral Drugs in Pregnant HIV-1-Infected Women for Maternal Health and Interventions to Reduce Perinatal HIV Transmission in the United States September 14, 2011 http://www.aidsinfo.nih.gov/ContentFiles/PerinatalGL.pdf *Evidence-based document that outlines guidelines for the management of pregnant HIV-infected women. This document covers preconception management to postpartum management of the HIV-infected pregnant woman.*

Shaheen F, Sison AV, McIntosh L, et al. Analysis of HIV-1 in the cervicovaginal secretions and blood of pregnant and nonpregnant women. *J Hum Virol* 1999;2(3):154–166. *Plasma VL showed significant correlation with the detection of HIV-1 RNA in the cervicovaginal lavage. This is important since the plasma HIV RNA VL serves as a surrogate marker for the vaginal VL.*

The European Collaborative Study*. Maternal viral load and vertical transmission of HIV-1: an important factor but not the only one. *AIDS* 1999;13(11):1377–1385. *Vertical transmission increased with increasing RNA levels, but there was no threshold below which transmission did not occur. Mother-to-child transmission of HIV-1 is multifactorial with high RNA load as a very important determinant.*

II   Viral Hepatitis

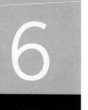

Diagnosis of Viral Hepatitis

Zhi Q. Yao

Viral hepatitis refers to a group of viral infections that primarily cause liver inflammation. The most common types include hepatitis A, hepatitis B, and hepatitis C. Hepatitis D occurs in the presence of hepatitis B. Hepatitis E, like hepatitis A, is transmitted by the fecal-oral route and only leads to an acute hepatitis. The differential diagnosis of liver inflammation is broad:

Differential Diagnosis

Viral hepatitis: A, B, C, D, and E
Other infections: Epsterin-Barr Virus (EBV), cytomegalovirus (CMV), herpes
    simplex virus (HSV), leptospirosis, tuberculosis (TB), and toxoplasmosis
Autoimmune hepatitis
Drug-induced hepatitis: acetaminophen, alcohol, isoniazid, azoles, and statins
Hemodynamic liver injury: sepsis, ischemia, heart failure, and vascular occlusion
Nonalcoholic fatty liver disease (NAFLD)
Cholestatic liver disease: primary biliary cirrhosis, primary sclerosing
    cholangitis, gallstones, and acute cholecystitis
Metabolic/genetic: hemochromatosis, Wilson disease, and α_1-antitrypsin
    deficiency
Pregnancy-related liver diseases
Hepatic tumors, cysts, abscesses, and biliary tract neoplasms

HEPATITIS A

- Hepatitis A virus (**HAV**) causes approximately half of the cases of acute hepatitis in the United States. Major routes of infection include ingestion of contaminated food or water and close contact with an infected person. Persons at high risk include men who have sex with men and those who travel to endemic areas. Typical incubation period is 2 to 3 weeks.
- Clinically, patients infected with hepatitis A may or may not exhibit the following typical symptoms or signs: fatigue, anorexia, jaundice, and nonspecific gastrointestinal symptoms such as nausea, poor appetite, and abdominal pain that are indistinguishable from other causes of hepatitis.
- The diagnosis of acute hepatitis A depends on serology: detecting an IgM anti-HAV; positive IgG anti-HAV antibody indicates prior infection and immunity, while the presence of both IgM and IgG antibodies suggests infection within the prior 2 to 6 months; the absence of both IgM and IgG anti-HAV antibodies indicates susceptibility to HAV.
- There is no chronic state of HAV infection.

HEPATITIS B

- An estimated 350 million persons worldwide are infected with hepatitis B virus (**HBV**), a double-strained DNA virus that is coated with a surface antigen (HBsAg) and has a central core (with HBV core and e antigens) containing the HBV DNA. HBV causes approximately one-third of acute viral hepatitis and approximately 15% of cases of chronic viral hepatitis in the United States.
- Hepatitis B is transmitted parenterally by percutaneous exposure; by sharing needles in drug use; by intimate person-to-person contact with an infected person, including sexual contact; and by mother-to-infant vertical transmission. The virus is found in blood as well as in body fluids such as saliva, milk, urine, or stool.
- The incubation period of HBV infection ranges from 6 weeks to 6 months after exposure. Symptoms are similar to those of hepatitis A and may include other nonspecific constitutional complaints.
- In most adult patients (>90%), the acute infection resolves within 6 months, whereas most infant HBV infection (>90%) leads to a chronic carrier status.
- Patients with persistent HBsAg positivity beyond 6 months are deemed a chronic infection. Patients with established chronic infection must be monitored for the development of cirrhosis and hepatocellular carcinoma (HCC) with ultrasonography and measurement of serum α-fetoprotein at an interval of every 6 to 12 months.
- The diagnosis of hepatitis B depends on accurately interpreting serologic tests according to the natural history of infection. The patient with **immune-tolerance**– acquired HBV perinatally will be HBeAg positive and have high levels of HBV DNA; the risk for active hepatitis increases with age.
- The patient with detectable HBeAg, high HBV DNA, elevated serum ALT levels, and inflammation on liver biopsy is in a phase of **immune clearance**, that is, the phase when the immune system is attempting to eliminate the virus. In this phase, elevations in liver enzymes may indicate the onset of HBeAg seroconversion.
- The **inactive carrier** is a patient in whom spontaneous seroconversion to HBeAg negativity occurs. Patients with positive HBsAg but absence of HBeAg may harbor HBV variants in the precore or promoter regions. In these patients, there is low HBV DNA with little or no inflammation on liver biopsy. However, periodic reversions back to HBeAg positivity may occur and be associated with elevation of liver enzymes and an increase in HBV DNA levels.
- There have been rare cases characterized by negative HBsAg but anti-HBc (alone) positive; most of these persons have a negative HBV DNA and are not infectious.

Interpretation	HBsAg	α-HBs	IgM α-HBc	IgG α-HBc	HBeAg	α-HBe	HBV DNA
Acute infection	+	−	+	−	+	−	+
Chronic infection/ active replication	+	−	−	+	+	−	+
Chronic infection/ inactive replication	+	−	−	+	−	+	+/−
Immune, prior infection	−	+	−	+/−	−	−	−

HEPATITIS C

- Hepatitis C virus (**HCV**) is a single-stranded RNA virus classified as a separate genus in the Flaviviridae family. HCV infection is the most prevalent blood-borne infection in the United States, affecting an estimated 4 million persons.
- Patients at risk for hepatitis C include persons who have ever injected illegal drugs, have received hemodialysis, or were born to an infected mother; health care workers who have sustained needlestick accidents are at risk.
- Most patients acutely infected with HCV are asymptomatic and do not clear the infection spontaneously; approximately 85% develop chronic infection, with mildly elevated liver enzymes or remain asymptomatic.
- Of patients with chronic infection, 20% develop cirrhosis over 20 years; of patients who develop cirrhosis, the risk for HCC is approximately 5% per year. Chronic HCV infection has become the leading cause for HCC and liver transplantation.
- Anti-HCV antibody is the screening test for at-risk persons and usually develops within 2 to 6 months following exposure; a positive test in a person with one of the risk factors confirms exposure to the virus. HCV RNA testing is required to determine active infection and the need for follow-up with antiviral therapy.
- Distinct HCV genotypes (6 major genotypes and over 100 subtypes) have been identified that differ in their clinical outcomes in response to therapy.
- Liver biopsy is useful in some patients (such as those with genotype 1, who experience poorer responses to treatment) to determine the extent of fibrosis and degree of inflammation; this provides the option to either treat or forgo therapy and observe.

HEPATITIS D

- Hepatitis D virus (**HDV** or delta agent) infection depends upon the presence of HBsAg for its replication. Patients with a history of injection drug use are at greatest risk for acquiring HDV infection. Diagnosis depends on anti-HDV serology.
- In an HBV-infected patient, HDV infection may present as an acute hepatitis (in which case it is a coinfection) or an exacerbation of preexisting chronic hepatitis (in which case it is a superinfection).

HEPATITIS E

- Hepatitis E virus (**HEV**) infection, like HAV, is spread by fecal-oral transmission and can produce an acute hepatitis.
- HEV infection most likely to occur in residents of or recent travelers to underdeveloped nations, notably India and the Middle East.
- Diagnosis is by detection of IgM antibody (available through CDC).
- Pregnant woman with acute HEV infection are at greatest risk for developing severe hepatitis or liver failure.

SUGGESTED READINGS

The A, B, Cs of Viral Hepatitis www.health.ny.gov/diseases/communicable/hepatitis/*Cached*
CDC DVH—Division of Viral Hepatitis Home Page www.cdc.gov/hepatitis
Ghany MG, et al. Diagnosis, management, and treatment of hepatitis C: an update. *Hepatology* 2009;49:1335.

This excellent review summarizes diagnostic methods and the emergence of novel therapies for HCV infection.

Klevins RM, et al. The evolving epidemiology of hepatitis A in the United States: incidence and molecular epidemiology from a population-based surveillance, 2005–2007. *Arch Intern Med* 2010;180:1811.

Martin A, Lemon SM. Hepatitis A virus: from discovery to vaccines. *Hepatology* 2006;43:S164.
This review gives an outstanding overview of hepatitis A infection.

Centers for Disease Control and Prevention. Recommendations for the prevention and control of hepatitis C virus (HCV) infection and HCV-related chronic disease. *MMWR Recomm Rep* 1998;47:1.
These recommendations provide a thorough summary of hepatitis C infection, including diagnosis and prevention.

Viral Hepatitis Symptoms, Causes, Diagnosis, and Treatment by Dr. Dennis Lee www.medicinenet.com *Cached-Similar* You +1'd this publicly. Undo

Viral Hepatitis: A through E and Beyond—NIDDK digestive.niddk.nih.gov/ddiseases/pubs/viralhepatitis/ *Cached-Similar*

Treatment of Viral Hepatitis

Zhi Q. Yao

HEPATITIS A

- There is no specific therapy for HAV infection. Supportive therapy to maintain fluid and caloric intake is usually sufficient, and hospitalization is rarely required. Please see the chapter on Prevention for further guidance.

HEPATITIS B

- Management of acute hepatitis B consists of observation and follow-up testing. It is prudent to reassess the hepatitis B serologic profile every 1 to 3 months until the acute infection resolves.
- Acute hepatitis B may rarely cause severe illness with impaired liver function (fulminant hepatitis) that should be evaluated for liver transplantation and antiviral treatment.
- The goal of therapy for chronic hepatitis B is to suppress viral replication, to mitigate hepatic inflammation, and to prevent or slow the progression to cirrhosis, liver failure, and hepatocellular carcinoma (HCC).
- A number of antiviral agents are approved for treatment of chronic, replicative hepatitis B with liver injury, including interferon (IFN), lamivudine, adefovir, entecavir, and telbivudine.
- Drug resistance, low cure rates, and side effects have been problematic.
- The advantages of IFN are its limited duration of therapy, the lack of resistance, and the high response rate in terms of antigen clearance in comparison to oral agents. However, patients with advanced liver disease or decompensated cirrhosis should not be given IFN therapy because of the risk for decompensation of liver disease.
- In such patients, the oral agents are used but are limited in their ability to achieve a sustained suppression of viral replication, are costly, and have a propensity for drug resistance.

Drug Treatments for Chronic Hepatitis B Infection

Drug	Dose	Efficacy	Resistance	Comments
Pegylated IFN α2a	180 mcg SC/ week × 48 weeks	E Ag +: 32% lose HBeAg and suppress DNA to <20,000 IU/mL E Ag −: 43% suppress HBV DNA to <4,000 IU/mL	No viral resistance *per se*	Do not use in the setting of cirrhosis (Childs B or C).

Drug Treatments for Chronic Hepatitis B Infection *(Continued)*

Drug	Dose	Efficacy	Resistance	Comments
Tenofovir	300 mg daily	E Ag +: 76% suppress DNA to <69 IU/mL E Ag −: 93% suppress DNA to <69 IU/mL	Low rate detected	Can be given as an emtricitabine coformulation; emtricitabine similar to lamivudine. (not FDA approved)
Entecavir	0.5 mg daily	E Ag +: 67% suppress DNA to <300 copies/mL; 22% lose E Ag	Not detected	
Lamivudine	100 mg daily	E Ag +: 32% lose HBeAg and 44% suppress DNA to <20,000 IU/mL	High rate noted (15%/year)	Hepatitis may flare upon cessation of therapy.
Telbivudine	600 mg daily	E Ag +: 35% lose HBeAg and 56% suppress DNA to undetectable	High rate in individuals who do not suppress HCV DNA to <1,000 copies/mL by 24 weeks	Duration remains unclear.
Adefovir	10 mg daily	E Ag +: 24% lose HBeAg and 21% suppress DNA to undetectable. E Ag −: 71% suppress DNA to <1,000 copies/mL	Not common	

HEPATITIS C

- Therapy for hepatitis C infection consists of the combination of pegylated interferon (IFN) and ribavirin (RBV).
- The goal of therapy is to achieve a sustained virologic response (SVR), which is defined as undetectable hepatitis C virus (HCV) RNA beyond 6 months after the end of treatment.
  - Treatment responses vary with the infecting HCV genotype, viral load, and host genetics
  - Patients infected with genotype 1 have an approximately 50% SVR if treated for 48 weeks

- Patients who achieve an undetectable HCV RNA by the 4th week rapid virological response (RVR) or 12th week early virological response (EVR) have a higher likelihood (~90% or 66%, respectively) of achieving an SVR
- Failure to achieve at least 2-log reduction of HCV RNA titer by the 12th week of therapy should lead to cessation of treatment
- Patients with genotypes 2 and 3 have an SVR rate in excess of 80% and require only 24 weeks of therapy; the dosage of RBV can also be reduced in these patients.
- Liver biopsy prior to therapy has been recommended for genotype 1 infection; controversial with genotypes 2/3 where SVRs are high (76% to 82%).
- Most patients treated with pegylated IFN and RBV experience side effects, which include a flu-like illness, bone marrow suppression, depression, and thyroid inflammation.
- Contraindications to therapy include severe preexisting bone marrow suppression, severe depression, autoimmune hepatitis, and advanced liver disease.
- An increasing number of specific antiviral agents are now available for treatment of hepatitis C.
  - Boceprevir and telaprevir have been approved in combination with pegIFN/RBV therapy for genotype 1 HCV infection and demonstrate promising SVRs (66% to79%).
  - Treatment durations are determined by response.

Drug Treatments for Chronic Hepatitis C Infection

Drug	Standard Dose	Side Effects	Comments
Pegylated IFN α 2a	180 mcg SC weekly	Flu-like symptoms, depression, fatigue, hair thinning, bone marrow suppression, cognitive changes	Support cytopenias with growth factors as needed.
Pegylated IFN α 2b	1.5 mcg/kg SC weekly	Flu-like symptoms, depression, fatigue, hair thinning, bone marrow suppression, cognitive changes	Support cytopenias with growth factors as needed.
Ribavirin	Weight-based PO b.i.d.	Hemolytic anemia, teratogenic	Dose reduction indicated once hemoglobin falls to <10 g/dL
Boceprevir	800 mg PO t.i.d. to start 4 weeks after IFN/RBV started	Anemia (greater than with IFN/RBV alone), fatigue, dysgeusia, nausea, headache	Duration of IFN/RBV dependent upon response at 8 or 24 weeks treatment
Telaprevir	750 mg PO t.i.d. with IFN/RBV for 12 weeks	Rash, pruritus, anemia (greater than with IFN/RBV alone)	Duration of IFN/RBV dependent upon response at 4 or 12 weeks treatment

SUGGESTED READINGS

The A, B, Cs of Viral Hepatitis www.health.ny.gov/diseases/communicable/hepatitis/*Cached*

Butt AA, Kanwal F. Boceprevir and telaprevir in the management of hepatitis C virus-infected patients. *Clin Infect Dis* 2012;54(1):96–104.

This recent review provides an excellent overview of the new drug therapies available for HCV infection.

CDC DVH—Division of Viral Hepatitis Home Page www.cdc.gov/hepatitis

Fried MW, et al. Peginterferon alfa-2a plus ribavirin for chronic hepatitis C virus infection. *N Engl J Med* 2002;347:975.

Ghany MG, et al. Diagnosis, management, and treatment of hepatitis C: an update. *Hepatology* 2009;49:1335.

Hézode C, et al. Telaprevir and peginterferon with or without ribavirin for chronic HCV infection. *N Engl J Med* 2009;360:1839.

This study demonstrated that a combination regimen of peginterferon α-2a and RBV for 12 weeks, followed by peginterferon α-2a and RBV for 12 more weeks, resulted in a response rate of 69% in genotype 1 HCV infection.

McHutchison JG, et al. Telaprevir with peginterferon and ribavirin for chronic HCV genotype 1 infection. *N Engl J Med* 2009;360:1827.

McHutchison JG, et al. Peginterferon alfa-2b or alfa-2a with ribavirin for treatment of hepatitis C infection. *N Engl J Med* 2009;361:580.

This study demonstrated equivalent but low response rates for genotype 1 infection using either pegIFN α 2a or 2b (≈40%).

Viral Hepatitis: A through E and Beyond—NIDDK digestive.niddk.nih.gov/ddiseases/pubs/viralhepatitis/*Cached-Similar*

Viral Hepatitis Symptoms, Causes, Diagnosis, and Treatment by Dr. Dennis Lee www.medicinenet.com*Cached-Similar*

Prevention of Viral Hepatitis

Zhi Q. Yao

HEPATITIS A

- Since hepatitis A is transmitted primarily by the fecal-oral route, on contaminated hands, or in food and water sources, personal hygiene is critical in prevention of viral spread.
- An inactivated HAV vaccine was licensed in 1995, and the FDA recommends that all children should be vaccinated starting at 1 year of age.
- HAV vaccine efficacy after two doses is 94% to 100%, with protection lasting for at least 20 years.
- Emergency prevention of hepatitis A consists of hepatitis A immune globulin and hepatitis A vaccine, which should be given to all nonimmune contacts exposed to an infected person.
- Persons at high risk should also be vaccinated
  - Chronic liver disease
  - Men who have sex with men
  - Travelers to areas of high incidence

Hepatitis A Vaccine Adult Schedule

Vaccine	Dose	Interval	Comment
Havrix	1 mL IM	0 and 6–12 months	
Vaqta	1 mL IM	0 and 6–18 months	
Twinrix (Hep A/Hep B)	1 mL IM in deltoid	0, 1, and 6 months	Alternative schedule: 0, 7 days, 21–30 days, and 1 year

HEPATITIS B

- Prevention of hepatitis B is predicated on providing prophylaxis and immunization to patients recently exposed or at risk for exposure.
- It is now universal practice to provide the hepatitis B vaccine to all newborns.
  - Infants whose mothers are HBV infected should also be given hepatitis B immune globulin at birth, which can result in a 95% reduction in prenatal transmission.
- Persons who were born before the onset of universal vaccination should be offered vaccination, especially if they are at risk of being exposed, including the following:
  - All children and adolescents who did not get the vaccine when they were younger
  - Sex partners of people infected with HBV
  - Men who have sex with men
  - Individuals who inject street drugs
  - Individuals with more than one sex partner

- Individuals with chronic liver or kidney disease
- People with occupations that expose them to human blood
- Household contacts of people infected with HBV
- People who travel to countries where HBV is common
- People with HIV infection
- Response:
  - >95% in the young and in healthy adults
  - <75% in HIV, renal disease, liver disease
  - Response = HBSAb level >10 mIU/mL >1 month after third dose

If someone is suspected of having been exposed to HBV and has not been previously vaccinated, that patient should receive passive immunization with hepatitis B immune globulin followed by the vaccination series as soon as possible.

Hepatitis B Vaccine Adult Schedule

Vaccine	Dose	Interval	Comments
Recombivax	10 mcg/mL IM	0, 1, and 6 months	40 mcg/mL for patients on hemodialysis and other immunocompromising conditions (e.g., HIV)
Engerix-B	20 mcg/mL IM	0, 1, and 6 months	Can be given at 0, 1, 2, and 12 months; given two doses (total 40 mcg) for patients on hemodialysis
Twinrix	1 mL IM in deltoid	0, 1, and 6 months	Alternative schedule: 0, 7 days, 21–30 days, and 1 year

HEPATITIS C

- No vaccine is available yet for HCV infection.
- In general, patients with chronic HCV infection should be counseled to avoid alcohol and liver toxicity medications and be immunized against hepatitis A and B.
- Individuals exposed to hepatitis C should be followed serologically, and converters should be offered therapy.
  - Average seroconversion rate after needlestick injury from an HCV-infected individual is 1.8%.
  - Baseline testing should include antibody to HCV and ALT.
  - Follow-up testing may include repeat antibody to HCV 4 to 6 months after exposure and/or HCV RNA testing at 4 to 6 weeks.
  - Limited data suggest that treatment of HCV early in infection may lead to higher rates of sustained virologic responses but no formal recommendations exist.

SUGGESTED READINGS

The A, B, Cs of Viral Hepatitis www.health.ny.gov/diseases/communicable/hepatitisCached

Advisory Committee on Immunization Practices (ACIP). Prevention of hepatitis A through active or passive immunization: recommendations of the Advisory Committee on Immunization Practices (ACIP). *MMWR Recomm Rep* 2006;55:1.

This ACIP publication presents the recommendations for immunization with hepatitis A vaccine.

Centers for Disease Control and Prevention (CDC). Use of hepatitis B vaccination for adults with diabetes mellitus: recommendations of the Advisory Committee on Immunization Practices (ACIP). *MMWR Morb Mortal Wkly Rep* 2011;60:1709.

Centers for Disease Control and Prevention. Recommendations for prevention and control of hepatitis C virus (HCV) infection and HCV-related chronic disease. *MMWR Recomm Rep* 1998;47:1.

CDC DVH - Division of Viral Hepatitis Home Page: www.cdc.gov/hepatitis

Mast EE, et al. A comprehensive immunization strategy to eliminate transmission of hepatitis B virus infection in the United States: recommendations of the Advisory Committee on Immunization Practices (ACIP) part 1: immunization of infants, children, and adolescents. *MMWR Recomm Rep* 2005;54:1

This ACIP publication presents the recommendations for immunization with hepatitis B vaccine, primarily in the young.

Viral Hepatitis: A through E and Beyond–NIDDK www.digestive.niddk.nih.gov/diseases/pubs/viralhepatitisCached-Similar

III Sexually Transmitted Diseases

Syphilis

Lamis Ibrahim and James W. Myers

INTRODUCTION

Syphilis is a systemic disease caused by the spirochete *Treponema pallidum* subspecies pallidum. It has been known as the "Great Imitator."

EPIDEMIOLOGY

- Modes of transmission:
  - **Sexual**
  - Vertical (causing congenital syphilis)
  - Rarely, by blood transfusion.
- Average age of diagnosis is 15 to 30 in females and 15 to 54 in males.
- Highest incidence in USA is in Southeast and Southwest regions.
- **Incubation period**: about 3 weeks (range 10 to 90 days).

PATHOGENESIS

- Main underlying pathology is endarteritis obliterans.
- Starts with local inoculation at site of contact, then erosion→ulcer. It then spreads to lymph nodes and hematogenously→immune complex formation→systemic manifestations and then goes into *latent period* and then *tertiary syphilis* if untreated.
- Spontaneous clearing can occur in about *2/3 of people without* treatment.

CLINICAL MANIFESTATIONS

Syphilis passes through four stages: primary, secondary, latent, and tertiary.
Primary syphilis: chancre or ulcer stage

- Appears **10 to 90** days after exposure
- Usually single, **painless ulcer**
- **Indurated** with **clean** base
- May be multiple, especially in human immunodeficiency virus (HIV) patients
- "Kissing" lesions can occur on opposing labial surfaces
- Usually seen over genital areas (penis, labia, cervix)
- Extragenital areas: lips, anal and perianal areas
- Regional **lymph nodes** may become enlarged, unilateral or bilateral, firm and painless, mobile, with no overlying skin changes
- May go unnoticed and can heal *spontaneously in 2 to 8* weeks
- Patient is *highly infectious* in this stage.

Secondary syphilis: occurs **2 to 18** weeks after contact

- Presents with systemic symptoms
- Fever, malaise, decreased appetite
- **Generalized lymphadenopathy**
- Rash: maculopapular, may be pustular. It starts in the trunk and then spreads, to involve palms and soles. It is usually symmetrical, nonpruritic, and painless.
- Mucocutaneous lesions.
- **Condyloma lata** (papilloma-like heaped-up lesions).
- Less common manifestations: alopecia, uveitis, retinitis, meningitis, osteitis,, hepatitis, glomerulonephritis
- Also **highly infectious** stage!

LATENT SYPHILIS

1. *Early latent is within 1 year* of infection.
   - Twenty-five percent can have relapses during this period.
   - Early latent period is extended to 4 years for pregnant women.
2. Late latent: >1 year after infection
   - Patients are considered noninfectious.
   - Evaluate for clinical evidence of tertiary disease and syphilitic ocular disease.
   - The diagnosis is made by serology. **The nontreponemal test may revert to normal, but the treponemal tests usually remain positive**.
   - *CSF exam needed* if there are neurologic or ophthalmologic signs or symptoms, evidence of active tertiary disease such as aortitis or gumma, or treatment failure (defined as failure of a fourfold decline in rapid plasma reagin (RPR) titer 6 months after treatment), HIV-infected persons with late latent or of unknown duration.

TERTIARY SYPHILIS

- **3 to 10 years** after infection
- Gummas: granulomatous-like, seen mainly of the skin, but can involve, nose, palate, liver, spleen, bone (palate perforations, saddle-shaped nose)
- Cardiovascular: aortitis→aortic aneurysm, aortic regurgitation, **10 to 30 years** after infection
- Neurologic: can be meningovascular or parenchymal
  - Meningovascular
    ○ May present as a stroke; usually **4 to 7 years** after infection
  - Parenchymal disease usually appears later.
    ○ General paresis (deterioration in cognitive function and psychiatric symptoms then progresses to neurologic signs like pupillary problems, hypotonia, weakness, tremors).
    ○ Tabes dorsalis starts with lightning pains of the lower extremities, followed by decreased sensation and progressive ataxia, impaired position, and vibration sensation. Up to 50% of patients have **Argyll Robertson** pupil (small, irregular pupils that are unreactive to light but react to accommodation). Later patients may present with visceral problems that mimic an acute abdomen.

- Note that central nervous system (CNS) involvement can occur during any stage and can be asymptomatic or present with cognitive impairment, motor or sensory deficits, ophthalmologic or auditory problems, cranial nerve palsies, meningitis, syphilitic eye disease (uveitis, iritis, optic neuritis, neuroretinitis).
- Obtain CSF examination and serology on all suspect cases.
  - CSF findings in neurosyphilis include pleocytosis, elevated protein, decreased glucose, or a reactive CSF Venereal Disease Research Laboratory (VDRL).

DIAGNOSIS

Direct Visualization of the Spirochete

- Dark field microscopy: gold standard for diagnosis in primary syphilis
  - Performed on a transudate from a chancre, mucocutaneous lesion of secondary syphilis or an aspirate of lymph nodes
  - Sensitivity, 74% to 86%; specificity, 86% to 100%
  - Considered to be truly negative if there are three negative samples
- DFA has 73% to 100% sensitivity; specificity, 89% to 100%
- PCR: not readily available

Serology: Nontreponemal and Treponemal

Nontreponemal: VDRL/RPR; more sensitive, less specific

- Can be negative in primary syphilis in up to 30% but almost always positive in secondary syphilis
- Fourfold changes are considered significant
- Can be used to monitor response to therapy
- Correlates with disease activity, but titers can persist for a long period of time and define a condition known as a "serofast reaction."
- In primary syphilis, they usually become negative at 12 months, and 24 months in secondary syphilis after appropriate treatment. If not, it may indicate persistent infection or a false positive.
- Causes of false-positive results: physiologic (pregnancy, old age), infections (HIV, herpes viruses infections, hepatitis, mycoplasma, TB, leprosy, leptospirosis, Lyme disease), vaccination, autoimmune disease, chronic liver disease, intravenous drug usage (IVDU), malignancy, and others.

Treponemal test: MHA-TP, FTA-ABS, TPHA, TPPA, EIA

- Directed against *specific treponemal* antigens
- More specific than nontreponemal test and mainly used **for confirmation**
- Some labs, however, started using these as "screening" tests as follows:
  - Anybody with a positive treponemal screening test should have a quantitative nontreponemal test done for further decision making.
  - If the nontreponemal test is negative, then a different treponemal test (based on different antigens than the first test) is used to confirm the results.
  - If a second treponemal test is positive, and the patient has history of previous treatment, then no further management is needed unless there is possibility of reexposure. But if there is no history of treatment for syphilis, then treatment should be offered.
  - If the second treponemal test is negative, then no treatment is indicated.
- Once positive, these usually remain positive for life but 15% to 25% of patients if treated in primary stage may become serologically nonreactive in 2 to 3 years.

TREATMENT

Parenteral Penicillin G is the preferred drug for treatment of **all syphilis** stages. The dosage and the length of treatment depend on the stage and clinical manifestations of the disease as below:

Nonpregnant, Non-HIV		
Stage	**Preferred Treatment**	**Alternative Treatment/ PCN Allergy**
Early (primary, secondary, early latent)	**Benzathine penicillin G** 2.4 million units IM in a single dose	Doxycycline 100 mg orally twice daily for **14 days** Tetracycline (500 mg four times daily for **14 days**) Azithromycin as a single **2-g** oral Ceftriaxone 1 g IV/IM for 10–**14 days**
Late Latent/ latent on unknown duration	**Benzathine penicillin G** 7.2 million units total, administered as **3 doses** of 2.4 million units IM each at **1-week intervals**	Doxycycline (100 mg orally twice daily) for **28 days** Tetracycline (500 mg orally four times daily), for **28 days**. Ceftriaxone may be effective
Tertiary (gumma and cardiovascular **but no** Neurosyphilis)	**Benzathine penicillin G** 7.2 million units total, administered as 3 doses of 2.4 million units IM each at 1-week intervals	
Neurosyphilis	**Aqueous crystalline penicillin G** 18–24 million units per day, administered as 3–4 million units IV every 4 hours or continuous infusion, for **10–14 days**	**Procaine penicillin** 2.4 million units IM once daily PLUS **Probenecid** 500 mg orally four times a day, both for 10–14 days. PCN Allergy: Ceftriaxone 2 g daily IM/IV for 10–14 days

FOLLOW-UP

1. For primary and secondary syphilis:
   • Clinical and serologic evaluation is usually performed at *6 and 12* months after treatment for primary and secondary syphilis.
     • Fourfold decline in titer of nontreponemal tests within 6 to 12 months is indicative of treatment response.

- If symptoms recurred or persisted, or if there is sustained increase in titer, then it is either **treatment failure or reinfection**. Such patients should be revaluated for HIV, should also undergo CSF examination, and be retreated.
- Retreatment includes weekly injection of benzathine penicillin G 2.4 million units IM for **3 weeks, unless CSF indicates** treatment for neurosyphilis.

2. Latent syphilis:
   - Serologic tests should be performed at 6, 12, *and 24 months*.
     - Fourfold decline in titers is expected at **12 to 24** months
   - Any patient with latent syphilis who has any neurologic symptoms (meningitis, stroke, altered mental status, cranial nerve, **ophthalmology, or auditory** involvement) or has evidence of tertiary syphilis or treatment/serologic failure should undergo CSF exam.
     - If patient misses any of the weekly doses, with >14 days between doses, **then should restart the sequence of injections**.

3. Neurosyphilis:
   - If initial CSF showed **pleocytosis**, then CSF exam should be performed **every 6** months till normalization of the cell count.
   - Serial CSF also can follow changes in CSF VDRL and protein although changes of these parameters *occur more slowly*.
   - **If CSF cell count is not decreased in 6 months or CSF protein or VDRL is not normal in 2 years, then patient should be retreated**.

HIV AND SYPHILIS

- Any patient diagnosed with syphilis should be tested for HIV.
- Syphilis enhances transmission of HIV.
- HIV patients can have **more number of chancres** in primary syphilis, more protracted course, accelerated ulceration, and rapid progression of disease.
- HIV patients can have **unusual serologic responses**. Usually have higher titers, yet false-negative results or delayed seropositivity can occur.
- HIV patients are at increased risk of neurologic complication and higher rates of treatment failure.

Stage	Preferred Treatment	Alternative Treatment/PCN Allergy
Primary/ secondary/ early latent	**Benzathine penicillin G** 2.4 million units IM in **a single** dose	Desensitization and PCN treatment in **noncompliant** patients. Doxycycline 100 mg orally twice daily for 14 days Tetracycline (500 mg four times daily for 14 days)
Late latent/ or unknown duration	**Benzathine penicillin G** 7.2 million units total, administered as **3 doses** of 2.4 million units IM each at 1-week intervals	Desensitization and PCN treatment in noncompliant patients. **Doxycycline/tetracycline like in non-HIV patients but efficacy is not well studied and such patients need very close follow-up.**

(Continued)

Stage	Preferred Treatment	Alternative Treatment/PCN Allergy
Neurosyphilis	**Aqueous crystalline penicillin G** 18–24 million units per day, administered as 3–4 million units IV every 4 hours or continuous infusion, for 10–14 days	Ceftriaxone 2 g daily IM/IV for 10–14 days **may be effective** alternative according to some observational studies

FOLLOW-UP FOR HIV PATIENTS

- Any patient with neurologic symptoms should have CSF exam like HIV-negative patients.
- In primary and secondary stages, clinical and serologic evaluation should be performed at a different schedule of *3, 6, 9, 12, and 24* months following treatment.
- In latent stages, follow-up should be done at *6, 12, 18, and 24* months.
- HIV patients in latent stages should probably undergo CSF exam.
- **Follow-up in neurosyphilis is the same as in non-HIV patients**.

SYPHILIS IN PREGNANCY

- All pregnant females should be screened for syphilis in early pregnancy.
- Patient with **high risk** should have serologic tests **done twice in third** trimester.
- Treatment is with PCN regimens according to stage as for nonpregnant adults. *In PCN allergic patients, desensitization and PCN treatment should be done.*
- If syphilis is diagnosed in second half of pregnancy, then **fetal US** should be done to look for congenital syphilis.
- Follow-up serology should be done at 28 to 32 weeks and at delivery.

CONGENITAL SYPHILIS

- Vertical transmission can occur at any stage of syphilis during pregnancy especially during early stages of disease and with titers >1:16.
- Seventy percent of untreated woman can transmit to fetus for up to **4 years**.
- Pregnant women should be screened at the first prenatal visit, at 28 weeks, and at the time of delivery in areas with high rates of syphilis
- May be asymptomatic at birth
- Early manifestations: rhinitis, rash (exfoliative, vesicular, bullous). Osteochondritis, anemia, hepatosplenomegaly, lymphadenopathy, neurologic symptoms, and nephritic syndrome.
- Late specific features: frontal bossing, small maxilla, saddle shaped nose, interstitial keratitis, high palatal arch and possible perforation of palate and nasal septum, Hutchinson incisors, eighth nerve deafness, and painless swelling of knees.

EVALUATION OF NEONATES FOR CONGENITAL SYPHILIS

- Maternal IgG antibodies can be transferred transplacental and persist up to 1 year
- Any child born to mother with positive serology for syphilis and no documentation of receiving treatment at least 4 weeks before delivery, or if non–PCN-based regimens were used for treatment of seropositive moms or if suspicion of reinfection is present, then the child should be screened and evaluated for congenital syphilis as such:
- Physical exam for any signs or symptoms of congenital syphilis
- X-rays for long bone to rule out periostitis
- CSF exam
- Direct fluorescent microscopy (DFM) or direct fluorescent antibody (DFA) of lesions or body fluids

A child is considered to have a **confirmed case** of congenital syphilis if a spirochete was seen by DFM or DFA performed on lesion, body fluid, placenta, and umbilical cord.

A **presumptive diagnosis** is considered if seropositive mother was not treated or inappropriately treated at delivery regardless of any stigmata seen in newborn or if a child has positive treponemal test with: signs and symptoms of congenital syphilis, radiograph suggestive of syphilis, positive CSF VDRL, elevated WBC in CSF, or positive FTA-ABS IGM using fractionated serum. Infection can be **suggested** if the serum of the neonate is fourfold higher than the mother's test.

JARISCH-HERXHEIMER REACTIONS

- Occurs **1 to 2 hours after** effective treatment of syphilis especially during the secondary stage.
- Presents with: fever, chills, HA, myalgia, tachycardia, tachypnea, hypotension, and obtundation.
- Can persist for 24 hours.
- It is self-limited.
- Can probably be avoided or treated with NSAIDS or steroids.

MANAGEMENT OF CONTACTS

1. Persons exposed within *90 days before the diagnosis* of primary, secondary, or early latent syphilis in a sex partner may be infected *even if seronegative*. These should be treated presumptively.
2. Those exposed **>90 days before the diagnosis** of primary, secondary, or early latent syphilis in a sex partner should be treated presumptively if serology *is not available immediately and follow-up is uncertain.*
3. Long-term sex partners of patients with latent syphilis should be **evaluated clinically and serologically for syphilis** and treated accordingly.
4. Sexual partners of infected patients are considered at risk and provided treatment if they have had sexual contact with the patient within 3 months plus the duration of symptoms for those diagnosed with primary syphilis, 6 months plus duration of symptoms for patients with secondary syphilis, and 1 year for patients with early latent syphilis.

SUGGESTED READINGS

Centers for Disease Control Guidelines:

CDC. Sexually Transmitted Diseases Treatment Guidelines, 2010. Available at http://www.cdc.gov/std/treatment/2010/STD-Treatment-2010-RR5912.pdf

CDC. Guidelines for the laboratory diagnosis of gonorrhea, chlamydia and syphilis. Available at http://www.aphl.org/aphlprograms/infectious/std/Pages/stdtestingguidelines.aspx.

Association of Public Health Laboratories (APHL). Laboratory Diagnostic Testing for *Treponema pallidum*. Expert Consultation Meeting Summary Report, January 13–15, 2009, Atlanta, GA. Available at http://www.aphl.org/aphlprograms/infectious/std/Documents/LaboratoryGuidelinesTreponemapallidumMeetingReport.pdf

CDC. Syphilis testing algorithms using treponemal tests for initial screening–four laboratories, New York City, 2005–2006. *MMWR Morb Mortal Wkly Rep* 2008;57:872–875.

Articles:

Goh BT. Syphilis in adults. *Sex Transm Infect* 2005;81(6):448–452.

Marra CM, Maxwell CL, et al. Cerebrospinal fluid abnormalities in patients with syphilis: association with clinical and laboratory features. *J Infect Dis* 2004;189(3):369–376.

> *In multivariate analyses, serum RPR titer > or =1: 32 increased the odds of neurosyphilis 10.85-fold in HIV-uninfected subjects and 5.98-fold in HIV-infected subjects. A peripheral blood CD4+ T cell count < or =350 cells/ mL conferred 3.10-fold increased odds of neurosyphilis in HIV-infected subjects. Similar results were obtained when neurosyphilis was more stringently defined as a reactive CSF VDRL test result.*

Wendel GD Jr, Sheffield JS, et al. Treatment of syphilis in pregnancy and prevention of congenital syphilis. *Clin Infect Dis* 2002;35(suppl 2):S200–S209.

> *Antepartum screening remains a critical component of congenital syphilis prevention, even in the era of syphilis elimination.*

10 Gonorrhea

James W. Myers and Lamis Ibrahim

INTRODUCTION

- Gonorrhea (GC) is the **second most** commonly reported bacterial sexually transmitted disease (STD).
- In the United States, an estimated 700,000 new infections occur each year.
- The majority of infections are symptomatic in **males but can be asymptomatic in females**.

MICROBIOLOGY

- Nonmotile, gram-negative diplococci.
- GC can use glucose but not maltose, sucrose, or lactose.
- Chocolate agar containing vancomycin, colistin, nystatin, and trimethoprim is known as **Thayer-Martin** media.
  - It should be used to plate specimens from nonsterile sites only.
  - Should be sent to the lab to be incubated quickly.
  - The sensitivity of culture ranges from 70% to 95%.
- GC is known to be fastidious and to require aerobic conditions with increased carbon dioxide atmosphere.

EPIDEMIOLOGY

- Transmitted both sexually and perinatally.
- The transmission rate of GC to females after a single sexual encounter is about 50%.
- Rates are highest in these groups.
  - **Ages 15 to 24**
  - **Men who have sex with men (MSM)**
  - African Americans
  - Lower socioeconomic classes
  - Those with less education
  - Residents in the southeastern part of the country
  - Single patients
  - Drug users
- **Forty-six percent had concurrent chlamydia detected**.
- GC facilitates the transmission of HIV.

CLINICAL MANIFESTATIONS

1. *Genital infections in males*:
   - Uncomplicated infection:

- Acute urethritis is the most common presentation.
- Incubation period **2 to 5 days** but can be 10 days.
- Dysuria
  - Purulent urethral discharge
  - Most infections resolve in several weeks even without antimicrobials.
- Acute epididymitis is the most common localized complication seen with GC.
- Other less common presentations include prostatitis and strictures.

2. *Genital infections in females*:
- Cervicitis
  - It is the most common presentation.
  - Urethral infection is less common.
  - Accessory gland infection can also occur.
  - **Many can be asymptomatic, up to 50%**
  - Usually presents with vaginal discharge, dysuria, bleeding, purulent cervical discharge, cervical swelling, and friability on exam.
- Pelvic inflammatory disease
  - Incidence of approximately 20% in females who have cervicitis.
  - Endometritis, salpingitis, tuboovarian abscess, perihepatitis, and peritonitis.
  - Patients may present with lower abdominal pain, nausea, vomiting, fever, and chills.
  - They will have **cervical motion tenderness**, adnexal tenderness, and lower abdominal pain on physical exam.
  - Laboratory testing will often show an elevated sedimentation rate (ESR), C-Reactive protein (CRP), and leukocytosis.
  - Perihepatitis can be a complication with GC or chlamydia, but infertility is more common with chlamydia infection.
- Gonorrhea and Pregnancy
  - It is associated with increased fetal mortality, preterm labor, and abortion.
  - Pelvic inflammatory disease (PID) and perihepatitis seldom occur after the first trimester.

3. *Infection in males and females*:
- Gonococcal pharyngitis
  - Oral sex is the major risk factor.
  - Usually asymptomatic but when present can be severe.
  - More common in **females and MSM** than in heterosexual men.
  - Rarely would be the only infection site.
  - Can be source for disseminated infection.
  - Nucleic acid amplification tests (NAATs) are **not FDA approved** for pharyngeal swabs.
  - Some recommend MSM or HIV (receptive oral sex) patient screening.
- Gonococcal conjunctivitis
  - Autoinoculation
  - Purulent exudate
  - Photophobia and pain
  - Corneal ulceration
- Gonococcal proctitis
  - Occurs in both females and homosexual men secondary to anal receptive intercourse.
  - Can be asymptomatic at times.
  - Mucopurulent discharge can be seen.

- Tenesmus or bleeding can occur.
- Disseminated gonococcal infection
  - A consequence of bacteremia or from immune complex formation.
  - Three percent of cases
  - **Presents with arthritis-dermatitis syndrome in most patients**.
  - Starts with asymmetrical arthralgia/arthritis of the knees, elbows, and distal joints and is associated with tenosynovitis.
  - Fifty percent of patients may have positive blood or synovial fluid cultures.
  - Skin lesions can be sent for gram stain and cultures can be done.
  - Test for GC at mucosal surfaces as well.
  - Other rare manifestations of disseminated disease include endocarditis, meningitis, osteomyelitis, and septic shock.
  - Up to 13% of cases of DGI are associated with complement deficiency, and patients with **repeated episodes of gonococcal bacteremia** should be evaluated for such.
  - Skin manifestations occur in up to 75% of patients and usually occur on the extremities.
    - Papules and pustules
    - Hemorrhagic lesions
4. *Neonatal infection*
  - Ophthalmia neonatorum (Gonococcal conjunctivitis).
  - Occurs secondary to perinatal transmission
  - Routine screening and treatment of pregnant women before term
  - Prophylaxis with antibiotics or a 1% aqueous solution of silver nitrate into the conjunctivae soon after delivery prevents infection. **Silver nitrate itself can cause a chemical conjunctivitis**.
  - It develops quickly, within few days of delivery, and it is diagnosed by finding GC in conjunctival secretions.
  - Septicemia and arthritis can occur as well.

DIAGNOSIS

- Gram stain:
  - Symptomatic in men.
    - A gram stain of urethral specimen showing polymorphonuclear cells (PMNS) with *intracellular* gram-negative diplococci is considered diagnostic!
    - Specificity (>99%) and sensitivity (>95%)
  - Gram staining of endocervical specimens, pharyngeal, or rectal specimens is ***not recommended***.
- Other diagnostic methods: culture, nucleic acid hybridization tests, and NAATs
  - Culture and nucleic acid hybridization tests are usually done on endocervical or male urethral swabs.
  - Cultures are also used to assess **antibiotic susceptibilities** if drug resistance is suspected.
  - NAATs are FDA cleared to be performed on specimens like endocervical swabs, vaginal swabs, urethral swabs (men), and urine (from both men and women)
  - **NAAT tests are not FDA cleared for use on rectal, pharyngeal, and conjunctival specimens.**
  - Some laboratories have performance specifications for using NAAT on rectal and pharyngeal swab specimens.

PREVENTION

- Screening of sexually active women, including those who are pregnant, is recommended for those at increased risk for infection (e.g., women with previous GC infection, other STDs, new or multiple sex partners, and inconsistent condom use; those who engage in commercial sex work and drug use; women in certain demographic groups; and those living in communities with a high prevalence of disease).
- **Screening for GC in men and women who are at low risk for infection is not recommended**.

ANTIMICROBIAL RESISTANCE

- Quinolone-resistant *Neisseria gonorrhoeae* strains are now widely disseminated.
- **Quinolones are not recommended anymore in the United States for the treatment of GC and PID**.
- Decreased susceptibility to ceftriaxone or cefixime has remained very low over time, but overall decreased susceptibility will continue to spread.
- MICs to cephalosporins increased from 0.2% in 2,000 to 1.4% in 2010 for cefixime and from 0.1% in 2,000 to 0.3% in 2010 for ceftriaxone.
- **When patients experience treatment failure, then specimens should be sent for culture and susceptibility and this should be reported to CDC**.

TREATMENT OF GC

- **Dual therapy for GC and chlamydia is the standard of care** if chlamydia is not ruled out.
- See the treatment tables for specific details

FOLLOW-UP

- No need for test of cure after treatment of uncomplicated gonococcal urogenital and rectal infection.
- Patients **with pharyngeal GC should have a test of cure 3 to 5** days after treatment
- If symptoms persist, check culture with susceptibility.
- Retest in **3 months after treatment** or any time in the following 3 to 12 months due to possibility of **reinfection as opposed to test of cure**.

MANAGEMENT OF SEX PARTNERS

- Sex partners of patients with *N. gonorrhoeae* within 60 days before symptoms or diagnosis should be evaluated and treated for *N. gonorrhoeae* and *Chlamydia trachomatis* infections.
- No sexual intercourse until therapy is completed and until patients and their sex partners have no more symptoms.

Treatment Tables: (GC) (Tables 10-1 to 10-5).

Table10-1	Treatment of Uncomplicated Urogenital and Rectal Infections

Recommended Regimen (Any of the Following)
- Ceftriaxone 250 mg IM in a single dose
- Cefixime 400 mg orally in a single dose
- Other injectable cephalosporins:
- ceftizoxime (500 mg, administered IM),
- cefoxitin (2 g, administered IM with probenecid 1 g orally)
- cefotaxime (500 mg, administered IM)
- (all above regimens should be *given PLUS azithromycin 1g orally in a single dose OR doxycycline 100mg* orally twice a day for 7 days)

Alternative Regimen
- Cefpodoxime 400 mg orally
- Cefuroxime axetil 1 g orally
- Spectinomycin: *not available in USA*, expensive, injectable, and is used in persons who cannot tolerate cephalosporins
- Azithromycin 2 g orally. *(should be limited for use as solitary due development of resistance of GC to macrolides)*

RX IN PREGNANCY

- Pregnant women should be treated with a recommended or alternate cephalosporin regimen mentioned before.
- Azithromycin 2 g orally can be considered for women who cannot tolerate a cephalosporin

RX IN HIV: SAME AS HIV NEGATIVE

Table 10-2	Treatment of GC at Other Body Sites

Rx of Pharyngeal Gonococcal Infection
- Ceftriaxone 250 mg IM in a single dose PLUS azithromycin 1 g orally in a single dose OR doxycycline 100 mg orally twice a day for 7 days.
- Oral cephalosporins and other injectable cephalosporins have limited efficacy for pharyngeal infection

Rx of Gonococcal Conjunctivitis
- *Ceftriaxone 1g IM* in a single dose
- Treat partners
- Treat for concurrent chlamydia

Table 10-3	Rx of Disseminated Gonococcal Infection (DGI)

Recommended Regimen
- Ceftriaxone 1 g IM or IV every 24 hours

Alternative Regimen
- Cefotaxime 1–g IV every 8 hours or Ceftizoxime 1 g IV every 8 hours

Continue above regimens for at least 24 to 48 hours and evidence of improvement and then switch to oral regimen of cefixime 400 mg PO b.i.d. for total of 1 week.
Treat associated meningitis for 10 to 14 days and endocarditis for 4 weeks.

Table 10-4	Treatment of PID: Parenteral Regimens

Recommended Regimen A
- Cefotetan 2g IV every 12 hours
- OR
- Cefoxitin 2g IV every 6 hours
- Plus Doxycycline 100 mg orally or IV every 12 hours

Recommended Regimen B
- Clindamycin 900 mg IV every 8 hours
- PLUS
- Gentamicin loading dose (2 mg/kg of body weight), followed by a maintenance dose (1.5 mg/kg) every 8 hours.
- Single daily dosing (3–5 mg/kg) can be substituted.

Alternative Parenteral Regimen
- Ampicillin/Sulbactam 3g IV every 6 hours
- Plus Doxycycline 100 mg orally or IV every 12 hours

Indications for Parenteral Regimens
Surgical emergencies
Pregnancy
No response to oral antimicrobial therapy;
Inability to tolerate an outpatient oral regimen
Severe illness, nausea and vomiting, or high fever
Tubo-ovarian abscess.
Parenteral therapy is continued 24 to 48 hours then stepped down to oral regimen.

Table 10-5	Oral Regimens (Any of the Following) for PID

- Ceftriaxone 250 mg IM in a single dose
PLUS
- Doxycycline 100 mg orally twice a day for 14 days
WITH or WITHOUT
- Metronidazole 500 mg orally twice a day for 14 days

- Cefoxitin 2 g IM in a single dose and probenecid, 1 g orally administered concurrently in a single dose
PLUS
- Doxycycline 100 mg orally twice a day for 14 days
WITH or WITHOUT
- Metronidazole 500 mg orally twice a day for 14 days

- Other parenteral third-generation cephalosporin (e.g., ceftizoxime or cefotaxime)
PLUS Doxycycline 100 mg orally twice a day for 14 days
WITH or WITHOUT
- Metronidazole 500 mg orally twice a day for 14 days

SUGGESTED READINGS

CDC. Sexually Transmitted Diseases Treatment Guidelines, 2010. Available at http://www.cdc.gov/std/treatment/2010/STD-Treatment-2010-RR5912.pdf

CDC. Guidelines for the laboratory diagnosis of gonorrhea, chlamydia and syphilis. Available at http://www.aphl.org/aphlprograms/infectious/std/Pages/stdtestingguidelines.aspx

CDC. Update to CDC's sexually transmitted diseases treatment guidelines, 2006: fluoroquinolones no longer recommended for treatment of gonococcal infections. *MMWR Morb Mortal Wkly Rep* 2007;56:332–336.

Cephalosporin susceptibility among *Neisseria gonorrhoeae* isolates—United States, 2000–2010. *MMWR Morb Mortal Wkly Rep* 2011;60(26):873–877.

Neisseria gonorrhoeae with reduced susceptibility to azithromycin—San Diego County, California, 2009. *MMWR Morb Mortal Wkly Rep* 2011;60(18):579–581.
Continued surveillance for antibiotic resistance and effective control efforts are critical for GC prevention.

Deguchi T, Nakane K, et al. Emergence and spread of drug resistant *Neisseria gonorrhoeae. J Urol* 2010;184(3):851–858; quiz 1235.
Clinicians should effectively treat patients with GC, always being conscious of local trends of drug resistance in N. gonorrhoeae, and should perform culture and antimicrobial susceptibility testing in those with persistent GC after treatment.

Fung M, Scott KC, et al. Chlamydial and gonococcal reinfection among men: a systematic review of data to evaluate the need for retesting. *Sex Transm Infect* 2007;83(4):304–309.

Hosenfeld CB, Workowski KA, et al. Repeat infection with *Chlamydia and gonorrhea* among females: a systematic review of the literature. *Sex Transm Dis* 2009;36(8):478–489.
High rates of reinfection with chlamydia and GC among females, along with practical considerations, warrant retesting 3 to 6 months after treatment of the initial infection. Further research should investigate effective interventions to reduce reinfection and to increase retesting.

Lyss SB, Kamb ML, et al. *Chlamydia trachomatis* among patients infected with and treated for *Neisseria gonorrhoeae* in sexually transmitted disease clinics in the United States. *Ann Intern Med* 2003;139(3):178–185.

The frequent presence of chlamydia among patients at STD clinics who received treatment for GC, including sex partners of GC-infected patients, supports continuing current recommendations for cotreatment.

Schachter J, Chernesky MA, et al. Vaginal swabs are the specimens of choice when screening for *Chlamydia trachomatis* and *Neisseria gonorrhoeae*: results from a multicenter evaluation of the APTIMA assays for both infections. *Sex Transm Dis* 2005;32(12):725–728.

Vaginal swabs identified as many infected patients as endocervical swabs and more than FCUs and may well be the specimen of choice for screening.

Schachter J, Moncada J, et al. Nucleic acid amplification tests in the diagnosis of chlamydial and gonococcal infections of the oropharynx and rectum in men who have sex with men. *Sex Transm Dis* 2008;35(7):637–642.

Further analyses with larger pharyngeal samples are needed, but clearly NAATs can improve our ability to diagnose rectal and oropharyngeal infection with CT or GC in MSM.

Tapsall JW. Antibiotic resistance in *Neisseria gonorrhoeae*. *Clin Infect Dis* 2005;41(suppl 4): S263–S268.

Without continued commitment and effort, GC may well become untreatable.

Walker CK, Sweet RL. Gonorrhea infection in women: prevalence, effects, screening, and management. *Int J Womens Health* 2011;3:197–206.

The Centers for Disease Control and Prevention recommend treatment of GC with a single class of drugs, i.e., the cephalosporins.

Workowski KA, Berman SM, Douglas JM Jr. Emerging antimicrobial resistance in *Neisseria gonorrhoeae*: urgent need to strengthen prevention strategies. *Ann Intern Med* 2008;148:606–613.

Chlamydia Trachomatis

James W. Myers and Lamis Ibrahim

INTRODUCTION

- Most frequently reported infectious disease.
- Causes **multiple complications, especially in females**.
  - PID
  - Ectopic pregnancy and infertility, and infant pneumonia.
  - Facilitates HIV transmission.

MICROBIOLOGY

- They are similar in many ways to gram-negative bacteria (contain LPS) but they are obligate intracellular parasites.
- Need tissue culture to grow in the laboratory.
- **Grow within a specialized vacuole in eukaryotic cells known as an "inclusion."**
- Exist in two forms: an infectious form, elementary body [EB], and an intracellular noninfectious form, the reticulate body (RB) that multiplies by binary fission.
- No long-lived immunity following infection.
- Serovars D-K cause genital tract chlamydia.
- Serovars L1-L3 cause lymphogranuloma venereum (LGV).

EPIDEMIOLOGY

- CDC estimated approximately 4 million new *C. trachomatis* infections per year in the United States.
  - Increased prevalence in women.
  - Incidence of approximately 15% of sexually active young women.
- Risk Factors:
  - Adolescents and young adults
  - Unmarried
  - African Americans
  - Those with multiple sex partners or a recent new sex partner
  - Inconsistent use of barrier contraceptives
  - Evidence of mucopurulent cervicitis or cervical ectopy
  - History of previous STD
  - Lower socioeconomic status or a lower level of education.
- Up to **70% of females** and 40% of men are asymptomatic.

CLINICAL MANIFESTATIONS

1. *Genital infections in males*:
   - **Urethritis**:
     - *C. trachomatis* causes 30% to 50% of cases of symptomatic nongonococcal urethritis (NGU), and it is more common than gonococcal urethritis.
       - Risk factors: young age <20 years, African American, and heterosexual orientation.
       - **Incubation period is usually 7 to 14 days. Often coinfected with gonorrhea, which has a shorter incubation period. Treatment for GC alone will miss the postgonococcal urethritis caused by chlamydia.**
       - Dysuria
       - Mucoid or watery urethral discharge, worse in the am.
       - Gram stain of a **urethral swab** specimen shows **five or more PMNs** in case of urethritis.
       - **Ten or more white blood cells** per high-power field in a first-catch **urine specimen** or **positive urine leukocyte** esterase test are also suggestive of urethritis.
   - **Epididymitis/Prostatitis**
     - *C. trachomatis* and *Neisseria gonorrhoeae* are the most common causes of epididymitis in men younger than 35 years, with gonorrhea being more common.
     - Fever
     - In young men, an associated urethritis is usually present, but they can be asymptomatic.
   - **Usually unilateral swelling and pain**.
2. *Genital infection in females*:
   - **Cervicitis and Urethritis**
     - **Seventy percent of women are asymptomatic**.
     - Symptoms include vaginal discharge, bleeding, postcoital bleeding, mild abdominal pain, or dysuria.
     - Dysuria usually secondary to associated urethritis.
     - Cervix may appear erythematous, friable, and swollen with a mucopurulent discharge but can be normal in appearance.
     - Cervical ectopy
     - Cofactor in cervical neoplasia?
   - **Endometritis and Salpingitis/PID**
     - Twenty percent incidence of PID.
       - Asymptomatic to severe in symptoms.
       - Fever
       - Abdominal pain, cervical motion tenderness.
       - Uterine and adnexal tenderness.
   - **Chlamydia and Pregnancy**:
     - Chlamydia is associated with **increased risk of miscarriage, premature rupture of membranes, preterm labor, low birth weight, and infant mortality**.
     - Without treatment, up to 50% of infants will develop conjunctivitis and up to 20% may develop pneumonia.
     - Long-term complications of PID include tubal infertility, ectopic pregnancy, and chronic pelvic pain syndrome. Treatment improves outcomes.
   - **Perihepatitis (Fitzhugh-Curtis syndrome)**:
     - Complicates approximately 15% of PID cases.
     - Normal LFTs.

- Acute onset
- Right upper-quadrant pain and tenderness aggravated by breathing, coughing, or movement, and may be referred to the right shoulder as well.
- "Violin string" adhesions.
- Treatment: NSAIDS/Supportive

3. *Infections in both males and females*
   - **Proctitis and Proctocolitis**:
     - Gay males predominate.
     - Females can also acquire this by either anal intercourse or from the cervico-vaginal route.
     - Mucopurulent rectal discharge. Leukocytes on Gram stain.
     - Pruritus, pain.
     - **Note that LGV strains may cause proctocolitis as well as proctitis. More severe in MSM who are HIV positive.**
   - **Sexually Reactive Arthritis**
     - One percent of NGU patients develop an acute aseptic arthritis syndrome referred to as sexually reactive arthritis, formerly known as Reiter syndrome.
     - **One-third of these patients have the complete manifestations (arthritis, uveitis, and urethritis) of this syndrome.**
   - **Conjunctivitis**:
     - Characteristically, this is a unilateral, acute inclusion conjunctivitis resulting from **autoinoculation** with infected genital secretions.
     - No permanent scarring.

4. Chlamydia neonatal infection:
   - Chlamydia can cause neonatal conjunctivitis or pneumonia.
     - Preventable by screening programs.
     - **Ocular prophylaxis with silver nitrate or antibiotics doesn't prevent chlamydia ophthalmia but prevents gonorrhea.**
     - **Conjunctivitis occurs at 5 to 12 days, and pneumonia at 1 to 3 months after infection.**
     - Diagnosis: culture is the gold standard, nucleic acid amplification tests (NAAT).
     - Rx; erythromycin for 14 days. A second course might be required in 20% of cases.

DIAGNOSIS

- Culture
  - McCoy or HeLa cells are incubated for up to 72 hours.
  - Detected by immunofluorescent staining with monoclonal antibodies against LPS.
  - Requires special handling of the specimens.
  - **Hundred percent specific** but much less sensitive.
  - NAAT: Nucleic acid amplification tests
  - **More sensitive than culture** and are nearly as specific as culture. Can detect 1 to 10 EBs as opposed to 10 to 100 for culture.
  - Can be used in legal matters. Culture is also sometimes used for this purpose.
  - NAATs can be used to detect *C. trachomatis* in **urine, self-collected vaginal swabs, endocervical/urethral swabs**.
  - **Not FDA approved for rectal and oropharyngeal swabs**.
  - Some laboratories have performance specifications for using NAAT on rectal and pharyngeal swab specimens.

- Serology: Not recommended.
  - **Group**-reactive complement-fixation antibodies.
  - Microimmunofluorescence test can identify the species. Possibly useful in infected infants with pneumonia.
- Antigen detection
  - Less sensitive (70%) and specific than NAATs.
  - EIA against the common LPS.
  - DFA
  - RNA probes
  - Can be falsely positive in low-risk populations. Cannot be used to self-collect a specimen, unlike NAATs.

PREVENTION

Screening Guidelines for Chlamydial Infection, U.S. Preventive Services Task Force, 2007

Screen all sexually active women ≤25 years old.
Screen **other high-risk women** (women ≤25 years old, or older females who are unmarried, African American, with history of prior sexually transmitted disease, have new or multiple sexual partners, have cervical ectopy, and have inconsistent use of barrier contraceptives)
Screen pregnant women ≤25 years old
Screen older high-risk pregnant women
Insufficient evidence to recommend male screening at present

Treatment
- Treat patients and their sex partners.
- Treatment of pregnant females prevents transmission to the fetus.
- Treat anyone who tests positive.
- Treatment should be dispensed on site with direct observation of first dose.
- No sexual intercourse for 7 days after single-dose regimen or until completion of the 7-day course, and until all partners are treated.

Recommended Regimens
- Azithromycin 1 g orally in a single dose, or doxycycline 100 mg orally twice a day for 7 days.
- Cure rate is 98% and 97% with these regimens.

Alternative Regimens
- Erythromycin base 500 mg orally four times a day for 7 days
- Erythromycin ethylsuccinate 800 mg orally four times a day for 7 days
- Levofloxacin 500 mg orally once daily for 7 days
- Ofloxacin 300 mg orally twice a day for 7 days

Follow-up
- Test of cure (which is defined as a repeat test 3 to 4 weeks after treatment) is not routinely recommended except for **pregnant females**, if patient is not complaint, has persistent symptoms, or there is suspicion of reinfection.
- Repeat infection increases risk for PID/complications.

- **Retest 3 months after treatment** or any time patient seeks medical care in the following 3 to 12 months after treatment because there is a high risk of reinfection in these patients.
- High rates of reinfection are associated with younger age, history of previous STDs, or risky sexual behaviors.

Sex Partner Management

Sex partners in the past **60 days** should be evaluated and treated.

Rx in Pregnancy

- **Recommended Regimens**: Either one.
  - Azithromycin 1 g orally in a single dose
  - **Amoxicillin** 500 mg orally three times a day for 7 days
- **Alternative Regimens**: Any.
  - Erythromycin base 500 mg orally four times a day for 7 days
  - Erythromycin base 250 mg orally four times a day for 14 days
  - Erythromycin ethylsuccinate 800 mg orally four times a day for 7 days
  - Erythromycin ethylsuccinate 400 mg orally four times a day for 14 days
- Test of cure is recommended in pregnant females. **It is done 3 to 4 weeks after treatment**.
  - If she is <25 years old and high risk, retest in third trimester too.
  - Pregnant women diagnosed with a chlamydial infection during the first trimester should not only receive a test to document chlamydial eradication but also be retested 3 months after treatment.

Rx in HIV

Same as in non–HIV patients.

LGV: LYMPHOGRANULOMA VENEREUM

Caused by the LGV serovars of *C. trachomatis*.
Three stages:
- **First stage**:
  - The primary lesion is a small papule or ulcer. Often unnoticed by the patient. Heals completely.
  - 3- to 30-day incubation period.
  - Can have an associated symptomatic urethritis, cervicitis, or proctitis.
- **Secondary stage**:
  - Occurs **days to weeks** after the primary lesion.
  - **Lymphadenopathy is a predominant finding**.
    - Unilateral
    - Tender
    - Erythematous
    - Abscesses and sinus tracts can complicate this stage.
  - Fever
  - Meningitis may occur.
  - **Groove sign** is characteristic.
    - Formed by the inguinal ligament dividing between the femoral and inguinal nodes.
    - Proctitis and proctocolitis can be seen.

- **Third stage**:
  - External genitalia ulceration, hypertrophy, and granulomatous inflammation.
  - Elephantiasis may occur secondary to lymphatic obstruction.

Diagnosis:
- Clinical symptoms, positive chlamydial serology, NAAT, isolation of LGV from infected tissue, or histopathology.

Treatment
- Note that in contrast to serovars D-K, you prescribe 21 days of doxycycline 100 mg twice daily for LGV.
- Erythromycin or sulfisoxazole are alternative regimens.

CDC guidelines:
Sexually Transmitted Diseases Treatment Guidelines, 2010. Available at http://www.cdc.gov/std/treatment/2010/STD-Treatment-2010-RR5912.pdf.

Guidelines for the laboratory diagnosis of gonorrhea, chlamydia, and syphilis. Available at http://www.aphl.org/aphlprograms/infectious/std/Pages/stdtestingguidelines.as

SUGGESTED READINGS

Bradshaw CS, Tabrizi SN, et al. Etiologies of nongonococcal urethritis: bacteria, viruses, and the association with orogenital exposure. *J Infect Dis* 2006;193(3):336–345.

Chernesky MA, Hook EW III, et al. Women find it easy and prefer to collect their own vaginal swabs to diagnose *Chlamydia trachomatis* or *Neisseria gonorrhoeae* infections. *Sex Transm Dis* 2005;32(12):729–733.
Self-collected vaginal swabs were easy to collect, and patients preferred them over urine and cervical swabs.

Chernesky MA, Martin DH, et al. Ability of new APTIMA CT and APTIMA GC assays to detect Chlamydia trachomatis and Neisseria gonorrhoeae in male urine and urethral swabs. *J Clin Microbiol* 2005;43(1):127–131.
The ACT and AGC assays performed on noninvasive specimens such as FCU effectively identified C. trachomatis or N. gonorrhoeae infections in symptomatic and asymptomatic men and should be suitable for screening male populations.

Fung M, Scott KC, et al. Chlamydial and gonococcal reinfection among men: a systematic review of data to evaluate the need for retesting. *Sex Transm Infect* 2007;83(4):304–309.
This study aimed to systematically review and describe the evidence on chlamydia and gonorrhoea reinfection among men and to evaluate the need for retesting recommendations in men. Retesting recommendations in men are appropriate, given the high rate of reinfection. To optimise retesting guidelines, further research to determine effective retesting methods and establish factors associated with reinfection among men is suggested.

Harkins A L, Munson E. Molecular Diagnosis of sexually transmitted Chlamydia trachomatis in the United States. *ISRN Obstet Gynecol* 2011;2011:279149.
The development of future molecular testing could address conundrums associated with confirmatory testing, medicolegal testing, and test of cure.

Hosenfeld CB, Workowski KA, et al. Repeat infection with Chlamydia and gonorrhea among females: a systematic review of the literature. *Sex Transm Dis* 2009;36(8):478–489.

Lau CY, Qureshi AK. Azithromycin versus doxycycline for genital chlamydial infections: a meta-analysis of randomized clinical trials. *Sex Transm Dis* 2002;29(9):497–502.
Azithromycin and doxycycline are equally efficacious in achieving microbial cure and have similar tolerability.

Lindan C, Mathur M, et al. Utility of pooled urine specimens for detection of *Chlamydia trachomatis* and *Neisseria gonorrhoeae* in men attending public sexually transmitted infection clinics in Mumbai, India, by PCR. *J Clin Microbiol* 2005;43(4):1674–1677.

Compared to individual FCU results, pooling for C. trachomatis and N. gonorrhoeae had an overall sensitivity of 96.1% (50/52). Specificity was 96.5% (83/86) in that three pools required single testing that failed to identify a positive specimen. Pooling missed two positive specimens, decreased the inhibition rate, and saved 50.3% of reagent costs. In this resource-limited setting, the use of pooling to detect C. trachomatis and N. gonorrhoeae by PCR proved to be a simple, accurate, and cost-effective procedure compared to individual testing.

Miller KE. Diagnosis and treatment of *Chlamydia trachomatis* infection. *Am Fam Physician* 2006;73(8): 1411–1416.

Moncada J, Schachter J, et al. Evaluation of self-collected glans and rectal swabs from men who have sex with men for detection of *Chlamydia trachomatis* and *Neisseria gonorrhoeae* by use of nucleic acid amplification tests. *J Clin Microbiol* 2009;47(6):1657–1662.

Self-collected glans swab specimens may not be appropriate for the detection of C. trachomatis or for the detection of N. gonorrhoeae in low-risk or asymptomatic patients by AC2 and SDA, and we would not recommend their use on the basis of our results. Further studies are needed.

Orellana MA, Gomez-Lus ML. Which is the best empirical treatment in patients with urethritis? *Rev Esp Quimioter* 2011;24(3):136–142.

N. gonorrhoeae showed a level of resistance to tetracycline and ciprofloxacin higher in the second period, being significant for ciprofloxacin. Quinolone resistance was higher in MSM. *Haemophilus* spp. showed a level of resistance to ampicillin, ciprofloxacin, and tetracycline higher in the second period, being significant for tetracycline. *Ureaplasma urealyticum* showed high level of resistance to ciprofloxacin (80.7%) and ofloxacin (32.4%) and low level of resistance to doxycycline (0.8%) and tetracycline (3.5%).

Rahangdale L, Guerry S, et al. An observational cohort study of *Chlamydia trachomatis* treatment in pregnancy. *Sex Transm Dis* 2006;33(2):106–110.

Schachter J, Chernesky MA, et al. Vaginal swabs are the specimens of choice when screening for *Chlamydia trachomatis* and *Neisseria gonorrhoeae*: results from a multicenter evaluation of the APTIMA assays for both infections. *Sex Transm Dis* 2005;32(12):725–728.

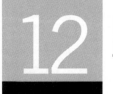

12 Genital Herpes Simplex

Lamis Ibrahim and James W. Myers

INTRODUCTION

- Herpes simplex virus (HSV) **is the most prevalent cause of genital ulcer** disease among sexually active people.
- It is a chronic, lifelong viral infection and so presents with recurrent episodes.
- HSV2 is almost always sexually transmitted.
- HSV1 is usually acquired during childhood through nonsexual contacts.
- Infections can be asymptomatic or unrecognized, but the **patient can still shed the virus** and transmit the disease.

EPIDEMIOLOGY

- About 50 million people have genital herpes in the United States.
- HSV2 is more common to cause genital infections (30% HSV1, 70% HSV2), although the incidence of HSV1 genital infection is probably increasing.
- **HSV2 is more likely to cause recurrent episodes**.
- Prior HSV1 infection can alleviate symptoms of subsequent HSV2 infection, and it can increase the chances of asymptomatic HSV2 infection by threefold.
- Transmission occurs **most commonly from asymptomatic** patients or from those with unrecognized infection.
- Risk of transmission increases with male source and with negative HSV antibodies.
- Male latex condoms might reduce the risk for genital herpes transmission.
- It increases risk of HIV acquisition and transmission.
- HSV perinatal transmission can be associated with fetal mortality and morbidity.

CLINICAL MANIFESTATIONS

Primary Infection

- Can be **asymptomatic**, subclinical, mild, or severe.
- Incubation period is normally from 2 to 12 days.
- **Painful** vesicular lesions/painful ulcers, and tender lymphadenopathy occur.
- Lesions are usually **multiple**.
- Fever, dysuria, and mucoid discharge can occur especially in females.
- Can cause urethritis and cervicitis, which cannot be distinguished clinically from chlamydia and gonorrhea.
- **Usually more severe infections occur in female**.

Recurrent Infection

- Usually **less severe and with fewer** lesions than primary infection.
- Has shorter duration of symptom and shorter duration of shedding.
- Lesions may be preceded by a **prodrome** of tingling or pain.

- Risk of frequent recurrences is higher with more severe and longer initial episode, in immunosuppressed, and with HSV2 compared to HSV1.
- More common in males than females.
- Median recurrence rates are **four to five episodes per year**, then a gradual decrease in rate over the years.

Proctitis
- Especially in MSM (men who have sex with men).
- Causes rectal pain, discharge, and tenesmus.
- A perianal lesion may be present.

COMPLICATIONS

- Aseptic meningitis and Mollaret syndrome (more common **with HSV2**)
- Transverse myelitis especially in immunosuppressed patients.
- Distant or extragenital lesions: more common **with HSV1** infection.
  - Can be secondary to autoinoculation or reactivation. Can appear on buttocks, thigh, or face.
- Autonomic dysfunction.
- Superinfection (bacterial/fungal).
- Disseminated infection.

DIAGNOSIS

1. **Culture**
   - Is the gold standard.
   - Highest yield with vesicular lesions.
   - Has **low sensitivity** (about 50%).
   - Typing should be done to detect the type of HSV when positive if possible.
2. **PCR**
   - Is *more sensitive* and is superior to virus isolation and culture.
   - Is not FDA approved.
   - Allows differentiation between HSV1 and HSV2.
   - Can detect asymptomatic shedding of the virus.
3. **Type-specific serology**
   - These are based upon glycoprotein G (G2 for HSV2 and G1 for HSV1)
   - Appear within the **first week of infection and remain** for life.
4. **Cytological changes:** nonspecific.

MANAGEMENT

Antiviral therapy controls signs and symptoms but does **not eradicate** the virus. It does not affect risk or frequency of recurrence after medication is stopped.

Treatment Regimens: See *Table 12.1*
- Treatment can be extended if healing is incomplete in 10 days.
- **Suppressive therapy for recurrent infections: see** *Table 12.1.*
  - Decreases recurrence by 70% to 80%, and decreases transmission to partners
  - Improves quality of life, and is preferred over episodic therapy.
  - Does **not reduce** the increased risk for HIV acquisition associated with HSV infection.

Table 12-1	Treatment of HSV in non-HIV patients	

Regimens for First Episode: (Any of the Following)	Regimens for Suppressive Therapy (Any of the Following)	Regimens for Episodic Therapy (Any of the Following)
• **Acyclovir** 400 mg orally three times a day for 7–10 days • **Acyclovir** 200 mg orally five times a day for 7–10 days • **Famciclovir** 250 mg orally three times a day for 7–10 days • **Valacyclovir** 1 g orally twice a day for 7–10 days	• **Acyclovir** 400 mg orally twice a day • **Famcyclovir** 250 mg orally twice a day • **Valacyclovir** 500 mg orally once a day • **Valacyclovir** 1 g orally once a day	• **Acyclovir** 400 mg orally three times a day for 5 days • **Acyclovir** 800 mg orally twice a day for 5 days • **Acyclovir** 800 mg orally three times a day for 2 days • **Famciclovir** 125 mg orally twice daily for 5 days • **Famciclovir** 1,000 mg orally twice daily for 1 day • **Famciclovir** 500 mg once, followed by 250 mg twice daily for 2 days • **Valacyclovir** 500 mg orally twice a day for 3 days • **Valacyclovir** 1 g orally once a day for 5 days

- **Episodic therapy: see** *Table 12.1*
  - Should be started within 1 day of the start of symptoms or during prodrome.
  - Doesn't prevent risk of transmission to partners!

Valacyclovir appears to be somewhat better than famciclovir for suppression of genital herpes and its associated shedding. Further comparative trials of antiviral drugs for various indications should be performed as acyclovir and penciclovir appear to have different ability to abrogate HSV reactivation.

Severe Disease/Complicated/CNS Involvement

- Treat with IV acyclovir 5 mg/kg IV every 8 hours for 2 to 7 days or until clinical improvement and then step down to oral antiviral therapy to complete at least 10 days of total therapy.
- Adjust for creatinine clearance and watch for possible crystallization in the urine and monitor kidney function.
- Use 10 mg/kg IV q 8 hours for CNS if creatinine allows.

Management of Partners

- Sex partners should be informed.
- Type-specific serologic testing of the asymptomatic partners is recommended to determine if they are already HSV seropositive or they are at risk of acquiring infection.
- No sexual activity with uninfected individuals till lesions and prodromal symptoms resolve.

HSV and Pregnancy
- Neonatal infection is the major problem.
- It is mainly transmitted to fetus from exposure to **vaginal secretions** during delivery.
- Can be transmitted by ascending route or transplacentally but not common.
- Twenty two percent of pregnant females are HSV2 seropositive.
- Risk of transmission is **30% to 50% when genital infection is acquired in third** trimester
- Must avoid infection during pregnancy.
- Do not expose the infants to lesion during delivery!
- Females at risk can be detected by checking type-specific antibodies.
- Females with genital lesion at delivery should have C-section, but if there are no signs or symptoms of HSV at delivery, they may have a vaginal delivery.
- Treatment is with acyclovir.

Neonatal Herpes
- Infants born to women with genital HSV near labor should be followed and tested.
- Acyclovir can be given when risk of infection is high even before manifestations start.
- Treatment is with acyclovir for 14 days if there is **limited disease**.
- Acyclovir should be given for 21 days if **disseminated**.

HIV and HSV
- Usually have **prolonged and severe** episodes of genital, perianal, or oral herpes.
- Can have more frequent recurrences and have more **atypical presentations**.
- Have more HSV shedding.
- Antiretroviral therapy reduces the severity and frequency of symptomatic infection.
- Suppressive or episodic therapy can decrease the clinical manifestations of HSV.
- If lesions recur or persist while on treatment, then HSV resistance should be ruled out.
- **Treatment: see** *Table 12.2.*

Table 12-2	Treatment of HSV in HIV patients	
Regimens for First Episode	**Regimens for Suppressive Therapy**	**Regimens for Episodic Therapy**
• Same as non-HIV patients	• **Acyclovir** 400–800 mg orally twice to three times a day OR • **Famciclovir** 500 mg orally twice a day OR • **Valacyclovir** 500 mg orally twice a day	• **Acyclovir** 400 mg orally three times a day for 5–10 days OR • **Famciclovir** 500 mg orally twice a day for 5–10 days OR • **Valacyclovir** 1 g orally twice a day for 5–10 days

SUGGESTED READINGS

Abudalu M, Tyring S, et al. Single-day, patient-initiated famciclovir therapy versus 3-day valacyclovir regimen for recurrent genital herpes: a randomized, double-blind, comparative trial. *Clin Infect Dis* 2008;47(5):651–658.
Single-day famciclovir (1,000 mg administered twice daily) was similar to 3-day vala-cyclovir (500 mg administered twice daily) in both efficacy and safety, representing a more convenient treatment for immunocompetent adults with recurrent genital herpes.

Bonnar PE. Suppressive valacyclovir therapy to reduce genital herpes transmission: good public health policy? *Mcgill J Med* 2009;12(1):39–46.
This article discusses the pros and cons of suppressive valacyclovir for genital herpes transmission. Seventy-two references.

CDC. Sexually Transmitted Diseases Treatment Guidelines, 2010. Available at http://www.cdc.gov/std/treatment/2010/STD-Treatment-2010-RR5912.pdf

Celum C, Wald A, et al. Acyclovir and transmission of HIV-1 from persons infected with HIV-1 and HSV-2. *N Engl J Med* 2010;362(5):427–439.
Daily acyclovir therapy did not reduce the risk of transmission of HIV-1, despite a reduction in plasma HIV-1 RNA of 0.25 log(10) copies per milliliter and a 73% reduction in the occurrence of genital ulcers due to HSV2.

Cernik C, Gallina K, et al. The treatment of herpes simplex infections: an evidence-based review. *Arch Intern Med* 2008;168(11):1137–1144.
In this review, data from all sources are tabulated to provide a handy clinical reference.

Conant MA, Schacker TW, et al. Valaciclovir versus aciclovir for herpes simplex virus infection in HIV-infected individuals: two randomized trials. *Int J STD AIDS* 2002;13(1):12–21.
Valacyclovir is a safe, effective, and convenient alternative to acyclovir for HSV infection in HIV-infected individuals.

Corey L, Wald A, et al. Once-daily valacyclovir to reduce the risk of transmission of genital herpes. *N Engl J Med* 2004;350(1):11–20.
Landmark article. Once-daily suppressive therapy with valacyclovir significantly reduces the risk of transmission of genital herpes among heterosexual, HSV2-discordant couples.

Emmert DH. Treatment of common cutaneous herpes simplex virus infections. *Am Fam Physician* 2000;61(6):1697–1706, 1708.
Review article. Several good tables and references.

Hollier LM, Wendel GD. Third trimester antiviral prophylaxis for preventing maternal genital herpes simplex virus (HSV) recurrences and neonatal infection. *Cochrane Database Syst Rev* 2008;(1):CD004946.
The risks, benefits, and alternatives to antenatal prophylaxis should be discussed with women who have a history and prophylaxis initiated for women who desire intervention.

Jones CW, Snyder GE. Mollaret meningitis: case report with a familial association. *Am J Emerg Med* 2011;29(7):840.e1–2.
Mollaret meningitis is a syndrome characterized by recurrent bouts of meningitis that occur over a period of several years in an affected patient. Also known as recurrent lymphocytic meningitis, this entity involves repeated episodes of headache, stiff neck, fever, and cerebrospinal fluid pleocytosis.
Herpes simplex virus type 2 is the most frequently implicated causative agent, and treatment involves the use of antiviral medications.

The authors described a case of Mollaret meningitis in a 47-year-old man who presented to the emergency department with his eighth episode of meningitis during a period of 20 years. Cerebrospinal fluid polymerase chain reaction testing for herpes simplex virus type 2 was positive, and further testing excluded other common viral, bacterial, and inflammatory causes of meningeal irritation. The patient's family history was significant for a brother who also had multiple episodes of aseptic meningitis during a period of several years. This represents the first published report of a possible familial association involving Mollaret meningitis.

Kang SH, Chua-Gocheco A, et al. Safety of antiviral medication for the treatment of herpes during pregnancy. *Can Fam Physician* 2011;57(4):427–428.
Studies have shown that the use of acyclovir or valacyclovir is not associated with an increase in birth defects.

Kim HN, Wald A, et al. Does frequency of genital herpes recurrences predict risk of transmission? Further analysis of the valacyclovir transmission study. *Sex Transm Dis* 2008;35(2):124–128.
Though patients with frequent recurrences are most likely to benefit clinically from suppressive therapy, frequency of recurrences is not helpful in identifying persons who are most likely to transmit HSV2.

Leone P, Abudalu M, et al. One-day famciclovir vs. placebo in patient-initiated episodic treatment of recurrent genital herpes in immunocompetent Black patients. *Curr Med Res Opin* 2010;26(3):653–661.
Famciclovir has proven efficacy and safety in the overall RGH population. Further understanding of the efficacy of antiherpes therapy in black patients with recurrent genital herpes may be warranted.

Pasternak B, Hviid A. Use of acyclovir, valacyclovir, and famciclovir in the first trimester of pregnancy and the risk of birth defects. *JAMA* 2010;304(8):859–866.
In this large nationwide cohort, exposure to acyclovir or valacyclovir in the first trimester of pregnancy was not associated with an increased risk of major birth defects.

Piret J, Boivin G. Resistance of herpes simplex viruses to nucleoside analogues: mechanisms, prevalence, and management. *Antimicrob Agents Chemother* 2011;55(2):459–472.
Foscarnet and cidofovir are useful in treating acyclovir-resistant HSV infections. Good overall review.

Romanowski B, Marina RB, et al. Patients' preference of valacyclovir once-daily suppressive therapy versus twice-daily episodic therapy for recurrent genital herpes: a randomized study. *Sex Transm Dis* 2003;30(3):226–231.

Song B, Dwyer DE, et al. HSV type specific serology in sexual health clinics: use, benefits, and who gets tested. *Sex Transm Infect* 2004;80(2):113–117.
Type-specific serology should be recommended for the management of couples where one has genital herpes and the other apparently does not and in individuals with genital complaints suggestive of herpes.

Stone KM, Reiff-Eldridge R, et al. Pregnancy outcomes following systemic prenatal acyclovir exposure: conclusions from the international acyclovir pregnancy registry, 1984-1999. *Birth Defects Res A Clin Mol Teratol* 2004;70(4):201–207.
The observed rates and types of birth defects for pregnancies exposed to acyclovir did not differ significantly from those in the general population.

Wald A, Huang ML, et al. Polymerase chain reaction for detection of herpes simplex virus (HSV) DNA on mucosal surfaces: comparison with HSV isolation in cell culture. *J Infect Dis* 2003;188(9):1345–1351.

Wald A, Selke S, et al. Comparative efficacy of famciclovir and valacyclovir for suppression of recurrent genital herpes and viral shedding. *Sex Transm Dis* 2006;33(9):529–533.

Valacyclovir appears to be somewhat better than famciclovir for suppression of genital herpes and associated shedding. Further comparative trials of antiviral drugs for various indications should be performed as acyclovir and pencyclovir appear to have different abilities to abrogate HSV reactivation.

Watson-Jones D, Weiss HA, et al. Effect of herpes simplex suppression on incidence of HIV among women in Tanzania. *N Engl J Med* 2008;358(15):1560–1571.

These data show no evidence that acyclovir (400 mg twice daily) as HSV suppressive therapy decreases the incidence of infection with HIV.

Xu F, Sternberg MR, et al. Trends in herpes simplex virus type 1 and type 2 seroprevalence in the United States. *JAMA* 2006;296(8):964–973.

These data show declines in HSV2 seroprevalence, suggesting that the trajectory of increasing HSV2 seroprevalence in the United States has been reversed. Seroprevalence of HSV1 decreased but the incidence of genital herpes caused by HSV1 may be increasing.

HPV Infections

James W. Myers and Emmanuel Okon

INTRODUCTION

Human papillomaviruses (HPV) are icosahedral nonenveloped dsDNA viruses belonging to the family papillomaviruses. HPVs are the commonest cause of sexually transmitted infection in the world and the third most common cause of cancer in women worldwide. Clinical manifestations of infection include anogenital disease and other types of disease (e.g., respiratory papillomatosis and focal epithelial hyperplasia of the oral cavity).

An association exists between oncogenic HPV infection and squamous intraepithelial lesions of the cervix, anus, vulva, penis, and vagina. Fifteen percent of HPV infections will progress to cervical intraepithelial neoplasia or carcinoma within 2 to 3 years if left untreated. Risk factors for persistent infection include multiple sexual partners, age of first intercourse, history of STDs, and smoking. Sixty-five percent of sexual contacts will develop an infection. Most people who become infected with HPV do not even know they have it.

CLINICAL MANIFESTATIONS

- Genital HPV infections can be divided into **low-risk** infections (genital warts) and **high-risk** infections (cervical and other cancers).
- The presence of genital warts is not an indication for HPV testing, a change in the frequency of Pap tests, or cervical colposcopy.
- Incubation period: 3 weeks to 8 months (3 months average).
- Up to 90% will clear the infection in about 2 years. Genital warts usually clear with treatment in about 6 months. Up to 30% clear spontaneously in 4 months. A minority of those infected will go on to malignant disease.
- **Genital warts** appear as a small bump or groups of bumps in the genital area. They can be small or large, raised or flat, or shaped like a cauliflower.
- Warts can appear within **weeks or months** after sexual contact with an infected partner—even if the infected partner has no signs of genital warts.
- HPV testing is not indicated for partners of persons with genital warts.
- HPV transmission—4.9 from penis to cervix, and 17.4 from cervix to penis events per 100 person months.
- If left untreated, genital warts might go away, remain unchanged, or increase in size or number. They will not turn into cancer.
- **Cervical cancer** usually does not have symptoms until it is quite advanced. For this reason, it is important for women to get regular screening. The interval between infection and cancer is about 10 to 20 years. Given a peak prevalence of HPV infection in women in their early 20s, screening is most effective for those patients between 30 and 40 years of age.

- **Other HPV-related cancers** might not have signs or symptoms until they are advanced and hard to treat. These include cancers of the vulva, vagina, penis, anus, and head and neck.
- **RRP (recurrent respiratory papillomatosis)** causes warts to grow in the throat. It can sometimes block the airway, causing a hoarse voice or troubled breathing.
  - Follows exposure during a vaginal birth.
  - May first appear between 6 months and 10 years of age.
  - Adults may get it from oral-genital contact.
  - Treatment: endoscopic cryotherapy or laser surgery

DIAGNOSIS

Diagnostic Tests[a]	Findings
Clinical evaluation	Speculum examination is needed for anogenital warts + Anoscopy for women with perianal and perineal warts.
Acetic acid	3%–5% acetic acid is applied, used to delineate disease prior to biopsy. **Look for characteristic acetowhite appearance**.
Cytology	Pap smear to detect HPV disease in the cervix, vagina, and sometimes in the anus, especially in homosexual men and women with HPV genitourinary tract lesions. **Look for koilocytes + nuclear atypia + delayed maturation**.
Histology	Biopsy is indicated in atypical cases and when the benign nature of the lesion is unclear, that is, Bowenoid or giant condylomas. **Look for papillomatosis accompanied by the characteristic features of acanthosis, parakeratosis, hyperkeratosis, and koilocytosis**.
Molecular-based methods	**Two HPV DNA detection tests, the Hybrid Capture II (Digene Corporation) and the Cervista HPV HR and HPV 16/18 (Hologic Inc.) assays, are approved by the U.S. Food and Drug Administration (FDA) for the triage of ASC-US Pap smears and for the primary screening of cervical cancer** in combination with cytology.

[a]See the Internet Resources table for an excellent algorithm for screening with Pap smears and HPV detection tests available from the American Society for Colposcopy and Cervical Pathology.

No recommended uses of the HPV test to diagnose HPV infection in **sex partners** have been established. HPV infection is commonly transmitted to partners but usually goes away on its own.

TREATMENT

- The response to treatment will depend on the following:
  - Duration of lesions more than 1 year.
  - >10 lesions
  - Dry skin heals less often than moist lesions.
  - Tobacco smoking and contraceptive use are adverse factors as well.
- The natural history of genital warts is usually benign, but recurrence of genital warts within the first several months after treatment is common.

- Treatment of genital warts can reduce HPV infection, but whether the treatment results in a reduction in risk for transmission of HPV to sex partners is unclear. The duration of infectivity after wart treatment is not clear at this time.
- Examination of sex partners is **not necessary** for the management of genital warts because reinfection plays no role in recurrences !

Self-Applied Therapies

Treatment	Mechanism of Action	Directions	Adverse Reactions
Podofilox (podophyllotoxin)	Unknown? Mitotic toxin.	Apply with a cotton-tipped applicator (solution) or finger (gel) q 12 hours for 3 days, then none for 4 days. May repeat in 1 week for up **to four cycles**.	Chemical burns, neurologic, hematologic, and febrile complications, sometimes leading to death, and allergic sensitization. *Therefore, areas larger than 10 cm² should not be treated. Total volume should be >0.5 mL/day.* **Contraindicated in pregnancy.**
Imiquimod	Induces the production of interferon-α and other cytokines. Likely mechanism of action involves binding to the toll-like receptors 7 and possibly 8 of dendritic cells	Three times/week at bedtime. Apply until gone or up to **16 weeks** maximum. Wash with soap and water, 6–10 hours after application.	Itching and burning sensations, erythema, erosions, and swelling. Safety **not** established in pregnancy. Might weaken condoms and vaginal diaphragms. Lactation safety unknown.
Polyphenon E, or sineatechin ointment	Contains green tea catechins. These compounds have some antiviral and anticarcinogenic activities.	Apply a 0.5 cm strand of ointment with a finger three times a day on the lesions until complete disappearance, but for **no more than 16** weeks. Do not wash off.	Erythema, pruritus, pain, and ulceration. **Contraindicated in pregnancy. Might weaken condoms too. Efficacy in HIV not established.** The red stain of the substance and its frequency of administration are potential drawbacks.

Provider-Applied Therapies:

Treatment	Directions	Side Effects.
Podophyllin resin	Apply with a cotton-tipped applicator (1–2 mL). No open lesions. Allow to air dry and then wipe off after 1–4 hours. May repeat in 1 week.	Similar to podofilox. **Pregnancy category X**
Trichloroacetic acid	Trichloroacetic acid in a 10%–90% solution is used topically at **weekly** intervals. Commonly used by gynecologists for the treatment of genital warts.	The application is painful and can cause ulcers. The unreacted acid should be removed with talcum powder or bicarbonate of soda. **Safe in pregnancy**.
5-Fluorouracil	It is used topically as a 5% cream applied daily. Best results **with intraurethral warts. Rarely used**.	It is used topically as a 5% cream applied daily. **Unsafe in pregnancy**
Cryotherapy	Lesions are frozen every 1 or 2 weeks with liquid nitrogen or cryoprobe.	Burning, which resolves within a few hours, and ulceration, which heals in 7–10 days with little or no scarring. **Safe in pregnancy**.
Conventional surgery or electrosurgery.	Refer to a specialist	Recurrences, and scarring, typically limited to some skin discoloration.

Special Circumstances:

RECOMMENDED REGIMENS FOR URETHRAL MEATUS WARTS

• Cryotherapy with liquid nitrogen
• Podophyllin 10% to 25% in compound tincture of benzoin. This treatment can be repeated weekly, if necessary.

RECOMMENDED REGIMENS FOR ANAL WARTS

• Cryotherapy with liquid nitrogen
• TCA or BCA 80% to 90% applied to warts. This treatment can be repeated weekly, if necessary.
• Surgery

PREGNANCY

• Imiquimod, podophyllin, sinecatechins, and podofilox should not be used during pregnancy.

- Cesarean delivery should *not be performed solely* to prevent transmission of HPV infection to the newborn.
- Cesarean delivery **is indicated for women with genital warts if** the pelvic outlet is obstructed or if vaginal delivery would result in excessive bleeding.

HIV

- No data suggest that treatment modalities for external genital warts should be different for HIV infected.
- Anal cytology can be *considered*.

PREVENTION

Male condoms can lessen the odds of giving or getting genital HPV, but such use is less than fully protective, because the virus infects areas that are not covered by a condom.

HPV VACCINE

- A quadrivalent vaccine, Gardasil, FDA approved in June 2006 for the prevention of several genital HPV diseases, including cervical cancer. It is directed against HPV types 6, 11, 16, and 18, thus aiming at 80% to 90% of the agents of genital warts and 70% of the agents of cervical cancer.
- The Advisory Committee on Immunization Practices (ACIP) recommendation is vaccination for girls aged 11 through 12 years and a catch-up immunization for ages 13 to 26-years.
- The vaccine is given as an IM injection (0.5 mL) at months 0, 2, and 6. No booster is needed, and protection lasts for about 5 years.
- Syncope may occur after the immunization; observation of the subject for 15 minutes after the injection is recommended.
- Other side effects include pain at the injection site (85%) and swelling (26%) as well as fever.
- Contraindications include yeast allergy *(Saccharomyces cerevisae)* or a prior allergic reaction to the vaccine or its components.
- Pregnancy is a contraindication.
- Should the series of three immunizations be interrupted, one should complete the series whenever possible.
- Because this is an inert, noninfectious vaccine, it is not contraindicated for patients with immunodeficiency or immunosuppression.
- Vaccine efficacy in these populations is unknown as there are no data available.
- Patients are advised to continue cervical cancer screening.
- **Gardasil is also licensed, safe, and effective for males aged 9 through 26 years. CDC recommends Gardasil for all boys aged 11 or 12 years, and for males aged 13 through 21 years, who did not get any or all of the three recommended doses when they were younger. All men may receive the vaccine through age 26, and should speak with their doctor to find out if getting vaccinated is right for them.**
  - **The vaccine is also recommended for gay and bisexual men (or any man who has sex with men) and men with compromised immune systems (including HIV) through age 26, if they did not get fully vaccinated when they were younger.**

Useful Internet Sites:

	Description	Link
CDC HPV	Main Web Site	http://www.cdc.gov/std/hpv/
CDC HPV	STD treatment Guidelines	http://www.cdc.gov/std/treatment/2010/hpv.htm
CDC HPV	STD-Warts	http://www.cdc.gov/std/treatment/2010/genital-warts.htm
CDC HPV	HP Resources	http://www.cdc.gov/hpv/resources.html
CDC HPV	Fact Sheet for Patients	http://www.cdc.gov/std/HPV/STDFact-HPV.htm
CDC HPV	Cervical Cancer Screening	http://www.cdc.gov/cancer/cervical/basic_info/screening.htm
CDC HPV	Brochure	http://www.cdc.gov/std/hpv/hpv-clinicians-brochure.htm
CDC HPV	Gardasil	http://www.cdc.gov/vaccines/pubs/vis/downloads/vis-hpv-gardasil.pdf
CDC HPV	Cervarix	http://www.cdc.gov/vaccines/pubs/vis/downloads/vis-hpv-cervarix.pdf
CDC HPV	Vaccines	http://www.cdc.gov/hpv/vaccine.html
CDC HPV	Self Study Module	http://www2a.cdc.gov/stdtraining/self-study/hpv.asp
Geneva Foundation	Acetic Acid	http://www.gfmer.ch/Books/Cervical_cancer_modules/Aided_visual_inspection_atlas.htm
About.com	Pap Smear Video for pts	http://video.about.com/womenshealth/ObGyn-PAP-Smear—Check-up.htm
Pap smear	Pap pictures	http://www.pap-smear.info/pap-smear-pictures.shtml
Colposcopy Society	Algorithm	http://www.asccp.org/LinkClick.aspx?fileticket=uUGOqspsCBU%3d&tabid=5964
Merck	Gardasil	http://www.merckvaccines.com/Products/Gardasil/Pages/home.aspx
GSK	Cervarix	http://www.cervarix.com/
LWW	Atlas	http://www.lww.com/product/Atlas-Infectious-Diseases-Female-Genital-Tract/?978-0-7817-5583-2
Expert Consult	Mandell Chapter	http://expertconsultbook.com

SUGGESTED READINGS

Abbas A, Yang G, et al. Management of anal cancer in 2010. Part 1: overview, screening, and diagnosis. *Oncology (Williston Park)* 2010;24(4):364–369.

There is a general consensus that high-risk individuals may benefit from screening. Nearly half of all patients with anal cancer present with rectal bleeding. Pain or sensation of a rectal mass is experienced in 30% of patients, whereas 20% have no tumor-specific symptoms.

Agorastos T, Sotiriadis A, et al. Can HPV testing replace the pap smear? *Ann N Y Acad Sci* 2010;1205:51–56.

Overall, available evidence convincingly shows that HPV testing is superior to traditional screening for the detection of high-grade cervical lesions, and efforts are focused on improving its sensitivity, either by increasing its cutoff for positivity or by selecting those subgroups where HPV testing is expected to have higher positive predictive value for cervical disease, or by seeking to optimize triage tests after a positive HPV result.

Barroso LF II, Wilkin T. Human papillomavirus vaccination in males: the state of the science. *Curr Infect Dis Rep* 2011;13(2):175–181.

This review focuses on HPV disease in men, existing data on HPV vaccination in men, and various factors associated with the decision to vaccinate boys and young men, as well as the timing of vaccination.

Bean SM, Chhieng DC. Anal-rectal cytology: a review. *Diagn Cytopathol* 2010;38(7):538–546.

Either conventional or liquid-based anal-rectal cytology specimens are acceptable, but liquid-based specimens are preferred. Specimens may be collected by health care professionals or by patients. Sensitivity and specificity of a single anal-rectal cytology specimen is comparable with that of a single cervical cytology test, but cytologic interpretations do not always correlate with lesion severity.

de Pokomandy A, Rouleau D, et al. HAART and progression to high-grade anal intraepithelial neoplasia in men who have sex with men and are infected with HIV. *Clin Infect Dis* 2011;52(9):1174–1181.

Human immunodeficiency virus (HIV)-seropositive men who have sex with men (MSM) are at risk for anal intraepithelial neoplasia (AIN) and cancer.

Conclusion. HPV16 and HPV18 infections and a low nadir CD4+ cell count increase the risk of AIN-2,3. Receiving the same HAART regimen for >4 years may contribute some benefit against AIN-2,3.

Domza G, Gudleviciene Z, et al. Human papillomavirus infection in pregnant women. *Arch Gynecol Obstet* 2010;284(5):1105–1112.

This study showed the high prevalence of HPV infection in pregnant women in Lithuania. The majority of pregnant women's HPV infection was cleared during the pregnancy. Only in a few cases was a new HPV infection detected.

Garland SM, Hernandez-Avila M, et al. Quadrivalent vaccine against human papillomavirus to prevent anogenital diseases. *N Engl J Med* 2007;356(19):1928–1943.

A phase 3 trial was conducted to evaluate the efficacy of a prophylactic quadrivalent vaccine in preventing anogenital diseases associated with HPV types 6, 11, 16, and 18. The coprimary composite end points were the incidence of genital warts, vulvar or vaginal intraepithelial neoplasia, or cancer and the incidence of cervical intraepithelial neoplasia, adenocarcinoma in situ, or cancer associated with HPV type 6, 11, 16, or 18. The quadrivalent vaccine significantly reduced the incidence of HPV-associated anogenital diseases in young women.

Garland SM, Smith JS. Human papillomavirus vaccines: current status and future prospects. *Drugs* 2010;70(9):1079–1098.

Both vaccines translate to protection of cervical cancer in the order of 70% to 75%, which represents the percentage of invasive cancers attributable to HPV-16 and -18.

Giuliano AR, Palefsky JM, et al. Efficacy of quadrivalent HPV vaccine against HPV Infection and disease in males. *N Engl J Med* 2011;364(5):401–411.

Quadrivalent HPV vaccine prevents infection with HPV-6, 11, 16, and 18 and the development of related external genital lesions in males 16 to 26 years of age.

Harper DM. Current prophylactic HPV vaccines and gynecologic premalignancies. *Curr Opin Obstet Gynecol* 2009;21(6):457–464.

Studies of the HPV vaccines, Cervarix and Gardasil, provide strong evidence for the recommendation that HPV vaccines may minimize the incidence of cervical cancer over time.

Hernandez BY, Wilkens LR, et al. Transmission of human papillomavirus in heterosexual couples. *Emerg Infect Dis* 2008;14(6):888–894.

The overall rate of HPV transmission from the penis to the cervix was 4.9/100 person months, which was substantially lower than that from the cervix to the penis (17.4/100 person months). Couples who transmitted HPV were more sexually active and used condoms less frequently.

Juckett G, Hartman-Adams H. Human papillomavirus: clinical manifestations and prevention. *Am Fam Physician* 2010;82(10):1209–1213.

Excellent review article. Contains several good tables and references. **Highly recommended. References 2, 16, 27, 32, 34, 41, 43, 47, 48, and 49 are especially noteworthy in my opinion.**

Lajer CB, von Buchwald C. The role of human papillomavirus in head and neck cancer. *APMIS* 2010;118(6–7):510–519.

Patients with HPV-positive HNSCC tend to be younger and have a lower intake of tobacco and alcohol. HPV-positive HNSCC show an affinity for the oropharynx, especially the tonsils and the base of the tongue, and tend to show low differentiation histopathologically.

There is a better prognosis regardless of the treatment regimen for HPV-positive HNSCC. Whether the new vaccines for HPV will protect not only against cervical cancer but also against HPV-positive HNSCC remains unknown.

Lebwohl MG, Rosen T, et al. The role of human papillomavirus in common skin conditions: current viewpoints and therapeutic options. *Cutis* 2010;86(5):suppl 1–11; quiz suppl 12.

This article explores the role of HPV in 2 common disorders associated with considerable morbidity: external genital and perianal warts (EGWs) and actinic keratosis (AK). It also has been suggested that HPV may increase the severity of AK lesions and contribute to their recurrence following therapy.

Markowitz LE, Dunne EF, et al. Quadrivalent Human Papillomavirus Vaccine: Recommendations of the Advisory Committee on Immunization Practices (ACIP). *MMWR Recomm Rep* 2007;56(RR-2):1–24.

These recommendations represent the first statement by the Advisory Committee on Immunization Practices (ACIP) on the use of a quadrivalent HPV vaccine licensed by the U.S. Food and Drug Administration on June 8, 2006.

1. Genital HPV is the most common sexually transmitted infection in the United States; an estimated 6.2 million persons are newly infected every year. Although the majority of infections cause no clinical symptoms and are self-limited, persistent infection with oncogenic types can cause cervical cancer in women. HPV infection also is the cause of genital warts and is associated with other anogenital cancers.

2. The licensed HPV vaccine is composed of the HPV L1 protein, the major capsid protein of HPV. Expression of the L1 protein in yeast using recombinant DNA technology produces noninfectious virus-like particles (VLP) that resemble HPV virions. The quadrivalent HPV vaccine is a mixture of four HPV type-specific VLPs prepared from the L1 proteins of HPV 6, 11, 16, and 18 combined with an aluminum adjuvant.

3. Clinical trials indicate that the vaccine has high efficacy in preventing persistent HPV infection, cervical cancer precursor lesions, vaginal and vulvar cancer precursor lesions, and genital warts caused by HPV types 6, 11, 16, or 18 among females who have not already been infected with the respective HPV type.

4. No evidence exists of protection against disease caused by HPV types with which females are infected at the time of vaccination. However, females infected with one or more vaccine HPV types before vaccination would be protected against disease caused by the other vaccine HPV types.

5. *The vaccine is administered by intramuscular injection, and the recommended schedule is a three-dose series with the second and third doses administered 2 and 6 months after the first dose. The recommended age for vaccination of females is 11 to 12 years. Vaccine can be administered in children as young as age 9 years.*

6. *Catch-up vaccination is recommended for females aged 13 to 26 years who have not been previously vaccinated. Vaccination is not a substitute for routine cervical cancer screening, and vaccinated females should have cervical cancer screening as recommended.*

Psyrri A, Gouveris P, et al. Human papillomavirus-related head and neck tumors: clinical and research implication. *Curr Opin Oncol* 2009;21(3):201–205.

It has now become clear that a subset of HNSCC is a sexually transmitted disease with distinct pathogenesis and clinical/pathological features. This review summarizes the epidemiology, clinical presentation, molecular pathogenesis, diagnosis, and therapy of HPV-associated HNSCC; it also summarizes how a better understanding of the molecular pathogenesis of HPV-associated HNSCC is expected to change treatment.

Winer RL, Hughes JP, et al. Condom use and the risk of genital human papillomavirus infection in young women. *N Engl J Med* 2006;354(25):2645–2654.

In women reporting 100% condom use by their partners, no cervical squamous intraepithelial lesions were detected in 32 patient-years at risk, whereas 14 incident lesions were detected during 97 patient-years at risk among women whose partners did not use condoms or used them less consistently.

14 Vaginitis

Emmanuel Okon and James W. Myers

- The term "vaginitis" refers to inflammation of the vagina.
- Symptoms include itching, irritation, and abnormal vaginal discharge.
- The presence of abnormal discharge, vulvovaginal discomfort, or both is required for the diagnosis of vaginitis.
- It accounts for an estimated 3 million office visits.

EPIDEMIOLOGY

Most common causes of Infectious Vaginitis	Bacterial vaginosis (BV) (40%–50%) Candidiasis (20%–25%) Trichomonal vaginitis (15%–20%)
Uncommon causes of infectious vaginitis	Foreign body with secondary infection Desquamative inflammatory vaginitis (DIV) (**clindamycin responsive**) Streptococcal vaginitis (group A), Staphylococcus, human immunodeficiency virus (HIV), Gonorrhea, chlamydia/herpes simplex virus (HSV).
Noninfectious vaginitis	Chemical/irritant (soap, tampons, sanitary napkins, condoms, spermicidal gels, diaphragms, and dyes). Allergic, hypersensitivity, and contact dermatitis (lichen simplex) Neurodermatitis, traumatic, postpuerperal atrophic vaginitis Atrophic vaginitis. Idiopathic, malignancy. Postpuerperal atrophic vaginitis Desquamative inflammatory vaginitis (corticosteroid responsive). Erosive lichen planus. Collagen vascular disease, Behçet syndrome, pemphigus syndromes.

PREDISPOSING FACTORS

- Increasing age
- Sexual activity
- Hormonal status
- Poor hygiene
- Immunologic status
- Anatomy of the genital area
- Underlying skin diseases
- Other factors including damp or tight-fitting clothing, scented detergents and soaps, feminine sprays.

MOST COMMON CAUSES OF VAGINITIS

1. **Bacterial Vaginosis (BV)**
   - This is usually a *result of disruption of normal vaginal flora* leading to changes in the concentrations of various microorganisms including a depletion of lactobacilli and a proliferation of other anaerobic bacteria like *Gardnerella vaginalis*, *Prevotella*, *Mobiluncus* spp., *Mycoplasma hominis*, and *Atopobium vaginae* (***Atopobium* species** are anaerobic bacteria, gram-positive, rod-shaped, or elliptical found as single elements or in pairs or short chains.) Nevertheless, a positive culture for *G. vaginalis should not be considered diagnostic* of BV unless other evidence of BV (abnormal pH, odor with 10% KOH, clue cells) are found.
   - There is an increase in vaginal pH caused by decrease in hydrogen peroxide–producing lactobacilli.
   - Anaerobes produce amines, which cause the characteristic *fishy* odor.
   - 50% of women are **asymptomatic**.
   - BV is less likely to occur in virgins but still does. Can occur in lesbian couples as well.
   - Prevalence is higher at **earlier stages** of menstrual cycle.
   - There is an associated increased risk of ***adverse obstetrical and gynecologic clinical outcomes*** such as preterm delivery, low birth weight, upper genital tract infections, and pelvic inflammatory disease (PID).
     - Treat **symptomatic** pregnant women.
     - Consider screening and treating those who have a high risk of prematurity.
     - Decreases risk of prematurity in those who have BV and a history of prematurity in some studies but not others.
     - Treatment for BV **before abortion or hysterectomy** significantly decreases the risk of postoperative infectious complications.
   - It also *increases the risk of acquiring HIV*, HSV2, gonorrhea, and chlamydial infection.
2. **Candidiasis**
   - It is most common in women of childbearing age. Second most common cause of vaginitis. Often precipitated by antibiotic use, pregnancy, diabetes, oral contraceptives, or menses but can occur without any of these factors.
   - 75% of women will have at least one episode.
   - Intractable disease in 5%.
   - *Candida albicans* is commonly isolated; however, in immunocompromised individuals with complicated (recurrent) candidiasis, C. glabrata have been isolated.
   - The nonalbicans species are found in 10% to 20% of patients.
3. **Trichonomiasis.**
   - The etiologic agent is Trichomonas vaginalis(TV).
   - 7.3 million new cases are estimated each year.
   - Coexistence of other sexually transmitted diseases (STDs) is very common.
   - It is a facultative anaerobe, 5 to 15 μm, pear-shaped, motile, flagellated protozoan parasite that exists in the trophozoite stage only.
   - Several deoxyribonucleic acid (DNA) probes and rapid antigen detection are commercially available, and are replacing culture (Affirm VP, Trichomonas Rapid Test).
   - Trichomoniasis can facilitate HIV transmission.
   - Trichomoniasis is probably a risk factor for acquiring posthysterectomy cellulitis, tubal infertility, cervical neoplasia, and PID.
   - Treatment of symptomatic disease in pregnancy is indicated.

The clinical findings, diagnosis, and treatment of the above entities are summarized in the table below.

	Bacterial Vaginosis	Candidiasis	Trichonomiasis
Vaginal discharge	Homogeneous, white to gray, **with a fishy odor coating** the vaginal wall. Pruritus +	Scant to moderate, white, clumped or **curd-like, adhering** to vaginal walls, with little or no odor. **Pruritus ++.**	**Profuse**, yellow-green to gray, homogeneous, with or without a mild fishy odor. Pruritus +
Vaginal/Cervical appearance	**Minimal or no erythema.** Cervix is normal.	Erythematous often with mucosal swelling. Cervix with infrequent ectocervical erythema.	Vulvovaginal area is usually erythematous. Cervix: "strawberry cervix," which is caused by punctate hemorrhages, infrequently seen but pathognomonic.
pH	>4.5	≤4.5	>4.5
Lab diagnosis	Wet mount–**clue cells** and few polymorphonuclear leukocytes (PMNs). 10% KOH gives a **positive "whiff" test.**	Wet mount–budding yeast, pseudohyphae, and few PMNs. 10% KOH slide–negative "whiff" test.	Wet mount–motile trichomonads and increased PMNs (ratio of PMNs to vaginal epithelial cells >1:1 ± positive whiff test.
Treatment	**Metronidazole** 500 mg PO daily × 7 days; **metronidazole gel** 0.75%, one full applicator (5 g) intravaginally, once daily × 5 days; **clindamycin** cream, 2%, 1 full applicator (5 g) intravaginally qhs × 7 days. Less effective, alternative treatments include: clindamycin 300 mg PO twice daily × 7 days; clindamycin ovules 100 g intravaginally qhs × 3 days.	Fluconazole 150 mg PO × 1 dose. Several topical agents available can be used between 3–7 days.	Metronidazole or tinidazole 2 g PO × 1 dose. Alternative treatment: Metronidazole 500 mg PO twice daily × 7 days.

FOLLOW-UP

- Uncomplicated cases of BV and candidiasis typically resolve after one standard treatment.
- BV that does not resolve after one treatment may be treated with a second course of the same agent or another agent.
  - Treatment is suboptimal with cure rates of only 60% to 80% and high recurrence/reinfection rates.
  - **Two new alternative BV treatment regimens**: Tinidazole 2 g orally once daily for 2 days or tinidazole 1 g orally once daily for 5 days are options for patients who do not tolerate metronidazole or have difficulty with compliance.
  - Concurrent treatment of male partner is controversial, an option used by some clinicians if BV is recurrent.
  - Unresponsive BV might respond to intravaginal boric acid, 600 mg at bedtime, twice a week. Long-term (4 to 6 month) biweekly antibiotic courses are used occasionally as well.
- Patients with recurrent candidiasis should be screened for immunosuppression i.e. HIV infection, diabetes mellitus (DM), leukemia, or other immunologic dysfunction. Complicated cases might require 10 to 14 days of azole therapy and possible long-term suppression.
- Unlike in candidiasis and BV, all current sexual partners of patients with trichomoniasis should be treated to prevent reinfection, and all previous sexual partners **within 90 days of sexual contact** should be referred for evaluation and possible treatment.
- Increased doses of metronidazole and longer duration of therapy are used to treat unresponsive TV patients.
  - Oral metronidazole of 2 to 4g/day for 10 to 14 days.
  - Intravenous metronidazole.
  - Tinidazole 1 to 4g/day for 14 days has been tried.
  - Some clinicians use topical paramomycin.
- All patients should be tested for coinfection with other STDs and are advised to avoid sexual intercourse until treatment is complete, partners have been treated as well, and both are free of symptoms.

Images

Clue cells	http://www.youtube.com/watch?v=ScJcyfEIWFs
Trichomonas	http://www.youtube.com/watch?v=UJ3yjJmBhY8&feature=related
Strawberry cervix	http://www2a.cdc.gov/stdtraining/self-study/vaginitis/vaginitis7.asp

SUGGESTED READINGS

Achkar JM, Fries BC. Candida infections of the genitourinary tract. *Clin Microbiol Rev* 2010;23(2):253–273.

Good review article.

Donders G, Bellen G, et al. Individualized decreasing-dose maintenance fluconazole regimen for recurrent vulvovaginal candidiasis (ReCiDiF trial). *Am J Obstet Gynecol* 2008;199(6):613 e611–e619.

Individualized, degressive, prophylactic maintenance therapy with oral fluconazole is an efficient treatment regimen to prevent clinical relapses in women with recurrent vulvovaginal candidiasis.

Falagas ME, Betsi GI, et al. Probiotics for prevention of recurrent vulvovaginal candidiasis: a review. *J Antimicrob Chemother* 2006;58(2):266–272.

The authors conclude that despite the promising results of some studies, further research is needed to prove the effectiveness of probiotics in preventing the recurrences of VVC and to allow their wide use for this indication.

Klebanoff MA, Carey JC, et al. Failure of metronidazole to prevent preterm delivery among pregnant women with asymptomatic Trichomonas vaginalis infection. *N Engl J Med* 2001;345(7):487–493.

Treatment of pregnant women with asymptomatic trichomoniasis does not prevent preterm delivery. Routine screening and treatment of asymptomatic pregnant women for this condition cannot be recommended.

Mammen-Tobin A, Wilson, JD. Management of metronidazole-resistant Trichomonas vaginalis—a new approach. *Int J STD AIDS* 2005;16(7):488–490.

Although a variety of total doses of tinidazole were used in these patients, based on their findings, and those of others, they would recommend giving tinidazole 2 g twice daily for 14 days (total dose 56 g).

Sobel JD, Wiesenfeld HC, et al. Maintenance fluconazole therapy for recurrent vulvovaginal candidiasis. *N Engl J Med* 2004;351(9):876–883.

Long-term weekly treatment with fluconazole can reduce the rate of recurrence of symptomatic vulvovaginal candidiasis. However, a long-term cure remains difficult to achieve.

Stockdale CK. Clinical spectrum of desquamative inflammatory vaginitis. *Curr Infect Dis Rep* 2010;12(6):479–483.

DIV is a rare chronic clinical syndrome of unknown etiology characterized by profuse purulent vaginal discharge, diffuse exudative vaginitis, epithelial cell exfoliation, and pain. A diagnosis of DIV is often missed by even experienced practitioners owing to its rarity and its clinical and laboratory presentation similar to other inflammatory vulvovaginal disorders. Although DIV is difficult to treat and often requires long-term therapy for maintenance, successful therapy has been reported with topical steroids and clindamycin.

U.S. Preventive Services Task Force. Screening for bacterial vaginosis in pregnancy to prevent preterm delivery: U.S. Preventive Services Task Force recommendation statement. *Ann Intern Med* 2008;148(3):214–219.

Current evidence is insufficient to assess the balance of benefits and harms of screening for BV in pregnant women at high risk for preterm delivery.

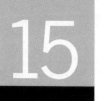

Other STDs

Lamis Ibrahim and James W. Myers

DONOVANOSIS

Introduction

- Also known as *Granuloma inguinale*.
- Causative agent is *Klebsiella granulomatis* (or *Calymmatobacterium granulomatis*), which is a gram-negative, pleomorphic bacterium.
- Large mononuclear cells containing inclusion bodies *(Donovan bodies)* are characteristic.
- It is not common in the United States.
- Much more common in tropical, subtropical, and developing countries.
- It is primarily transmitted sexually.
  - Less commonly through fecal contamination.
  - Rarely transmitted by passage through an infected birth canal.
- It is mostly seen in sexually active people aged 20 to 40 years
- It is more common in blacks in the United States.

Clinical Manifestations

- **Incubation period** is uncertain, but it might even be up to a year. Probably ranges from 3 days up to 80 days in most patients.
- Starts as a nodule and then ulcerates.
- Classically there are four types of donovanosis:
  1. ulcerogranulomatous: most common type, *painless, beefy red ulcer that is highly vascular and bleeds easily*.
  2. hypertrophic or verrucous ulcer: dry ulcer with irregular edges.
  3. necrotic ulcer: deep destructive ulcer with a foul smell.
  4. cicatricial ulcer: lesion with scar tissue.
- No lymphadenopathy is typically seen but may resemble pseudobuboes in the inguinal region.
- Can disseminate to extra-abdominal organs, nose, neck, or bones.
- May be complicated by stenosis of the urethral, vaginal, anal, and rectovaginal fistulas.

Diagnosis

1. Direct visualization of intracellular organism in macrophages (Donovan bodies) on biopsy or tissue crush preparation or smear.
2. Special stains such as a Warthin-Starry, Wright-Giemsa.
3. Bipolar staining giving a "safety-pin" appearance.
4. PCR more sensitive but mainly a research tool.
5. Culture: difficult to grow this organism.
6. IFA: less accurate.

Table 15-1	Treatment of Donovanosis^a	

Regimens for recommended therapy^b	Regimens for alternative therapy (any of the following)
• Doxycycline 100 mg orally twice a day for at least 3 weeks is the traditional therapy. • Azithromycin 1 g orally once per week for at least 3 weeks is becoming the preferred regimen by some authors.	• Ciprofloxacin 750 mg orally twice a day for at least 3 weeks • Erythromycin base 500 mg orally four times a day for at least 3 weeks • Trimethoprim-sulfamethoxazole one double-strength (160/800 mg) tablet orally twice a day for at least 3 weeks

^aAll of the above regimens should be given for at least 3 weeks or until lesions heal.
^bAminoglycoside (gentamicin 1 mg/kg IV every 8 hours) can be added if there is no evidence of improvement.

Management

- Treatment prevents progression of lesions.
- Usually prolonged till healing occurs.
- Relapses *can still occur despite* appropriate therapy, especially in the first 2 years.
- Regimens used: see **Table 15-1**

Follow-Up and Management of Sex Partners

- Patients should be followed till resolution of symptoms and healing of lesions.
- Sex partners of patients within the *past 60 days* should be evaluated and treated.

Donovanosis and HIV

- HIV patients are treated with same regimen as HIV negative.
- Lesion might take longer to heal in HIV patients.

Donovanosis and Pregnancy

- **Pregnant females should be treated with erythromycin regimen.**
- Doxycycline and ciprofloxacin are contraindicated, and sulfonamides are relatively contraindicated.

Complications

- Pseudoelephantiasis: most common complication (females, up to 5% >males) and requires surgical intervention.
- Hematogenous dissemination: unusual and may be fatal.
- Autoinoculation: cause of "kissing lesions" on adjacent skin.
- Possible association with squamous cell carcinoma of the penis.

CHANCROID

Introduction

- Not commonly found in the United States, but it is common in developing countries.
- Twenty-four cases reported to CDC in 2010.
- Prevalence decreasing worldwide.

- Risk factor for HIV transmission.
- Causative agent is *Haemophilus ducreyi,* which is a highly infectious, fastidious gram-negative organism.
- Seen more commonly in African Americans, heterosexuals, prostitutes, and in the southern part of the Unites States.
- Up to 10% **coinfected with syphilis;** therefore, you must consider treatment for both!

Clinical Manifestations

- Incubation period is from 4 to 10 days. It starts out as a papule that becomes a pustule, which evolves into a **painful ulcer** with associated **tender** lymph nodes.
- Ulcers:
  - Painful
  - Shaggy edges.
  - Not undurated.
  - Purulent base.
- Lymph nodes:
  - Usually unilateral.
  - Found more commonly in men.
  - Often fluctuant.
  - May rupture and drain.
- Scarring can occur after infection.

Diagnosis

- *Definite diagnosis* by CDC requires i**solation** of organisms from lesions.
- *Probable diagnosis* per CDC showed meet below criteria:
  1. The patient has *one or more* painful genital ulcers.
  2. The patient has no evidence of *T. pallidum* infection by dark-field microscopic examination of ulcer exudate, or by serology done at least 7 days after ulcers appear.
  3. Typical clinical presentation for chancroid.
  4. HSV testing of the ulcer exudate is negative.
- Culture: requires specific media
- Organism is difficult to isolate
- No FDA-approved PCR for diagnosis. Multiplex PCRs have been studied.

Management

- HIV and uncircumcised patients don't respond as well to treatment as others do.
- Rule out coinfection with HIV and syphilis.
- Fluctuant lymph nodes may require incision and drainage.
- Treatment: See *Table 15-2*
- **Treat for syphilis due to high rates of coinfection.**

Follow-Up and Sex Partner Management

- Reexamine in 3 to 7 days to check response to therapy.
- If no improvement, then rule out other STD including HIV, and rule out a resistant organism.
- Sex partners of the index case in the **past 10 days** should be evaluated and treated.

Table 15-2	Treatment of Chancroid

Regimens for Chancroid Treatment: (any of the following)
- Azithromycin 1 g orally in a single dose
- Ceftriaxone 250 mg IM in a single dose
- Ciprofloxacin 500 mg orally twice a day for 3 days
- Erythromycin base 500 mg orally three times a day for 7 days
- Ciprofloxacin is contraindicated for pregnant and lactating women.

HIV and Chancroid
- Ulcers take longer to heal in HIV-infected patients.
- HIV patients may have treatment failure.
- HIV patients may require prolonged therapy.
- Treat HIV patients with same regimen as non-HIV patients, but **be certain that there is follow-up for potential failure.**

Pregnancy and Chancroid
- Ciprofloxacin is contraindicated in pregnancy.
- No reported adverse outcome of pregnancy with chancroid.

MYCOPLASMA GENITALIUM/MYCOPLASMA HOMINIS/ UREAPLASMA UREALYTICUM

Introduction
- Many healthy asymptomatic adults have genitourinary colonization with Mycoplasma or Ureaplasma species.
- Colonization is more common in females.
- They are the smallest free-living organisms.
- Can't be seen by gram stain as they have no cell wall.
- Need special media to grow.

Clinical
- *M. genitalium* has been associated in women with several disorders:
  - Cervicitis
  - Endometritis
  - Nongonococcal urethritis
  - PID.
  - Infertility?
- Ureaplasmas have been suggested to be associated with several conditions as well:
  - Chorioamnionitis.
  - Spontaneous abortion.
  - Preterm birth.
  - Low birth weight.
  - Postpartum fever.
- Both of the above are associated with NGU in men.
- These organisms do not cause vaginitis.

- *M hominis* has been found in the endometria and in the fallopian tubes of approximately 10% of women with salpingitis.
- *M hominis* has been isolated from the upper urinary tract of patients with symptoms of acute pyelonephritis.
- *M hominis* has been detected in the blood in 10% of women with postpartum or postabortal fever, but not from afebrile women who had abortions or from healthy women who are pregnant.
- Infected patients generally present with symptoms milder than gonorrhea infection and more like chlamydia infection.

Diagnosis
- Difficult to diagnose, usually treated empirically.
- Specimens usually sent for both culture and PCR.
  - Culture: difficult, not all labs are prepared to perform it
  - PCR: not readily available, more sensitive than culture.

Treatment
- *Mycoplasma genitalium* is usually susceptible to macrolides more than tetracyclines and quinolones. Resistance to macrolides has been increasing.
- *Mycoplasma hominis* is usually susceptible to tetracyclines and quinolones, but resistant to macrolides.
- *Ureaplasma urealyticum* is susceptible to tetracyclines, macrolides, and quinolones.
- Resistance to macrolides, tetracyclines, and quinolones has been increasing. Moxifloxacin might be more active than the other quinolones.

SUGGESTED READINGS

Arevalo Morles C, Hernandez I, et al. Donovanosis: treatment with azithromycin. *Int J STD AIDS* 1997;8(1):54–56.

Bradshaw CS, Jensen JS, et al. Azithromycin failure in Mycoplasma genitalium urethritis. *Emerg Infect Dis* 2006;12(7):1149–1152.
In vitro evidence supported reduced susceptibility of M. genitalium to macrolides. Moxifloxacin administration resulted in rapid symptom resolution and eradication of infection in all cases. These findings have implications for management of urethritis.

Carter J, Bowden FJ, et al. Diagnostic polymerase chain reaction for donovanosis. *Clin Infect Dis* 1999;28(5):1168–1169.

CDC. Sexually Transmitted Diseases Treatment Guidelines, 2010. Available at http://www.cdc.gov/std/treatment/2010/STD-Treatment-2010-RR5912.pdf.

Freinkel AL, Dangor Y, et al. A serological test for granuloma inguinale. *Genitourin Med* 1992;68(4):269–272.
An indirect immunofluorescence technique may prove valuable for the diagnosis of individual cases of granuloma inguinale and as an epidemiologic tool in studies of the disease.

Ito S, Shimada Y, et al. Selection of Mycoplasma genitalium strains harbouring macrolide resistance-associated 23S rRNA mutations by treatment with a single 1 g dose of azithromycin. *Sex Transm Infect* 2011;87(5):412–414.

Jensen JS, Bradshaw CS, et al. Azithromycin treatment failure in Mycoplasma genitalium-positive patients with nongonococcal urethritis is associated with induced macrolide resistance. *Clin Infect Dis* 2008;47(12):1546–1553.
The genetic basis for the drug resistance was shown to be mutations in region V of the 23S rRNA gene, which is well described in other Mollicutes. These findings raise

concern about the use of single-dose azithromycin treatment of nongonococcal urethritis of unknown etiology.

Lewis DA. Chancroid: clinical manifestations, diagnosis, and management. *Sex Transm Infect* 2003;79(1):68–71.

Liu AY, Jiang MJ, et al. Detection of pathogens causing genital ulcer disease by multiplex polymerase chain reaction. *Chin Med Sci J* 2005;20(4):273–275.

Manhart LE, Holmes KK, et al. Mycoplasma genitalium among young adults in the United States: an emerging sexually transmitted infection. *Am J Public Health* 2007;97(6):1118–1125.

M genitalium was more prevalent than Neisseria gonorrhoeae but less prevalent than Chlamydia trachomatis, and it was strongly associated with sexual activity.

Mena LA, Mroczkowski TF, et al. A randomized comparison of azithromycin and doxycycline for the treatment of Mycoplasma genitalium-positive urethritis in men. *Clin Infect Dis* 2009;48(12):1649–1654.

A single 1-g dose of azithromycin is more effective than multidose doxycycline for the treatment of M. genitalium–associated urethritis in men. M. genitalium may be an important cause of recurrent nongonococcal urethritis after administration of the treatment regimens currently recommended by the Centers for Disease Control and Prevention.

Nassar FA, Abu-Elamreen FH, et al. Detection of Chlamydia trachomatis and Mycoplasma hominis, genitalium and Ureaplasma urealyticum by polymerase chain reaction in patients with sterile pyuria. *Adv Med Sci* 2008;53(1):80–86.

Testing of sterile pyuria showed a significant number of C. trachomatis, Mycoplasma, and Ureaplasma infections. Consequently, PCR is recommended for the detection of those microorganisms in the urine samples of sterile pyuria patients.

O'Farrell N. Donovanosis. *Sex Transm Infect* 2002;78(6):452–457.

O'Farrell N, Moi H. European guideline for the management of donovanosis, 2010. *Int J STD AIDS* 2010;21(9):609–610.

Petrikkos GL, Hadjisoteriou M, et al. PCR versus culture in the detection of vaginal Ureaplasma urealyticum and Mycoplasma hominis. *Int J Gynaecol Obstet* 2007;97(3):202–203.

Ross JD, Jensen JS. Mycoplasma genitalium as a sexually transmitted infection: implications for screening, testing, and treatment. *Sex Transm Infect* 2006;82(4):269–271.

Short VL, Totten PA, et al. Clinical presentation of Mycoplasma genitalium Infection versus Neisseria gonorrhoeae infection among women with pelvic inflammatory disease. *Clin Infect Dis* 2009;48(1):41–47.

Because symptoms might be mild, women with M. genitalium infection might not seek PID treatment. Further studies are needed to assess the potential reproductive tract sequelae of M. genitalium infection of the upper genital tract.

Taylor-Robinson D. Infections due to species of Mycoplasma and Ureaplasma: anupdate. *Clin Infect Dis* 1996;23(4):671–682; quiz 683–674.

Yokoi S, Maeda S, et al. The role of Mycoplasma genitalium and Ureaplasma urealyticum biovar 2 in postgonococcal urethritis. *Clin Infect Dis* 2007;45(7):866–871.

IV Central Nervous System Infections

16 Cerebrospinal Fluid Analysis

James W. Myers and Sunanda Mangraj

INTRODUCTION

Cerebrospinal fluid (CSF) analysis is a very important diagnostic tool in evaluation of central nervous system (CNS) infections and other conditions.

CSF is usually obtained from the lumbar subarachnoid space via a spinal tap at the L3-4 or L4-5 interspace, with the patient in the lateral decubitus position. In some cases, it is easier to perform lumbar puncture (LP) with the patient in a sitting position.

Contraindications to Performing a Lumbar Puncture
- Increased intracranial pressure
- Possible intracranial mass, especially in the posterior fossa
  - A spinal tap can precipitate herniation of the tonsils of the cerebellum through the foramen magnum.
  - If you suspect a possible intracranial mass lesion, or if you find papilledema during a patient's exam, LP should be deferred until CT of the head has ruled out possible herniation. Seizures and focal neurologic signs are suggestive of a mass lesion.
- Vertebral changes such as scoliosis are a relative contraindication.
- Infection at the site of LP overlying skin or epidural abscess can introduce the organism into the underlying subarachnoid space.
- Coagulation disorders (<50,000 platelets, patients with hemophilia, vitamin K deficiency)
  - Bleeding may complicate the procedure.
  - LP should be performed under these circumstances only if necessary.
- Improper specimen handling
  - Cells will begin to lyse within an hour of collection. Transport as soon as possible to the laboratory.
  - Refrigeration helps to slow this process.
  - If there is going to be a significant delay, the fluid should be transported in ice.

Opening Pressure
- CSF opening pressure (OP) is measured in the *lateral decubitus position* with the legs and neck in a neutral position. The meniscus will fluctuate between 2 and 5 mm with the patient's pulse and between 4 and 10 mm with respirations.
- Normal OP in adults ranges from 70 to 180 mm of H_2O.
- **Elevated pressure** would clearly be over 200 to **250** mm for most patients.
  - Normal OP may be up to 250 in some obese patients.
- Straining or coughing can falsely increase OP.
- Hyperventilation may lower OP.

- OP over 200 mm of H_2O is suggestive of elevated intracranial pressure, which can be seen in many conditions including meningitis, subarachnoid hemorrhages, and space-occupying lesions.
- When OP is found to be elevated, slowly remove just enough CSF until pressure reaches 50% of the original OP.

Appearance

- Normal CSF is clear.
- Greater than 200 white blood cells (WBCs) per mm^3, or 400 red blood cell (RBC) per mm^3 will give CSF a *turbid* appearance.
- **Xanthochromia (yellow, orange, or pink discoloration)** is present in the majority of cases of subarachnoid hemorrhage and in a few other conditions as listed in Table 16-1.
  - If the RBCs found after a spinal tap are from a bleed, they would have been present long enough to be metabolized into the yellow-green pigment bilirubin, as well as oxyhemoglobin and methemoglobin, *unlike those that are only present because of a traumatic tap.*
- Discoloration begins after RBCs have been in spinal fluid for at **least 2 hours**, and remains for 2 to 4 weeks.

Cell Counts

Normal cell count in CSF is up to 5 WBC per mm^3 in adults. Please see Table 16-2 for a comparison of cell counts by cause of meningitis.

- **In neonates,** it can be as many as 20 WBC per mm.
- As many as 30% of patients may exhibit CSF pleocytosis **after a generalized or focal seizure.** Generally these counts are <10 to 20 cells.
- Over 90% of the patients with bacterial meningitis will have more than 100 mm^3 WBC with neutrophil predominance.
- WBC counts <100 mm^3 are seen more commonly in patients with viral meningitis.
- **Estimated correction for WBCs from a traumatic tap.**
  - *Peripheral blood in CSF after traumatic tap will result in artificial increase in CSF WBC count by 1 WBC for every 750 to 1,000 RBC.*

Table 16-1	Cerebrospinal Fluid Appearance and Associated Conditions
Color of CSF Supernatant	**Conditions or Causes**
Yellow (Xanthochromia)	Blood breakdown products
	CSF protein >150 mg/dL
	>100,000 RBCs
	Hyperbilirubinemia
Orange	Blood breakdown products
	Excessive carrot ingestion
Pink	Blood breakdown products
Green	Hyperbilirubinemia, purulent CSF
Brown	Melanomatosis of the meninges.

Table 16-2	CSF Findings in Various Types of Meningitis			
Test	Bacterial	Viral	Fungal	Tubercular
Opening Pressure	Usually elevated	Usually normal	Variable	Variable
WBC Count / mm³	500–10,000, usually >1,000	6–1,000, usually <100	Variable	Variable
Cell Differential	PMN predominance[a]	Lymphocytic predominance[b]	Lympho-cytic predom-inance[b]	Lymphocytic predominance[b]
Glucose Level	Usually low <40 mg/dL.	Normal Mumps may be low.	Low	Low
Protein Level	Elevated>45mg/dL	Normal to elevated	Elevated	Elevated

[a]Lymphocytosis present in 10%.
[b]PMN may predominate early in the course.

- **Formula for added WBCs**
  - *WBCs added = WBC (blood) × RBC(CSF) / RBC(blood).*
  - *The blood WBC count is multiplied by the ratio of the cerebrospinal fluid RBC count to blood RBC count.*
  - *The result is the number of artificially introduced WBCs.*
  - *The true CSF white cell count is then calculated by subtracting the artificially introduced WBCs from the actual CSF WBC count.*
- If the **RBC count** remains stable in **three consecutive** tubes, then it is most likely secondary to *subarachnoid bleed.*
  - A falling count is attributed to a traumatic tap.
  - A higher RBC count in CSF can also be seen in herpes simplex virus (HSV) encephalitis.

Cell Differential

- Normal adult CSF cell count:
  - Seventy percent lymphocytes
  - **Thirty percent monocytes.**
- Lymphocytic predominance.
  - Viral, fungal, and tubercular meningitis.
  - Note that a polymorphonuclear (PMN) predominance *can be seen in early* stages of these infections.
- In bacterial meningitis PMNs predominate.
  - Note that in up to 10% cases of bacterial meningitis, a lymphocytic predominance can be seen.
  - Some patients may have a lymphocytic pleocytosis in response to antibiotic therapy.
- **Eosinophilic meningitis** (EM) is defined as more than 10 eosinophils per mm³ or a total CSF count made up of more than **10% eosinophils.**

- Parasitic infections.
  - *Angiostrongylus cantonensis*, a natural parasite of rats, has traditionally been found in the Pacific region, but it has been more recently found in North America because of the intercontinental spread of infected rats.
  - *Baylisascaris procyonis*, a parasite of raccoons, may also cause this.
- Other causes include
  - Myelography or pneumoencephalography
  - Tuberculous (TB), fungal meningitis (*Coccidioides immitis*) and neurosyphilis
  - Ventriculoperitoneal shunts, malignancy, and adverse drug reactions

Glucose

- Normal range for glucose in CSF is 50 to 80 mg/dL, which is normally 60% to 70% of the serum glucose obtained within a few hours of the spinal tap. CSF glucoses seldom go over 300 mg/dL.
- Glucose levels may remain subnormal for up to 2 weeks after successful treatment.
- A CSF glucose below 40 mg/dL (or a CSF to serum glucose ratio of <0.5) is abnormal.
- In bacterial meningits, the CSF to serum glucose ratio is typically below 0.4.
- **Low CSF glucose** may be associated with several other diseases:
  - Tubercular and fungal meningitis
  - Amoebic meningitis, cysticercosis, and trichinosis
  - **Mumps meningitis and** herpes simplex encephalitis
  - Syphilis.
  - Sarcoidosis, meningeal carcinamatosis, subarachnoid hemorrhage, and hypoglycemia can cause this on occasion.
- Several hours are required for CSF glucose to reach equilibrium with serum glucose concentrations; so prior administration of D 50 prior to a LP will *not change* the CSF glucose to any significant degree.

Protein

- **Traumatic tap correction formula**:
  - *For every 1,000 RBCs/mm in the CSF the protein level will increase by 1 mg/dL.*
  - *Must use same tube for both.*
- Elevated protein concentrations (>0.45 g/dL) are seen in majority of patients with bacterial, fungal, and tubercular meningitis and Lyme disease.
- In viral meningitis/encephalitis protein concentrations are not as high. The concentration in HSV encephalitis is normal in half of patients during the first week of the illness.
- Other conditions with elevated protein:
  - Intracranial hemorrhage
  - Multiple sclerosis, Guillain Barre (no cells, increased protein)
  - Leptomeningeal metastases
  - Some spinal tumors.

Microscopic Examination

- A Gram stain of CSF is positive in 60% to 90% of untreated cases.
- Sensitivity of the Gram stain:
  - *S. pneumoniae,* **90%**
  - *H. influenzae,* 85%

- *N. meningitidis,* 75%
- GNRs, 50%
- **Note that for** *L. monocytogenes,* it is <50% sensitive.
- Gram stain is positive in up to 97% of cases when there are 10^{x5} or more organisms per milliliter, as opposed to around 25% when there are 10^{x3} or fewer organisms per milliliter.
- **Acid-fast staining** should be done if tuberculosis is clinically suspected.
  - Only a small percentage, 37%, of initial smears will be positive for acid-fast bacilli (AFB).
  - This result can be increased to 87% if **four or more smears** are done.
  - Sensitivity also can be increased by examining the CSF sediment for AFB.
- *Cryptococcus* may be identified up to 50% of the time on an **India ink** preparation. Experience may be needed to be sure and not misread artifacts as yeast organisms. The India Ink smear does not need to be either too thick or too thin.

Cultures

- Positive in 70% to 85% of cases overall but they are <50% if you have been given antibiotics. In fact, most patients' cultures are negative by 24 to 48 hours after antibiotics have been started, if not sooner.
- Blood cultures may be positive in 40% to 90% of cases depending on the organism.
- For culture, blood and chocolate agar are used.
  - *N. menigitidis* and *H influenzae* grow best in *chocolate agar.*
- Cultures are examined at 24 to 48 hours but plates should be kept up to 7 days, especially if antibiotics are given first or a fastidious organism is expected.
- Larger volumes (15 to 50 mL) of CSF may improve yields especially for fungal and tubercular meningitis.
  - Fifty percent positive with one specimen for TB versus 80% for four.
  - *Cryptococcus* is positive in 95% of cases.

Rapid Diagnostic Tests

- Latex agglutination (LA) test for bacterial antigens are not routinely used by most labs because of **problems with false-positive and false-negative** results. They have fallen out of favor in most recent reviews.
  - *Antigen testing may be useful when the CSF Gram stain and culture are negative because of prior antibiotic use:*
- Limulus amebocyte lysate assay:
  - A rapid diagnostic test for detection of **gram-negative endotoxin** in CSF
  - Sensitivity is 97% and specificity is 99%.
  - Does not distinguish between specific gram-negative organisms, and a negative test result does *not rule out* the diagnosis of gram-negative meningitis
  - Not routinely recommended
- Procalcitonin, LDH isoenzymes, C-reactive protein (CRP), and CSF lactate have also been used as adjunctive tests in meningitis.
  - CSF lactate is elevated in cerebral malaria.
  - Elevated CSF lactate concentrations may be useful in differentiating bacterial from nonbacterial meningitis in patients who have not received prior antimicrobial therapy but other factors (hypoxia, vascular compromise) can affect it; so, it is *not routinely recommended* for community-acquired bacterial meningitis.

- Some experts recommended that in a postoperative neurosurgical patient, initiation of empirical antimicrobial therapy should be considered if CSF lactate concentrations are approximately 4.0 mmol/L.
- A normal CRP has a high *negative predictive value* in the diagnosis of bacterial meningitis.
- In adults, serum concentrations of procalcitonin >0.2 ng/mL had a sensitivity and specificity of up to 100% for the diagnosis of bacterial meningitis.
- Patients with suspected meningitis in whom the CSF Gram stain is negative and serum concentrations of CRP or procalcitonin are normal, can probably be observed *without initiation of antimicrobial therapy*.

Polymerase Chain Reaction

- Mostly used for viral infections
  - Polymerase chain reaction (PCR) of the CSF has a sensitivity of 95% to 100% for HSV type 1, Epstein-Barr virus (EBV), and Enterovirus.
  - PCR shows promise in the diagnosis of bacterial meningitis. Perhaps useful in patients with negative grams stains, or in those patients who may have been pretreated with antibiotics but they are not routinely available at this time.
  - CSF PCR for West Nile virus (WNV) is highly specific, but less sensitive than serologic studies.
    - May be useful early in infection
    - Immunocompromised hosts

CSF FINDINGS IN SELECTED CNS INFECTIONS

Neurosyphilis

- Treponemal tests
  - A positive *serum* treponemal test may indicate past infection and may remain reactive even after treatment. So these tests are not helpful in diagnosing CNS involvement by themselves.
  - **Blood contamination can make CSF versions of these tests unreliable or difficult to interpret.** Their value may be best in ruling out disease. A *negative* CSF treponemal test *rules out* active neurosyphilis in patients with late disease but not in those with early disease.
  - To test for local central nervous system (CNS) production of antibodies, one can compute a Treponema pallidum hemagglutination (TPHA) index where CSF (TPHA)/albumin quotient (CSF albumin × 103/serum albumin). A value >100 is suggestive of neurosyphilis.
- A serum rapid plasma reagin (RPR) titer of 1:32 seems to be the best cutoff point to decide whether or not to perform an LP.
  - CSF findings suggestive of neurosyphilis include >5 to 20 WBC/mm³ (usually lymphocytic),elevated protein, elevated gamma globulin concentration, and normal glucose.
- Venereal Disease Research Laboratory (VDRL) is the test of choice for CSF and **when positive is strongly suggestive** of neurosyphilis. The CSF VDRL is insensitive (30% to 70 %) but highly specific. A negative test, therefore, **does not** rule out CNS disease.

- False-positive VDRLs are rare. Sometimes the CSF VDRL may be reactive by contamination of seropositive blood during a traumatic tap. Usually this is visible blood contamination.
- For patients who had prior abnormalities in their spinal fluid, **repeating LPs every 6 months until resolution of all abnormalities** has been suggested.
- CSF VDRL results may take years to become normal after successful treatment. So a more useful marker is normalization of *CSF pleocytosis* to monitor the response to therapy.
- If there is worsening of CSF parameters or persistent abnormalities after 2 years, **retreatment** should be considered.
- PCR tests for neurosyphilis appear to be specific *but not sensitive* at this time.

Viral Meningitis/Encephalitis

- The typical profile of viral CNS infection include lymphocytic pleocytosis (10 to 500 cell/mm³),normal or slightly elevated protein (rarely over 0.95 g/dL), and a normal glucose.
- Gram stain, AFB, and india ink stain are negative for organisms.
- PMN pleocytosis can be seen up to **48 hours** in many viral infections including mumps, Eastern equine encephalitis, and West nile virus.
- PCR of viral-specific deoxyribonucleic Acid (DNA) or ribonucleic Acid (RNA) has become the most important diagnostic test for viral CNS infections. It is widely used for CNS infections caused by Cytomegalovirus (CMV), HSV, EBV, varicella-zoster virus (VZV), human herpesvirus 6 (HHV-6), and enteroviruses.
- Viral culture has limited use in diagnosis of viral CNS infections.
- For some viruses including mumps virus and arboviruses such as **West Nile** virus (WNV) serologic studies are a crucial diagnostic tool. Serologic tests are not useful for viral infections with high seroprevalence rate in general populations like HSV, VZV etc. For viruses with low seroprevalence rate these tests can be used. **WNV encephalitis is diagnosed by demonstration of WNV IgM in the CSF.**

Tubercular Meningitis

- If TB is suspected, a large volume of CSF should be obtained for adequate culture.
- Usually CSF will show lymphocytic predominance, though in early course up to 30% patients may have PMN predominance.
- Only 37% of the initial smears will be positive, and this can be increased up to 87% if four smears are done.
- Sensitivity of the test can also be increased by examining CSF sediments.
- Culture sensitivity also can be increased if multiple samples are cultured. The culture can take up to 6 to 8 weeks to become positive.
- **Adenosine deaminase (ADA) levels** are elevated in CSF in patients with tubercular meningitis. Xu et al showed the sensitivity of ADA measurement is 79% and specificity is 91%.
- CSF PCR for diagnosis of TB is not the standard of care at this time. A negative test *does not* conclusively rule out TB meningitis.

PML

- CSF is typically normal; however, in up to 25% cases pleocytosis (<25 cells/mm)³ with monocytic predominance and mild protein elevation may be seen
- PCR amplification (sensitivity of 60% to 90%, and a specificity of 90% to 100%) of the JC virus in the CSF is the important diagnostic test.
- Patients with negative PCR may require brain biopsy for definitive diagnosis.

SUGGESTED READINGS

Carbonnelle E. Laboratory diagnosis of bacterial meningitis: usefulness of various tests for the determination of the etiological agent. *Med Mal Infect* 2009;39(7–8):581–605.

Markers like CRP, procalcitonin, or sTREM-1 may be very useful for the diagnosis and to differentiate between viral and bacterial meningitis. Bacterial meningitis diagnosis and management require various biological tests and a multidisciplinary approach.

Cruickshank A, Auld P, et al. Revised national guidelines for analysis of cerebrospinal fluid for bilirubin in suspected subarachnoid haemorrhage. *Ann Clin Biochem* 2008;45 (Pt 3):238–244.

Centrifuge the specimen at >2,000 rpm for 5 minutes as soon as possible after receipt in the laboratory. Store the supernatant at 4°C in the dark until analysis. An increase in CSF bilirubin is the key finding, which supports the occurrence of SAH but is not specific for this. In most positive cases, bilirubin will occur with oxyhemoglobin.

Debiasi RL, Tyler KL, Molecular methods for diagnosis of viral encephalitis. *Clin Microbiol Rev* 2004;17(4):903–925, table of contents.

Dubos F, Moulin F, et al. Serum procalcitonin and other biologic markers to distinguish between bacterial and aseptic meningitis. *J Pediatr* 2006;149(1):72–76.

PCT and CSF protein had the best predictive value to distinguish between bacterial and aseptic meningitis in children.

Fishman R. *Cerebrospinal fluid in diseases of the nervous system.* Philadelphia, PA: WB Saunders; 1992.

Garcia P, Grassi B, et al. Laboratory diagnosis of Treponema pallidum infection in patients with early syphilis and neurosyphilis through a PCR-based test. *Rev Chilena Infectol* 2011;28(4):310–315.

Although the sensitivity of the PCR in CSF was low, it may be useful to support clinical diagnosis.

Huy NT, Thao NT, et al. Cerebrospinal fluid lactate concentration to distinguish bacterial from aseptic meningitis: a systemic review and meta-analysis. *Crit Care* 14(6):R240.

To distinguish bacterial meningitis from aseptic meningitis, CSF lactate is a good single indicator and a better marker compared to other conventional markers.

Johansen IS, Lundgren B, et al. Improved sensitivity of nucleic acid amplification for rapid diagnosis of tuberculous meningitis. *J Clin Microbiol* 2004;42(7):3036–3040.

The new pretreatment procedure with the ProbeTec assay described here provides a rapid, simple, and sensitive tool for the diagnosis of TBM.

Kamei S, Takasu T, et al. Cerebrospinal fluid findings in 108 Japanese cases of herpes simplex encephalitis. *Rinsho Shinkeigaku* 1989;29(2):131–137.

Kanegaye JT, Soliemanzadeh P, et al. Lumbar puncture in pediatric bacterial meningitis: defining the time interval for recovery of cerebrospinal fluid pathogens after parenteral antibiotic pretreatment. *Pediatrics* 2001;108(5):1169–1174.

The present study demonstrates that CSF sterilization may occur more rapidly after initiation of parenteral antibiotics than previously suggested, with complete sterilization of meningococcus within 2 hours and the beginning of sterilization of pneumococcus by 4 hours into therapy. Lack of adequate culture material may result in inability to tailor therapy to antimicrobial susceptibility or in unnecessarily prolonged treatment if the clinical presentation and laboratory data cannot exclude the possibility of bacterial meningitis.

Marra CM, Maxwell CL, et al. Normalization of serum rapid plasma reagin titer predicts normalization of cerebrospinal fluid and clinical abnormalities after treatment of neurosyphilis. *Clin Infect Dis* 2008;47(7):893–899.

In most instances, normalization of serum RPR titer correctly predicts success of treatment of neurosyphilis, and follow-up lumbar puncture can be avoided.

Marra CM, Tantalo LC, et al. CXCL13 as a cerebrospinal fluid marker for neurosyphilis in HIV-infected patients with syphilis. *Sex Transm Dis* 2010;37(5):283–287.

CSF CXCL13 concentration may be particularly useful for diagnosis of neurosyphilis in HIV-infected patients because it is independent of CSF pleocytosis and markers of HIV disease.

Moskophidis M, Peters S, Comparison of intrathecal synthesis of Treponema pallidum-specific IgG antibodies and polymerase chain reaction for the diagnosis of neurosyphilis. *Zentralbl Bakteriol* 1996;283(3):295–305.

The findings suggest that the intrathecal production of T. pallidum-specific IgG antibodies is an important indicator for the diagnosis of neurosyphilis. In addition, a positive result by PCR performed in CSF establishes a diagnosis of active neurosyphilis.

Nussinovitch M, Finkelstein Y, et al. Cerebrospinal fluid lactate dehydrogenase isoenzymes in children with bacterial and aseptic meningitis. *Transl Res* 2009;154(4):214–218.

The LDH isoenzyme pattern may be of clinical diagnostic value in meningitis, particularly when culture results are pending.

Pai M, Flores LL, et al. Diagnostic accuracy of nucleic acid amplification tests for tuberculous meningitis: a systematic review and meta-analysis. *Lancet Infect Dis* 2003;3(10):633–643.

On current evidence, commercial NAA tests show a potential role in confirming tuberculous meningitis diagnosis, although their overall low sensitivity precludes the use of these tests to rule out tuberculous meningitis with certainty.

Saravolatz LD, Manzor O, et al. Broad-range bacterial polymerase chain reaction for early detection of bacterial meningitis. *Clin Infect Dis* 2003;36(1):40–45.

Broad-range bacterial PCR may be useful for excluding the diagnosis of meningitis, and the results may influence the decision to initiate or discontinue antimicrobial therapy.

Seehusen DA, Reeves MM, et al. Cerebrospinal fluid analysis. *Am Fam Physician* 2003;68(6):1103–1108.

Excellent review article. Several good tables. Has 25 references, many of them are classics in the field.

Slom T, Johnson S. Eosinophilic Meningitis. *Curr Infect Dis Rep* 2003;5(4):322–328.

Steroid therapy without specific anthelmintic treatment is safe and effective in control of headache of adult patients with A. cantonensis-associated EM.

Thomson RB. Jr, Bertram H. Laboratory diagnosis of central nervous system infections. *Infect Dis Clin North Am* 2001;15(4):1047–1071.

Good Review Article.

Welinder-Olsson C, Dotevall L, et al. Comparison of broad-range bacterial PCR and culture of cerebrospinal fluid for diagnosis of community-acquired bacterial meningitis. *Clin Microbiol Infect* 2007;13(9):879–886.

PCR is particularly useful for analysing CSF from patients who have been treated with antibiotics before lumbar puncture.

Xu HB, Jiang RH, et al. Diagnostic value of adenosine deaminase in cerebrospinal fluid for tuberculous meningitis: a meta-analysis. *Int J Tuberc Lung Dis* 2010;14(11):1382–1387.

Author's data suggest that ADA in the CSF can be a sensitive and specific target and a critical criteria for the diagnosis of TBM.

Zanusso G, Fiorini M, et al. Cerebrospinal fluid markers in sporadic creutzfeldt-jakob disease. *Int J Mol Sci* 2011;12(9):6281–6292.

While the 14-3-3 assay and tau protein levels were the most sensitive indicators of sCJD, the highest sensitivity, specificity, and positive predictive value were obtained when all the above markers were combined. The latter approach also allowed a reliable differential diagnosis with other neurodegenerative dementias.

17 Acute Infections of the Central Nervous System: Meningitis and Brain Abscess

Jonathan P. Moorman

Central nervous system dysfunction is common and characterized by a broad differential diagnosis. Rapid diagnosis and treatment are often necessary to prevent morbidity or mortality. Primary factors that drive the brain's susceptibility to damage from infection are (i) inadequate room for expansion when inflammation is present, (ii) poor immune function within the blood-brain barrier, (iii) difficulty in achieving adequate antimicrobial concentrations in the cerebrospinal fluid (CSF) and parenchyma, and (iv) inability of the brain to regenerate neural tissue once cell death has occurred.

INITIAL EVALUATION

- Patients with CNS infections can present with minimal signs and symptoms of CNS irritation or with obtundation and shock.
- If suspicion for CNS infection is high, blood cultures should be drawn and empiric antimicrobials should be immediately administered, preferably within 1 hour of presentation and prior to lumbar puncture (LP) if any delay is expected
  - The sensitivity of Gram stain and culture is decreased when antibiotics are given before LP, but the effect is small if LP is performed within 1 to 2 hours of antibiotics
  - Sensitivities as high as 38% have been reported when LP was delayed for 24 hours.
- Patients who have altered mental status or focal neurologic signs or seizures must undergo brain imaging prior to LP.

History and Physical Examination

- A thorough history and physical examination is essential and helps to determine if the suspected infection is acute or chronic, community-acquired or nosocomial, primary or metastatic
- It is common to find a history of fever, headache, stiff neck, and confusion
  - frequently not all present, especially in the elderly or immunocompromised.
  - review of symptoms necessary for determining the source; sinus pain, otorrhea, productive cough, abdominal pain, or dysuria may point to a primary focus of infection and help determine selection of initial antimicrobials.
- Exposure to individuals with known infections suggests a common pathogen.
- Past medical history alerts the clinician to underlying illnesses that may predispose to a particular CNS infection or organism
  - prior CNS infections or neurosurgical procedures (*Staphylococcus* and aerobic gram-negative bacilli)
  - immunosuppression (*Toxoplasma*, fungi, and mycobacteria)
  - diabetes (fungi)

- head trauma (*Staphylococci* and *Streptococci*)
- alcoholism (*Streptococcus pneumoniae* and *Listeria monocytogenes*)
- when brain abscess or subdural empyema is considered, a history of chronic ear, sinus, and dental infections is supportive.
- Social history should determine homelessness, ethanol or drug abuse, animal or insect exposure, employment, and HIV risk factors.
- Medication list should be reviewed with special attention to new medications, as signs and symptoms of CNS infection can be mimicked by many medications.
- Physical exam helps confirm the hemodynamic and neurologic stability of the patient, and helps to target suspicions about a primary source of infection.
  - classically, meningitis presents with fever and headache accompanied by meningeal signs such as Kernig and Brudzinski signs. Encephalitis (covered in an accompanying chapter) is much more likely to appear with cognitive dysfunction and personality changes.
  - sinus tenderness or otitis, or dental infection suggests intracranial extension from these sites.
  - focal findings on auscultation of the lungs suggest pneumococcal pneumonia and meningitis.
  - a new murmur accompanied by peripheral stigmata suggests endocarditis with intracranial complications.
  - rash may suggest *meningococcal, rickettsial*, or viral etiologies, among others.

Laboratory Evaluation

- If there is any question of meningitis, LP is warranted.
- Computed tomography (CT) of the brain has been used to predict intracranial hypertension and the risk for brainstem herniation from LP.
  - when focal neurologic signs, seizures, or signs of elevated intracranial pressure on physical examination are present, a CT scan of the brain is indicated.
  - otherwise, preprocedure radiography is generally not indicated and may increase time to appropriate antibiotic therapy and increase costs of care.
  - the absence of the following factors has a high negative predictive value for abnormalities on head CT: age older than 60, immunocompromised state, history of a CNS lesion such as a tumor, recent seizure, altered mental status/cognition, and focal neurologic findings.
- The most common complication of LP is headache, which occurs in 10% to 30% of patients.
- Spinal hematoma occurs in <1% of procedures and is almost always associated with anticoagulation or a platelet count <50,000/mL.
- De novo infection resulting from LP is rare.
- CSF pressure should be measured during every diagnostic LP.
- CSF analysis (please refer to the chapter on CSF Analysis for a thorough discussion):
  - four tubes of CSF are obtained: Tube 1 is sent for Gram stain and culture, tube 2 for protein and glucose, tube 3 for cell count and differential, and at least one additional tube is set aside for further testing as indicated
  - more fluid may be required, however, depending mostly on the number of cultures and DNA studies desired, and on whether cytology will be ordered.
  - forty milliliters can be removed safely during one procedure.
  - when mycobacteria or fungi infections are considerations, 10 to 20 mL may be required. In patients with potential AIDS-related diagnoses, CSF testing for cryptococcal antigen and VDRL should be considered.

Table 17-1	CSF Findings Indicative of Meningitis		
Parameter	**Normal CSF**	**Acute bacterial**	**Viral**
Opening pressure	6–20 cm H$_2$O	Elevated	Often normal
CSF WBCs/ mm^3	0–5 (lymphocytes)	Hundreds-thousands (PMNs predominate)	Few to several hundred[a] (lymphocytes predominate, but early on may see PMNs)
Protein (mg/dL)	18–45	100–500 (occasionally >1,000)	Often normal or only slightly elevated
Glucose (mg/dL)	45–80, or 0.6 × serum glucose	Often 5–40, or <0.3 × serum glucose	Usually normal, can be depressed in mumps and HSV
Miscellaneous	For traumatic LP, add one WBC and 1 mg/dL protein for each 1,000 RBCs	Gram stain (+) in 60%–80% cases, somewhat organism specific, and related to prior use of antimicrobials	Usually not necessary to identify specific etiology of viral meningitis

[a]Lymphocytes >5,000 commonly noted with lymphocytic choriomeningitis (LCM).
Adapted from Choi CK. Bacterial meningitis in aging adults. *Clin Infect Dis* 2001;33:1380–1385.

- the results of CSF testing are used to determine whether a septic or an aseptic process is operative (Table 17-1).
- results suggesting septic inflammation include an elevated CSF opening pressure, several hundred to many thousands of mostly polymorphonuclear (PMN) WBCs, protein levels generally higher than 100 mg/dL, and glucose levels of 5 to 40 mg/dL or <30% of the serum glucose.
- an aseptic picture includes a normal or only slightly elevated opening pressure, several hundred cells mostly of mononuclear lineage, normal or slightly elevated protein, and a normal glucose concentration.
- the CSF profile of many patients may be mixed and caused by a large group of diagnoses, including parameningeal foci, infective endocarditis, rheumatologic disorders, early aseptic meningitis, partially treated septic meningitis, medication-induced disease, and postsurgical inflammation.

Etiology and Antimicrobial Treatment of Specific CNS Syndromes
Acute Bacterial Meningitis
- Fifty percent of cases of community-acquired bacterial meningitis are due to *S. pneumoniae*, 25% to *Neisseria meningitidis*, 13% to group B streptococci, 8% to *L. monocytogenes*, and 7% to *Hemophilus influenzae*.
- Nosocomially acquired meningitis may also be associated with enteric gram-negative bacilli in up to 33% of cases.

- Mortality rates for bacterial meningitis in adults remain at approximately 20% but rise to at least 40% among those older than age 60.
- Classic presentation of bacterial meningitis is fever, headache, and meningismus, with or without altered mental status.
  - a recent evidence-based review demonstrated that one of three findings—fever, neck stiffness, or altered mental status—was present in nearly all patients with the disease.
  - presence of at least one of these three findings was 99% sensitive for acute bacterial meningitis; absence of all three signs has a high negative predictive value.
  - Kernig and Brudzinski signs are present in 50% of adults.
- A CSF WBC count of more than 3,000/mL consisting predominately of PMN cells is highly suspicious for bacterial infection
  - the WBC count is higher than 2,000/mL in 38% of bacterial cases
  - a low glucose is classic but occurs in only 50% of cases
  - CSF/serum glucose ratio of <0.4 is 80% sensitive and 96% specific for acute bacterial meningitis (as opposed to acute viral meningitis), and a ratio of <0.25 is found in <1% of cases of viral meningitis.
  - CSF protein level of more than 100 mg/dL is 82% sensitive and 98% specific for acute bacterial meningitis (as opposed to acute viral meningitis).
  - Gram stain is positive in up to 85% of cases of untreated bacterial meningitis, and CSF culture is positive in up to 85% of cases.
  - Blood culture identifies the causative organism in 80% to 95% of cases.
- CSF bacterial antigen testing is most useful when antibiotics have been given prior to LP. Negative tests are generally not helpful, but positive tests are considered diagnostic for a particular organism.
- Because penicillin-resistant *S. pneumoniae* has become more common, empiric treatment has changed (Table 17-2).

Table 17-2	Recommended Empiric Antibiotic Therapy for Bacterial Meningitis Based on Age[a]		
Age	**Major pathogens**	**Antibiotic regimens**	**Alternatives**
3 months–18 years	*N. meningitidis, S. pneumoniae, H. influenzae*	Ceftriaxone or cefotaxime plus vancomycin	Meropenem or chloramphenicol plus vancomycin
18–50 years	*S. pneumoniae, N. meningitidis, H. influenzae*	Same as above	Same as above
>50 years	*S. pneumoniae, L. monocytogenes,* enteric gram-negative bacilli	Ampicillin plus ceftriaxone or cefotaxime plus vancomycin	Ampicillin plus fluoroquinolones plus vancomycin

[a]Dexamethasone 10 mg IV qh × 4 days recommended 15–20 minutes prior to or simultaneous with first antibiotic dose for cases of suspected pneumococcal meningitis.
Adapted from Tunkel et al. Practice guidelines for the management of bacterial meningitis. *Clin Infect Dis* 2004;39:1267–1284; and Brouwer et al. Epidemiology, diagnosis, and antimicrobial treatment of acute bacterial meningitis. *Clin Microbiol Rev* 2010;23(3):467–492.

- current recommendations in immunocompetent hosts younger than age 50 includes ceftriaxone (2 g IV every 12 hours) or cefotaxime (2 g IV every 6 hours) plus vancomycin (1 g IV every 12 hours). This regimen covers sensitive and resistant *S. pneumoniae, N. meningitidis, H. influenzae,* group B streptococci, and many Enterobacteriaceae.
- in the elderly or immunocompromised, ampicillin (2 g IV every 4 hours) is added for coverage of *L. monocytogenes.*
- in penicillin-allergic individuals, trimethoprim-sulfamethoxazole (10 mg/kg [trimethoprim component] IV every 12 hours) is recommended.
- if a specific organism is found, the regimen should be narrowed based on sensitivities. Duration of therapy is generally 10 to 14 days for *S. pneumoniae,* and up to 21 days for *L. monocytogenes, Streptococcus agalactiae,* and Enterobacteriaceae. One week of antibiotics is sufficient for meningitis caused by *N. meningitidis;* most recent data suggest that 3 days is acceptable. Table 17-3 presents a list of the antimicrobials mentioned in this chapter and appropriate dosing regimens for treating CNS infections.
- Use of corticosteroids has historically been controversial but is currently recommended to be administered prior to the first dose of antibiotics in all patients in whom acute bacterial meningitis is suspected.
- Tuberculous meningitis may have a CSF profile identical to that in classic acute septic meningitis in 25% of cases, particularly early in the course.

Table 17-3	Recommended Dosages of Antimicrobial Agents for Central Nervous System Infections in Adults[a]	
Agent	**Daily dosage**	**Dosing interval (hours)**
Ampicillin	12 g	4
Cefepime	6 g	8
Cefotaxime	8–12 g	4–6
Ceftazidime	6 g	8
Ceftriaxone	4 g	12
Chloramphenicol	4–6 g	6
Gentamicin	3–5 mg/kg	8
Imipenem	2 g	6
Meropenem	6 g	8
Metronidazole	30 mg/kg	6
Nafcillin	9–12 g	4
Penicillin	24 million units	4
Piperacillin/Tazobactam	13.5 g	6
Pyrimethamine	50–75 mg (oral)	24
Sulfadiazine	4–6 g	6
Ticarcillin/clavulanate	12.4 g	6
Trimethoprim-sulfamethoxazole	10–20 mg/kg[b]	6–12
Vancomycin	2–3 g[c]	8–12

[a]Patients with normal renal and hepatic function. All doses are intravenous.
[b]Dosage based on trimethoprim component.
[c]Need to monitor trough serum concentrations.
Adapted from Mandell G, Bennett J, Dolin R. *Mandell, Douglas, and Bennett's principles and practice of infectious diseases.* 7th ed. Philadelphia, PA: Churchill Livingstone; 2010.

- lymphocytic predominance is usual, however, and decreased CSF glucose is often noted
- large volumes (10 to 20 mL) of CSF may need to be removed on up to four separate occasions to increase the sensitivity of staining and culture above 75%
- PCR testing for *Mycobacterium tuberculosis* DNA has become standard where available
- management is best left to an infectious disease specialist, but standard three- and four-drug regimens are usually used.

Acute Aseptic Meningitis

- Aseptic meningitis represents inflammation of the meninges with no bacterial cause identifiable on initial assessment
- The annual number of cases is 8,300 to 12,700; most are caused by enteroviruses
- Aseptic meningitis caused by such agents can present in a fashion identical to bacterial meningitis, causing great confusion when patients are first evaluated
- Herpes simplex virus (HSV) accounts for 1% to 3% of all cases of aseptic meningitis, and HSV-2 is associated with meningitis in 11% to 33% of all primary genital infections. However, most have a more protracted and subacute course than those with bacterial meningitis.
- Etiologies other than viruses include parameningeal foci (brain or epidural abscess), partially treated bacterial meningitis, infection with HIV, hematologic malignancies, and metastatic solid cancers
- Treatable organisms that may present with an aseptic picture include *M. tuberculosis, L. monocytogenes, Mycoplasma pneumoniae, Rickettsia rickettsii, Ehrlichiae, Borrelia burgdorferi, Treponema pallidum, Leptospira* species, *Bartonella* species, *and Brucella* species. In the immunocompromised patient, *M. tuberculosis*, fungal infections, *Toxoplasma gondii, T. pallidum*, Epstein-Barr virus (EBV), cytomegalovirus (CMV), varicella-zoster virus (VZV) or HSV should be considered.
- A variety of noninfectious diseases (e.g., collagen vascular and autoimmune diseases) and medications can also be implicated. Of medications, nonsteroidal antiinflammatory drugs, antibiotics (particularly trimethoprim-sulfamethoxazole) and intravenous immunoglobulins are the most frequent offenders. Treatment is discontinuation of the agent. Table 17-4 lists infectious and noninfectious causes of meningitis that can present with CSF profiles that are consistent with aseptic meningitis.

Brain Abscess

- Brain abscess is a focal intracerebral collection of pus that often presents as a mass lesion with localized neurologic defects related to the area involved
- Up to 2,500 cases are treated in the United States annually and it affects males more often than females
- It occurs most commonly in those who are aged 30 to 40
- The advent of antibiotics, enhanced brain imaging, and stereotactic drainage techniques have decreased the mortality to near zero when cases are optimally managed.
- The primary source of abscess is often cryptogenic.
  - fifty percent are caused by contiguous spread from the middle ear, paranasal sinuses, or dentition.
  - twenty percent of cases are thought to occur after hematogenous spread from heart or lung.
  - penetrating head trauma and immunosuppression are other predisposing conditions.

Table 17-4	Common Causes of Aseptic Meningitis

Infectious

Bacterial: M. tuberculosis, parameningeal infection, acute or subacute
  bacterial endocarditis, Brucella, Listeria
Fungal: Candida albicans, Coccidioides immitis, Cryptococcus neoformans,
  Histoplasma Capsulatum
Mycoplasmal: M. pneumoniae, M. hominis (in neonates)
Protozoal: T. gondii, Plasmodium spp., amoebas, visceral larva migrans
Rickettsial: Rocky Mountain spotted fever, Q fever, typhus
Spirochetal: Syphilis, leptospirosis, Lyme disease
Viral: Enteroviruses, mumps virus, lymphocyte choriomeningitis agent, EBV,
  arboviruses, CMV, VZV, HSV, HIV

Malignant

Primary medulloblastoma, metastatic leukemia, lymphoma, Hodgkin disease,
  metastatic carcinomatosis, craniopharyngioma

Noninfectious

Autoimmune disease: Guillain-Barré syndrome
Collagen-vascular disease: systemic lupus erythematosus, Sjögren syndrome
Direct toxin exposure: Intrathecal injections of contrast media, spinal anesthesia
Granulomatous disease: Sarcoidosis
Poisoning: Lead, mercury
Trauma: Subarachnoid hemorrhage, traumatic LP, neurosurgery

Medications

Sulfamethoxazole, trimethoprim, nonsteroidal anti-inflammatory agents,
  carbamazepine, isoniazid, penicillin

Vaccinations

Mumps, measles

Miscellaneous

Behçet syndrome, Kawasaki disease, Mollaret meningitis, multiple sclerosis

Adapted from Nelsen S, Sealy D, Schneider E. The aseptic meningitis syndrome. *Am Fam Phys* 1993;48:809–815.

- The clinical presentation of brain abscess is variable.
  - with virulent organisms such as *S. aureus*, initial headache or fever may be followed rapidly by deteriorating mental status and focal neurologic signs.
  - alternatively, patients may have an indolent course spanning more than 1 month, with only a headache as a complaint.
  - headache is the most common presenting complaint, occurring in approximately 70% of cases.
  - fever is noted in about 50% of patients.
  - other signs or symptoms include mental status changes, focal neurologic deficits, seizures, nausea, vomiting, and nuchal rigidity.
  - mortality is highest in patients who report having more than 4 days of these signs and symptoms.

- Diagnosis of brain abscess is based on a high index of suspicion plus brain imaging.
  - leukocytosis is frequently absent, so that absence of fever, leukocytosis, or other signs of inflammation should not deter evaluation when suspicion exists.
  - blood cultures are positive in only 10% of cases.
  - because intracranial pressure is elevated in many patients, LP is generally contraindicated when brain abscess is suspected (up to 20% die of complications).
  - the imaging modality of choice is gadolinium-enhanced MRI.
    ○ Characteristic changes over time are often noted. During the first week (acute cerebritis stage), only mild edema or microhemorrhages may be seen. After 7 days, the late cerebritis stage begins, characterized by a focus or foci of necrotic tissue, separated from normal brain by a thin rim of vascular granulation tissue. Local mass effect is usually present. After approximately 2 weeks, a capsular stage characterized by a maturing collagenous capsule filled with liquefied debris occurs. It is here that drainage should be considered. Earlier drainage is unlikely to yield pus but more likely to result in bleeding.
    ○ If allowed to become chronic and untreated, brain abscesses continue to enlarge, causing death from brain-stem herniation or from rupture into the subarachnoid space or ventricular system.
- Abscess location helps to indicate the primary infection.
  - temporal lobe and cerebellar lesions suggest chronic otitis media or mastoiditis.
  - frontal lobe lesions suggest complications of paranasal sinusitis.
  - multiple lesions at the gray-white matter interface suggest hematogenous spread.
- Aspiration of one or more of the lesions is indicated to both determine microbiology and to rule out alternative diagnoses, such as glioblastoma, metastasis, infarct, or demyelination.
  - generally, lesions larger than 2.5 cm in diameter should be aspirated.
  - the microbiology of a brain abscess is dictated by the location of the primary source, and the majority are bacterial, with 60% of cases being polymicrobial.
  - Streptococcal species are found in 70% of cases, most commonly *Streptococcus milleri* group. *S. aureus* is noted in up to 20% of cases, most commonly associated with hematogenous spread or penetrating or neurosurgical trauma. Enteric gram-negative bacilli and anaerobic bacteria are found in up to 20% and 50% of cases, respectively, with *Bacteroides* and *Fusobacterium spp.* the most common anaerobes.
- After initial evaluation, antibiotics may be indicated. In nonemergent situations, aspiration of the abscess should occur before empiric antimicrobial therapy, and Gram stain results may aid with an initial regimen. This should be based in part on the suspected primary source of infection.
  - if there is a complication of otitis, metronidazole and an antipseudomonal penicillin or advanced-generation cephalosporin can be used.
  - metronidazole plus a third-generation cephalosporin is effective for a suspected source in the paranasal sinuses.
  - suspected dental sources can be covered with penicillin or a third-generation cephalosporin plus metronidazole.
  - for patients who have undergone neurosurgical procedures or have sustained penetrating skull trauma, vancomycin can be added to an extended-spectrum penicillin or cephalosporin with antipseudomonal activity.
  - when there is no history to guide therapy, vancomycin with metronidazole and a third-generation cephalosporin, or vancomycin with an extended-spectrum penicillin/β-lactamase inhibitor combination can generally be used.

- the duration of therapy is dictated by clinical and radiographic response but generally continues for 4 to 8 weeks, depending on the adequacy of initial drainage. Brain imaging should be repeated within several weeks after antibiotics have been initiated—and periodically thereafter—to gauge response.
- A complication of brain abscess is rupture into the ventricular system with resultant bacterial meningitis.
  - focal neurologic findings are common and patients appear toxic.
  - their presence should cause the clinician to suspect a ruptured brain abscess or subdural empyema.
  - mortality approaches 100% and LP is frequently performed in these cases, especially when an antecedent brain abscess is not known to exist.
  - therapy consists of high-dose parenteral antimicrobials, intensive support, and, occasionally, neurosurgical intervention.

Subdural Empyema

- Infection in this space is uncommon but associated with up to 20% mortality, even with prompt neurosurgical and antibiotic therapy.
- Most common in young males and complicates paranasal sinus infections (60% to 70%) and middle ear infections (20%) most commonly
- In 80% of cases, both hemispheres become involved.
- Most patients are toxic and febrile and 75% demonstrate focal neurologic signs and have meningismus.
- Focal seizures occur in up 50% of cases. Presence of focal neurologic disturbances should prompt rapid imaging, as these are unusual in uncomplicated meningitis.
- Mortality is closely associated with mental status level at initiation of treatment.
- Contrast-enhanced MRI represents the best imaging modality. Osteomyelitis or epidural abscess is present in up to 50% of cases.
- LP should not be performed because intracranial pressure is frequently significantly elevated, and because CSF findings are generally not helpful.
- The bacteriology of subdural empyema is similar to that of brain abscess, and empiric antimicrobial therapy should follow the same guidelines.
- Urgent surgical drainage is mandatory.
- Most patients are treated with intravenous therapy for at least 4 weeks after drainage.

SUGGESTED READINGS

Attia J, et al. Does this adult patient have acute meningitis? *JAMA* 1999;282:175–181.
Brouwer MC, Tunkel AR, van de Beek D. Epidemiology, diagnosis, and antimicrobial treatment of acute bacterial meningitis. *Clin Microbiol Rev.* 2010;23(3):467–92.
   This excellent and comprehensive review discusses all aspects of bacterial meningitis, including pathogen-specific disease patterns and virulence factors.
Choi CK. Bacterial meningitis in aging adults. *Clin Infect Dis* 2001;33:1380–1385.
Chowdhury MH, Tunkel AR. Antibacterial agents in infections of the central nervous system. *Infect Dis Clin North Am* 2000;14:391–408.
Dill SR, et al. Subdural empyema: analysis of 32 cases and review. *Clin Infect Dis* 1995;20: 372–386.
   The authors divide patients with subdural empyema into those resulting from sinusitis, trauma, or miscellaneous. Sinusitis was the most common cause and was generally associated with streptococci and anaerobes. Cases resulting from trauma (including

neurosurgery) were more likely to harbor gram-negative bacilli or S. aureus. Surgical drainage plus at least 1 month of antibiotics is considered appropriate therapy.

Hasbun R, et al. Computed tomography of the head before lumbar puncture in adults with suspected meningitis. *N Engl J Med* 2001;345:1727–1733.

The authors prospectively studied 301 adults with suspected meningitis to determine the clinical characteristics that would predict abnormalities on head CT prior to LP. The absence of all the following characteristics yielded a negative predictive value of 97%: age older than 60 years, immunocompromise, a history of CNS disease, a history of seizure <1 week, an abnormal level of consciousness, an alteration in cognition, and a focal neurologic exam. Even patients with mass effect on CT, but without any of these characteristics, could safely undergo LP.

Heilpern KL, Lorber B. Focal intracranial infections. *Infect Dis Clin North Am* 1996;10: 879–898.

Mandell G, Bennett J, Dolin R. *Mandell, Douglas, and Bennett's principles and practice of infectious diseases.* 5th ed. Philadelphia, PA: Churchill Livingstone; 2000:973.

Motis G, Garcia-Monaco JC. The challenge of drug-induced aseptic meningitis. *Arch Intern Med* 1999;159:1185–1194.

This is a comprehensive review that focuses on the clinical characteristics, CSF profiles, related underlying conditions, differential diagnoses, and most common offending drugs.

Nelsen S, Sealy D, Schneider E. The aseptic meningitis syndrome. *Am Fam Phys* 1993;48: 809–815.

Schuchat A, et al. Bacterial meningitis in the United States in 1995. *N Engl J Med* 1997;337:970.

The authors review the epidemiology of bacterial meningitis in the United States before and after the introduction of the H. influenzae vaccine. They estimate that the total number of cases of bacterial meningitis has been halved and the median age at diagnosis nearly doubled since the vaccine's introduction. This demographic shift was caused by a 94% decrease in H. influenzae meningitis.

Spack D, Jackson L. Bacterial meningitis. *Neurol Clin* 1999;17:711–735.

Thomson RB Jr, Bertram H. Laboratory diagnosis of central nervous system infections. *Infect Dis Clin North Am* 2001;15:1047–1071.

A complete review of the various tests used to diagnose bacterial, viral, fungal, protozoal, and parasitic infections of the CNS. Information is included on the volume of CSF required for each test. The optimal methods of transport and assay are detailed.

Tunkel AR, et al. Practice Guidelines for the Management of Bacterial Meningitis. *Clin Infect Dis* 2004;39:1267–1284.

These IDSA guidelines provide recommendations for management of acute bacterial meningitis and are an excellent source for a complete understanding of specific antimicrobial therapy and adjunctive therapies.

van de Beek D, et al. Steroids in adults with acute bacterial meningitis: a systematic review. *Lancet Infect Dis* 2004;4:139–143.

The authors perform a systematic review of the benefits and risks of using dexamethasone for this disease. Compared with placebo, the relative risk (RR) for both death and neurologic sequelae was 0.6 (both statistically significant). When stratified by causative organism, a significant mortality benefit was found only for pneumococcal meningitis (RR 0.5). A reduction in neurologic sequelae was not significant for any specific organism. Dexamethasone was not associated with excessive adverse events. The authors recommend initiating dexamethasone (10 mg IV every 6 hours) before or concurrent with the first dose of parenteral antibiotics in all patients with suspected bacterial meningitis.

Wong J, Quint D. Imaging of central nervous system infections. *Semin Roentgenol* 1999;34: 123–143.

18 Encephalitis

Lamis Ibrahim and James W. Myers

INTRODUCTION

Encephalitis is an *inflammatory process of the brain* in association with clinical evidence of neurologic dysfunction. Viruses are the most common cause of this condition.
  Causes: both infectious and noninfectious.

- Noninfectious causes include postinfectious, postinflammatory, vasculitis, collagen vascular disorder, malignancy, paraneoplastic or drug, and toxin induced.
- United States—Herpes simplex virus-1 (HSV-1), West Nile virus (WNV), and the enteroviruses are most common.

CLINICAL FEATURES

Important history taking should include travel, geography, insect exposure, season, contact with animals or rodents, occupation, immunization, and sexual history:

- Recent vaccination—Acute disseminated encephalitis (up to 14 days after vaccination) (Table 18-1).
- Location
  - Russia—Tickborne encephalitis (TBE)
  - Africa—West Nile, trypanosomes, plasmodia
  - Australia—West Nile, Japanese encephalitis (JE), Hendra
  - Europe—TBE
  - India—Rabies, malaria, JE
  - Middle East—West Nile, malaria
  - Central America—Eastern equine encephalitis (EEE), St. Louis encephalitis (SLE), Venezuelan Equine Encephalitis virus (VEE), Rocky Mountain spotted fever (RMSF), rabies, malaria
  - Southeast Asia—JE, TBE, malaria, Nipah, Gnathostoma
  - South America—Rickettsia, SLE, EEE, VEE, Western equine encephalitis (WEE), bartonella, malaria
- Swimming—Naegleria
- Tsetse flies—Trypanosoma brucei gambiense, Trypanosoma brucei rhodesiense (Africa)
- Rodents—LCM, leptospirosis
- Bats—Rabies, Nipah virus
- Sexual activity—HIV, HSV 2
- Birds—West Nile, EEE, WEE, VEE, JE, SLE
- Horses—EEE, WEE, VEE, Hendra
- Swine—JE, Nipah.
- Raccoon—*Baylisascaris procyonis*
- Mosquitoes—EEE, SLE, WEE, VEE, JE, Murray Valley, La Crosse

Table 18-1	Vector Borne Viruses That Cause Encephalitis			
Virus	**Epidemiology/Transmission**	**Manifestations**	**Diagnostic tests**	**Treatment**
Colorado tick fever virus	Western USA, Canada. Vector: wood tick, seasonal from March to September. Also can be transmitted by blood transfusion.	**Saddleback temperature curve.** Prodromal stage is followed by a petechial or maculopapular rash. 5%–10% have encephalitis	Serology/PCR	Supportive
Eastern equine encephalitis virus	Sporadic, **severe course.** Mosquito is the vector, birds/rodents reservoir. Summer or fall season. Atlantic/gulf states in north America are endemic. **Affects children and old population disproportionately.**	Can be subclinical. Symptomatic infections **usually acute with rapid progression** from headache, seizures to coma. Brain stem involvement is common and is associated with gaze palsies, nystagmus, and pupillary abnormalities. **High mortality.**	MRI-Thalamus, basal ganglia, and brain stem involvement. CSF: higher WBC /neutrophil counts than other viruses. Protein, RBCs elevated, low glucose. CSF IgG and IgM positive. Also serum serology positive. Decreased serum sodium.	Only supportive.
Japanese encephalitis virus	Birds/swine are reservoir, vector is mosquito. Southeast Asia, Japan, China, Korea, Taiwan, India, and Australia.	Can cause a flaccid paralysis, seizures, or Parkinson-like symptoms. Nearly 1/3 mortality rate.	Serology. CSF IgM or antigen tests.	Supportive. **Vaccine available**
La Crosse virus	Seasonal from July–September. Mosquito vector, **squirrel and chipmunk are reservoirs.** Affects school-age children. Areas affected are eastern, Midwest USA.	Most commonly subclinical course but can progress to fulminant fatal stage	Serology. CSF IgM. CSF may have increased WBCs with a PMN predominance.	Supportive

Virus	Epidemiology	Clinical features	Diagnosis	Treatment
Murray Valley encephalitis virus	Australia, New Guinea. Affects children. **Birds are reservoirs** and mosquitoes are vectors	Rapid progression to spastic paresis and coma	Serology	Supportive
Powassan virus	Seen in New England, Canada. Has tick vector and **rodent reservoir.**	Can have GI symptoms	Serum or CSF IgM	Supportive
St. Louis encephalitis virus	Usually affects **older adults (>50 years of age).** Birds are the reservoir, with Culex mosquitoes as the vectors. Found in the United States, in addition to being found in South-Central America.	Presents early with **urinary symptoms.** Can have **severe course with older age** and can cause seizures and paresis. SIADH can occur.	Serum or CSF IgM	Supportive. interferon alpha 2b's role.
Tick-borne encephalitis virus	Spring-summer season. Biphasic course. Found in Central Europe, Far East. Rodents are reservoir. Tick vector	Can cause myelitis, **flaccid paralysis,** in addition to encephalitis	Serology. CSF IgM Viral culture in blood in early phase	Supportive. **Effective vaccine in Europe.**
Venezuelan Equine Encephalitis virus	In South and Central America, and southeastern USA (Florida). Reservoirs are rodents, horses, and birds, and vectors are mosquito. Occupational hazard, bioterrorism risk?	Usually subclinical. Respiratory symptoms, myalgia can occur. Rarely fatal unless encephalitis occurs (20%).	Serology. Blood/pharyngeal culture. CSF IgM, PCR tests.	Supportive.
Western equine encephalitis virus	West of Mississippi, Canada, Argentina. Bird reservoir, mosquito vector.	**Mainly subclinical course.** The case-fatality rate is approximately 4%–10%, but is higher in **infants and the elderly.**	Serology IgM or CSF IgM.	Supportive

- Ticks—Powassan, TBE, Lyme, *Anaplasma phagocytophilum,* and rickettsial illnesses
- Parturient cats and farm animals—Q fever
- Fall—Arboviruses and enteroviruses
- Winter—Influenza

SIGNS AND SYMPTOMS

Fever, cognitive and focal neurologic signs, possible seizures, possibly preceded by flu-like prodrome.

On physical exam, patient may have confusion, AMS, nerve palsies, aphasia, balance problems, motor or sensory deficits, altered behavior, and personality changes (Table 18-2).

- Oculomasticatory–Whipples
- Parkinsonian—SLE, West Nile, JE, Nipah
- Polio-like paralysis—West Nile, TBE, JE, and Enterovirus 71
- Retinitis—West Nile, Cytomegalovirus (CMV), bartonella, treponemes
- Rash—Zoster, West Nile, human herpes virus (HHV) 6, Herpes B, RMSF, enteroviruses, mycoplasma
- Respiratory symptoms—Hendra, Nipah, VEE, mycoplasma, Q fever
- Urinary—SLE
- Cerebellar ataxia—SLE, Varicella

DIAGNOSIS

MRI, CT, cerebrospinal fluid (CSF) analysis, serology, culture, and PCR are the most frequent tests ordered

- **MRI is the most sensitive radiographic study**. Diffusion-weighted MRI is probably superior to conventional MRI for the detection of early signal abnormalities in viral encephalitis caused by HSV and some other viruses (Table 18-3).
  - Arteritis—Varicella-zoster virus (VZV), Nipah virus
  - Focal abnormalities:
    - Focal lesions in basal ganglia, thalamus, and/or brain stem
      - EEE, SLE, JE, WNV, enterovirus 71, Epstein-barr virus (EBV), Murray Valley
    - Temporal and/or frontal lobe involvement
      - HSV, varicella-zoster virus, HHV 6, WNV, enteroviruses
  - Subependymal enhancement—CMV
- Paired serum samples may not be useful in establishing the cause during the acute presentation but they are frequently useful for the retrospective diagnosis.
  - For WNV, detection of intrathecal IgM antibody is both specific and sensitive.
  - Note that there is significant cross-reactivity among the flaviviruses.
  - Plaque-reduction neutralization can help distinguish among the different flaviviruses that cross-react with WNV.
- Many viruses cannot be cultured from the CSF, so PCR is very useful.
  - Note that false-negative PCR tests can occur **within the first 72 hours** and that a repeat HSV PCR on a second sample of CSF from later in the disease course should be performed if your suspicion is high enough.
- Brain biopsy might be useful in HSV, rabies, and parasitic infections.

Table 18-2	Other Viral Causes of Encephalitis[a]

Virus	Information
HSV	Sporadic, can affect any age. Presents with fever, head-ache, AMS, memory, language, behavioral impairment. Check CSF PCR MRI: May show temporal lobe predilection. RX—Acyclovir
VZV	More likely in immunocompromised hosts. May occur even without rash. Presents with focal neurologic deficits. Vasculitis reported frequently. CSF PCR MRI may show arteritis, ischemic changes. Acyclovir
CMV	Immunocompromised patients, other organ involvement. CSF PCR. Ganciclovir or foscarnet
EBV	Encephalitis, myelitis, cerebellar involvement. CSF PCR. Supportive, ? steroids.
HHV6	Immunocompromised, skin rash, seizures. Serology, PCR. Ganciclovir or foscarnet
Rabies	Animal bite (bats), organ donation. Hydrophobia/agitation, delirium then goes into stupor and coma. RT-PCR of saliva, nuchal biopsy specimen. Rx: supportive, postexposure prevention.
Hendra virus	Australia, transmitted through exposure to horse's excretion or body fluid. Starts as flu-like symptoms that progress to drowsiness, coma. Rx is supportive.
Enterovirus	More likely to be a meningitis than encephalitis. CSF PCR, supportive care.
Nipah	Exposure to infected pigs and bats. South Asia. Fever, AMS, myoclonus. Serology or CSF culture. Rx: supportive or ? ribavirin.

[a]Other viruses would also include Adenovirus, Influenza, JC virus, herpes B virus, poliovirus, measles, mumps, or HIV.

- Herpes simplex encephalitis will manifest as a temporal lobe focus with periodic lateralizing epileptiform discharges (PLEDs).
- CSF analysis will usually show a lymphocytic predominance in most cases, but this will vary greatly based on the final diagnosis, uUsually <1,000 cells.
  - If the patient is tapped early on, the **CSF pleocytosis may be absent or there may be an elevation in neutrophils.**
- The CSF protein concentration is usually <100 to 200 mg/dL, CSF glucose concentration is typically normal.

Table 18-3	Protozoa[a]
Acanthamoeba	Immunocompromised, subacute presentation. Serology. Rx: TMP-SMX plus rifampin plus ketoconazole or other drugs.
Naegleria fowleri	Swimming in brackish water, may notice a change in smell and taste first then follows the meningitis picture, with subsequent progression to coma. Trophozoites can be seen in CSF. Amphotericin B plus rifampin plus other agent ?
Toxoplasma gondii	Reactivation in immunocompromised patients. Focal deficits. MRI: ring-enhancing lesions. CSF PCR not that sensitive.

[a]Other protozoa include malaria, *Trypanosoma brucei*, baylisascaris, Gnathostoma species, cysticercosis as well.

TREATMENT

Will often be primarily supportive, but use directed therapy if available.

SELECTED ENTITIES

West Nile Virus

Epidemiology
- It is a RNA flavivirus. Serology may cross-react.
- Transmission
  - **Mosquito bite**s are the usual means.
    - *Primarily Culex (Culex pipiens* and *Culex restuans) but others may be involved as well.*
  - Blood transfusion, organ donation, transplacental, and breast-feeding are less frequently implicated.
- **Wild Birds** such as crows and blue jays are main reservoir or amplifying hosts, as **humans and horses are dead-end hosts**.
- Endemic in the United States
- Seasonality is usually in the summer or fall.
- Severe disease in old patients and immunosuppressed. Ten percent mortality in older patients.

Clinical Findings
- West Nile infection can be *asymptomatic* or can cause West Nile fever or meningo-encephalitis, in addition to less common manifestations like myocarditis, hepatitis, and ocular symptoms.
- **One in five people infected with WNV develops fever and of that only about 1 in 150 develops CNS disease.**
- **Incubation period** is from 3 to 14 days but is usually 2 to 6 days.
- In one study, half of hospitalized patients still had a functional deficit at discharge, and only one-third had recovered fully by 1 year.

1. **West Nile fever**:
   - Usually self-limited
   - May be influenza-like in presentation
     - Associated with headache, myalgia, arthralgia, fatigue, and decreased appetite like many other viral syndromes
     - Can also be associated with eye pain, pharyngitis, lymphadenopathy, and GI symptoms
     - Occasional hepatosplenomegaly
   - May last from 3 to 6 days
   - Rash can occur in up to 50% of patients. The rash is usually maculopapular, and found on the trunk, chest, and extremities. More common in children.
2. **CNS disease**
   - WNV can cause meningitis, encephalitis, or **flaccid paralysis** or any combination of these.
   - Patients typically have a febrile prodrome of 1 to 7 days, which may even be biphasic.
   - Encephalitis occurs in 2/3 of CNS presentations.
     - More likely to occur in older people
     - Can progress to severe encephalopathy and coma
     - Other presentation include extrapyramidal symptoms, Parkinson-like symptoms, and mycoclonus/seizures symptoms.
   - Acute flaccid paralysis syndrome (myelitis) may or may not be associated with encephalitis.
     - An asymmetric, poliomyelitis-like syndrome
     - Caused by invasion of the anterior horn of the spinal cord
     - Very poor long-term prognosis for recovery of this syndrome.
   - Cranial nerve palsy can occur, and may lead to respiratory failure
   - Optic neuritis, seizures, and ataxia are less common
3. **Meningitis**
   - Headache, meningeal signs occur in one-third of cases.

Diagnosis
- Made by the finding of **IgM antibody to WNV in serum or CSF** collected within 8 days of illness using the IgM antibody capture ELISA
  - Subsequent plaque reduction neutralization test (PRNT) confirmation
  - PCR is not the mainstay of diagnosis for this disease.
- Fifteen percent lymphopenia
- Forty percent leukocytosis
- Imaging Studies
  - MRI may show high signal intensities in the **thalamus** in T2-weighted images and diffusion-weighted images.
    - Later finding in severe cases
  - Electroencephalograms show diffuse slowing or rarely seizures.
- Nerve conduction studies
  - Will show reduced motor axonal amplitudes consistent with **anterior horn** cell damage
- CSF: pleocytosis (usually a lymphocytic predominance but polymorphonuclear cells (PMN) predominance can occur in early infection), increased protein, normal glucose. CSF IgM/IgG positive.

Treatment
1. Supportive care is the rule.
2. In CNS disease, rule out HSV infection as it can be treated.
3. Some drugs like Ribavirin, hyperimmune globulin, and interferon alpha 2b have been studied but with inconclusive results. Not the standard of care.

Prevention.
Mosquito control, repellents, and screening of organ and blood products are the main measures used.

Hendra and Nipah Viruses

Epidemiology
- Two outbreaks of previously unrecognized zoonotic disease (Hendra) **affecting horses and animals in Australia** were reported within 1 month of each other in Brisbane (southeast Queensland) and Mackay (central Queensland) in 1994.
  - A third event involving a single fatal equine case occurred near Cairns (North Queensland) in 1999.
- Nipah was responsible for an outbreak of severe febrile encephalitis in humans in Malaysia in 1998 to 1989.
  - The outbreak was associated with **respiratory illness in pigs** and was initially considered to be JE because of the epidemiology.
  - Other outbreaks occurred in Bangladesh and India.
- The N genes of HeV and NiV have 78% nucleotide homology, but the two viruses have no more than 49% similarity with any other members of the *Paramyxovirinae.*
- **Fruit bats** of the genus *Pteropus* are considered to be the reservoir hosts for both.

Clinical Findings
- The incubation period for NiV and HeV ranges from 4 to 18 days.
- Onset of disease may be influenza-like with high fevers and myalgia.
- Sore throat, dizziness, and drowsiness and disorientation can occur.
- Mortality is about 50%.
- Both viruses grow well in Vero cells.
  - A cytopathic effect usually develops within 3 days in most cases.
  - Requires a level 4 lab
  - Positive virus neutralization tests, only in a level 4 lab, are demonstrated by the inhibition of cytopathic effect (CPE) production by sera.
    o ELISA tests are less sensitive.
  - PCR available
- These can be spread by the aerosol route, so care should be exercised as NiV has been isolated in the respiratory secretions and urine of patients identified as having Nipah virus encephalitis in Malaysia and Bangladesh.
- No vaccines or treatment are available at the time of this publication.

SUGGESTED READINGS

Centers for Disease Control and Prevention (CDC). West Nile virus disease and other arboviral diseases—United States, 2010. *MMWR Morb Mortal Wkly Rep* 2011;60(30):1009–1013.
States with the highest incidence were Arizona (1.60), New Mexico (1.03), Nebraska (0.55), and Colorado (0.51). After WNV, the next most commonly reported cause of neuroinvasive arboviral disease was California serogroup viruses (CALV), with

68 cases, followed by eastern equine encephalitis virus (EEEV), 10 cases, St. Louis encephalitis virus (SLEV), 8 cases, and Powassan virus (POWV), 8 cases.

Granerod J, Tam CC, et al. Challenge of the unknown. A systematic review of acute encephalitis in non-outbreak situations. *Neurology* 2010;75(10):924–932.

This review highlights research areas that might lead to a better understanding of the causes of encephalitis and ultimately reduce the morbidity and mortality associated with this devastating condition.

Long SS. Encephalitis diagnosis and management in the real world. *Adv Exp Med Biol* 2011;697:153–173.

Petersen LR, Marfin AA, et al. West Nile virus. *JAMA* 2003;290(4):524–528.

Solomon, T. Flavivirus encephalitis. *N Engl J Med* 2004;351(4):370–378.

Trevejo RT, Eidson M. Zoonosis update: West Nile virus. *J Am Vet Med Assoc* 2008;232(9): 1302–1309.

Tunkel AR, Glaser CA, et al. The management of encephalitis: clinical practice guidelines by the Infectious Diseases Society of America. *Clin Infect Dis* 2008;47(3):303–327.

Excellent review article with excellent tables throughout the article!

Tyler KL. Herpes simplex virus infections of the central nervous system: encephalitis and meningitis, including Mollaret's. *Herpes* 2004;11(suppl 2):57A–64A.

Good review.

Whitley RJ, Lakeman F. Herpes simplex virus infections of the central nervous system: therapeutic and diagnostic considerations. *Clin Infect Dis* 1995;20(2):414–420.

Prevention and Treatment of Herpes Zoster and Postherpetic Neuralgia

Lamis Ibrahim and James W. Myers

INTRODUCTION

Varicella-zoster virus (VZV) causes chicken pox as primary infection, and then it resides in sensory ganglia in latent stage. Reactivation of the latent virus causes zoster infection especially when VZV cell-mediated immunity declines.

- Herpes zoster (HZ) presents with vesicular, painful rash that follows a dermatomal distribution and usually lasts 1 week to 10 days.
- Thoracic dermatomes are most commonly affected.
- It can be transmitted through direct contact with skin lesions till they epithelize or through airborne transmission if disseminated infection is present
- In immunocompromised patients, it can cause disseminated skin infection and may involve other organs especially the nervous system.
- A significant complication of zoster is pain. Pain is divided into three stages: **acute pain** (occurs within 30 days of onset of rash), **subacute pain** (occurs within 30 to 120 days of rash), and postherpetic neuralgia (**PHN**) which is persistent pain beyond 120 days after zoster rash onset.

PHN

- May persist for months or years.
- It can be extremely incapacitating and can result in insomnia, weight loss, and an inability to perform daily tasks of living.
- Its effect on quality of life may be similar to that of other chronic diseases like diabetes, depression, and congestive heart failure.
- Pathophysiology is not very well understood.
  - Pathologic studies have demonstrated damage to the sensory nerves, the sensory dorsal root ganglia, and the dorsal horns of the spinal cord in patients with this condition.
  - The pain of HZ results from a sequence of changes in neuronal sensitivity starting at the point of neural damage in the periphery and moving centrally to affect one cell after another within the pain pathway.
  - Once central sensitization occurs, attempts to reduce the pain purely by influencing peripheral nociceptor function are unlikely to be successful.
  - Furthermore, once established, such neuropathic pain is notoriously difficult to control.
- Risk factors include old age, severity of acute pain, female sex, and possibly ophthalmic distribution.

Table 19-1	Antiviral Therapy of Zoster	
Medication	**Dose**	
ACV	800 mg orally five times daily for 7–10 days 10 mg/kg IV every 8 hours for 7–10 days 500 mg orally three times daily for 7 days	Antiviral therapy has been shown to be beneficial only when patients are treated within 72 hours of onset of the HZ rash
Famciclovir Valacyclovir	1,000 mg orally three times daily for 7 days	
Prednisone	30 mg orally twice daily on days 1 through 7; then 15 mg twice daily on days 8 through 14; then 7.5 mg twice daily on days 15 through 21	Prednisone used in conjunction with ACV has been shown to reduce the pain associated with HZ but probably is ineffective for PHN. Probably more useful for those patients older than age 50

Treatment of HZV: see Table 19-1
Treatment of PHN: Table 19-2

PHARMACOLOGIC AGENTS

1. **Anticonvulsants:**
   - **Gabapentin**:
     - Is structurally related to the neurotransmitter GABA (gamma-aminobutyric acid). The mechanism by which gabapentin exerts its analgesic action is unknown.
     - It is demonstrated to provide significant benefits when compared with placebo.
   - Studies showed that treatment with gabapentin at daily doses of 1,800 to 3,600 mg was associated with a statistically significant reduction in daily pain ratings as well as improvements in sleep, mood, and quality of life.
   - It may cause dizziness, somnolence, and other symptoms and signs of CNS depression and can cause or exacerbate gait and balance problems and cognitive impairment in elderly patients
   - To reduce side effects and increase patient compliance with treatment, gabapentin should be initiated at low dosages and then titrated, as tolerated.
   - Dosing information can also be found on the Internet at www.rxlist.com/cgi/generic/gabapent.htm
   - **Lyrica (pregabalin):**
     - Is a modulator of voltage-gated calcium channels, designed to affect neurologic transmission.
     - For the treatment of PHN, recommended initial dosing is 75 mg twice daily or 50 mg thrice daily (in patients with creatinine clearance>60 mL/min), with escalation to 150 mg twice daily or 100 mg thrice daily (in patients with creatinine clearance>60 mL/min) permissible.

Table 19-2	Treatment Options for PHN

Medication	Dosage
Topical Agents	
Capsaicin cream (Zostrix)	Apply to affected area three to five times daily
Lidocaine (Xylocaine) patch	Apply to affected area every 4–12 hours as needed (http://www.endo.com/PDF/lidoderm_pack_insert.pdf)
Tricyclic Antidepressants	
Amitriptyline (Elavil)	25 mg orally at bedtime; increase dosage by 25 mg every 2–4 weeks until response is adequate, or to maximum dosage of 150 mg/day
Nortriptyline (Pamelor)	25 mg orally at bedtime; increase dosage by 25 mg every 2–4 weeks until response is adequate, or to maximum dosage of 125 mg/day
Desipramine (Norpramin)	25 mg orally at bedtime; increase dosage by 25 mg every 2–4 weeks until response is adequate, or to maximum dosage of 150 mg/day
Anticonvulsants	
Gabapentin (Neurontin)	100–300 mg orally at bedtime; increase dosage by 100–300 mg every 3 days until dosage is 300–900 mg three times daily or response is adequate
Lyrica	Start with 75 mg b.i.d. and titrate dose.

Adapted from Stankus SJ, et al. Management of herpes zoster (shingles) and postherpetic neuralgia. *Am Fam Physician* 2000;61:2437–2444, 2447–2448.

2. **Opioid Analgesics:**
   - In one double-blind study, compared with placebo, oxycodone resulted in pain relief and reductions in steady pain, allodynia, and paroxysmal spontaneous pain. Global effectiveness, disability, and masked patient preference all showed superior scores with oxycodone relative to placebo.
   - In another study, a comparison between the analgesic and cognitive effects of opioids with those of tricyclic antidepressant (TCA) and placebo in the treatment of PHN was done. Treatment with opioids and TCA resulted in greater pain relief compared with placebo, but more patients completing all three treatments preferred opioids than TCA.
   - Evaluation by a pain specialist may be considered when high doses of opioids are needed.

3. **Antidepressants: TRICYCLIC ANTIDEPRESSANTS**
   - These agents most likely lessen pain by inhibiting the reuptake of serotonin and norepinephrine neurotransmitters
   - They have showed established efficacy for treatment of PHN.
   - They are best tolerated when they are started in a low dosage and given at bedtime.

- Patients at risk of increased toxicity with this class of drugs include those with a history of cardiovascular disease, glaucoma, urinary retention, and autonomic neuropathy.
- These drugs should be titrated for effect
- Because TCAs do not act quickly, a clinical trial of at least 3 months is required to judge a patient's response.
- The onset of pain relief using TCAs may be enhanced by beginning treatment early in the course of HZ infection in conjunction with antiviral medications.

4. **Topical treatment: lidocaine patch 5%:**
- Topical local anesthetics have shown promise in both uncontrolled and controlled studies.
- In one study, lidocaine-containing patches significantly reduced pain intensity at all time points 30 minutes to 12 hours, compared with no-treatment observation, and at all time points 4 to 12 hours compared with vehicle patches. The highest blood lidocaine level measured was 0.1 mcg/mL, indicating minimal systemic absorption of lidocaine.
- Treatment with the lidocaine patch 5% consists of the application of a maximum of three patches per day for a maximum of 12 hours applied directly to the area of maximal PHN-associated pain and allodynia, which typically overlaps the primary affected dermatome.
- It should not be used for patients with open lesions, because the available formulation is not sterile.
- Satisfactory relief from lidocaine patch 5% usually will be apparent within 2 weeks, and time-consuming dose escalation is not required.
- Further dosing information can be found on the Internet at www.endo.com/healthcare/products/lidoderm.html and www.endo.com/PDF/lidoderm_pack_insert.pdf.

5. **Interventional therapy:**
- Sympathetic and epidural nerve block:
- Some patients who don't respond to combination pharmacologic therapy may be referred for nerve block therapy.
- Epidural steroid injection and local anesthetics are sometimes used to treat severe acute pain, but there is no evidence that this would prevent PHN. In addition, such therapy is not always feasible.

PREVENTION

Zoster Vaccine
- It is a **live attenuated** vaccine. It is given as a one-time subcutaneous injection.
- It contains up to 60,000 virus units. *This is much more than the varicella vaccine.*
- In 2006, ACP recommended Zoster vaccine for adults 60 years old and up. It was proven to be well tolerated and immunogenic in adults ≥60 years old
- One study showed that the use of zoster vaccine decreased the incidence of PHN by 66.5 %, and that of HZ by 51.3 %.
- Zoster vaccine, compared to placebo, also decreased the duration and severity of illness when zoster occurred.
- In 2011, FDA approved it for adults 50 to 59 years of age too, but ACIP do not recommend it for this age group because of limited supply for the higher-risk age group>60.
- **In a recent study, vaccine efficacy for preventing HZ in age group 50 to 59 was 69.8%, and the vaccine was well tolerated.**

- It can be given *regardless of prior zoster episodes*, or varicella infection.
- It is generally a safe vaccine.
  - Major side effects is secondary to site injection reaction (swelling, pain)
- Duration of immunity is not known, but patient may require a booster in about 20 years.
- There are limited data on administration of zoster vaccine with other inactivated vaccines, although it has been accepted to administer multiple inactivated vaccine with no impairment of the immune response
- **Contraindications to the vaccine**: anaphylaxis to vaccine component like gelatin or neomycin, pregnant patients, patients with immunodeficiencies (primary or acquired)

SUGGESTED READINGS

Ali NM. Does sympathetic ganglionic block prevent postherpetic neuralgia? Literature review. *Reg Anesth* 1995;20:227–233.

Considering the degree of uncertainty and the seriousness of PHN, sympathetic block in addition to treatment with ACV should be considered early during acute HZ. Large controlled trials are needed to provide the necessary scientific evidence.

Alper BS, Lewis PR. Does treatment of acute herpes zoster prevent or shorten postherpetic neuralgia? *J Fam Pract* 2000;49:255–264.

There is limited evidence that current interventions prevent or shorten PHN. Famciclovir and valacyclovir have been shown to reduce the duration of PHN in single published trials.

Alper BS, Lewis PR. Treatment of postherpetic neuralgia: a systematic review of the literature. *J Fam Pract* 2002;51:121–128.

No single best treatment for PHN is known. TCAs, topical capsaicin, gabapentin, and oxycodone are effective for alleviating PHN; however, long-term, clinically meaningful benefits are uncertain and side effects are common. Patients with PHN refractory to these therapies may benefit from intrathecal methylprednisolone. Little evidence is available regarding treatment of PHN of less than 6 months' duration.

Backonja M, Glanzman RL. Gabapentin dosing for neuropathic pain: evidence from randomized, placebo-controlled clinical trials. *Clin Ther* 2003;25:81–104.

Based on available data, it appears that treatment should be started at a dose of 900 mg/day (300 mg/day on day 1,600 mg/day on day 2, and 900 mg/day on day 3). Additional titration to 1,800 mg/day is recommended for greater efficacy. Doses up to 3,600 mg/day may be needed in some patients. The effective dose should be individualized according to patient response and tolerance.

Bernstein JE, et al. Topical capsaicin treatment of chronic postherpetic neuralgia. *J Am Acad Dermatol* 1989;21:265–270.

After 6 weeks, almost 80% of capsaicin-treated patients experienced some relief from their pain.

Boivin G, Jovey R, et al. Management and prevention of herpes zoster: a Canadian perspective. *Can J Infect Dis Med Microbiol* 2010;21(1):45–52.

A live, attenuated zoster vaccine has been recently shown to significantly decrease HZ incidence, PHN, and the overall burden of illness when administered to adults older than 60 years of age.

Bowsher D. Factors influencing the features of postherpetic neuralgia and outcome when treated with tricyclics. *Eur J Pain* 2003;7:1–7.

This paper retrospectively reviews features of PHN in up to 279 personal patients in relation to treatment outcome when treated with TCAs. Factors affecting characteristics of PHN: (1) Patients with allodynia (89%) and/or burning pain (56%) have a *much higher visual analog pain intensity score than those withou t it; (2) ACV given for acute shingles (HZ) does not reduce the incidence of subsequent PHN, but reduces the pain intensity in PHN patients with allodynia; (3) ACV given for acute HZ reduces the incidence of burning pain in subsequent PHN, but not of allodynia; (4) ACV given for acute HZ reduces the incidence of clinically detectable sensory deficit in subsequent PHN. Factors affecting outcome of TCA-treated PHN: (1) The point in time at which TCA treatment is commenced is by far the most critical factor: started between 3 and 12 months after acute HZ onset, more than two-thirds obtain pain relief (NNT = 1.8); between 13 and 24 months, two-fifths (41%) (NNT = 3.6); and more than 2 years, one-third (NNT = 8.3). Background and paroxysmal pain disappears earlier and is more susceptible to relief than allodynia. (2) Twice as many (86%) of PHN patients without allodynia obtain pain relief with TCA treatment than those with it (42%); (3) The use of ACV for acute HZ more than halves the time-to-relief of PHN patients by TCAs; (4) PHN patients with burning pain are significantly less likely to obtain pain relief with TCAs than those without it (p< 0.0001).*

Dworkin RH, et al. Postherpetic neuralgia: impact of famciclovir, age, rash severity, and acute pain in herpes zoster patients. *J Infect Dis* 1998;178(suppl 1):S76–S80.

The results of these analyses indicated that greater age, rash severity, and acute pain severity are risk factors for prolonged PHN. In addition, they demonstrated that treatment of acute HZ patients with famciclovir significantly reduces both the duration and prevalence of PHN.

Gammaitoni AR, et al. Safety and tolerability of the lidocaine patch 5%, a targeted peripheral analgesic: a review of the literature. *J Clin Pharmacol* 2003;43:111–117.

The safety, tolerability, and efficacy of the lidocaine patch 5% (Lidoderm), a targeted peripheral analgesic with a Food and Drug Administration (FDA)–approved indication for the treatment of PHN, has been well established. The lidocaine patch provides a treatment option that carries a relatively low systemic adverse event and drug-drug interaction risk burden, even with continuous application of up to four patches per day.

Kotani N, et al. Intrathecal methylprednisolone for intractable postherpetic neuralgia. *N Engl J Med* 2000;343:1514–1519.

There is no effective treatment for intractable PHN. In the patients who received methylprednisolone, interleukin-8 concentrations decreased by 50%, and this decrease correlated with the duration of neuralgia and the extent of global pain relief (p< 0.001 for both comparisons). The results of this trial indicate that the intrathecal administration of methylprednisolone is an effective treatment for PHN.

Oxman MN, Levin MJ. Vaccination against Herpes Zoster and Postherpetic Neuralgia. *J Infect Dis* 2008;197(suppl 2): S228–S236.

The Shingles Prevention Study demonstrated that HZ vaccine significantly reduced the morbidity due to HZ and PHN in older adults.

Raja SN, et al. Opioids versus antidepressants in postherpetic neuralgia: a randomized, placebo-controlled trial. *Neurology* 2002;59:1015–1021.

Opioids effectively treat PHN without impairing cognition. Opioids and TCAs act through independent mechanisms and with varied individual effect.

Rowbotham MC, et al. Lidocaine patch: double-blind controlled study of a new treatment method for post-herpetic neuralgia. *Pain* 1996;65:39–44.

This study demonstrates that topical 5% lidocaine in patch form is easy to use and relieves PHN.

Sanford M, Keating GM. Zoster vaccine (Zostavax): a review of its use in preventing herpes zoster and postherpetic neuralgia in older adults. *Drugs Aging* 2010;27(2):159–176.

Over a mean HZ surveillance period of 3.1 years, zoster vaccine reduced the HZ-related burden of illness by 61%, reduced the incidence of HZ by 51%, and reduced the incidence of PHN by 67%. Zoster vaccine recipients who developed HZ had a shorter illness duration and severity than placebo recipients who developed HZ. Zoster vaccine had continuing efficacy in a Shingles Prevention Study subpopulation followed for 7 years after vaccination. Zoster vaccine was generally well tolerated in older adults.

Santee JA. Corticosteroids for herpes zoster: what do they accomplish? *Am J Clin Dermatol* 2002;3:517–524.

Oral corticosteroids may confer a slight benefit for initial symptoms as long as the patient is not at risk for complications resulting from corticosteroid therapy. Two controlled, blinded trials investigating the use of intrathecal corticosteroid administration for intractable PHN suggest that corticosteroid administration results in a significant improvement in pain. Despite this, several authors have voiced concern over possible serious adverse events with the intrathecal administration of corticosteroids. Intrathecal corticosteroids may provide a benefit for intractable PHN, but because of risks of serious complications, this is a last-line option and should only be administered by experienced personnel.

Schmader KE, Levin MJ, et al. Efficacy, safety, and tolerability of herpes zoster vaccine in persons aged 50–59 years. *Clin Infect Dis* 2012;54(7):922–928.

The ZV reduced the incidence of HZ (30 cases in vaccine group, 1.99/1,000 person-years vs. 99 cases in placebo group, 6.57/1,000 person-years). Vaccine efficacy for preventing HZ was 69.8% (95% confidence interval, 54.1–80.6). AEs were reported by 72.8% of subjects in the ZV group and 41.5% in the placebo group, with the difference primarily due to higher rates of injection-site AEs and headache.

Stankus SJ, et al. Management of herpes zoster (shingles) and postherpetic neuralgia. *Am Fam Physician* 2000;61:2437–2444, 2447–2448.

Good overall review article with useful references.

Vermeulen JN, Lange JM, et al. Safety, tolerability, and immunogenicity after one and two doses of zoster vaccine in healthy adults≥60 years of age. *Vaccine* 2012;30(5):904–910.

ZV was generally well tolerated and immunogenic in adults≥60 years old. A second dose of ZV was generally safe, but did not boost VZV-specific immunity beyond levels achieved postdose 1.

V Travel-Related Infections

Prophylaxis of Infection in Travelers

James W. Myers and Paras Patel

INTRODUCTION

If possible, the initial consultation about travel abroad should occur at least 6 weeks to 2 months before the patient's departure date to allow adequate time to give the appropriate immunizations and for assessment of any serious reactions.

- Patients may have special needs that require additional pretravel interventions or cause modifications to their itineraries.
  - For example travel, particularly to developing countries, can carry significant risks for exposure to opportunistic pathogens for HIV-infected travelers, especially those who are severely immunosuppressed.
  - Also counseling about preventing sexually transmitted diseases (STDs) may be helpful, given that many travelers may acquire a STD abroad.
- The pretravel history should include information about the places the patient plans to visit, the season of the year, and the duration of the trip.
- Ideally, one should review the patient's vaccination status at this time.
- Routine immunizations that need to be evaluated would include the pneumococcal vaccine, measles, mumps and rubella, polio, tetanus, varicella, and influenza.
- Recommendations for adult vaccinations may be found on the Centers for Disease Control and Prevention (CDC) Web site listed in Table 20-1.
- Issues regarding safe consumption of water need to be addressed at the pretravel visit.
- Only boiled water, hot beverages (such as coffee or tea), canned or bottled carbonated beverages, beer, and wine can be considered safe.
- **A common error committed by travelers is to add ice to their soft drinks.**
  - Ice may be made from unsafe water and should be avoided if possible.
  - As an alternative to boiling, chemical disinfection can be achieved with either iodine or chlorine.
- **As a general rule, if you can peel fruit yourself, it is safe.**
- Foods that are more worrisome include salads, uncooked vegetables and fruit, unpasteurized milk and milk products, raw meat, and shellfish.
- The traveler is at risk to acquire salmonellosis, toxoplasmosis, trichinosis, or cysticercosis from inadequately cooked meat; salmonellosis, shigellosis, leptospirosis, amebiasis, giardiasis, dracunculiasis, or hepatitis A from contaminated ice cubes or drinking water; brucellosis, salmonellosis, campylobacteriosis, or tuberculosis from unpasteurized milk or milk products, including cheese and ice cream; and salmonellosis, hepatitis A, fish roundworm infection, gnathostomiasis, or infection with liver or lung flukes from raw or undercooked fish or shellfish.

Table 20-1	Useful Web Sites
Adult vaccination	http://www.cdc.gov/mmwr/preview/mmwrhtml/mm5140a5.htm
DEET	http://www.deet.com
Travel vaccines	http://www.cdc.gov/travel/vaccinat.htm
Mosquito protection	http://www.cdc.gov/travel/bugs.htm
Destination information	http://www.cdc.gov/travel/destinat.htm
Specific information for travel-related infections	http://www.cdc.gov/travel/destinat.htm
Safe food and water	http://www.cdc.gov/travel/foodwater.htm
Travel clinics	http://www.cdc.gov/travel/travel_clinics.htm
International Society of Travel Medicine	http://www.istm.org/
The American Society of Tropical Medicine and Hygiene	http://www.astmh.org/
U.S. State Department	http://travel.state.gov/
WHO	http://www.who.int/en/
CDC malaria site	http://www.cdc.gov/travel/yb/index.htm
Special travel needs	http://www.cdc.gov/travel/spec_needs.htm
Alternate CDC malaria site	http://www.cdc.gov/malaria/
Malaria pocket guide	http://www.vnh.org/Malaria/Malaria.html
Diarrhea site	http://www.travelhealthline.com/z_diarrhea.html

• Some fish are not guaranteed to be safe even when cooked because of the presence of toxins in their flesh. Some species of fish and shellfish can contain poisonous biotoxins, even when well cooked. The most common type of biotoxin in fish is ciguatoxin. The barracuda and puffer fish are usually toxic, and should be avoided. Tropical reef fish, red snapper, amber jack, grouper, and sea bass can occasionally be toxic as well.

DIARRHEA

Please see chapter on diarrhea for information on this subject.

INSECTS

• Many travel-related illnesses, such as malaria and dengue fever, are transmitted by insect vectors. Precautions against infection include the use of insect repellents, mosquito netting, and screened windows.
• Insect repellents should be applied only to exposed skin and should be washed off as soon as possible after exposure.

- They should contain DEET (30% to 35% diethylmethylbenzamide). The DEET concentration alone may not predict toxicity, but a standard maximum concentration of 10% for children and 30% for adults usually provides hours of safe protection without significant toxicity. Light, long-sleeved clothing and long pants should be worn where appropriate, and pants should be tucked into socks.
- Permethrin-coated clothing and bed nets provide additional protection against insects.
- DEET is far less toxic than many people believe.
- Adverse effects, though documented, are infrequent and are generally associated with gross overuse of the product.
- The risk of DEET-related adverse effects pales in comparison with the risk of acquiring vector-borne infection in places where such diseases are endemic.
- More information about DEET can be found in Table 20-1.

VACCINATIONS

- General information about vaccination requirements for adults can be found on the CDC Web site. Specific requirements for certain countries can be found there as well. Pretravel counseling is a good time to do routine health maintenance, including vaccination status for some patients.
- See Table 20-2 for list of recommended vaccines, dose, and indication.

Table 20-2	Drugs for the Prevention of Malaria	
Drug	**Dose**	**Other**
Mefloquine	The adult dosage is 250 mg salt (one tablet) once a week. Take the first dose of mefloquine 1 week before arrival in the malaria-risk area, once a week, on the same day of the week, in the malaria-risk area, and once a week for 4 weeks after leaving the malaria-risk area. Mefloquine should be taken on a full stomach, for example, after dinner.	See Table 20-3 for adverse reactions to Larium.
Doxycycline	The adult dosage is 100 mg once a day. Take the first dose of doxycycline 1 or 2 days before arrival in the malaria-risk area, once a day, at the same time each day, in the malaria-risk area, and once a day for 4 weeks after leaving the malaria-risk area.	Potential for photosensitivity. Avoid in pregnancy. Potential drug interactions.

Table 20-2	Drugs for the Prevention of Malaria *(Continued)*	
Drug	**Dose**	**Other**
Malarone	The adult dosage is one adult tablet (250 mg atovaquone/100 mg proguanil) once a day. Take the first dose of Malarone 1 to 2 days before travel in the malaria-risk area. Take Malarone once a day in the malaria-risk area. Take Malarone once a day for 7 days after leaving the malaria-risk area. Take the dose at the same time each day with food or milk.	Malarone is a combination of two drugs (atovaquone and proguanil) and is an effective alternative for travelers who cannot or choose not to take doxycycline or mefloquine.
Chloroquine	The adult dosage is 500 mg (salt) chloroquine phosphate once a week. Take the first dose of chloroquine 1 week before arrival in the malaria-risk area, once a week on the same day of the week in the malaria-risk area, and once a week for 4 weeks after leaving the malaria-risk area. Chloroquine should be taken on a full stomach, for example, after dinner, to minimize nausea.	Potential for ocular toxicity, drug interactions, marrow suppression, skin eruptions, and resistance.

Adapted from http://www.cdc.gov/travel/malariadrugs2.htm.

HEPATITIS A AND B

• Hepatitis A and B can be prevented by vaccines, and both have widely overlapping epidemiologic distribution.

• The disease endemicity in the travel destination, the duration and frequency of travel, the activities to be undertaken, and the purpose of the travel are the risk factors for hepatitis A virus (HAV) and HBV infection in the travelers.

• Travelers requiring medical care while traveling are at increased risk for blood-borne virus, such as HBV.

• The risk of hepatitis A in nonimmune travelers to developing countries has been estimated at **1 per 1,000 travelers per week for most tourists, but as high as 1 per 200 per week for backpackers**.

As a result, the CDC recommends hepatitis A vaccine be given for all international travelers except those going to **low-risk countries such as Canada, Australia, New Zealand, Japan, or most of western Europe.**

• Hepatitis A and B vaccines are available either as monovalent formulations or in various combinations.

- HAVRIX is formulated with 2-phenoxyethanol as a preservative, unlike VAQTA, which is formulated without a preservative.
  - These two vaccines are available in pediatric (ages 2 to 18) and adult (older than age18) formulations, administered intramuscularly in a two-dose schedule.
  - Also a combination hepatitis A and hepatitis B vaccine (TWINRIX, GlaxoSmith-Kline) is available, and it contains 720 ELU of HAV antigen and 20 μg of recombinant hepatitis B surface antigen.
- Unlike the previous vaccines, the combination vaccine is given as a three-dose schedule.
- Hepatitis B vaccine is produced by two manufacturers in the United States, Merck (Recombivax HB) and GlaxoSmithKline Pharmaceuticals (Engerix-B). Both vaccines are available in both pediatric and adult formulations.
- Hepatitis B vaccine is recommended for international travelers to regions with high or intermediate levels (HBsAg prevalence of 2% or higher) of endemic HBV infection and persons with HIV infection.
- The standard primary course of hepatitis B vaccination consists of three doses, with doses administered at 0, 1, and 6 months. A short 0-, 1-, and 2- month schedule and an accelerated 0-, 7-, and 21-day schedule also exist, with a fourth dose recommended at 12 months in both schedules.
- Immune globulin (IG) is effective, providing 85% to 90% protection, but provides only short-term (i.e., months) protection.
  - In general, even a single dose of the vaccine induces higher levels of antibodies than achieved with use of IG, but lower than levels induced by natural infection.
  - However, levels of neutralizing antibodies are lower immediately after active immunization than after administration of IG.
  - Antibody production is somewhat slower and antibody levels are lower when IG and vaccine are given simultaneously, but still reach protective levels in healthy adults.
- Testing for antibodies to hepatitis A after vaccination to assess for adequacy of response is not recommended.
- Commercially available tests for hepatitis A antibodies were developed to assess immunity to natural infection, so the vaccine does not cause a long-lasting false-positive result or diagnostic dilemmas.
- Protection from the vaccine is expected to be long lasting.
- Exposure to wild virus after receiving the vaccine will most likely lead to a booster effect.
- Mathematical models have predicted that protective levels of antibodies will persist for 24 to 47 years, with an average annual decrease of 25% in anti-HAV.
- Nevertheless, long-term follow-up studies are required to assess duration of protection.

MENINGOCOCCAL MENINGITIS

- There are five major meningococcal serogroups, A, B, C, Y, and W-135, that are associated with disease.
- It is transmitted from person to person by close contact with respiratory secretions or saliva.
- Vaccine is indicated in people traveling to the "meningitis belt" of sub-Saharan Africa during December to June as well as Mecca during the annual Hajj and Umrah pilgrimages.

- Serogroup A infection predominates in the meningitis belt, although serogroups C, X, and W-135 are also found.
- Two quadrivalent meningococcal polysaccharide-protein conjugate vaccines (Men-ACWY) (Menactra, Menveo) are licensed for use in the United States.
- A one-dose primary series of MenACWY-D (Menactra) is licensed for people aged 2 to 55 years; a two-dose primary series of MenACWY-D is licensed for children aged 9 to 23 months. MenACWY-Crm (Menveo) is licensed for people aged 2 to 55 years.
- Quadrivalent meningococcal polysaccharide vaccine (MPVS4) (Menomune) is licensed for use among people aged ≥2 years. These vaccines protect against meningococcal disease caused by serogroups A, C, Y, and W-135.
- Approximately, 7 to 10 days are required after vaccination for development of protective antibody levels.
- MenACWY-D is the only meningococcal vaccine licensed for children aged 9 to 23 months.
- Using either one of the MenACWY vaccines is preferred for people aged 2 to 55 years; MPSV4 should be used for people >55 years.
- There is no licensed vaccine for infants <9 months in the United States.

RABIES

- Rabies is a disease caused by neurotropic viruses in the family Rhabdoviridae and present with an acute, progressive, fatal encephalomyelitis.
- Travelers to rabies-enzootic countries should be warned about the risk of acquiring rabies and educated in animal bite–prevention strategies.
- Travelers should avoid stray animals, be aware of their surroundings so that they do not accidentally surprise a stray dog, avoid contact with bats and other wildlife, and not carry or eat food while nonhuman primates are near.
- Rabies is a disease of both domestic and wild mammals, particularly dogs and related species, raccoons, mongooses, skunks, and bats.
- Although often thought of as being a domestic illness, rabies prevention should be part of pretravel counseling.
- In Asia, Africa, Russia, Latin America, and other countries, dogs are the vector of rabies.
- Preexposure rabies vaccine may be recommended, based on the prevalence of rabies in the country to be visited, the availability of appropriate antirabies biologics, intended activities, and duration of stay.
- A decision to receive preexposure rabies immunization may also be based on the likelihood of repeat travel to at-risk destinations or taking up residence in a high-risk destination.
- Preexposure vaccination may be recommended for veterinarians, animal handlers, field biologists, cavers, missionaries, and certain laboratory workers
- Preexposure vaccination may be used for those who may come in contact with the virus or rabid animals
- Travelers should be aware that appropriate postexposure prophylaxis (PEP) treatment might unfortunately not be available in most of the third world.
- Also, neurologic complications associated with Semple (sheep brain-derived) vaccine may be as high as 1 case per 200 recipients.
- Postexposure management includes immediate wound washing, followed by the use of human or equine rabies immunoglobulin (HRIG or ERIG) and a World Health Organization (WHO)–approved vaccination series.

- The postexposure regimen recommended in the United States and by WHO is rabies immune globulin (RIG) on day 0 and human diploid cell rabies vaccine (HDCV) on each of days 0, 3,7 and 14; 1 mL of vaccine is administered intramuscularly in the deltoid area only.
- To be optimally effective, RIG must be injected into and around wounds to neutralize virus before it enters peripheral nerves, where, once established, it is in an immune-protected environment.
- Vaccines require up to 10 days to induce detectable neutralizing antibodies in most patients.
- Because chloroquine may cause interference with the immune response, WHO recommends that preexposure treatment should be administered intramuscularly when a patient is receiving malaria prophylaxis concurrently.
- Those who have received prior preexposure or postexposure treatment with a cell-culture vaccine, or those who have proven viral neutralizing antibody (VNA) to rabies after other vaccines, should receive an intramuscular injection on each of days 0 and 3, without RIG.

JAPANESE B ENCEPHALITIS

- The risk of Japanese B encephalitis (JE) virus infection appears to be *very low* for most travelers despite the fact that almost 50,000 cases are reported annually.
- JE is a mosquito-transmitted viral infection that is endemic in rural parts of Asia.
- **The risk is felt to be highest in China, Korea, the Indian subcontinent, and Southeast Asia, especially in areas where pig farming is common.**
- Occasionally, cases have been reported in Japan, Hong Kong, southeastern Russia, Singapore, Malaysia, the Philippines, Taiwan, and parts of Oceania.
- **Most infections are asymptomatic, but among people who develop a clinical illness, the case-fatality rate can be as high as 30%.**
- Neuropsychiatric sequelae are reported in 50% of survivors. A higher case-fatality rate is usually reported in older persons.
- Both *domestic pigs and wild birds* serve as the reservoirs of this infection, with *Culex* mosquitoes being the principal vectors.
- This species of mosquito feeds outdoors beginning at dusk and during evening hours until dawn. Larvae are typically found in flooded rice fields, marshes, and small stable collections of water around cultivated fields.
- In temperate zones, the vectors are present in greatest numbers from June through September and are inactive during winter months.
- **Individuals visiting endemic areas for stays of longer than 30 days are candidates for vaccination.**
- Short-term travelers who engage in outdoor activities with exposure to mosquito bites and long-term travelers going to endemic areas for more than 1 month should follow personal insect precautions, including the use of bed nets and insect repellents when outdoors.
- At the time of this publication, only one JE vaccine is licensed in the United States.
  - It is an inactivated Vero cell-culture–derived vaccine (Ixiaro).
  - This vaccine is made by Novartis Vaccines
  - It was approved in March 2009 for use in people **aged ≥17 years.**
  - JE-Vax, an **inactivated mouse brain–derived** vaccine with significant side effects has been discontinued. Pain and tenderness are the most common side effects of the Ixiaro vaccine, as it is much better tolerated than the older vaccine.

- The primary immunization schedule for Ixiaro is **two doses administered intramuscularly on days 0 and 28.** The dose is 0.5 mL for people aged ≥17 years, and the two-dose series should be completed **≥1 week before travel**. If the primary series of Ixiaro was administered ≥1 year previously, a **booster dose** should be given prior to potential reexposure.

YELLOW FEVER

Yellow fever occurs in tropical regions of Africa and South America**, but it has never emerged in Asia, and vaccination for travel is currently not indicated for travel there.**

- Yellow fever is a zoonotic infection, maintained in nature by wild nonhuman primates and diurnally active mosquitoes.
- In a study of 103 patients, the average stay in hospital for surviving patients was 14 days and the average duration of acute illness was 17 days.
- Serologic diagnosis is accomplished principally by measurement of IgM antibodies by enzyme-linked immunosorbent assay (ELISA).
- A certificate of vaccination is required under the International Health Regulations for entry into yellow fever-endemic countries or travel from endemic countries to *Aegypti*-infested countries at risk of introduction. Information on vaccination requirements can be obtained from travel clinics and on the CDC Web site (www.cdc.gov/travel).
- **Yellow fever 17D is a highly effective, well-tolerated live, attenuated vaccine produced from embryonated eggs. As a result, egg-allergic patients should not be immunized or should be skin tested and desensitized.**
- Protective levels of neutralizing antibody are found in 90% of vaccinees within 10 days and in 99% within 30 days.
- Most likely, vaccination provides lifelong protection after a single dose, **but revaccination after 10 years is required under International Health Regulations** for a valid travel certificate.
- The vaccine may be simultaneously administered with measles, polio, DPT, hepatitis B, hepatitis A, oral cholera, and oral or parenteral typhoid.
- The vaccine is very well tolerated; in practice, few patients complain of side effects.
- Adverse events may be more likely in older persons.

CONTRAINDICATIONS

1. Allergy to the vaccine.
2. Age <6 months.
3. Symptomatic HIV infection or CD4+ T-lymphocytes <200/mm3.
4. Thymus disorder associated with abnormal immune function.
5. Primary immunodeficiencies.
6. Malignant neoplasms.
7. Transplantation.
8. Immunosuppressive and immunomodulatory therapies.
9. Yellow fever vaccine is **contraindicated during pregnancy and breast feeding, but pregnant women who inadvertently get vaccinated should be reassured that there is no** risk to themselves and no or low risk to the fetus. However, they should be followed up to determine the outcome of pregnancy.

Reactions to yellow fever vaccine are usually mild, but serious events can follow yellow fever vaccination.

- Anaphylaxis (2 per 100,000).
- Yellow fever vaccine–associated viscerotropic disease (YEL-AVD)
  - YEL-AVD appears to occur after the first dose of yellow fever vaccine.
  - The onset of illness averaged 3 days (range, 1 to 8 days) after vaccination.
  - **The case-fatality ratio for reported YEL-AVD cases is 65%.**
  - Resembles "wild type" illness.
  - The rate is higher for people aged ≥60 years, with a rate of 1.0 per 100,000 doses in people aged 60 to 69 years and 2.3 per 100,000 doses in people aged ≥70 years.
  - The pathogenesis of YEL-AVD is unknown but older age and thymic dysfunction as well as genetic factors may play a role in disease.
- Yellow fever vaccine–associated neurologic disease (YEL-AND).
  - Meningoencephalitis
  - Guillain-Barré syndrome
  - Acute disseminated encephalomyelitis,
  - Bulbar palsy and Bell palsy
  - Usually occurs in first time vaccine recipients, 3 to 28 days after vaccination.
  - The rate is higher in people aged ≥60 years, with a rate of 1.6 per 100,000 doses in people aged 60 to 69 and 2.3 per 100,000 doses in people aged ≥70 years.
  - Rarely fatal.

TYPHOID FEVER

- Typhoid is the **second most common vaccine-preventable** disease affecting travelers.
- Estimates of risk for contracting typhoid for short-stay travelers have ranged from 1 in 30,000 to 10 in 30,000 for trips to North Africa, India, and Senegal.
- CDC recommends typhoid vaccine for travelers to areas where there is an increased risk of exposure to *S. Typhi*. The typhoid vaccines do not protect against *Salmonella* Paratyphi infection.
- Two vaccines are recommended in the United States, **both of which give only about 70% protection and typhoid fever could still occur.**
- The newer vaccines became available during the 1990s and, although they do not result in improved vaccine efficacy, they do offer better ease of administration and fewer adverse reactions.
- A **parenteral Vi capsular polysaccharide vaccine** (Typhim Vi) given in a single intramuscular dose will give protection for **2 years**.
- An oral, live attenuated vaccine (Vivotif Berna) is administered in capsules, with one capsule taken every other day for 4 days; **a booster series is required every 5 years for those still at risk. It is not licensed for children younger than age 6 in the United States,** and administration of this vaccine may be limited by the ability of small children to ingest capsules.
- The oral vaccine results in fever or headache in up to 5% of recipients.
- In general, either the oral vaccine or the Vi capsular polysaccharide vaccine is the vaccine of choice for all individuals except for children between the ages of 6 months and 2 years, for whom the whole-cell vaccine is the only option available.
- **The oral typhoid vaccine is a live virus preparation and cannot be given to those travelers with HIV infection.**

- Growth of the live Ty21a strain is *inhibited by some antimicrobial agents and by the antimalarial agent* **mefloquine,** so the series should be completed before beginning antimalarials, or doses of each should be separated by at least 24 hours.
- Fortunately, chloroquine does not inhibit the growth of Ty21a.
- Vaccine may be administered at the same time as IG.
- The safety of vaccines against typhoid during pregnancy **has not** been established.

ANTIMALARIAL CHEMOPROPHYLAXIS

- Travelers should be aware that the peak biting time of mosquitoes is between dusk and dawn. Travelers should be advised to wear light-colored, long-sleeved clothing and socks and pants to minimize exposure.
- Also DEET may be used in combination with barrier protection, and mosquito netting should be used if possible.
- In general, *Anophelines* prefer to bite the lower extremities, often the ankles.
- Apart from those remaining areas with chloroquine-sensitive strains, mefloquine is usually the drug of choice for prevention.
- See Table 20-2 for information about the dosing of antimalarial drugs.
- Mefloquine has a very long half-life, and is recommended for prophylaxis and therapy in chloroquine-resistant areas.
- Resistance to mefloquine appears to depend on export by the pfmdr1 transporter protein. Pfmdr1 amplification is associated with mefloquine resistance (Table 20-3).
- Resistance to mefloquine is seen in much of Southeast Asia, although it appears to be effective in Africa.
- Mefloquine also has been used as solo treatment in much of Southeast Asia, although high levels of resistance have been noted.
- Mefloquine is still effective in most African countries and can be used in areas of chloroquine resistance.
- Mefloquine and halofantrine show a high degree of in vitro cross-resistance, and although evidence of in vivo cross-resistance is limited, it indicates that increasing levels of resistance to mefloquine may limit the effective chemotherapy lifetime of both mefloquine and halofantrine (Table 20-3).
- Mefloquine has been the subject of much controversy regarding its side effects but six randomized, double-blind trials and seven prospective comparative studies failed to find significant differences in the rates of adverse events or drug discontinuation between subjects taking mefloquine and those taking other antimalarial drugs.
- If mefloquine cannot be tolerated, an alternative is daily doxycycline.
- Doxycycline is the preferred agent for persons unable to take mefloquine and for those traveling to areas where there is mefloquine resistance, that is, the western provinces of Cambodia and the border regions between Thailand and Cambodia and between Thailand and Myanmar (Burma).
- Regional information regarding antimalarial resistance can be found on the Internet (www.cdc.gov/travel/regionalmalaria/index.htm).
- See Table 20-5 for geographic distribution of drug-resistant malaria
- An alternative for travelers who are unable to take mefloquine or doxycycline is the combination of weekly chloroquine plus daily proguanil (the product is not available in the United States).
- However, chloroquine plus proguanil is significantly less effective than doxycycline or mefloquine in areas where these agents have been studied.

Table 20-3	Side Effects of Mefloquine

Adverse Reactions

The most frequently reported adverse events are nausea, vomiting, loose stools or diarrhea, abdominal pain, dizziness or vertigo, loss of balance, and neuropsychiatric events, such as headache, somnolence, and sleep disorders (insomnia, abnormal dreams). These are usually mild and may decrease despite continued use.

Halofantrine must not be given simultaneously with or subsequent to Lariam, because significant, potentially fatal prolongation of the QTc interval of the electrocardiogram may result.

Concomitant administration of Lariam and quinine or quinidine may produce cardiographic abnormalities. Administration of Lariam with quinine or chloroquine may increase the risk of convulsions.

Mefloquine may cause psychiatric symptoms in a number of patients, ranging from anxiety, paranoia, and depression to hallucinations and psychotic behavior. On occasions, these symptoms have been reported to continue long after mefloquine has been stopped. Rare cases of suicidal ideation and suicide have been reported, although no relationship to drug administration has been confirmed. To minimize the chances of these adverse events, mefloquine should not be taken for prophylaxis in patients with active depression or with a recent history of depression, generalized anxiety disorder, psychosis, or schizophrenia or other major psychiatric disorders. Lariam should be used with caution in patients with a previous history of depression.

Lariam may increase the risk of convulsions in patients with epilepsy. Caution should be exercised with regard to activities requiring alertness and fine motor coordination, because dizziness, a loss of balance, or other disorders of the central or peripheral nervous system have been reported during and following the use of Lariam.

Periodic liver function tests and ophthalmic examinations are recommended during prolonged administration.

Lariam should be used during pregnancy only if the potential benefit justifies the potential risk to the fetus or nursing infant. Women of childbearing potential should be warned against becoming pregnant while taking Lariam.

Mefloquine is excreted in human milk. Because of the potential for serious adverse reactions in nursing infants, a decision should be made whether to stop taking Lariam, taking into consideration the importance of the drug to the mother.

Adapted from http://www.lariam.com/about_lariam.asp#safety_info and http://www.fda.gov/cder/foi/label/2003/19591s19lbl_Lariam.pdf.

Table 20-4	Vaccines for Travelers	
Vaccine	**Adult Dose**	**Indication**
Hepatitis A	1 mL IMBooster in 6 to 12 months.	Endemic area
HAV/SIG	2 mL IM staying <3 month 5 mL IM staying ≥3 months	Age ≥40
Hepatitis B	Three dose series	Travel to endemic area (≥2 prevalence of HBsAg serology)
Measles/MMR	0.5 mL SQ	Born after 1956 In all international travelers
Poliomyelitis	IPV	Last dose ≥5 years Eastern hemisphere one lifetime booster post primary series
Tetanus/ Diphtheria	Td Tdap	Every 10 years One time
Typhoid	one oral live four caps, taken one cap every other day 0.5 mL IM	Age ≥6 years Booster q 5years Booster q 2 years
Varicella vaccine	0.5 mL SQ × 2	Not immune,≥12 months old.
Japanese B encephalitis	IM on days 0 and 28. Newer Ixiaro vaccine.	Rural Asia in summer (visiting for more than 30 days in Encephalitis-endemic area)
Meningococcal	0.5 mL SQ	Epidemic area, SS Africa/ Mecca, Dec-June
Rabies	0,7, 21, or 28 days (three doses IM)	Endemic area for more than 3 months
Yellow fever	0.5 mL SQ Booster q 10 years	Endemic area, South subsaharan Africa, South America

- Primaquine is aimed at the preerythrocytic stage and thus may be a potential causal-prophylactic treatment that can abolish the need for long postexposure therapy.
- A potential advantage of primaquine, because of its activity against the liver stages of parasites, is that prophylaxis may be discontinued 1 week after the recipient has left the endemic area. Primaquine is not yet approved for this indication.
- For prophylaxis against *Plasmodium falciparum* malaria, primaquine has an efficacy and toxicity competitive with those of standard agents.
- Potential side effects include oxidant-induced hemolytic anemia and methemoglobinemia; its use is contraindicated in pregnant women and in persons with glucose-6-phosphate dehydrogenase deficiency.

Table 20-5	Geographic Distribution of Drug-Resistant Malaria	
Drug resistance	**Geographic Area of Drug-Resistant Malaria**	**Alternative Drug**
Mefloquine	Borders of Thailand with Burma (Myanmar) and Cambodia, western provinces of Cambodia, the eastern states of Burma on the border between Burma and China, along the borders of Laos and Burma, the adjacent parts of the Thailand-Cambodia border, and southern Vietnam	Atovaquone-proguanil, doxycycline.
Chloroquine	All areas with *P. falciparum* malaria except the Caribbean, Central America west of the Panama Canal, and some countries in the Middle East.	Atovaquone-proguanil, doxycycline, mefloquine.
Sulfadoxine-pyrimeth-amine	Amazon River Basin area of South America, much of Southeast Asia, other parts of Asia, and in large parts of Africa.	Mefloquine,- atovaquone-proguanil or doxycycline.

- It appears that the addition of chloroquine did not increase the prophylactic efficacy of primaquine.
- In combination with proguanil, the ability of atovaquone to inhibit parasitic mitochondrial electron transport is markedly enhanced.
- Evidence suggests that this drug combination has activity against a liver stage of the malaria parasite, allowing travelers to discontinue it 1 week after leaving a malarious area. Atovaquone/proguanil is highly effective against drug-resistant strains of *P. falciparum,* and cross-resistance has not been observed between atovaquone and other antimalarial agents. Halofantrine, artemisinin derivatives, and azithromycin should not be considered as first-line agents for prevention of malaria.
- The use of doxycycline or primaquine is contraindicated during pregnancy, but chloroquine is safe in all trimesters.
- Mefloquine may be considered for use during pregnancy when exposure to chloroquine-resistant *P. falciparum* is anticipated. Also the combination of chloroquine plus proguanil is considered to be safe.
- Please see Table 20-1 for information about useful Web sites (JWM).

SUGGESTED READINGS

Compendium of Animal Rabies Prevention and Control, 2001. National Association of State Public Health Veterinarians, Inc. *MMWR Recomm Rep* 2001;50:1–9.
The purpose of this compendium is to provide rabies information to veterinarians, public health officials, and others concerned with rabies prevention and control. Vaccination procedure recommendations are contained in Part I; all animal rabies vaccines licensed by the United States Department of Agriculture (USDA) and marketed in the United States are listed in Part II; Part III details the principles of rabies control.

Advice for travelers. *Med Lett Drugs Ther* 2002;44:33–8.

Abell L, et al. Health advice for travelers. *N Engl J Med* 2000;343:1045–1046.

Altekruse SF, et al. Factors in the emergence of food borne diseases. *Vet Clin North Am Food Anim Pract* 1998;14:1–15.
This article examines these factors and briefly addresses prevention and control of foodborne diseases.

Caeiro JP, et al. Oral rehydration therapy plus loperamide versus loperamide alone in the treatment of traveler's diarrhea. *Clin Infect Dis* 1999;28:1286–1289.
Administration of loperamide plus oral rehydration therapy (ORT) for the management of traveler's diarrhea, in cases in which subjects were encouraged to drink ad libitum, offered no benefit over administration of loperamide alone.

Camus D, et al. Clinical studies using the combination atovaquone-proguanil as malaria prophylaxis in non-immune adult and child travelers. *Med Trop (Mars)* 2002;62:225–228.
The combination of atovaquone/proguanil (Malarone) could provide an answer as it is not only effective on multiresistant strains of P. falciparum but also simplifies the conditions of administration and shows good tolerance in adults and children.

Cetron MS, et al. Yellow fever vaccine. Recommendations of the Advisory Committee on Immunization Practices (ACIP), 2002. *MMWR Recomm Rep* 2002;51:1–11; quiz 1–4.

Dick L. Travel medicine: helping patients prepare for trips abroad. *Am Fam Physician* 1998;58:383–398; 401–402.
Excellent review article. One-third of persons who travel abroad experience a travel-related illness, usually diarrhea or an upper respiratory infection. Medical advice for patients planning trips abroad must be individualized and based on the most current expert recommendations.

Dumont L, et al. Health advice for travelers. *N Engl J Med* 2000;343:1046.

Eichmann A. Sexually transmissible diseases following travel in tropical countries. *Schweiz Med Wochenschr* 1993;123:1250–1255.
Travel to tropical countries is an important factor in the spread of STDs. In spite of intensive anti-AIDS campaigns, some 30% of Swiss tourists have casual sexual contacts abroad.

Ericsson CD, et al. Treatment of traveler's diarrhea with sulfamethoxazole and trimethoprim and loperamide. *JAMA* 1990;263:257–261.
The combination of sulfamethoxazole-trimethoprim plus loperamide can be highly recommended for the treatment of most patients with traveler's diarrhea.

Fradin MS, Day JF. Comparative efficacy of insect repellents against mosquito bites. *N Engl J Med* 2002;347:13–18.
Currently available non-DEET repellents do not provide protection for durations similar to those of DEET-based repellents and cannot be relied on to provide prolonged protection in environments where mosquito-borne diseases are a substantial threat.

Freedman DO, Woodall J. Emerging infectious diseases and risk to the traveler. *Med Clin North Am* 1999;83:865–883, v.
This article examines the relationship between travel and emerging infections. The authors also discuss several novel pathogens, such as Ebola virus, that are clearly of insignificant or minimal risk to travelers, but are the subject of frequent questions from patients requesting pretravel advice from medical providers.

Fryauff DJ, et al. Randomised placebo-controlled trial of primaquine for prophylaxis of falciparum and vivax malaria. *Lancet* 1995;346:1190–1193.

Malaria prophylaxis with primaquine was evaluated in Irian Jaya for 1 year in Javanese men who were not deficient in glucose-6-phosphate dehydrogenase (G-6-PD). One hundred twenty-six volunteers were randomized to receive 0.5 mg/kg primaquine base or placebo daily (double-blinded), or 300 mg chloroquine base weekly (open). When used daily for 1 year by men with normal G-6-PD activity, primaquine was well tolerated and effective for prevention of malaria.

Glandt M, et al. Enteroaggregative *Escherichia coli* as a cause of traveler's diarrhea: clinical response to ciprofloxacin. *Clin Infect Dis* 1999;29:335–338.

This study provides additional evidence that enteroaggregative Escherichia coli (EAEC) should be considered as a cause of antibiotic-responsive traveler's diarrhea.

Heppner DG Jr, et al. Primaquine prophylaxis against malaria. *Ann Intern Med* 1999;130:536; author reply 536–537.

Hogh B, et al. Atovaquone-proguanil versus chloroquine-proguanil for malaria prophylaxis in non-immune travellers: a randomised, double-blind study. Malarone International Study Team. *Lancet* 2000;356:1888–1894.

Chloroquine plus proguanil is widely used for malaria chemoprophylaxis despite low effectiveness in areas where multidrug-resistant malaria occurs. Studies have shown that atovaquone and proguanil hydrochloride is safe and effective for prevention of falciparum malaria in lifelong residents of malaria-endemic countries, but little is known about nonimmune travelers. METH-ODS: "In a double-blind equivalence trial, 1,083 participants traveling to a malaria-endemic area were randomly assigned to two treatment groups: atovaquone-proguanil plus placebos for chloroquine and proguanil; or chloroquine, proguanil, and placebo for atovaquone-proguanil. Overall the two preparations were similarly tolerated. However, significantly fewer adverse gastrointestinal events were observed in the atovaquone-proguanil group than in the chloroquine-proguanil group."

Jong EC. Immunizations for international travel. *Infect Dis Clin North Am* 1998;12:249–266.

Immunization recommendations for international travelers is a complex subject that takes into consideration the geographic destination, planned activities during travel, health conditions at destination, length of trip, and underlying health status of the traveler.

Jong EC. Travel immunizations. *Med Clin North Am* 1999;83:903–922, vi.

An updated approach to selecting and prioritizing immunizations for the international traveler is presented. This article addresses vaccines against yellow fever, typhoid fever, cholera, meningococcal meningitis, rabies, tetanus, diphtheria, measles, mumps, rubella, polio, varicella, and influenza. Vaccine preparations, dosing regimens, efficacy, adverse effects, indications, and contraindications are discussed in the context of pretravel preparation.

Kain KC, et al. Imported malaria: prospective analysis of problems in diagnosis and management. *Clin Infect Dis* 1998;27:142–149.

Imported malaria is an increasing problem in many countries. The diagnosis of malaria was initially missed in 59% of cases. Community-based microscopic diagnosis provided incorrect species identification in 64% of cases. After presentation, the average delay before treatment was 7.6 days for falciparum malaria and 5.1 days for vivax malaria. Overall, 7.5% of P. falciparum-infected patients developed severe malaria, and in 11% of all cases, therapy failed. Patients who come to a center that has no expertise in tropical medicine receive suboptimal treatment. Improvements in recognition, diagnosis, and treatment of malaria are essential to prevent morbidity and death among travelers.

Laursen SB, Jacobsen E. Air travel and deep venous thrombosis. *Ugeskr Laeger* 1998;160:4079–4080.

A case of deep venous thrombosis (DVT) in a woman with polio sequelae is reported. Guidelines for air travelers to prevent the economy class syndrome are presented.

Lavelle O, Berland Y. Travel and renal insufficiency. *Med Trop (Mars)* 1997;57:449–451.

Traveling can be dangerous for subjects with kidney insufficiency. Pretravel evaluation is necessary to determine metabolic, nutritional, and immune status. Subjects with kidney insufficiency and transplanted kidneys should be informed of the dangers and appropriate action in case of trouble.

Lemon SM, et al. Immunoprecipitation and virus neutralization assays demonstrate qualitative differences between protective antibody responses to inactivated hepatitis A vaccine and passive immunization with immune globulin. *J Infect Dis* 1997;176:9–19.

These results are best explained by differences in the affinity of antibodies for virus following active versus passive immunization.

Magill AJ. The prevention of malaria. *Prim Care* 2002;29:815–842, v–vi.

In this article, the author focuses on practical uses of currently available prevention tools.

Maiwald H, et al. Long-term persistence of anti-HAV antibodies following active immunization with hepatitis A vaccine. *Vaccine* 1997;15:346–348.

Seventy-one anti-HAV-negative volunteers were immunized against hepatitis A. The annual decrease of anti-HAV titers was 25%. Based on these data, the antibody persistence was calculated over time. Geometric mean titers (GMTs) at protective levels higher than 20 mIU/mL can be expected to persist for at least 15 years.

McKeage K, Scott L. Atovaquone/proguanil: a review of its use for the prophylaxis of *Plasmodium falciparum* malaria. *Drugs* 2003;63:597–623.

In combination with proguanil, the ability of atovaquone to inhibit parasitic mitochondrial electron transport is significantly enhanced. Both atovaquone and proguanil are effective against hepatic stages of P. falciparum, which means that treatment need only continue for 7 days after leaving a malaria-endemic region. Atovaquone/proguanil was generally well tolerated and was associated with fewer gastrointestinal adverse events than chloroquine plus proguanil and fewer neuropsychiatric adverse events than mefloquine. Thus, atovaquone/proguanil provides effective prophylaxis of P. falciparum malaria and, compared with other commonly used antimalarial agents, has an improved tolerability profile. Overall, it offers a more convenient dosage regimen, particularly in the posttravel period.

Mileno MD, Bia FJ. The compromised traveler. *Infect Dis Clin North Am* 1998;12:369–412.

Compromised travelers represent a diverse and challenging group of individuals. These patients are also at greater risk for acquisition of tuberculosis, severe community-acquired pneumonia, urinary tract infections, and pyomyositis. Older travelers present both the infectious disease and travel medicine specialist with issues such as malignancy-related infections, myocardial infarction, and other forms of cardiopulmonary compromise, which the authors address in this article.

Miltgen J, N'Guyen G, et al. Travel and patients with allergies. *Med Trop (Mars)* 1997;57: 469–472.

By changing their surroundings and lifestyle, travelers with allergic conditions exposed themselves to new risks. Travelers with allergic conditions should carry alert identification cards and medications for routine as well as emergency treatment including self-injectable adrenaline.

Monath TP. Yellow fever: an update. *Lancet Infect Dis* 2001;1:11–20.

Yellow fever, the original viral hemorrhagic fever, was one of the most feared lethal diseases before the development of an effective vaccine. Today, the disease still affects as many as 200,000 persons annually in tropical regions of Africa and South America and poses a significant hazard to unvaccinated travelers to these areas. New applications of yellow fever 17D virus as a vector for foreign genes hold considerable promise as a means of developing new vaccines against other viruses, and possibly against cancers.

Mulhall BP. Sexually transmissible diseases and travel. *Br Med Bull* 1993;49:394–411.

STDs continue to be the most common notifiable infectious conditions worldwide. Their unacceptably high incidence is underlined by the recent emergence of a (presently) incurable and lethal STD, HIV infection, which merits its description as a pandemic, and with which other STDs interact in an epidemiologic synergy.

Ohrt C, et al. Mefloquine compared with doxycycline for the prophylaxis of malaria in Indonesian soldiers. A randomized, double-blind, placebo-controlled trial. *Ann Intern Med* 1997;126:963–972.

Mefloquine and doxycycline are the two drugs recommended for prophylaxis of malaria for visitors to areas where P. falciparum is resistant to chloroquine. Mefloquine and doxycycline were both highly efficacious and well tolerated as prophylaxis of malaria in Indonesian soldiers.

Ostroff SM, Kozarsky P. Emerging infectious diseases and travel medicine. *Infect Dis Clin North Am* 1998;12:231–241.

International movement of individuals, populations, and products is one of the major factors associated with the emergence and reemergence of infectious diseases as the pace of global travel and commerce increases rapidly. Because of the unique role of travel in emerging infections, efforts are under way to address this factor by agencies such as the CDC, WHO, the International Society of Travel Medicine, and the travel industry.

Overbosch D, et al. Atovaquone-proguanil versus mefloquine for malaria prophylaxis in nonimmune travelers: results from a randomized, double-blind study. *Clin Infect Dis* 2001;33:1015–1021.

Concerns about the tolerability of mefloquine highlight the need for new drugs to prevent malaria. Atovaquone-proguanil was better tolerated than was mefloquine, and it was similarly effective for malaria prophylaxis in nonimmune travelers.

Petruccelli BP, et al. Treatment of traveler's diarrhea with ciprofloxacin and loperamide. *J Infect Dis* 1992;165:557–560.

Although not delivering a remarkable therapeutic advantage, loperamide appears to be safe for treatment of nonenterotoxic Escherichia coli (ETEC) causes of traveler's diarrhea. Two of 54 patients with Campylobacter enteritis had a clinical relapse after treatment that was associated with development of ciprofloxacin resistance.

Pollack RJ, et al. Repelling mosquitoes. *N Engl J Med* 2002;347:2–3.

Ramzan NN. Traveler's diarrhea. *Gastroenterol Clin North Am* 2001;30:665–78, viii.

This article presents a review of causes, presentation, and diagnosis of traveler's diarrhea. Treatment and prevention of this common problem is described in some detail. Finally, a practical and cost-effective approach to evaluating and treating a returning traveler is presented.

Robert E, et al. Exposure to yellow fever vaccine in early pregnancy. *Vaccine* 1999;17:283–285.

Although the sample is too small to rule out a moderately increased risk of adverse reproductive effect of yellow fever vaccine, it gives no argument for such an effect and should help to reassure pregnant women who might be inadvertently vaccinated.

Ryan ET, Kain KC. Health advice and immunizations for travelers. *N Engl J Med* 2000;342:1716–1725.

Samuel BU, Barry M. The pregnant traveler. *Infect Dis Clin North Am* 1998;12:325–354.

The care of the pregnant traveler is both challenging and rewarding. A safety profile of commonly used travel medications, antibiotics, and antiparasitic drugs is reviewed.

Schwartz E, Regev-Yochay G. Primaquine as prophylaxis for malaria for nonimmune travelers: a comparison with mefloquine and doxycycline. *Clin Infect Dis* 1999;29:1502–1506.

Malaria prophylaxis for travelers is a controversial issue. Primaquine was shown to be a safe and effective prophylactic drug against both P. falciparum malaria and Plasmodium vivax malaria in travelers.

Shanks GD, et al. Effectiveness of doxycycline combined with primaquine for malaria prophylaxis. *Med J Aust* 1995;162:306–307, 309–310.

To assess the causal prophylactic activity (activity against the preerythrocytic liver stage) of a daily regimen of doxycycline combined with low-dose primaquine against malaria in Australian Defence Force personnel deployed to Papua New Guinea (PNG). Although doxycycline generally provides good protection against malaria infection, it cannot be relied on for causal prophylaxis, even when combined with low-dose primaquine. Because the malaria infections occurred only after return to Australia, doxycycline appears to be effective in suppressing malaria while the drug is being taken. Intense, repeated exposure to malaria may require an extended period of chemoprophylaxis on return from an endemic area.

Shanks GD, et al. Efficacy and safety of atovaquone/proguanil as suppressive prophylaxis for *Plasmodium falciparum* malaria. *Clin Infect Dis* 1998;27:494–499.

Both atovaquone/proguanil prophylactic regimens were as well tolerated as placebo. Thus, atovaquone/proguanil appears to be highly efficacious and safe as prophylaxis for P. falciparum malaria.

Shouval D, et al. Single and booster dose responses to an inactivated hepatitis A virus vaccine: comparison with immune serum globulin prophylaxis. *Vaccine* 1993;11(suppl 1): S9–S14.

Soto J, et al. Primaquine prophylaxis against malaria in nonimmune Colombian soldiers: efficacy and toxicity. A randomized, double-blind, placebo-controlled trial. *Ann Intern Med* 1998;129:241–244.

For prophylaxis against P. falciparum malaria, primaquine has an efficacy and toxicity competitive with those of standard agents. A potential advantage of primaquine is that prophylaxis may be discontinued 1 week after the recipient has left the endemic area.

Soto J, et al. Double-blind, randomized, placebo-controlled assessment of chloroquine/ primaquine prophylaxis for malaria in nonimmune Colombian soldiers. *Clin Infect Dis* 1999;29:199–201.

To improve upon the efficacy of primaquine prophylaxis for malaria (94%, P. falciparum malaria; 85%, P. vivax malaria), we administered chloroquine (300 mg weekly) in combination with primaquine (30 mg daily) to nonimmune Colombian soldiers during 16 weeks of patrol in a region of endemicity and for a further 1 week in base camp. Comparison of these data with data from a previous study indicates that the addition of chloroquine did not increase the prophylactic efficacy of primaquine.

Taylor DN, et al. Treatment of travelers' diarrhea: ciprofloxacin plus loperamide compared with ciprofloxacin alone. A placebo-controlled, randomized trial. *Ann Intern Med* 1991;114:731–734.

To compare the safety and efficacy of loperamide used in combination with ciprofloxacin or ciprofloxacin alone for the treatment of travelers' diarrhea. In a region where enterotoxigenic E. coli was the predominant cause of travelers' diarrhea, loperamide combined with ciprofloxacin was not better than treatment with ciprofloxacin alone. Loperamide appeared to have some benefit in the first 24 hours of treatment in patients infected with enterotoxigenic E. coli. Both regimens were safe.

Taylor WR, et al. Malaria prophylaxis using azithromycin: a double-blind, placebo-controlled trial in Irian Jaya, Indonesia. *Clin Infect Dis* 1999;28:74–81.

New drugs are needed for preventing drug-resistant P. falciparum malaria. Daily azithromycin offered excellent protection against P. vivax malaria but modest protection against P. falciparum malaria.

Virk A. Medical advice for international travelers. *Mayo Clin Proc* 2001;76:831–840.

Each year, approximately 30 to 40 million Americans travel outside the United States. This review primarily updates pretravel management of adults.

Wagner G, et al. Simultaneous active and passive immunization against hepatitis A studied in a population of travellers. *Vaccine* 1993;11:1027–1032.

Three hundred travelers, seronegative for hepatitis A, were enrolled into this study to evaluate a new inactivated hepatitis A vaccine. The slight inhibition of antibody production, induced by the concurrent administration of IG, does not affect the overall protection afforded by the vaccine. We conclude that simultaneous active and passive hepatitis A immunizations can be recommended.

Wiedermann G, et al. Estimated persistence of anti-HAV antibodies after single dose and booster hepatitis A vaccination (0–6 schedule). *Acta Trop* 1998;69:121–125.

Even when taking the minimum observed titers in the older age group into account, the duration of protection will be more than 10 years. Considering at the same time its good tolerability and compliance, the single-dose hepatitis A vaccination appears highly recommendable in travel medicine.

Wilde H, et al. Rabies update for travel medicine advisors. *Clin Infect Dis* 2003;37:96–100.

Rabies is a neglected disease in many developing countries. It is preventable, and the tools to prevent it are known. There is urgent need for more funding, for study of innovative dog population-control measures, and for sustainable canine immunization. Travelers who leave the safe environments of tourist hotels and buses in regions of Asia, Russia, Africa, and Latin America where canine rabies is endemic may be at risk of life-threatening exposure to rabies.

Wilson ME. Travel-related vaccines. *Infect Dis Clin North Am* 2001;15:231–251.

Studies on special and travel vaccines in older individuals are needed urgently to define how these vaccines should be used in older populations and whether alternative means for protection are needed.

21 Fever in Returning Travelers

Paras Patel and James W. Myers

INTRODUCTION

When patients are being evaluated, it is important to obtain a detailed history, perform a focused clinical examination, and obtain the appropriate lab tests to diagnose a travel-acquired infection.

- Important factors to consider would include the destination and the nature of the trip that was taken (business, leisure, and medical) as well as a description of accommodations, information about pretravel vaccinations or chemoprophylaxis during travel, a sexual history, and a list of exposures and risk factors.
- Knowledge of water and insect exposures, as well as what kind of human (sexual, medical) contacts occurred, can be used to help determine the degree of risk that exists for each patient.
- Seasonality and trip duration are important factors as well.
- Tables 21-1 and 21-2 may provide helpful clues to help determine an etiology.
- The incubation period of the illness often can help the physician formulate a differential diagnosis.

FEVER

- Infection is the most common cause of fever in the returned traveler, but other causes such as medications, thromboembolism, malignancy, and other noninfectious causes also need to be considered.
- Fever patterns, although classically described, are seldom useful in the clinical setting.
  - See Table 21-3 for specific details.
- Generally, a few illnesses account for the majority of diagnoses.
  - These would include malaria, dengue, typhoid, and viral hepatitis.
  - On the other hand, leptospirosis, amoebic liver abscess, viral meningitis, and relapsing fever are rare causes of febrile illness in the returning travelers.
  - Immunization history and compliance with antimalarial chemoprophylaxis are helpful clues to the etiology of fever.
  - Even though these measures clearly decrease the risk of acquiring malaria, no antimalarial chemoprophylactic regimen is completely protective.
  - Poor adherence with antimalarial drug regimens is well documented in travelers who contract malaria.
  - Malaria was the most common cause of hospital admissions in ill travelers in several studies from Europe, Australia, and Israel.
  - The most common illness that requires immediate treatment *is Plasmodium falciparum* malaria.

Table 21-1	Risk Factors for Infection after Travel

Exposure	Potential Diseases
Undercooked food	Cholera, salmonellosis, typhoid fever, *Escherichia coli*
Milk	*Brucella, Salmonella*, tuberculosis
Water exposure	Leptospirosis, schistosomiasis, dracontiasis
Infected animals	Brucellosis, plague, Q fever, rabies, tularemia, monkey pox, leptospirosis
Mosquitoes	Dengue fever, malaria, encephalitis
Ticks	Rickettsial diseases, tularemia, Colorado tick fever, relapsing fever, Babesia, typhus, Lyme, Crimean hemorrhagic fever
Reduviids	American trypanosomiasis
Tsetse flies	African trypanosomiasis
Sexual contacts	Chancroid, gonorrhea, hepatitis B, herpes, and HIV
Sick contacts	Meningococcal disease, tuberculosis, VHFs, severe acute respiratory syndrome (SARS)
Transfusion	Hepatitis, HIV, malaria, Chagas

- This should be urgently investigated with thick and thin blood smears. One of the most useful investigation for fever in returning travelers is a malaria film, which was positive in 45% of cases in which it was performed.
- The second largest group was assumed to have a nonspecific viral infection (25%).
- Cosmopolitan infections (urinary tract infection, community-acquired pneumonia, streptococcal sore throat, etc.) accounted for 9%.

Table 21-2	Incubation Periods

Less than 21 Days	More than 21 Days
Meningococcemia	Acute HIV infection
Nontyphoidal salmonellosis	Schistosomiasis
Plague	Epstein-Barr virus
Typhoid fever	Filariasis
Typhus	Secondary syphilis
VHFs	Amebic liver abscess
Yellow fever	Borreliosis (relapsing fever)
Campylobacter	Brucellosis
Toxigenic *E. coli*	Leishmaniasis
Influenza	Malaria
Rickettsial diseases	Rabies
Shigella	Tuberculosis
Measles	Viral hepatitis (A, B, C, D, E)
CMV	West African trypanosomiasis
East African trypanosomiasis	
Dengue fever	
Japanese encephalitis	
Leptospirosis	
Malaria	

Table 21-3	Fever Patterns	
Fever Patterns	**Illness**	**Comments**
Tertian	*P. vivax*	Fever spike every other day
Quartan	*P. malariae*	Spike every 3rd day
Saddleback	Dengue, yellow fever, and Colorado tick fever	Biphasic pattern. Febrile period between spikes
Relapsing	*Borealis* spp.	A period of days or weeks between spikes
Undulant	Brucellosis, visceral leishmaniasis	Moving like waves
Bradycardia	Typhoid and yellow fever	Relative to the temperature
Breakbone	Dengue	Severe myalgias

- Coincidental infections (schistosomiasis, filariasis, and intestinal helminths) were found in 16%.
- Serology was positive for HIV infection in 3%.
- Respiratory infections including influenza, diarrheal diseases, and urinary tract infections are, as a group, among the most common causes of fever in travelers.

RASH, SPLENOMEGALY, JAUNDICE, AND EOSINOPHILIA

- The presence of a rash often will alert the physician to a specific diagnosis (Table 21-4).
- A biopsy with pathologic analysis and culture can be very helpful.
- Splenomegaly and lymphadenopathy are often present as well (Table 21-5).

Table 21-4	Differential Diagnosis of Skin Lesions Associated with Travel				
Maculopapular	**Petechiae**	**Eschar**	**Chancre**	**Ulcers**	**Papular**
Dengue	Dengue	Anthrax	Syphilis	Leishman-iasis	Syphilis
Rubella	Leptospirosis			Mycobac-teria	Insect bites
Epstein-Barr virus (EBV)			African	Insect bites	Tungiasis
Rickettsia	Rickettsia	Rickettsia	Trypano-somiasis	STDs	Myiasis
Meningococ-cemia	Meningococ-cemia	Scrub typhus		Sporotri-chosis	Onchocer-ciasis
Rose spots in typhoid fever					
Measles					

Table 21-5	Diseases Associated with Lymphadenopathy and Splenomegaly		
Lymphadenopathy		**Splenomegaly**	
Localized	**Generalized**	**Bacterial**	**Nonbacterial**
Plague, tularemia African trypanosomiasis American trypanosomiasis, filariasis, toxoplasmosis Tuberculosis	Brucellosis, leptospirosis, melioidosis Dengue fever, Lassa fever, measles Visceral leishmaniasis HIV infection, secondary syphilis	Enteric fever, brucella, endocarditis, leptospirosis, typhus	EBV, CMV, HIV, malaria, visceral Leishmaniasis, trypanosomiasis, schistosomiasis

- The most common diseases in the tropics that present with fever and eosinophilia are acute schistosomiasis (Katayama fever) and ascariasis (Table 21-6).
- Diseases that may be associated with jaundice are noted in Table 21-7.

MALARIA

- Urgent evaluation of a potential *P. falciparum* malaria infection is required because it carries a high fatality rate of more than 20%. Attention should be given to the type of and compliance with any previously prescribed antimalarial medication.
- Perhaps out of a false sense of security, a greater prevalence of malaria is seen in residents of developing countries who have returned home to visit friends and relatives.

Table 21-6	Degree of Eosinophilia	
None to Rare	**Minimal to Moderate**	**Moderate to Significant**
Protozoa (Isospora, Toxoplasma rarely) Tapeworms	Filariasis Ascariasis Clonorchiasis Enterobiasis Trichuriasis Hydatid disease Cysticercosis	Trichinosis Loaiasis Strongyloidiasis Ascariasis Hookworm Paragonimiasis Onchocerciasis Fascioliasis Schistosomiasis Paragonimiasis Fasciolopsiasis Toxocariasis Angiostrongylus Gnathostomiasis

Table 21-7	Causes of Jaundice
Bacterial	**Nonbacterial**
Leptospirosis	Severe malaria
Typhus	Fascioliasis
Typhoid	Cytomegalovirus
	Viral hepatitis
	Yellow fever

- Regardless of whether antimalarial medication was taken, patients should have thick and thin smears (at least three over 48 hours) ordered for malaria.
- Symptoms of *P. falciparum* infection are usually apparent within 2 months of returning, but those caused by other species might take longer to present (several months). Some patients, such as immigrants and visitors from endemic areas and those taking chemoprophylaxis, may have delayed onset or atypical presentation.
- Almost all patients will report fever but not necessarily with classic fever pattern as noted in Table 21-3.
- They may also complain of malaise, headache, myalgias, and gastrointestinal symptoms. Jaundice and hepatosplenomegaly also may be seen as well.
- Rash and lymphadenopathy, however, are uncommon and should suggest another diagnosis. The World Health Organization (WHO) defines *severe malaria* as a parasitemic person (>5%) with one or more of the following: prostration, impaired consciousness, respiratory distress or pulmonary edema, seizures, circulatory collapse, abnormal bleeding, jaundice, hemoglobinuria, and anemia.
- Several complications of severe malaria can occur and include severe anemia, acute renal failure, respiratory failure, intravascular hemolysis, and cerebral malaria.
- Hematologic abnormalities are common, and liver function test results are often abnormal.
- An elevated bilirubin level in the face of a high lactate dehydrogenase level suggests hemolysis. Hypoglycemia and hyponatremia may be present as well.
- See Table 21-8 for details clinical manifestations of malaria.
- The thick blood film provides enhanced sensitivity of the blood film technique and is much better than the thin film for detection of low levels of parasitemia. As shown in Table 21-9, a thin smear is more useful for species identification than a thick smear.
  - A recognized way of estimating the number of parasites present in 1 μL of blood is to use a standard value for the white blood cell (WBC) count (8,000 WBC/μL).
  - Counting the number of parasites present until 200 WBCs have been seen and then multiplying the parasites counted by 40 will give the parasite count per microliter of blood.
  - The sensitivity for the examination of the thick blood film procedure is about 50 parasites/μL of blood, which is equivalent to 0.001% of red blood cells (RBC) infected.
  - The identification of the parasite to the species level is much easier and provides greater specificity.

Table 21-8 Clinical Manifestations of the Five Human Infections

Clinical Characteristics	P. vivax	P. ovale	P. malariae	P. falciparum	Plasmodium knowlesi
Incubation period	8–17 days	10–17 days	18–40 days	8–11 days	9–12 days
Fever pattern	Irregular (48 hours)	Irregular (48 hours)	Regular (72 hours)	Continuous remittent	Regular (24 hours)
Symptom periodicity	48 hours	48 hours	72 hours	36–48 hours	24–27 hours
Severity of disease	Moderate to severe	Mild	Moderate to severe	Severe	Moderate to severe
Fever, chills, malaise, fatigue, diaphoresis, headache, cough, anorexia, nausea, vomiting, abdominal pain, diarrhea, arthralgia, and myalgias	Presence	Presence	Presence	Presence	Presence
CNS manifestation	Rare	Possible	Rare	Very common	Possible
Nephrotic syndrome	Possible	Rare	Very common	Rare	Probably common
Pulmonary manifestation	Very common	Possible	Possible	Common	Rare
Hepatosplenomegaly	Possible	Possible	Possible	Possible	Not known
Anemia	Presence	Presence	Presence	Presence	Presence
Disseminated Intravascular coagulation	Rare	Rare	Very common	Rare	Rare

Table 21-9	Plasmodia in Giemsa-Stained Thin Blood Smears				
	P. vivax	*P. malariae*	*P. falciparum*	*P. ovale*	*P. knowlesi*
Shape and size of parasitized RBCs	1.5–2 times larger than normal; oval to normal; may be normal size until ring fills one-half of cell	Normal shape; size may be normal or slightly smaller	Both normal	60% of cells larger than normal and oval; 20% have irregular, frayed edges	Normal shape, size
Schuffner dots	Usually present	None	None; occasionally comma-like red dots are present (Maurer dots)	Present in all stages including early ring forms; dots may be larger and darker than in *P. vivax*	No true stippling; occasional faint dots
Infections of RBCs with multiple parasites	Occasional	Rare	Common	Occasional	Common
Ring	Large cytoplasm with occasional pseudopods and large chromatin dot	Dense cytoplasm and large chromatin dots	Delicate cytoplasm with one to two small chromatin dots	Dense cytoplasm and large chromatin dots.	Delicate cytoplasm; one to two prominent chromatin dots
Trophozoite	Large ameboid cytoplasm and chromatin with fine, yellowish-brown pigment	Compact, oval, band shaped, or nearly round cytoplasm almost filling cell with coarse, dark-brown pigment	Rarely seen in the peripheral blood	Compact with large chromatin; dark-brown pigment	Denser cytoplasm; large chromatin; occasional band forms; coarse, dark-brown pigment
Schizont	12–24 mature merozoites almost filling RBC with yellowish-brown, coalesced pigment	6–12 merozoites in rosettes or irregular clusters filling normal-sized cells	Not seen in peripheral blood	6–14 merozoites with large nuclei, clustered around mass of dark-brown pigment	Maximum of 16 merozoites with large nuclei, clustered around mass of coarse, dark-brown pigment; occasional rosettes
Gametocytes	Round to oval; homogeneous cytoplasm almost occupying RBC, diffuse delicate light brown pigment throughout parasite	Round to oval; compact may almost occupy RBC	Crescent or sausage shaped; chromatin in a single mass or diffuse, dark pigment mass	Smaller than *P. vivax*	Round to oval; compact; may almost occupy RBC.

- The thin blood film is often preferred for estimation of the parasitemia.
  - The parasitemia may be estimated by examination of a well-stained thin blood film. This is usually accomplished by noting the number of parasitized RBC (not individual parasites) seen in 10,000 RBC (equal to approximately 40 monolayer cell fields of a standard microscope using the 100× oil immersion objective; however, microscopists are advised to calculate the average number of cells per microscope field of view for their own microscopes) and expressing the number of parasitized cells seen as a percentage. The approximate numbers of parasites present in 1 μL of blood can be calculated by assuming that 1 μL of blood contains 5×10^6 RBC; therefore, a 1% parasitemia will contain 1 parasite/100 RBC or 50,000 parasites/μL of blood. Similarly, a 0.1% parasitemia will contain 5,000 parasites/μL of blood.
  - This may be corrected to exact counts if the total RBC count per microliter is known. See Table 21-10.
- **Polymerase chain reaction (PCR)** has been used to detect malaria as well. Its utility lies in its sensitivity, with the ability to detect five parasites or less per microliter of blood.
  - Nested and multiplex PCR methods can give valuable information when difficult morphologic problems arise during attempts to identify parasites to the species level.
- **Immunochromatographic dipsticks** offer the possibility of more rapid, nonmicroscopic methods for malaria diagnosis, thereby saving on training and time.
  - The new immunochromatographic antigen capture tests are capable of detecting more than 100 parasites/μL (0.002% parasitemia) and of giving rapid results (15 to 20 minutes).
  - They are commercially available in a kit with all the necessary reagents, and no extensive training or equipment is required to perform or interpret the results. The persistence of HRP-2 antigenemia beyond the clearance of peripheral parasitemia in certain cases reduces the usefulness of these assays for monitoring the response to therapy.
  - The overall sensitivity and specificity of rapid detection tests (RDTs) for the detection of *Falciparum* malaria are better than 90%. **However, sensitivity falls dramatically with low-level parasitemia, and at present, RDTs cannot be used alone to exclude malaria**.

Treatment of Malaria

- Uncomplicated malarial infections can usually be managed on an outpatient basis in the absence of other comorbidities. ***Plasmodium vivax and Plasmodium ovale infection treatment should be followed with eradication of liver hypnozoites to prevent relapse of infection***.
- Chloroquine is the drug of choice for treatment of the **erythrocytic forms for all nonfalciparum** species.
- Chloroquine resistance *P. vivax* (CRPV) has been known since the early 1990s, and it is an increasing problem, particularly in the regions of Papua New Guinea and Indonesia.
- Rare case reports of CRPV have also been documented in Burma (Myanmar), India, and Central and South America. Infections acquired anywhere except in Indonesia, East Timor, Papua New Guinea, and the Solomon Islands may be presumed to be chloroquine sensitive.
- Therapeutic options for CRPV include mefloquine, atovaquone-proguanil, or the combination of quinine plus tetracycline or doxycycline (Table 21-12).

Table 21-10   Available Techniques for Detection of Malarial Parasites in the Human

Technique	*Plasmodium* spp.	Limits of Detection (parasites per μL)	Sensitivity of Test (percent)	Specificity (percent)
Microscopy	Stains: Giemsa	Presence of *Plasmodium* spp. (thick film)	5–20	Excellent
		All *Plasmodium* spp. (thin smear)	50–200	Excellent
Fluorescent microscopy	Acridine orange	Presence of *Plasmodium* spp.	100	Poor
	Quantitative buffy coat	Presence of *Plasmodium* spp.	100	Poor
	Rhodamine 123	Presence of *Plasmodium* spp.	No data	Poor
	P. falciparum LDH detection	Specific for *P falciparum* and non-falciparum, principally *P. vivax*	100	88	88
Rapid diagnostic tests for antigen detection	HRP2 detection	*P falciparum, P vivax* or mixed nonfalciparum spp.	100	94	71
PCR test, limited to research use only.	Using primers encoding genus- and species-specific sequences	Presence of *Plasmodium* spp.	1–5	Poor	Poor

- Combination therapy of artemisinin such as dihydroartemisinin-piperaquine (DP) is suggested in areas where both *P. vivax* and *P. falciparum* are endemic and species diagnosis is unreliable.
- Pyronaridine plus artesunate versus mefloquine plus artesunate is being evaluated in the clinical trial for the treatment of *P. falciparum* and *P. vivax*.
- **Chloroquine also remains the treatment of choice for treatment of *P. ovale* and *Plasmodium malariae*.**
- First-line treatment of uncomplicated malaria due to chloroquine-resistant *P. falciparum* consists of one of the following agents: artemisinin derivative combinations atovaquone-proguanil, quinine-based regimen (in combination with doxycycline or clindamycin), and mefloquine (Lariam) in combination with artesunate or doxycycline.
- See Table 21-13 for details treatment of malaria.

See Tables 21-11 through 21-13 for information regarding treatment of malaria.

LEPTOSPIROSIS

- *Leptospirosis* is a bacterial zoonosis transmitted from animals to humans through contact with contaminated water or moist soil.
- It is caused by the spirochete, *Leptospira interrogans*, in the human host.

Table 21-11	CQ-Sensitive Strains			
Organism	**Treatment**	**Dose**	**Prevention**	**Comments**
Vivax, sensitive strains	Chloroquine (CQ) plus primaquine if sensitive.	1 g PO (600 mg of base) then 0.5 g at 6 hours and 0.5 g daily times 2 days. Total of 1,500 mg of base. *Give 30 mg of primaquine base/day times 14 days.*	CQ 500 mg (300 mg base) PO q week beginning 1–2 weeks before and continuing until 4 weeks after travel	For persons with borderline G6PD deficiency or as an alternate to the above regimen, primaquine may be given at the dose of 45 mg (base) orally one time per week for 8 weeks. Primaquine must not be used during pregnancy
Ovale	CQ plus primaquine	As above	As above	G6PD as above
Malariae	CQ	As above for CQ	As above	
Falciparum, sensitive strains	CQ	As above for CQ	As above	Haiti, Central America, Parts of Middle East

Table 21-12	Treatment of CQ-Resistant Organisms	
Organism	Treatment	Dose	Comments
Vivax, CQ resistant	Quinine sulfate plus doxycycline and primaquine, mefloquine (MQ) plus primaquine	(A) 542 mg of base (650 mg of salt) PO t.i.d. for 3–7 days. Doxycycline 100 mg PO b.i.d. times 7 days. Primaquine as above. (B) MQ 684 mg base (750 mg salt), then 456 mg base (500 mg salt) PO given 6–12 hours after initial dose for a total of 1,250 mg salt	Papua New Guinea and Indonesia and other areas occasionally atovaquone plus proguanil There are no adequate, well-controlled studies to support the use of atovaquone-proguanil to treat CRPV infections Less desirable is MQ 750 mg salt PO as an initial dose followed by 500 mg salt 6–12 hours later
Falciparum, resistant	(A) Atovaquone (250 mg) proguanil (100 mg). Known as Malarone (B) Artemether-lumefantrine (Coartem) (C) Quinine sulfate plus doxycycline (D) Mefloquine	(A) 4 tablets PO q day times 3 days. (B) **1 tablet = 20 mg artemether and 120 mg lumefantrine.** A 3-day treatment schedule with a total of six oral doses is recommended for both adult and pediatric patients based on weight. The patient should receive the initial dose, followed by the second dose 8 hours later, then one dose PO b.i.d. for the following 2 days. 5 to <15 kg: one tablet per dose. 15 to <25 kg: two tablets per dose. 25 to <35 kg: three tablets per dose. ≥35 kg: four tablets (C) 542 mg base (650 mg salt) PO t.i.d. times 7 days. (3 days for Africa) Plus 100 mg b.i.d. times 7 days for doxycycline (D) 684 mg base (=750 mg salt) PO as initial dose, followed by 456 mg base (=500 mg salt) PO given 6–12 hours.	
Severe Falciparum	Quinidine gluconate plus doxycycline (or clindamycin) times 7 days if necessary	Dose of quinidine is 6.25 mg base/kg loading dose IV over 2 hours, then 0.0125 mg base/kg minute continuous infusion times 24 hours	Once the parasitemia level is <1%, try oral quinine if possible

Table 21-13	Prevention of CQ-Resistant *Falciparum*		
Organism	**Prevention**	**Dose**	**Comments**
CQ-resistant Falciparum	(A) Atovaquone-proguanil daily (B) Doxycycline 100 mg daily (C) MQ (D) Primaquine	(A) One adult tablet orally, daily (B) 100 mg daily (C) 228 mg base (250 mg salt) orally, once/week 30 mg base daily	Atovaquone/proguanil primary prophylaxis should begin 1–2 days before travel to malarious areas and should be taken daily, at the same time each day, while in the malarious area, and daily for 7 days after leaving such areas (A) Doxycycline primary prophylaxis should begin 1–2 days before travel to malarious areas. It should be continued once a day, at the same time each day, during travel in malarious areas, and daily for 4 weeks after the traveler leaves such areas MQ primary prophylaxis should begin 1–2 weeks before travel to malarious areas. It should be continued once a week, on the same day each week, during travel to malarious areas, and for 4 weeks after the traveler leaves such areas Primaquine primary prophylaxis should begin 1–2 days before travel to the malaria-risk area. It should be continued once a day, at the same time each day, while in the malaria-risk area, and daily for 7 days after leaving the malaria-risk area For MQ resistance, use either atovaquone-proguanil or doxycycline. Most likely in parts of Burma, Cambodia or Thailand

- People who work close to where either rats or infected livestock contact water are at a higher risk of infection. Leptospirosis is an important cause of fever in travelers returning from the tropics.
- Prophylaxis with 200 mg of doxycycline per week can be considered for those at highest risk.
- Travelers will become ill within 1 to 2 weeks after a potential exposure.
- The majority of patients (90%) experience a mild febrile illness, but more severe forms can affect some patients.
- A biphasic course of illness is characteristic.
  - The initial or *septicemic* stage is characterized by the sudden onset of fever, retro-orbital headache, chills, myalgias, conjunctival suffusion, and skin rashes. In addition to the conjunctival injection seen in the primary stage, a uveitis can be seen in the secondary stage. Defervescence of fever occurs in 7 days in this phase and is usually followed by an interval afebrile period of 2 days.
  - The second or *immune phase* is heralded by the appearance of IgM antibodies. The organisms usually cannot be cultured from blood or cerebrospinal fluid (CSF) during this second immune phase but can be found in the urine for months. Symptoms may recur and meningitis is noted in about 50% of cases.
- Severe cases are characterized by renal failure, pulmonary hemorrhage, jaundice, and myocarditis.
- The treatment of choice is doxycycline, 100 mg orally twice a day for 7 days as an outpatient. Hospitalized patients with severe disease can be treated with intravenous penicillin (6 million units daily), doxycycline (100 mg twice daily), ceftriaxone (1 g every 24 hours), or cefotaxime (1 g every 6 hours).
- The clinical features and routine laboratory findings of leptospirosis are not specific, so a high index of suspicion must be maintained for the diagnosis.
- Usually the diagnosis is made serologically but can be made by culture of the organism on special media such as Fletcher, Stuart, Ellinghausen-McCullough-Johnson-Harris (EMJH), or Tween 80-albumin medium.
- Appropriate fluids to be cultured include blood and CSF during the first week of illness; urine should be cultured thereafter. Detection of leptospiral DNA by PCR is more sensitive than culture. The spirochetes can be demonstrated in tissue sections with silver stains as well.

DENGUE

- Also known as *breakbone fever*, this mosquito-borne illness is typically self-limited and nonfatal.
- It is caused by one of four single-stranded, positive-sense RNA viruses (dengue virus type 1 through dengue virus type 4) of the genus flavivirus (family Flaviviridae).
- Dengue viruses present in the urban or endemic areas where humans and mosquitoes are the only known hosts, where as in the forested areas, transmission of mosquito-borne viruses occurs between nonhuman primates and, rarely, from these primates to humans.
- After an **incubation period of about 1 week**, symptoms start suddenly and follow three phases:
  - An initial febrile phase, a critical phase around the time of defervescence, and a spontaneous recovery phase

- ○ The initial phase is characterized by high-grade fever associated with headache, retro-orbital pain, vomiting, myalgia, and arthralgia.
- ○ Transient macular rash and hepatomegaly may be noted on physical examination. Only minor hemorrhagic manifestations such as petechiae or bruising are present in most patients at venipuncture sites, but occasionally significant bleeding results from gastrointestinal ulcers may occur.
- ○ Mild to moderate leukopenia, thrombocytopenia and moderated elevation of hepatic aminotransferase not uncommon.
- Second phase of illness—critical phase of dengue hemorrhagic fever (DHF) characterized by ascites, pleural effusions, and spontaneous hemorrhages, including gastrointestinal hemorrhage, ecchymoses, and epistaxis.
  - ○ Capillary permeability and coagulation defects lead to hemorrhagic manifestations and, in more severe cases, to hypovolemic shock.
  - ○ The risk factors of hemorrhage in DHF/dengue shock syndrome (DSS) are prolonged shock with a normal or low hematocrit at the time of shock.
  - ○ DHF and DSS appear to have an immunologic basis and occur with subsequent episodes of dengue.
- Final recovery phase is characterized by healing of altered vascular permeability after 48 to 72 hours and improvement in the patient's symptoms.
  - ○ Mild maculopapular rash to severe itchy lesion suggesting leukocytoclastic vasculitis may appear during the recovery phase, which resolve with desquamation over a period of 1 to 2 weeks period.
- Laboratory diagnosis is confirmed with detection of viral nucleic acid in serum by means of reverse transcriptase-polymerase chain reaction (RT-PCR) assay or detection of the virus-expressed soluble nonstructural protein 1 (NS1) by means of enzyme-linked immunosorbent assay (ELISA) or the lateral-flow rapid test during febrile phase of dengue fever.
- Detection of high level of IgM in a single specimen obtained from a patient with a clinical syndrome of dengue fever widely used to establish a presumptive diagnosis.
- At present, there is no specific drug therapy for DHF beyond supportive care.
- A dengue fever vaccine ChimeriVax (Sanofi Pasteur), which is a tetravalent formulation of attenuated yellow fever 17D vaccine strains expressing the dengue virus prM and E proteins is being investigated.
  - There is a multicenter phase 2 to 3 clinical trials that are under way; those are designed to determine the efficacy of this three-dose vaccine.
- Other candidates in early phases of clinical development include vaccines containing live attenuated dengue viruses and recombinant subunit vaccines.

SUGGESTED READINGS

Advice for travelers. *Med Lett Drugs Ther* 2002;44:33–38.

Abell L, et al. Health advice for travelers. *N Engl J Med* 2000;343:1045–1046.

Antinori S, Galimberti L, Gianelli E, et al. Prospective observational study of fever in hospitalized returning travelers and migrants from tropical areas, 1997–2001. *J Travel Med* 2004;11:135–142.

Brown WM, Yowell CA, Hoard A, et al. Comparative structural analysis and kinetic properties of lactate dehydrogenases from the four species of human malarial parasites. *Biochemistry* 2004;43(20):6219.

Cetron MS, et al. Yellow fever vaccine. Recommendations of the Advisory Committee on Immunization Practices (ACIP), 2002. *MMWR Recomm Rep* 2002;51:1–11;quiz CE1–4.

This report updates Centers for Disease Control and Prevention's (CDC) recommendations for using yellow fever vaccine.

Cheng AC, Thielman NM. Update on traveler's diarrhea. *Curr Infect Dis Rep* 2002;4:70–77.

Fluoroquinolones effectively treat severe traveler's diarrhea, and even a single dose may be sufficient. However, with the emergence of resistance, particularly in Campylobacter infection, other agents are required; interest has focused on azithromycin and rifaximin.

Cristian Speil MD, Adnan Mushtaq MD, Alys Adamski BS, et al. Fever of unknown origin in the returning traveler. *Infect Dis Clin North Am* 2007; 21:1091–1113.

D'Acremont V, et al. Practice guidelines for evaluation of fever in returning travelers and migrants. *J Travel Med* 2003;10(suppl 2):S25–S52.

Although the quality of evidence was limited by the paucity of clinical studies, these guidelines established with the support of a large and highly experienced panel should help physicians to deal with patients coming back from the tropics with fever.

Doherty JF, Grant AD, Bryceson AD. Fever as the presenting complaint of travelers returning from the tropics. *QJM* 1995;88:277–281.

Dumont L, et al. Health advice for travelers. *N Engl J Med* 2000;343:1046.

DuPont HL. Treatment of travelers' diarrhea. *J Travel Med* 2001;8(suppl 2):S31–S33.

Eichmann A. Sexually transmissible diseases following travel in tropical countries. *Schweiz Med Wochenschr* 1993;12324:1250–1255.

Travel to tropical countries is an important factor in the spread of sexually transmitted diseases.

Ericsson CD. Rifaximin: a new approach to the treatment of travelers' diarrhea. Conclusion. *J Travel Med* 2001;8(suppl 2):S40.

Fradin MS, Day JF. Comparative efficacy of insect repellents against mosquito bites. *N Engl J Med* 2002;347:13–18.

Freedman DO, Woodall J. Emerging infectious diseases and risk to the traveler. *Med Clin North Am* 1999;83:865–883, v.

The authors also discuss several novel pathogens, such as Ebola virus, that are clearly of insignificant or minimal risk to travelers but are the subject of frequent questions from patients requesting pretravel advice from medical providers.

Freedman DO, Weld LH, Kozarsky PE, et al. Spectrum of disease and relation to place of exposure among ill returned travelers. *N Engl J Med* 2006;354:119–30.

Forney JR, Wongsrichanalai C, Magill AJ, et al. Devices for rapid diagnosis of Malaria: evaluation of prototype assays that detect *Plasmodium falciparum* histidine-rich protein 2 and a Plasmodium vivax-specific antigen. *J Clin Microbiol* 2003;41(6):2358.

Fryauff DJ, et al. Randomised placebo-controlled trial of primaquine for prophylaxis of falciparum and vivax malaria. *Lancet* 1995;346:1190–1193.

Isaacson M. Viral hemorrhagic fever hazards for travelers in Africa. *Clin Infect Dis* 2001;33: 1707–1712.

This short review covers six viral hemorrhagic fevers (VHFs) that are known to occur in Africa: yellow fever, Rift Valley fever, Crimean-Congo hemorrhagic fever, Lassa fever, Marburg virus disease, and Ebola hemorrhagic fever.

James WD. Imported skin diseases in dermatology. *J Dermatol* 2001;28:663–666.

The clinical characteristics, diagnostic tests, and therapeutic options for such imported tropical diseases are discussed.

Jong EC. Immunizations for international travel. *Infect Dis Clin North Am* 1998;12:249–266.

Jong EC. Risks of hepatitis A and B in the traveling public. *J Travel Med* 2001;8(suppl 1): S3–S8.

Joubert JJ, et al. Schistosomiasis in Africa and international travel. *J Travel Med* 2001;8: 92–99.

Leder K, et al. Travel vaccines and elderly persons: review of vaccines available in the United States. *Clin Infect Dis* 2001;33:1553–1566.

Consideration of potential age-related differences in responses to travel vaccines is becoming increasingly important as elderly persons more frequently venture to exotic destinations.

Lo Re V III, Gluckman SJ. Eosinophilic meningitis due to Angiostrongylus cantonensis in a returned traveler: case report and review of the literature. *Clin Infect Dis* 2001;33:e112–e115. *Angiostrongylus cantonensis, the rat lungworm, is the principal cause of eosinophilic meningitis worldwide. The increase in world travel and ship-borne dispersal of infected rat vectors has extended this parasite to regions outside of its traditional geographic boundaries.*

Magill AJ. Fever in the returned traveler. *Infect Dis Clin North Am* 1998;12:445–469. *Excellent review article.*

Magill AJ. The prevention of malaria. *Prim Care* 2002;29:815–842, v–vi.

Maiwald H, et al. Long-term persistence of anti-HAV antibodies following active immunization with hepatitis A vaccine. *Vaccine* 1997;15:346–348. *Geometric mean titers (GMTs) at protective levels higher than 20 mIU mL-L can be expected to persist for at least 15 years.*

Matteelli A, Carosi G. Sexually transmitted diseases in travelers. *Clin Infect Dis* 2001;32: 1063–1067. *Prevention of sexually transmitted diseases (STDs) is a low priority among travel clinic services, despite increasing evidence that travelers have an increased risk of acquiring such infections.*

Makler MT, Hinrichs DJ. Measurement of the lactate dehydrogenase activity of *Plasmodium falciparum* as an assessment of parasitemia. *Am J Trop Med Hyg* 1993;48(2):205.

Makler MT, Piper RC, Milhous WK. Lactate dehydrogenase and the diagnosis of malaria. *Parasitol Today* 1998;14(9):376.

Mileno MD, Bia FJ. The compromised traveler. *Infect Dis Clin North Am* 1998;12:369–412.

Monath TP. Yellow fever: an update. *Lancet Infect Dis* 2001;1:11–20.

Moody A. Rapid diagnostic tests for malaria parasites. *Clin Microbiol Rev* 2002;15:66–78. *Comparison of methods for diagnosing Plasmodium infection in blood. Table 21-3 is very informative*

O'Brien D, et al. Fever in returned travelers: review of hospital admissions for a 3-year period. *Clin Infect Dis* 2001;33:603–609.

Parola P, Soula G, Gazin P, et al. Fever in travelers returning from tropical areas: prospective observational study of 613 cases hospitalised in Marseilles, France, 1999–2003. *Travel Med Infect Dis* 2006;4:61–70.

Pollard AJ, Shlim DR. Epidemic meningococcal disease and travel. *J Travel Med* 2002;9:29–33.

Ramzan NN. Traveler's diarrhea. *Gastroenterol Clin North Am* 2001;30:665–678, viii. *This article presents a review of causes, presentation, and diagnosis of traveler's diarrhea. Treatment and prevention of this common problem is described in some detail. Finally, a practical and cost-effective approach to evaluating and treating a returning traveler is presented.*

Rueangweerayut R, Phyo AP, Uthaisin C, et al; Pyronaridine–Artesunate Study Team. Pyronaridine–artesunate versus Mefloquine plus Artesunate for Malaria. *N Engl J Med* 2012;366:1298–1309.

Rieder HL. Risk of travel-associated tuberculosis. *Clin Infect Dis* 2001;33:1393–1396.

Ryan ET, Calderwood SB. Cholera vaccines. *J Travel Med* 2001;8:82–91.

Sa-ngasang A, et al. Evaluation of RT-PCR as a tool for diagnosis of secondary dengue virus infection. *Jpn J Infect Dis* 2003;56:205–209. *Review of this diagnostic tool.*

Samuel BU, Barry M. The pregnant traveler. *Infect Dis Clin North Am* 1998;12:325–354. *A safety profile of commonly used travel medications, antibiotics, and antiparasitic drugs is reviewed.*

Simmons CP, Farrar JJ, Nguyen VV, et al. Dengue. *N Engl J Med* 2012;366:1423–1432.

Stienlauf S, Segal G, Sidi Y, et al. Epidemiology of travel-related hospitalization. *J Travel Med* 2005;12:136–141.

Steffen R. Immunization against hepatitis A and hepatitis B infections. *J Travel Med* 2001;8(suppl 1):S9–S16.

Taylor WR, et al. Malaria prophylaxis using azithromycin: a double-blind, placebo-controlled trial in Irian Jaya, Indonesia. *Clin Infect Dis* 1999;28:74–81.

Daily azithromycin offered excellent protection against P. vivax malaria but modest protection against P. falciparum malaria.

Virk A. Medical advice for international travelers. *Mayo Clin Proc* 2001;76:831–840.

This review primarily updates pretravel management of adults.

Wagner G, et al. Simultaneous active and passive immunization against hepatitis A studied in a population of travelers. *Vaccine* 1993;11:1027–1032.

The slight inhibition of antibody production induced by the concurrent administration of immunoglobulin does not affect the overall protection afforded by the vaccine. We conclude that simultaneous active and passive hepatitis A immunizations can be recommended.

22 Infectious Diarrhea
Jonathan P. Moorman and James W. Myers

Clinically, diarrhea is defined by the passage of three or more watery stools, or one or more bloody stools, in 24 hours. Viruses account for 50% to 70% of causes of acute infectious diarrhea, bacteria 15% to 20%, and parasites 10% to 15%, and it appears that 5% to 10% of cases are of unknown etiology. Definitions of the types of diarrhea are shown in Table 22-1. Specific indications for medical evaluation include profuse watery diarrhea with dehydration; dysentery; passage of many small-volume stools containing blood and mucus; fever (temperature of 38.5°C [101.3°F] or higher); passage of six or more unformed stools every 24 hours or a duration of illness longer than 48 hours; diarrhea with severe abdominal pain in a patient older than age 50; and diarrhea in the elderly (age 70 or older) or the immunocompromised patient (AIDS, after transplantation, or receipt of cancer chemotherapy). Note: *Clostridium difficile*–associated diarrhea is covered in an accompanying chapter dedicated to nosocomial infection.

DIAGNOSIS

- From a study at the University Hospital of Geneva, the culture positivity rate of 6.1% decreased to 2.7% when patients received antimicrobial agents ($p < 0.001$). The positivity rate for patients hospitalized for 3 days or fewer was 12.6%, whereas it dropped to 1.4% for patients hospitalized for longer than 3 days ($p < 0.001$).
- Stool studies will be more useful in those patients who have a history of bloody diarrhea; have traveled to an endemic area; or have recently had antibiotics, immunosuppression, or exposure to infants in day care centers.
- The bacterial enteropathogens identified by normal stool culture are *Shigella, Salmonella, Campylobacter, Aeromonas,* and usually *Yersinia.* As an alternative, a rectal swab can be placed in transport media and then cultured. Please note that some pathogens will not be detected by routine stool culture. One should alert the laboratory to look for these microbes: *Escherichia coli* 0157:H7 and other Shigatoxin-producing *E. coli, Vibrios cholerae,* other noncholera *Vibrios,* and possibly *Yersinia.*
- Positive fecal leukocyte, lactoferrin, and occult blood tests lend support toward using empiric antimicrobial therapy. Conversely, when negative, they will eliminate the need for stool cultures. The most commonly identified pathogens in patients with these positive test results include *Shigella, Salmonella, Campylobacter, Aeromonas, Yersinia,* noncholera *Vibrios,* and *C. difficile.*
- Several studies have shown that the *routine* ordering for ova and parasites is not cost-effective in severe acute diarrhea.
- A **travel history** is important to help define who might benefit from such testing. Infection by *Cryptosporidium, Giardia,* or both, should be suspected whenever one returns from Russia; *Cyclospora* should be considered in travelers to Nepal; and *Giardia* should be suspected in persons who have recently traveled to the mountainous areas of North America. In day care centers, *Giardia* and *Cryptosporidium* are

Table 22-1		Definitions of Types of Diarrhea
Entity	**Days**	**Comments**
Diarrhea		Defined as stool weight >200 g in 24 hours. The average stool output is 100 g of stool per day.
Acute	<14	
Persistent	>14	
Chronic	>30	
Severe		The patient will have one or more of the following: volume depletion, fever, six or more stools in 24 hours, an illness lasting longer than 48 hours, or be immunocompromised.

common causes of diarrhea. Also note that homosexual males will often have positive results for *Giardia* and *Entamoeba histolytica*. See Tables 22-2 and 22-3 for information about persistent and/or parasitic causes of diarrhea.

TREATMENT OF COMMON PATHOGENS

• In all patients with diarrhea requiring medical evaluation, fluid and electrolyte therapy and alteration of the diet should be part of the management.
• When nonspecific therapy is desired, loperamide is the drug of choice for most cases of diarrhea. Loperamide is the recommended agent for most cases of diarrhea because of its safety and efficacy of approximately 80%.
• Diphenoxylate possesses central opiate effects, which can be problematic. The antimotility drugs should not be given to patients with moderate to severe *C. difficile*–related diarrhea. Bismuth subsalicylate (BSS) is the preferred agent when vomiting is the important clinical manifestation of enteric infection. BSS, however, should not be given to immunocompromised patients with diarrhea to prevent the taking of excessive doses.
• In some cases of severe, refractory cases, octreotide may be effective. Consultation with a gastrointestinal (GI) specialist is advised. Table 22-4 includes information on treatment of common bacterial pathogens.

TRAVELER'S DIARRHEA

General Concerns

• The most common travel disease is traveler's diarrhea (TD), affecting between 20% and 75% of those who vacation abroad. The onset of TD usually occurs within the first week of travel but may occur at any time while traveling, and even after returning home.
• The risk of TD varies according to the itinerary of the tourist. Risk also varies according to the underlying health status and age of the host, with the highest incidence occurring in small children and young adults aged 20 to 30.
• Certain conditions may predispose patients to a higher risk of acquiring TD, including those with HIV and other immunocompromising conditions.
• Choice of cuisine also affects a traveler's risk. Particularly risky would be food bought from a street vendor. Higher risk foods include uncooked vegetables, salads,

Table 22-2	Acid-Fast Negative Protozoans				

Organism	Geography	Transmission	Clinical Features	Diagnosis	Treatment
Giardia lamblia	Anywhere but notably acquired in St. Petersburg, and the mountainous regions in North America	Waterborne and person to person Boil drinking water, or if not possible, use halogenated water purification tablets Patients with common variable immunodeficiency or x-linked agammaglobulinemia are at increased risk of infection	1–2 weeks incubation period. The clinical spectrum of giardiasis is broad, including asymptomatic cyst passage; acute, often self-limited diarrhea; and chronic severe diarrhea with malabsorption and weight loss. In addition to diarrhea, a majority of symptomatic patients report bloating, cramping, and foul-smelling, greasy stools	Identification of cysts or motile trophozoites in stool or duodenal aspirate. Sensitivity is around to 85%–90% after three stools. Newer antigen detection assays range in sensitivity from 85%–98%	Metronidazole 250–500 t.i.d. for 1–2 weeks Tinidazole 2 g PO × one dose Paromomycin 25–30 mg/kg/day in three doses for 5–10 days Avoid milk products if there is a transient lactase deficiency

(Continued)

Table 22-2	Acid-Fast Negative Protozoans *(Continued)*				
Organism	**Geography**	**Transmission**	**Clinical Features**	**Diagnosis**	**Treatment**
Microsporidia, Enterocytozoon bieneusi and Encephalitozoon (formerly Septata) intestinalis	Diverse locations	Any immunocompromised patient presenting with persistent unexplained diarrhea. HIV	Persistent diarrhea	Calcofluor White and Uvitex stains lack specificity Polymerase chain reaction techniques hold promise for improved detection of microsporidia in stool.	Albendazole 400–800 mg PO b.i.d. for 3 or more weeks Other therapies besides albendazole under study include metronidazole, atovaquone, thalidomide, and nitazoxanide Albendazole is not effective for *E. bieneusi*
E. histolytica	Diverse locations	Fecal-oral	Persistent diarrhea	Stool studies or serologic tests. Serologic tests such as enzyme-linked immunosorbent assay and agar gel diffusion are more than 90% sensitive, but these tests often become negative within a year of initial infection	Metronidazole, 750 mg t.i.d. × 5–10 days, plus either diiodohydroxyquin, 650 mg t.i.d. × 20 days, or paromomycin, 500 mg t.i.d. × 7 days

Table 22-3	Acid-Fast Organisms	
Parasite	**Treatment**	**Comments**
Cryptosporidium	If severe, consider paromomycin, 500 mg t.i.d. × 7 days	5 μm. Yellow under auramine. Fluorescence with monoclonal antibody to *Cryptosporidium*
Isospora spp	Bactrim DS, b.i.d. × 7–10 days	20–30 μm long containing two visible sporocysts that are acid-fast. Eosinophilia is possible.
Cyclospora	Bactrim DS b.i.d. × 7 days	10 μm in diameter. Bright blue under ultraviolet light

Table 22-4	Treatment of Common Bacterial Pathogens		
Etiology	**Treatment**	**Dose**	**Comments**
Shigellosis (febrile dysentery)	FQ (possibly Bactrim or azithromycin)	500 mg PO b.i.d. × 3 days. Bactrim DS PO b.i.d. × 3 days	Up to 10 days if immunocompromised
Moderate to severe TD	FQ	Cipro 500 mg PO b.i.d. × 3–5 days or Bactrim DS PO b.i.d. × 3 days	Treat for longer if ill enough. One dose may be helpful in mild cases.
Enteropathogenic *E. coli* diarrhea (EPEC)	Treat as febrile dysentery		
Enterotoxigenic *E. coli* diarrhea (ETEC)	Treat as for mod-severe TD		
Enteroinvasive *E. coli* diarrhea (EIEC)	Treat as for *Shigella*		
Enterohemorrhagic *E. coli* diarrhea (EHEC)	Avoid if possible. May increase HUS risk		Avoid antimotility agents
Salmonella	Cipro (Azithro and ceftriaxone also effective)	500 mg PO b.i.d. × 5–7 days.	Treat if immunocompromised or ill.
Campylobacteriosis	Azithromycin or Cipro (FQ)	500 mg q day × 3 days, or 500 mg b.i.d. × 3 days	FQ resistance occurs. Emycin may be used as well

Table 22-4	Treatment of Common Bacterial Pathogens *(Continued)*		
Etiology	**Treatment**	**Dose**	**Comments**
Aeromonas	FQ, Bactrim, or third-generation cephalosporin	Treat as febrile dysentery	
Yersinia	For most cases, treat as febrile dysentery, for severe cases give ceftriaxone	1 g IV q 24 hours for 5 days	
Listeria	Ampicillin (plus gentamicin if severe)	200 mg/kg/day IV, divided q 6 hours.	Bactrim is an alternative

FQ, Fluoroquinolone; HUS, Hemolytic-uremic syndrome.

unpeeled fresh fruit; and raw or undercooked meat or shellfish. Safe drinks include bottled carbonated beverages; beer or wine; and boiled or treated water. Tap water and unpasteurized milk carry an increased risk of infection.

- A common mistake is to put ice into a glass to cool a soft drink, thereby contaminating the beverage with infected water. Water should be brought to a boil or chemically purified using tincture of iodine (five drops per quart), tetraglycine hydroperiodide tablets, or iodinizing filters. To kill viruses at altitudes above 2,000 m (6,562 ft), water should be boiled for 3 minutes or chemical disinfection should be used after the water has boiled for 1 minute.

- Chemical disinfection with iodine is an alternative method of water treatment when it is not feasible to boil water. However, this method cannot be relied on to kill *Cryptosporidium* unless the water is allowed to sit for 15 hours before it is drunk. Two well-tested methods for disinfection with iodine are the use of tincture of iodine and tetraglycine hydroperiodide tablets (e.g., Globaline, Potable-Aqua, or Coghlan's). A guide to buying water filters for preventing cryptosporidiosis and giardiasis can be found at http://www.cdc.gov/parasites/crypto/gen_info/filters.html. These two organisms are either highly (*Cryptosporidium*) or moderately (*Giardia*) resistant to chlorine, so conventional halogen disinfection may be ineffective. Boiling water or filtration can be used as an alternative to disinfection.

- Many filters that remove parasites may not be able to kill or remove smaller organisms. More details are available at http://wwwnc.cdc.gov/travel/page/health-during-trip.htm.

Organisms that Cause Traveler's Diarrhea

- Bacterial enteropathogens cause approximately 80% of TD cases (See Table 22-5). Five major groups of *E. coli* cause enteric infections: enterotoxigenic *E. coli* (ETEC), enteropathogenic *E. coli* (EPEC), enterohemorrhagic *E. coli* (EHEC), enteroaggregative *E. coli* (EaggEC), and enteroinvasive *E. coli* (EIEC). Of the offending bacteria, ETEC accounts for the majority of infections, although *Shigella* species, *Campylobacter* species, *Salmonella* species, *Aeromonas* species, *Plesiomonas shigelloides*, and noncholera *Vibrios* all have been isolated from travelers.

Table 22-5	Traveler's Diarrhea			
Pathogen	**Clinical Symptoms**	**Stool Findings**	**Treatment**	**Other**
ETEC Heat-stable toxins (Sta; STb)	Abdominal cramps, headache, myalgias Vomiting Low-grade fever	Watery diarrhea. No WBCs	FQ if needed, rifaximin	Boil it, cook it, peel it-or forget it
EHEC	Blood, pain, and fever	Specialized testing	Probably avoid antibiotics and antimotility agents	Associated with hamburger consumption
Salmonella	Abdominal cramps, headache, myalgias Fever	Watery or inflammatory Culture serology[a]	FQ, cephalosporin	Beef, poultry, pork, eggs, dairy products, vegetables, fruit
Shigella	Abdominal cramps and bloody diarrhea Fever	Inflammatory or watery Culture	Loperamide decreases the number of unformed stools and shortens the duration of diarrhea in adults treated with ciprofloxacin	Potential reactive arthropathy or Reiter syndrome sequelae
Campylobacter	Abdominal cramps, bloody diarrhea, myalgias Fever	Watery or inflammatory	In patients who have moderate-to-severe dysentery, who are elderly, who are presumed to be bacteremic with chills and systemic symptoms, or who are at increased risk of complications, such as immunocompromised or pregnant patients, treatment may be of significant benefit FQ or azithromycin	Poultry is the primary source of Campylobacter
V. parahaemolyticus	Abdominal cramps, headache Bloody diarrhea on occasion	Inflammatory or watery	Doxycycline, TMP-SMX and quinolones	Raw or poorly cooked seafood Caribbean cruise ships and in people traveling in Asia

FQ, fluoroquinolone; WBC, white blood cells.
[a]Inflammatory may have fecal WBCs.

- **ETEC** produces a watery diarrhea, especially during warmer, wetter months. Diarrheal symptoms are associated with cramps and low-grade or no fever. ETEC is the most common cause of diarrhea in travelers to Latin America, whereas *Campylobacter jejuni* is relatively more common in Southeast Asia, particularly Thailand. *Vibrio parahaemolyticus* has been isolated with increased frequency in travelers to Southeast Asia.
- **EPEC** was the first recognized *E. coli* capable of causing outbreaks of diarrhea in infants. Effective treatment is important because of mortality rates of 25% to 50% and the potential for prolonged diarrhea. Unfortunately, resistance to trimethoprim-sulfamethoxazole (TMP-SMX) is increasing.
- **EaggEC** has been associated with prolonged diarrhea in children in developing countries and in HIV-infected adults. EaggEC has been shown to have significant resistance to TMP-SMX (57%) and ampicillin (65%).
- **EIEC** is closely related to *Shigella* and appears to respond to treatment directed against that organism. Resistance to TMP-SMX and ampicillin is common, unlike resistance to quinolones, which continues to be low at present.
- **EHEC**, especially *E. coli* O157:H7, are responsible for an estimated 20,000 infections each year in the United States, but unfortunately, studies do not support a role for antibiotic therapy, either in the treatment of the diarrheal syndrome or in the prevention of hemolytic-uremic syndrome.
- Clinically, features of **C. jejuni** infection range from an absence of symptoms to rare fulminant sepsis and death.
  - *Campylobacter* species are found in fowl and many wild and domestic animals, and most human infections probably result from contamination of milk and other animal food sources, especially poultry.
  - The most common clinical manifestation is diarrhea, but most patients also have fever, abdominal pain, nausea, and malaise.
  - Diarrhea lasts for about 1 week in most travelers without antimicrobial therapy, but symptoms may persist for 1 to 3 weeks in 20% of ill persons.
  - **Reactive arthritis** has been reported in association with this infection, and **Guillain-Barré syndrome** occurs about 1 to 3 weeks after the intestinal infection. However, no relation between the severity of the GI symptoms and the chance of developing Guillain-Barré syndrome has been demonstrated, and even asymptomatic infections can trigger Guillain-Barré syndrome.
  - Erythromycin is the drug of choice for most cases of *Campylobacter enteritis*, but clindamycin also can be used. Erythromycin has not altered the duration of GI symptoms in multiple clinical trials, although it does reduce the duration of fecal carriage of *Campylobacter*. In contrast, ciprofloxacin has been shown to reduce the duration of clinical symptoms and to eradicate *Campylobacter* from the stool, but resistance is a concern. Studies have shown azithromycin to be superior to ciprofloxacin in decreasing the excretion of *Campylobacter* spp. and as effective as ciprofloxacin in shortening the duration of illness.
  - Azithromycin therapy may be an effective alternative to ciprofloxacin therapy in areas where ciprofloxacin-resistant *Campylobacter* spp. are prevalent.
- **Norwalk virus, rotavirus, and enteric adenoviruses** have been isolated from between 2% and 27% of returning travelers with diarrhea. Among parasites:
  - **Giardia lamblia** is an important cause of diarrhea in travelers to St. Petersburg, Russia, and the mountainous regions of North America. Of note, *E. histolytica, Cryptosporidium parvum*, and *Cyclospora cayetanensis* are less common causes of diarrhea in travelers.
  - **Cyclosporiasis** especially should be considered in travelers returning from Peru and Nepal, whereas **cryptosporidiosis** occurs with increased frequency in travelers to

Russia. An important clue to a possible parasitic etiology is that a prolonged visit (longer than 2 months) is often required to acquire a parasite as opposed to a bacterial etiology.

Treatment of Traveler's Diarrhea

General Measures

- BSS (Pepto-Bismol), taken in the form of two 262-mg tablets four times a day with meals and qhs, lowers the attack rates of TD from 40% to 14% compared with a placebo. The dosage of two tablets of BSS four times daily (2.1 g/day) appears to be a safe and effective means of reducing the occurrence of TD among persons at risk for periods up to 3 weeks. Caution is advised for patients taking salicylate-containing medications or anticoagulants, as well as those with chronic renal insufficiency and gout. BSS may produce tinnitus and blackened stools and may also interfere with the absorption of doxycycline. Comparisons of BSS with loperamide have shown similar efficacy, but less stools are passed in those taking loperamide.
- Loperamide might also be beneficial when added to TMP-SMX or ciprofloxacin, particularly during the first 24 hours of therapy.
- *Lactobacillus* preparations have been used to prevent TD, but their efficacy remains uncertain. Diphenoxylate plus atropine (Lomotil) is not as effective as loperamide and may actually prolong symptoms of infection secondary to *Shigella*, and may cause urinary retention and central nervous system toxicity.

Antibiotic Prophylaxis

- Patients for whom antibiotic prophylaxis might be considered include those who are at increased risk of developing severe or complicated disease, such as the immuno-compromised, those with inflammatory bowel disease, insulin-dependent diabetics, and patients taking either diuretics or proton pump inhibitors.
- When used as prophylaxis, antibiotics should be taken daily as a single dose while in an area of risk and continued from 1 to 2 days after leaving. Quinolones have emerged as the drugs of choice, but resistance may limit their long-term usefulness. Ciprofloxacin given at a dose of 500 mg daily has been shown to be up to 95% effective in preventing diarrhea, but perhaps azithromycin should be considered if *Campylobacter* is endemic in the proposed destination.

Antibiotic Therapy of Traveler's Diarrhea

- For travelers with significant diarrhea (more than three stools during an 8-hour period, particularly if associated with nausea, vomiting, abdominal cramping, fever, or bloody stools), antibiotic therapy is recommended either with or without loperamide. Until recently, TMP-SMX was the drug of choice for the treatment of TD but resistance has limited its effectiveness, except in areas where *Cyclospora* is a significant cause of diarrhea.
- **Fluoroquinolones**, either alone or in combination with loperamide, reduce the duration of diarrhea by more than 50% compared with a placebo. In instances where the use of a fluoroquinolone is appropriate, a 3-day course is effective in most cases.
  - Single-dose therapy may be adequate in most cases; however, for bacteria such as *Campylobacter* and *Shigella dysenteriae*, concerns have been raised that single-dose therapy may be inadequate, especially if the potential for invasive disease exists.
  - In areas where fluoroquinolone-resistant *C. jejuni* has been found, azithromycin might be considered the drug of choice.
- **Rifaximin** 200 mg TID for three days has been approved for use in traveler's diarrhea caused by noninvasive strains of *E. coli.*

SUGGESTED READINGS

DuPont HL. Guidelines on acute infectious diarrhea in adults. The Practice Parameters Committee of the American College of Gastroenterology. *Am J Gastroenterol* 1997;92: 1962–1975.

DuPont HL, Ericsson CD. Prevention and treatment of traveler's diarrhea. *N Engl J Med* 1993;328:1821–1827.

DuPont HL, et al. Rifaximin: a nonabsorbed antimicrobial in the therapy of travelers' diarrhea. *Digestion* 1998;59:708–714.
   Discussion of a newer antibiotic for TD. Rifaximin shortened the duration of travelers' diarrhea compared with TMP/SMX and two earlier studied placebo-treated groups. A poorly absorbed drug, if effective in treating bacterial diarrhea, has pharmacologic and safety advantages over the existing drugs.

DuPont HL. Bacterial Diarrhea. *N Engl J Med* 2009;361:1560–1569.
   This review article summarizes the epidemiology and treatment of the most common bacterial causes of diarrhea.

Ericsson CD. Travelers' diarrhea. Epidemiology, prevention, and self-treatment. *Infect Dis Clin North Am* 1998;12:285–303.

Ericsson CD, et al. Single dose ofloxacin plus loperamide compared with single dose or three days of ofloxacin in the treatment of traveler's diarrhea. *J Travel Med* 1997;4:3–7.

Ericsson CD, et al. Treatment of traveler's diarrhea with sulfamethoxazole and trimethoprim and loperamide. *JAMA* 1990;263:257–261.
   The combination of sulfamethoxazole-trimethoprim plus loperamide is highly recommended for the treatment of most patients with TD.

Ericsson CD. Safety and efficacy of loperamide. *Am J Med* 1990;88:10S–14S.

Goldsweig CD, Pacheco PA. Infectious colitis excluding E. coli O157:H7 and C. difficile. *Gastroenterol Clin North Am* 2001;30:709–733.

Goodgame R. Emerging causes of traveler's diarrhea: *Cryptosporidium, Cyclospora, Isospora,* and *Microsporidia. Curr Infect Dis Rep* 2003;5:66–73.

Guerrant RL, et al. Practice guidelines for the management of infectious diarrhea. *Clin Infect Dis* 2001;32:331–351.
   Excellent review article summarizing consensus guidelines for managing infectious diarrhea.

Johnson PC, et al. Comparison of loperamide with bismuth subsalicylate for the treatment of acute travelers' diarrhea. *JAMA* 1986;255:757–760.

Kuschner RA, et al. Use of azithromycin for the treatment of Campylobacter enteritis in travelers to Thailand, an area where ciprofloxacin resistance is prevalent. *Clin Infect Dis* 1995;21:536–541.

LaRocque RC, Jentes ES. Health recommendations for international travel: a review of the evidence base of travel medicine. *Curr Opin Infect Dis.* 2011;24(5):403–409.

Okhuysen PC. Traveler's diarrhea due to intestinal protozoa. *Clin Infect Dis* 2001;33:110–114.
   The microbiology, epidemiology, clinical presentation, and treatment of the most common intestinal parasites found in travelers are presented in this minireview.

Oldfield EC III, Wallace MR. The role of antibiotics in the treatment of infectious diarrhea. *Gastroenterol Clin North Am* 2001;30:817–836.

Rendi-Wagner P, Kollaritsch H. Drug prophylaxis for travelers' diarrhea. *Clin Infect Dis* 2002;34:628–633.

Schlim DR. Update in travelers' diarrhea. *Infect Dis Clin North Am* 2005;19:137–149.
   This review article presents a summary of the most common mistakes made by travelers leading to infectious diarrhea. The article also summarizes the more recent data on treatment of diarrhea in travelers.

Thielman NM, Guerrant RL. Acute infectious diarrhea. *N Engl J Med* 2004;350:38–47.
   This excellent, thorough review article outlines a reasonable approach to the problem of acute diarrhea and describes appropriate treatment options.

VI Tickborne and Related Illnesses

23 Rocky Mountain Spotted Fever

Dima Youssef and James W. Myers

INTRODUCTION

- *Rickettsia rickettsii* affects the endothelial cells of small vessels. This infectious vasculitis causes microvascular injury and subsequent fluid leakage.
- Gram-negative coccobacilli of the Rickettsiaceae family.
- Obligate intracellular organisms.
- Incidence—two to four cases per million.

EPIDEMIOLOGY

- Incidence—four cases per million.
- Occurs in the Western hemisphere. Oklahoma, Tennessee, and North Carolina are the states that usually have the highest incidence. Note that RMSF has been described in nontraditional locations like Arizona and New York City on occasion.
- Humans become infected from the bite of an infected tick.
  - *Dermacentor variabilis* (American dog tick) in most of the USA
  - *Dermacentor andersoni* (Rocky Mountain wood tick) in the Rockies and Canada
  - *Rhipicephalus sanguineus* (brown dog tick) in Mexico *and Arizona*
  - *Amblyomma cajennense* (Cayenne tick) in Central and S. America
  - *Amblyomma areolatum* (yellow dog tick) in Brazil
- Most cases occur during the months of April through September.

RISK FACTORS

- Males > females
- Residence in a wooded area, with exposure to ticks or dogs with ticks.
- Children from 5 to 10 years old are at highest risk.

CLINICAL PRESENTATION

- The incubation period ranges from 2 to 14 days.
- Classic triad—fever, headache, and rash. May not be present on admission.
- No eschar. Bite is painless. Many do not recall a bite.
- Rash typically appears on the second or third day of illness.
- Rash begins as macules, then becomes petechial.
- Spreads from ankles and wrists to palms and soles and then the chest.
- No nuchal rigidity
- Can sometimes present with myalgias, abdominal findings mimicking appendicitis or cholecystitis, periorbital edema, conjuctival effusion, hand or foot edema, myocarditis, and hepatosplenomegaly.

- WBC count is often normal but can see thrombocytopenia.
- Mortality is 20% untreated and 5% treated (see Tables 23-1 and 23-2).

DIAGNOSIS

- The diagnosis of RMSF must be entertained before the onset of rash if possible as delays in therapy are associated with a much worse outcome.
- Laboratory diagnosis of RMSF may be achieved by isolation of *R. rickettsii* from the blood.
- Serology (Table 23-2).
  - Indirect fluorescent antibody (IFA) is 95% sensitive but takes at least 7 to 10 days to appear. A negative test early on does not rule out the diagnosis. Convalescent serology in 4 weeks with a fourfold increase is often the best way to make the diagnosis.
  - Greater than 1:64 is diagnostic.
- Polymerase chain reaction (PCR) amplification is not very useful at this time.
- Skin Biopsy
- Immunohistochemical staining is 100% specific but 70% sensitive.

DIFFERENTIAL DIAGNOSIS

- **Meningococcemia**, other Rickettsia, and viral illnesses are the main entities to be considered. Treatment with **ceftriaxone** in addition to doxycycline is often prescribed until the diagnosis of either is more secure.

DIAGNOSTIC LABORATORIES

ARUP	(Rocky Mountain Spotted Fever) Antibodies, IgG and IgM by IF 00050371 Test code	http://www.arupconsult.com/index.html
Specialty Labs	7896: *Rickettsia rickettsii* IgG and IgM Antibodies	http://www.specialtylabs.com/
Mayo Clinic Labs	Unit Code 84343: Rickettsia Antibody Panel, Spotted Fever and Typhus Fever Groups, Serum	http://www.mayomedical-laboratories.com/
Centers for Disease control (CDC)[a]	Skin biopsy diagnosis	http://www.cdc.gov/rmsf/ 1-800-CDC-INFO (1-800-232-4636) http://www.cdc.gov/rmsf/resources/CDC50_34_SpecimenSubmission.pdf

[a]Serologic tests for RMSF are available at commercial labs, state public health laboratories, and CDC. Early serologic tests (within 1 week of illness onset) frequently are negative, and testing of acute and convalescent phase serum samples is recommended to confirm diagnosis. Nucleic acid detection (e.g., by using PCR assay), immunohistochemical staining of formalin-fixed tissues, and cell culture of biopsy or autopsy specimens also can be used for diagnosis and are available at specialized research laboratories and CDC.

Table 23-1   Tick Diseases of Africa

Name	Vector	Eschar/Rash	Clinical Features
Rickettsia conorii subsp. conorii Mediterranean Spotted Fever	*Rhipicephalus sanguineus, R. simus, Haemaphysalis leachi*	Rash occurs in 97%. Single eschar	Cases generally sporadic. Single eschar. Case fatality ratio, approximately 2.5%.
Rickettsia africae	*Amblyomma hebraeum, A. variegatum, A. lepidum*	Eschars are often multiple in 54%. Maculopapular rash in 49%. May be vesicular in 24%.	Disease occurs in predominantly rural settings and is associated with international travelers returning from safari, hunting, camping, or adventure races. Outbreaks and clustered cases common (74%).
African Spotted Fever			Symptoms include fever (88%) and lymphadenopathy (43%) No fatalities reported.
Rickettsia sibirica subsp. *mongolitimonae* Lymphangitis-associated rickettsiosis	*Hyalomma truncatum*	Symptoms include eschar (75%), rash (63%).	Few described cases in South Africa. Patients have lymphangitis in (25%) of cases.
Rickettsia slovaca	*Dermacentor marginatus*	Fever and rash rare Typical eschar on the scalp with cervical lymphadenopathy; illness mild.	Tick-borne lymphadenopathy "TIBOLA" (1997), Dermacentor-borne necrosis and lymphadenopathy "DEBONEL"
Rickettsia helvetica	*Ixodes ricinus*	Rash and eschar seldom occur	Has been linked to perimyocarditis and sarcoidosis
Rickettsia aeschlimannii	*Hyalomma marginatum marginatum, H. marginatum rupifes, Rhipicephalus appendiculatus*	Symptoms include eschar and maculopapular rash	Few cases described in patients from Morocco and South Africa.
Rickettsia monacencis	*Ixodes ricinus*	Fever and maculopapular rash	
Rickettsia raoultii	*Dermacentor marginatus*	TIBOLA/DEBONEL	Typical eschar on the scalp with cervical lymphadenopathy

Table 23-2   Comparison of RMSF to Similar Illnesses

Name	Geography	Rash	Organism	Clinical Features
RMSF (Dog tick)	United States	Maculopapular	*R. rickettsii*	20% of cases do not develop rash
Rickettsialpox (house mouse mite)	Baltimore and New York	Eschar present Vesicular rash	*R. akari*	Rash distributed on the face, neck, trunk, and extremities and is easily confused with rash of varicella (chickenpox)
Bouto nneuse fever (*Rhipicephalus sanguineus* ticks)	Spain, Italy, and Israel	50% have a tache noire (black spot) develops	*R. conorii*	Rash is spotty and may persist for 2–3 weeks in some patients; often severe.
Louse-borne typhus (lice)	Ethiopia and Nigeria	Rash appears, spreading from trunk to extremities	*R. prowazekii*	Brill Zinser disease occurs later. Fever and intractable headache Flying squirrels
Tsutsugamushi disease (chiggers)	Japan and the Far East	Rash usually only around the trunk Usually a few eschars.	*O. tsutsugamushi*	Fever and headache Lymphadenopathy.1%–6% fatality rate.
Murine Typhus (Rat fleas, cat fleas and insect feces)	Texas and California	Flea-bite does not have an exchar.	*R. typhi* and *R. felis*	Associated with Opossums. Milder illness than louse borne. Rash spares palms and soles.
R. parkeri (*Amblyomma maculatum, the Gulf coast tick.*)	Southeast USA	Eschars are often present to differenti- ate this from RMSF.	*R. parkeri*	Probably less severe than RMSF.
TIBOLA (*Dermacentor marginatus* ticks)	Europe	The eschar site may have prolonged alopecia.	*R. slovaca in Europe*	eschar, typically on the scalp, and enlarged, often tender, draining cervical lymph nodes. Fewer than half of patients manifest a fever, and rash occurs rarely.

Table 23-3	Prevention of Tick Bites
DEET	http://www.deet.com
Environmental Protection Agency (EPA) Insect Repellants	http://cfpub.epa.gov/oppref/insect/
CDC Tick Avoidance	http://www.cdc.gov/ticks/avoid/ on_people.html
Tick Removal	http://www.cdc.gov/ticks/ removing_a_tick.html
MMWR Tick-borne	http://www.cdc.gov/mmwr/PDF/rr/ rr5504.pdf
Images of ticks	http://www.dpd.cdc.gov/DPDx/html/ ImageLibrary/S-Z/Ticks/body_ Ticks_il1.htm
CDC RMSF	http://www.cdc.gov/rmsf/
CDC RMSF rash	http://www.cdc.gov/rmsf/symptoms/ index.html#rash

TREATMENT

- The minimum duration of treatment is 5 to 7 days; longer courses of therapy may be warranted in patients with more severe illness.
- Doxycycline is the treatment of choice for treating RMSF in both adults **and children.**
- Give the **same dose** of doxycycline whether given PO (mild to moderate) or intravenously (severe cases).
  - For adults and children weighing >45kg: 100 mg orally every 12 hours.
  - For children <45 kg: 2.2 mg/kg every 12 hours.
- Delays in therapy, especially past 5 days are associated with a worse outcome.
- Chloramphenicol can also be used. **Note that it is the drug of choice for pregnant women. Use doxycycline only if it is not available.**

PREVENTION

- No vaccine.
- Reduce tick exposure.
  - *N, N*-diethyl-*m*-toluamide (DEET) is the most effective commercially available arthropod repellent.
  - Expeditious removal of attached ticks reduces the chance of acquiring the disease after a tick bite.
- **No role** for doxycycline prophylaxis for tick bites to prevent RMSF (please see Table 23-3 for more information about prevention of tick borne illnesses).

SUGGESTED READINGS

Archibald LK, Sexton DJ. Long-term sequelae of Rocky Mountain spotted fever. *Clin Infect Dis* 1995;20(5):1122–1125.
   Long-term neurologic sequelae included paraparesis; hearing loss; peripheral neuropathy; bladder and bowel incontinence; cerebellar, vestibular, and motor dysfunction;

and language disorders. Nonneurologic sequelae consisted of disability from limb amputation and scrotal pain following cutaneous necrosis.

Buckingham SC, Marshall GS, et al. Clinical and laboratory features, hospital course, and outcome of Rocky Mountain spotted fever in children. *J Pediatr* 2007;150(2):180–184, 184.e181.

Children with RMSF presented to study institutions after a median of 6 days of symptoms, which most commonly included fever (98%), rash (97%), nausea and/or vomiting (73%), and headache (61%); no other symptom or sign was present in >50% of children. Only 49% reported antecedent tick bites. Platelet counts were <150,000/mm³ in 59% of children, and serum sodium concentrations were <135 mEq/dL in 52%.

Cazorla C, Socolovschi C, et al. Tick-borne diseases: tick-borne spotted fever rickettsioses in Africa. *Infect Dis Clin North Am* 2008;22(3):531–544, ix–x.

Excellent review with several good tables.

Chen LF, Sexton DJ. What's new in Rocky Mountain spotted fever? *Infect Dis Clin North Am* 2008;22(3):415–432, vii–viii.

Good overall review.

Cunha BA. Clinical features of Rocky Mountain spotted fever. *Lancet Infect Dis* 2008;8(3):143–144.

This letter adds additional information about clincal features of RMSF.

Dantas-Torres F. Rocky Mountain spotted fever. *Lancet Infect Dis* 2007;7(11):724–732.

Good comprehensive review article with excellent references and pictures.

Demma LJ, Traeger MS, et al. Rocky Mountain spotted fever from an nexpected tick vector in Arizona. *N Engl J Med* 2005;353(6):587–594.

This investigation documents the presence of RMSF in eastern Arizona, with common brown dog ticks (R. sanguineus) implicated as a vector of R. rickettsii. The broad distribution of this common tick raises concern about its potential to transmit R. rickettsii in other settings.

Helmick CG, Bernard KW, et al. Rocky Mountain spotted fever: clinical, laboratory, and epidemiological features of 262 cases. *J Infect Dis* 1984;150(4):480–488.

Reviews 262 cases !

Holman RC, McQuiston JH, et al. Increasing incidence of Rocky Mountain spotted fever among the American Indian population in the United States. *Am J Trop Med Hyg* 2009;80(4):601–605.

The incidence of RMSF increased dramatically among American Indians disproportionately to trends for other race groups. Education about tick-borne disease and prevention measures should be addressed for high-risk American Indian populations.

Kaplan JE, Schonberger LB. The sensitivity of various serologic tests in the diagnosis of Rocky Mountain spotted fever. *Am J Trop Med Hyg* 1986;35(4):840–844.

IFA and indirect hemagglutination (IHA) appear to be the most sensitive serologic tests currently in use for the diagnosis of RMSF.

Kirkland KB, Marcom PK, et al. Rocky Mountain spotted fever complicated by gangrene: report of six cases and review. *Clin Infect Dis* 1993;16(5):629–634.

Skin necrosis and gangrene in association with RMSF are the extreme end on a continuum from reversible to irreversible skin and tissue damage caused by Rickettsia rickettsii. I have personally seen this in a patient of mine as well. She lacked any other skin findings but had an extremely high RMSF titer.

Kirkland KB, Wilkinson WE, et al. Therapeutic delay and mortality in cases of Rocky Mountain spotted fever. *Clin Infect Dis* 1995;20(5):1118–1121.

Patients with RMSF who received antirickettsial therapy within 5 days of the onset of symptoms were significantly less likely to die than were those who received treatment after the 5th day of illness. Three factors were independent predictors of failure by the physician to initiate therapy the first time a patient was seen: absence of a rash, presentation between 1 August and 30 April, and presentation within the first 3 days of illness.

Masters EJ, Olson GS, et al. Rocky Mountain spotted fever: a clinician's dilemma. *Arch Intern Med* 2003;163(7):769–774.

They examined the dilemmas facing the clinician who is evaluating the patient with possible RMSF, with particular attention to the following 8 pitfalls in diagnosis and treatment: (1) waiting for a petechial rash to develop before diagnosis, (2) misdiagnosing as gastroenteritis, (3) discounting a diagnosis when there is no history of a tick bite, (4) using an inappropriate geographic exclusion, (5) using an inappropriate seasonal exclusion, (6) failing to treat on clinical suspicion, (7) failing to elicit an appropriate history, and (8) failing to treat with doxycycline.

Raoult D, Parola P, Rocky Mountain spotted fever in the USA: a benign disease or a common diagnostic error? *Lancet Infect Dis* 2008;8(10):587–589.

Reviews difficulty in diagnosis.

Stallings SP. Rocky Mountain spotted fever and pregnancy: a case report and review of the literature. *Obstet Gynecol Surv* 2001;56(1):37–42.

Several conditions of pregnancy have similar presentations to the initial, often nonspecific manifestations of RMSF. Although doxycycline is the recommended therapy for children and nonpregnant women, chloramphenicol remains the recommended therapy for women during pregnancy. Vertical transmission of RMSF has not been documented in humans.

Walker DH. Rocky Mountain spotted fever: a disease in need of microbiological concern. *Clin Microbiol Rev* 1989;2(3):227–240.

Review article. Good table comparing diagnostic tests.

24 Human Granulocytic Anaplasmosis, Human Monocytic Ehrlichiosis, and *Ehrlichia ewingii* Ehrlichiosis

James W. Myers and Dima Youssef

INTRODUCTION

- *Anaplasma phagocytophilum* (*A. phagocytohilum*), *Ehrlichia chaffeensis* (*E. chaffeensis*), and *Ehrlichia ewingii* (*E. ewingii*) are tick-borne pathogens.
- They cause human granulocytic anaplasmosis (HGA), human monocytic ehrlichiosis, and *E. ewingii* ehrlichiosis, respectively.
- They cause illness in patients ranging from an asymptomatic seroconversion to mild, severe, or, rarely, fatal disease.
- Obligate intracellular bacterial pathogens of the family Anaplasmataceae
- Transmitted by Ixodes spp. or *Amblyomma americanum* ticks
- *Ehrlichia* and *Anaplasma* have the characteristic gram-negative cell wall structure but lack important cell membrane components including lipopolysaccharide and peptidoglycan.
- The ehrlichial cell wall is rich in cholesterol, which is derived from the host cell.
- Cholesterol-rich cell walls may function as ligands for stimulation of innate and acquired immune responses.

CLINICAL SYNDROMES

1. **Human monocytotropic ehrlichiosis: HME**

Epidemiology

- Tick-borne infectious disease transmitted by several tick species, especially ***Amblyomma*** species.
  - *E. chaffeensis* belongs to the family Anaplasmataceae.
  - The lone-star tick ***Amblyomma americanum*** is the main vector, but *Dermacentor variabilis* and *Ixodes pacificus* may play a smaller role as well.
    - *Amblyomma* ticks have three feeding stages (larval, nymph, and adult); each developmental stage feeds only once.
    - Transstadial (i.e., larva-nymph-adults) transmission of *Ehrlichia* occurs during nymph and adult feeding stages because larvae are uninfected.
    - *Ehrlichia* are *not maintained* by transovarial transmission.
  - **White-tailed deer**, *Odocoileus virginianus*, are the principal reservoir, but other species play a smaller role as well.
    - Dogs
    - Coyotes

  ○ Red foxes
  ○ Raccoons
  ○ Opossums
  ○ Birds
- Missouri, Oklahoma, Tennessee, Arkansas, and Maryland are higher incidence states.
- Some cases are reported from Asia, Europe, and Brazil, too.
- Rates of HME of 100 to 200 cases per a population of 100,000 in endemic areas
- Usually occur from April to September.
- The median age for HME is 50 years.
- Most of the patients are male.

Pathogenesis
- The **most frequently infected blood cells are monocytes**, but lymphocytes, atypical lymphocytes, promyelocytes, metamyelocytes, and band and segmented neutrophils have also been infected.
- Infected cells typically contain only one or two **morulae.**
- Following entry into mononuclear phagocytes, *E. chaffeensis* inhibits phagolysosome fusion involving genes controlled by a two-component regulatory system.
- *E. chaffeensis* also suppresses and induces host genes to facilitate their intracellular survival.
- Downregulation of Th1 cytokines such as IL-12 and IL-18, which are important inducers of adaptive Th1-mediated immune responses.
- Ehrlichial infection is curtailed by NKT, CD4, and CD8 T lymphocytes, antibodies, IFN-γ, IL-10, and TNF-α.
- The toxic shock manifestations of HME are related to proinflammatory cytokines, including interleukin-10 (IL-10) and tumor necrosis factor-α (TNF-α).

Frequent Pathologic Findings of HME
- Myeloid hyperplasia
- Megakaryocytosis in the bone marrow.
- Erythrophagocytosis
- Plasmacytosis
- Focal hepatocellular necrosis
- Hepatic granulomas
- Cholestasis
- Splenic and lymph node necrosis
- Diffuse mononuclear phagocyte hyperplasia of the spleen, liver, lymph node, and bone marrow
- Perivascular lymphohistiocytic infiltrates of various organs including kidney, heart, liver, meninges, and brain
- Interstitial mononuclear cell pneumonitis
- Lymphohistiocytic foci, centrilobular and/or coagulation necrosis, Kupffer cell hyperplasia, and marked monocytic infiltration.

General Clinical Features
- Incubation period ranges from 5 to 21 days with a mean of 7 days.
- HME is a more severe disease than HGA or human ewingii ehrlichiosis (HEE), with 42% of cases requiring hospitalization, and a case-fatality rate of 3%.

- Seventeen percent of patients develop life-threatening complications, especially if the patient is immunocompromised.
- Prodrome is characterized by malaise, low-back pain, or gastrointestinal symptoms, or the patient may develop sudden onset of fever (often >39°C).
- Fever (>95%)
- Headache (60% to 75%)
- Myalgias (40% to 60%)
- Nausea (40% to 50%)
- Arthralgias (30% to 35%)
- Malaise (30% to 80%)
- Cough, pharyngitis, lymphadenopathy, diarrhea, vomiting, abdominal pain, and changes in mental status (10% to 40%)
- A skin eruption is relatively common among children with HME, occurring in 66% of pediatric cases compared to 21% of adults.
- **Rash is seen in 10% of cases of HME**
  - Most often maculopapular.
  - Petechial
  - Erythroderma
  - Usually spares the face, palms, and soles of the feet.
- Less frequently reported: conjunctivitis, dysuria, and peripheral edema.
- Altered mental status and abdominal pain (in children and pregnant women).
- Complications with HME
  - Renal failure
  - Myocarditis
  - **Adult respiratory distress syndrome**
  - Disseminated intravascular coagulopathy
  - CNS disease
    - 20% incidence
    - Meningitis or meningoencephalitis is seen most often.
    - Seizures
    - Cranial nerve palsies are rare.
    - Long-term neurologic sequelae are uncommon.
    - CSF pleocytosis
      - Usually <100 cells
      - Mostly lymphocytes
      - Morula are uncommon.
    - Radiographic may show leptomeningeal enhancement.

2. Human granulocytic anaplasmosis: HGE

Epidemiology
- Reported most often in Connecticut, Wisconsin, Minnesota, and New York State.
- **Ten percent of patients with HGA have serologic evidence of coinfection with Lyme disease, or babesiosis**.
- A 50-year-old white male infected during the summer would be the most likely scenario.

Pathogenesis of HGA
- **Neutrophils are infected.**
- Inhibits phagosome-lysosome fusion and delays apoptosis

- Pathologic findings in patients with HGA:
  - Normocellular or hypercellular bone marrow
  - Erythrophagocytosis
  - Focal splenic necrosis
  - Mild interstitial pneumonitis
  - Pulmonary hemorrhage
  - **Thrombocytopenia, leukopenia, mild anemia.**
  - **Abnormal liver function tests (LFTS).**

Tick Vectors

- Ixodes scapularis in the northeastern and upper Midwest regions of the United States
- *I. pacificus* along the northern Pacific coast
- *I. ricinus* ticks in Europe
- **These ticks also transmit Borrelia burgdorferi, Babesia microti, and tick-borne encephalitis virus.**
- White-tailed deer (*Odocoileus virginianus*) and the white-footed mouse (*Peromyscus leucopus*) are both reservoirs.
- Both adult and nymphal Ixodes ticks can feed on humans who are dead-end hosts.

HGA General Clinical Features

- HGA resembles HME with respect to the frequency of fever, headache, and myalgias, **but rash is uncommon**.
- Concurrent Lyme disease probably accounts for most of the rashes seen.
- HGA ranges in severity from an asymptomatic seroconversion to a mild or severe febrile illness.
- **Leukopenia, thrombocytopenia, and elevations in transaminases are seen.**
- HGA tends to be a **less severe illness than HME**, although life-threatening complications including acute respiratory distress syndrome, acute renal failure, and hemodynamic collapse have been reported.
- Reported CSF abnormalities include lymphoctyic pleocytosis and moderate elevation in proteins but CNS disease is rare.
- **Fatalities associated with HGA occur in <1% of infections unlike the 3% rate seen with HME.**

3. Human ewingii ehrlichiosis

Epidemiology

- *E. ewingii* (a cause of granulocytic ehrlichiosis in dogs) can also infect humans.
- Similar to *E. chaffeensis, E. ewingii* is **transmitted by the lone-star tick.**
- White-tailed deer
- Most infections reported to date have occurred in patients with HIV or who were immunosuppressed following organ transplantation.
- Most cases of HEE have been reported in Tennessee, Missouri, and Oklahoma.

HEE General Clinical Features

- Clinical manifestations appear to be milder than HME. No fatalities
- Findings of leukopenia, thrombocytopenia, and abnormal LFTS are variably present.
- HEE may be associated with meningitis.

Diagnosis
- **Hematologic findings and abnormal LFTS suggest the diagnosis in most patients.**
- Hyponatremia in 50%.
- Other laboratory abnormalities such as increased serum creatinine, lactate dehy-drogenase, creatine phosphokinase, amylase, and electrolyte abnormalities includ-ing hypocalcemia, hypomagnesemia, hypophosphatemia, prolonged prothrombin times, increased levels of fibrin degradation products, metabolic acidosis, profound hypotension, and disseminated intravascular coagulopathy may be seen.
- See Table 24-1 for other diagnostic tests

Treatment
- The current recommended therapeutic regimen for HME, HGA, and *E. ewingii* ehrlichiosis is administration of doxycycline or tetracycline for 5 to 14 days. (If at risk for coinfection with *B. burgdorferi* then doxycycline therapy should continue for a full 14 days).

Table 24-1	Diagnostic Tests		
Test	**Sensitivity**	**Specificity**	**Comments**
A. phagocytophilum IFA serology *E. chaffeensis* IFA	82%–100% IgG 27%–37% IgM 88%–90% IgG 44% IgM	83%–100 %	Fourfold increase in titer or single titer >256 is diagnostic. Single titer >128 is probable. Often négative in the first week of Illness. Lower titers after therapy is started.
Wright stain for morula.	Sensitivity in week one: 25%–75% for *A. phagocytophi-lum.* 2%–38% for *E. chaffeensis.*		Morulae disappear after 24–72 hours of therapy.
PCR	60%–85% for *E.chaffeensis A. phagocyto-philum* 67%–90 %		Also useful for *E. ewingii.* Less sensitive in the CSF for all species.
Immunohistochemistry	Bone marrow, or autopsy.		Less useful after therapy is started.

Table 24-2	Recommended Adult and Pediatric Antibiotic Treatment for *Ehrlichia*		
Antibiotic	**Dose (Adults)**	**Dose (Children)**	**Duration (Days)**
Doxycycline hyclate	100 mg IV. or PO q12h	2.2 mg/kg PO q12h	5–14
Tetracycline hydrochloride	500 mg PO q6h	25–50mg/kg/ day PO in four divided doses	5–14
Rifampin	300 mg PO q12h	10 mg/kg PO q12h	7

- The clinical response to doxycycline or tetracycline is pronounced within 24 to 48 hours.
- Doxycycline is contraindicated in pregnant patients.
  - In this population, as well as in patients with a specific contraindication to doxycycline, rifampin (adults: 300 mg twice daily; children <100lb 10 mg/kg twice daily) may be substituted.
- Chloramphenicol is an alternative drug that has been considered for treatment of HGA or HME.
- Prophylactic antibiotic therapy for human ehrlichial infections **is not** recommended for patients who recall having been bitten by a tick and are not ill.
- See Table 24-2 for dosages of antibiotics.

Prevention
- Limit exposure to ticks.
  - Four to twenty-four hours of tick attachment are required.
  - Wearing protective clothing and using N-Diethyl-meta-toluamide (DEET) and permethrin.

SUGGESTED READINGS

Bakken JS, Dumler JS. Clinical diagnosis and treatment of human granulocytotropic anaplasmosis. *Ann N Y Acad Sci* 2006;1078:236–247.
  Excellent summary.
Bakken JS, Dumler S. Human granulocytic anaplasmosis. *Infect Dis Clin North Am* 2008;22(3):433–448, viii.
  This article focuses on the diagnosis and management of HGA caused by Anaplasma phagocytophilum.
Dumler JS. *Anaplasma* and *Ehrlichia* infection. *Ann N Y Acad Sci* 2005;1063:361–373.
  Human and animal infections by Anaplasmataceae are increasingly recognized as important and potentially fatal arthropod-transmitted diseases.
Dumler JS, Bakken JS. Ehrlichial diseases of humans: emerging tick-borne infections. *Clin Infect Dis* 1995;20(5):1102–1110.
  Therapy with doxycycline is highly efficacious.
Dumler JS, Madigan JE, et al. Ehrlichioses in humans: epidemiology, clinical presentation, diagnosis, and treatment. *Clin Infect Dis* 2007;45(Suppl 1):S45–S51.
  Once an ehrlichiosis is suspected on historical and clinical grounds, doxycycline treatment should be initiated concurrently with attempts at etiologic confirmation using

laboratory methods such as blood smear examination, polymerase chain reaction, culture, and serologic tests.

Ganguly S, Mukhopadhayay SK. Tick-borne ehrlichiosis infection in human beings. *J Vector Borne Dis* 2008;45(4):273–280.

Human monocytic ehrlichiosis is diagnosed by demonstration of a four-fold or greater change in antibody titer to E. chaffeensis antigen by IFA in paired serum samples, or a positive polymerase chain reaction (PCR) assay and confirmation of E. chaffeensis DNA, or identification of morulae in leukocytes and a positive IFA titer to E. chaffeensis antigen, or immunostaining of E. chaffeensis antigen in a biopsy or autopsy sample, or culture of E. chaffeensis from a clinical specimen.

Ismail N, Bloch KC, et al. Human ehrlichiosis and anaplasmosis. *Clin Lab Med* 2010;30(1):261–292.

This article reviews recent advances in the understanding of ehrlichial diseases related to microbiology, epidemiology, diagnosis, pathogenesis, immunity, and treatment of the two prevalent tick-borne diseases found in the United States, HME and HGA. Table 1 is an excellent table. Figures 2 and 3 demonstrates ehrlichial morula.

Paddock CD, Childs JE. *Ehrlichia chaffeensis*: a prototypical emerging pathogen. *Clin Microbiol Rev* 2003;16(1):37–64.

Excellent review article. Figure 6 has a life cycle diagram for E. chaffeensis.

Thomas RJ, Dumler JS, et al. Current management of human granulocytic anaplasmosis, human monocytic ehrlichiosis and *Ehrlichia ewingii* ehrlichiosis. *Expert Rev Anti Infect Ther* 2009;7(6):709–722.

Table 1 is a good summary table of HME, HGE, and HEE. Table 2 is excellent for recommending test based on the time interval for diagnosis. Figure 2 has very good pictures.

25 Babesiosis

Dima Youssef and James W. Myers

INTRODUCTION

Babesia infections have probably been occurring for centuries, but the first documented case of babesiosis in humans was in a splenectomized farmer in Yugoslavia who was diagnosed with a *B. bovis* in 1957. Clinical infection varies from a silent infection to a severe, life-threatening disease.

- Babesiosis parasites:
  - Tick-transmitted by Ixodid ticks or hard-bodied ticks (*Ixodes dammini [Ixodes scapularis]* and *Ixodes ricinus*).
  - Human infection usually follows a tick bite although two-thirds of patients may not recall the bite.
  - Note that it may occasionally occur after a blood transfusion or transplacental/perinatal infection. Overall, the risk of acquiring babesiosis from a blood transfusion is very low.
    - A transfused unit of packed red blood cells is about 0.17%. Platelet transfusion risk is even lower.
  - Those cases of transfusion-acquired babesiosis in the United States occurred with an incubation period varying from 17 days to 8 weeks.
  - Zoonotic disease
  - Infects a wide variety of vertebrate hosts
  - The parasites are intraerythrocytic.
  - They are called *piroplasms* due to the *pear-shaped* forms.
  - *Babesia microti* is the most common species infecting humans.
  - Both humoral and cellular factors are involved in immunity to babesiosis.

EPIDEMIOLOGY

- Babesiosis in Europe (30 cases) occurs only in *splenectomize*d patients (minus one case) and is caused by **Babesia divergens, a cattle pathogen. Forty-two percent** mortality rate is much greater than the 5% rate found in the United States found with *B. microti*.
- The tick vector of *B. divergens* is *Ixodes ricinus* and that of *B. microti* in England is *I. trianguliceps*.
- Two or more divergens-like pathogens occur in the United States (please see Table 25-1 for a comparison of species.)
  - A 73-year-old man who had had a splenectomy and had a fatal case of babesiosis. Indirect immunofluorescent antibody testing showed that the patient's serum had strong reactivity with *Babesia divergens*, which causes babesiosis in cattle and humans in Europe, but that it had minimal reactivity with *B. microti* and WA1. Known as MO1.

Table 25-1	Comparison of Species		
	B. divergens	*B. duncani* type organisms (WA, CA) and other species	*B. microti*
Splenectomy as a risk factor	Yes	Usually not but varies.	No
Ixodes tick vector	*Ixodes scapularis*	*Varies*	*Ixodes ricinus*
Host	Cattle	Varies	Mice
Treatment duration	6 weeks. (2 weeks after clearance)	Not well defined	10 days normally
Exchange transfusion used	Common	Perhaps	Rare
Atovaquone-azithromycin combination	No pentamidine and TMP-SMX might be an alternative.	Possible	Yes, for milder disease
Quinine-clindamycin regimen	Yes	Yes. Probably the best approach	Yes

- The second case was a 56-year-old man from Kentucky. He had a history of splenectomy, a Caribbean cruise 9 months earlier, and deer and rabbit hunting 4 weeks previously, but he had no recollection of a tick bite. He presented with a fever (temperature, 40°C), a hemoglobin level of 13.7 g per deciliter, a platelet count of 43,000 per cubic millimeter, and hemoglobinuria.
- A few cases of babesiosis in the western United States have been reported previously; all occurred in Washington or California. They were either tick borne or transfusion related.
- Rarely reported in other parts of the world, including China, Taiwan, Egypt, South Africa, and Mexico.

CHARACTERIZATION OF THE ORGANISM

Invertebrate Hosts

- Ixodid ticks are the vectors for *Babesia* spp.
- *B. microti* can only infect ticks from the genus *Ixodes*.
- Several tick vectors can carry more than one *Babesia* species.
- The nymphal stage of *I. dammini* and its interaction with *Peromyscus leucopus* (white-footed mouse) is essential for the maintenance of *B. microti*.
- The adult stages of *I. dammini* feed primarily on deer (*Odocoileus virginianus*) and then lay eggs.
- The eggs hatch in the summer, and the larvae feed primarily on mice during August and September.
- These infected larvae molt to become nymphs in the spring.
- The nymphs feed on hosts from May through July.

Vertebrate Hosts

- Almost any mammal that serves as a host for a *Babesia*-infected tick is a potential reservoir.
- Small terrestrial mammals to subhuman primates to humans for *B. microti* and from cattle to various rodents and to humans for *B. divergens*.
- Most white-footed mice (*P. leucopus*) in babesiosis-enzootic areas are parasitemic for life.

Events in the Vertebrate

- The longer the tick is attached, the more likely the sporozoites will be transmitted.
- Sporozoites invade the lymphocytes and then differentiate into multinucleate schizonts. These differentiate into merozoites, which lyse the cell to infect the erythrocytes.
- The merozoite invades the host erythrocyte through a process of invagination, forming a parasitophorous vacuole.
- Within the host erythrocytes, most merozoites become trophozoites and divide by binary fission; more merozoites get produced, and additional erythrocytes get infected.
- **Four parasites can form at the same time, leading to a Maltese cross form.**
- Rapid reproduction destroys the host cell and leads to hemoglobinuria in the host.
- Some trophozoites can become potential gametocytes that develop into gametes in the tick prior to leaving the erythrocytes within the tick gut.

Host Immune Responses

- Both humoral and cellular factors are involved in immunity to babesiosis.
- Parasitemia levels begin to decline approximately 10 days after infection after degeneration inside the erythrocyte and clearance by the spleen.
- Intraerythrocytic killing at the resolution stage requires T lymphocytes.
- NK cells might be mediating protection in the early stages of infection.
- NK cell activity is higher during peak parasitemia and the recovery phase.
- Marked increase in NK cells during the acute phase.
- Macrophage stimulation has been found to inhibit parasite growth in infected mice through the production of nitric oxide.
- TNF-α has also contributes to parasite death in babesiosis.

Symptoms in Humans

- Malaria-like infection. Please see Table 25-2 which compares these two parasitic illnesses.
  - One to nine weeks incubation period. Longer if by blood transfusion.
  - Symptoms depend on the level of parasitemia (1% to 80% range), but usually it takes 2 weeks to make a diagnosis.
  - Malaise, chills, myalgia, anemia, fatigue, and fever.
  - Nausea, vomiting, night sweats, weight loss, and hematuria.
  - Hepatomegaly and splenomegaly are common. May rupture or infarct
  - Neck stiffness, cough, abdominal pain, and petechiae.
  - **Hemolytic anemia can be sustained for several days to a few months. It occurs most commonly in asplenic or elderly hosts**.
  - Often asymptomatic or self-limited. Most patients respond quickly to antibiotics, but some patients relapse or take several months to recover.

Table 25-2	Comparison of Malaria and *Babesia* Parasites			
	Schizonts	Pigment	Extracellular Parasites	Maltese Cross
Babesia	No	No	Yes	Yes
Malaria	Yes	Yes	No	No

- Complications occur more often in immunocompromised patients (such as adult respiratory distress syndrome, congestive heart failure [CHF], and disseminated intravascular coagulation [DIC]).
- *B. divergens* infections seen in Europe (splenectomized) were more severe than those caused by *B. microti*.
- Elevated transaminases, alkaline phosphatases, unconjugated bilirubin, and lactic dehydrogenase in serum.
- Normochromia, normocytic anemia, thrombocytopenia, and *leukopenia* (possible coinfection) can be seen as well.

Host Susceptibility

- Most severe infections occur predominantly in the elderly and in splenectomized or immunocompromised hosts.
- There is a correlation between the severity of the infection and the age of the patient.
- **Coinfection with other tick-transmitted infectious agents can result in more severe manifestations**.
- Patients coinfected with *B. burgdorferi* (agent in Lyme disease) and *B. microti* have higher disease severity.
- Human immunodeficiency virus infection may increase the severity of symptoms.

DIAGNOSIS

Typical History

- Travel to an area where it is endemic, tick bite or exposure to a tick-infested area, recent blood transfusion, and splenectomy
- Serologic evaluation with indirect (immuno) fluorescent antibody tests (IFATs) and possibly polymerase chain reaction (PCR)
- Morphologic changes in the spleen may be identified with imaging in severe cases
- PCR is rapidly becoming the test of choice for confirmation of actual infection and for monitoring therapeutic responses.

Hematology

- Examination of thin blood smears stained with Wright or Giemsa stain for the presence of parasites within erythrocytes is the most frequently used technique
- The organisms appear in the red blood cells as darkly staining ring forms with light blue cytoplasm
- *B. microti* merozoites are approximately 1.5 to 2 μm, and *B. divergens* merozoites are variable (1 to 3 μm)

- Simple rings (annular), paired or single pear-shaped trophozoites (piriform), and the **rarely seen but often described Maltese cross**
- *B. microti* infections can have parasitemias that are detectable to levels as high as 85%.
- The duration of detectable parasitemia on blood smears varies from 3 to 12 weeks.
- The ring forms visible within erythrocytes can vary greatly and can be confused with *Plasmodium falciparum.*
- However, *Babesia* **does not form pigment** and does not cause alterations in red cell morphology or staining, such as the Maurer clefts of *P. falciparum* and the Schüffner dots of *P. vivax*
  - *Babesia* does not form schizonts.
- Anemia ranges from 6 to 12 g/dL in most patients.
- Serum haptoglobin levels may be reduced and the reticulocyte count increased.
- Total white blood cell counts are low or normal.
- Thrombocytopenia can be seen.

Serology and Immunology
- The IFAT is both specific and sensitive and is the current recommended serologic method.
- IFATs can be used to distinguish infections due to different *Babesia* species.
- The cutoff titer should be above 1:64 to be diagnostic.
- Titers of 1:128 to 1:256 are rarely associated with false positivity
- Antibody is usually detectable when patients are first diagnosed with infections of *B. microti.*
- Antibody titers can remain elevated for as long as 13 months to 6 years.
- There is cross-reactivity with other protozoa, generating false-positive results in *B. microti*
- *B. divergens* antibodies do not become detectable in serum until 7 to 10 days after the onset of hemoglobinuria.

Molecular Diagnostic Approaches
- The molecular diagnosis has become possible.
- PCR is *more sensitive than and equally specific* for the detection of acute cases as smear evaluation and hamster inoculation.
- Patients with detectable babesial DNA in their blood are likely to be parasitemic.
- Presence of DNA is probably reflective of an active infection.
- DNA clearance was directly related to a decline in the number of these organisms.

TREATMENT

- Most cases of *B. microti* infection are mild and usually resolve on their own
- In severe cases, a combination of **clindamycin and quinine** is administered as the standard treatment. Oral quinine 650 mg every 8 hours plus clindamycin 300 to 600 mg intravenously or intramuscularly every 6 hours (adult doses) for 7 to 10 days. Patients infected with *B. divergens* usually require longer periods, up to 6 weeks, of treatment along with exchange transfusion.
- Treatment reduces the duration of parasitemia.
- Babesial DNA persisted for 16 days in 22 acutely ill subjects who received clindamycin and quinine therapy ($p = 0.03$). Among the subjects who did not receive specific therapy, symptoms of babesiosis persisted up to 114 days.

- The potential for drug-related toxicity includes hearing loss, tinnitus, syncope, hypotension, and gastrointestinal distress.
- **In very serious cases, erythrocyte exchange transfusion can be beneficial or even lifesaving (>10% parasites).**
- In humans, a prospective, randomized study comparing the efficacy of clindamycin and quinine with that of atovaquone and azithromycin has been conducted. This study included 58 patients with non–life-threatening babesiosis. Forty received atovaquone and azithromycin, and 18 received clindamycin and quinine. The resolution of symptoms and parasitemia were similar between the two groups and both treatments were effective for all patients. However, 72% of the patients who received quinine and clindamycin suffered side effects from the antibiotics, compared with 15% of patients in the atovaquone and azithromycin group
- Patients with *B. divergens* infections require erythrocyte exchange transfusion with intravenous clindamycin and oral quinine.
- Pentamidine has been successful.
- Chloroquine, tetracycline, primaquine, sulfadiazine, and pyrimethamine had variable results.

HUMAN COINFECTION

- Coinfection with *B. microti* and other tick-borne pathogens, particularly *B. burgdorferi* (the causative agent of Lyme disease).
- Thirteen percent of Lyme disease patients in babesia-endemic areas are coinfected with *B. microti.*
- The increase in *B. microti* seropositivity is consistent with the increased incidence of Lyme disease.
- Coinfection with *B. divergens* and *B. burgdorferi sensu lato* in Europe.
- *B. microti* is transmitted by the same *Ixodes* tick that perpetuates the agents of Lyme disease and human granulocytic ehrlichiosis and possibly by a novel *Bartonella* species.
- The symptoms of babesiosis and Lyme disease overlap significantly.
- Like babesiosis, Lyme disease presents with nonspecific symptoms of fever, fatigue, and other flu-like symptoms.
- Patients coinfected with *B. microti* and *B. burgdorferi* experience more severe symptoms, resulting in fatality in rare cases and the persistence of postinfectious fatigue.
- Coinfection with babesiosis and Lyme disease may well affect the frequency of recognition of infections due to *B. microti.*
- Antibiotic therapy used for the treatment of Lyme disease is not likely to eradicate *B. microti.*
- A coinfected patient treated only for (early) Lyme disease could therefore still have a persistent babesial infection after therapy.

PREVENTION

- Use of tick repellents before entering a tick-infested area
- Avoidance of or minimization of exposure to tick-infested areas
- Thorough examination of skin after exposure.
- Ticks found after attachment should be removed to limit the possibility of transmission within 24 hours after attachment.

- At the present time, there are no vaccines for humans against babesial organisms.
- The use of living parasites to immunize cattle against the spread of babesiosis has been employed for a long time in livestock management.
- At the present time, there are no vaccines for humans against babesial organisms.

SUGGESTED READINGS

Conrad PA, Kjemtrup AM, et al. Description of Babesia duncani n.sp. (Apicomplexa: Babesiidae) from humans and its differentiation from other piroplasms. *Int J Parasitol* 2006;36(7):779–789.

The morphologic characteristics together with the phylogenetic analysis of two genetic loci support the assertion that B. duncani n.sp. is a distinct species from other known Babesia spp. for which morphologic and sequence information are available.

Herwaldt B, Persing DH, et al. A fatal case of babesiosis in Missouri: identification of another piroplasm that infects humans. *Ann Intern Med* 1996;124(7):643–650.

Although MO1 is probably distinct from B. divergens, the two share morphologic, antigenic, and genetic characteristics; MO1 probably represents a Babesia species not previously recognized to have infected humans. Medical personnel should be aware that patients in the United States can have life-threatening babesiosis even though they are seronegative to B. microti and WA1 antigen.

Herwaldt BL, de Bruyn G, et al. *Babesia divergens*-like infection, Washington State. *Emerg Infect Dis* 2004;10(4):622–629.

By indirect fluorescent-antibody testing, his serum reacted to B. divergens but not to B. microti or WA1 antigens. This case demonstrates that babesiosis can be caused by novel parasites detectable by manual examination of blood smears but not by serologic or molecular testing for B. microti or WA1-type parasites.

Homer MJ, Aguilar-Delfin I, et al. Babesiosis. *Clin Microbiol Rev* 2000;13(3):451–469.

Best overall review of this topic. A must read. Several good tables, pictures and figures.

Krause PJ, Gewurz BE, et al. Persistent and relapsing babesiosis in immunocompromised patients. *Clin Infect Dis* 2008;46(3):370–376.

Immunocompromised people who are infected by B. microti are at risk of persistent relapsing illness. Such patients generally require antibabesial treatment for ≥6 weeks to achieve cure, including 2 weeks after parasites are no longer detected on blood smear.

Krause PJ, Lepore T, et al. Atovaquone and azithromycin for the treatment of babesiosis. *N Engl J Med* 2000;343(20):1454–1458.

For the treatment of babesiosis, a regimen of atovaquone and azithromycin is as effective as a regimen of clindamycin and quinine and is associated with fewer adverse reactions.

Krause PJ, Spielman A, et al. Persistent parasitemia after acute babesiosis. *N Engl J Med* 1998;339(3):160–165.

When left untreated, silent babesial infection may persist for months or even years. Although treatment with clindamycin and quinine reduces the duration of parasitemia, infection may still persist, and recrudescence and side effects are common. Improved treatments are needed.

Loa CC, Adelson ME, et al. Serological diagnosis of human babesiosis by IgG enzyme-linked immunosorbent assay. *Curr Microbiol* 2004;49(6):385–389.

These results indicate that the established ELISA methods could be utilized as an accurate measure for the clinical diagnosis of human babesiosis.

Mylonakis E. When to suspect and how to monitor babesiosis. *Am Fam Physician* 2001;63(10):1969–1974.

Good review article.

Persing DH, Mathiesen D, et al. Detection of *Babesia microti* by polymerase chain reaction. *J Clin Microbiol* 1992;30(8):2097–2103.

Swanson SJ, Neitzel D, et al. Coinfections acquired from ixodes ticks. *Clin Microbiol Rev* 2006;19(4):708–727.

Clinicians should consider the likelihood of coinfection when pursuing laboratory testing or selecting therapy for patients with tick-borne illness.

Vannier E, Gewurz BE, et al. Human babesiosis. *Infect Dis Clin North Am* 2008;22(3):469–488, viii-ix.

Babesial infections range from asymptomatic to severe and occasionally are fatal. Specific laboratory diagnosis of babesial infection is made by morphologic examination of Giemsa-stained blood smears, serology, and amplification of babesial DNA using PCR. The combination of atovaquone and azithromycin is the treatment of choice for mild-to-moderate illness, whereas clindamycin and quinine and exchange transfusion are indicated for severe disease.

Wudhikarn K, Perry EH, et al. Transfusion-transmitted babesiosis in an immunocompromised patient: a case report and review. *Am J Med* 2011;124(9):800–805.

Incidence of transfusion-transmitted babesiosis has increased over the past decade.

26 Q Fever

Dima Youssef and James W. Myers

INTRODUCTION

- *Coxiella burnetii* is a gram-negative intracellular, pleomorphic coccobacillus that undergoes phase variation. This variation is associated with changes in the lipopolysaccharide of the outer membrane.
- The virulent **phase I** exists in nature, but the **avirulent phase II** form is found following repeated passage of phase I bacteria in embryonated chicken eggs.
- *C. burnetii* can be found in arthropods (ticks) rodents, birds, and fish.
- The infected ticks can transmit it to sheep, goats, and cattle.
- Acute Q fever, which develops after an incubation period of a few weeks, is usually characterized by a nonspecific febrile illness, pneumonitis, or hepatitis. On the other hand, chronic Q fever may present months to years after initial infection, usually manifesting as culture-negative endocarditis.

EPIDEMIOLOGY

Sources of Human Infection

- Milk
  - The pasteurization process of commercial milk may reduce transmission of *C. burnetii* from cattle to humans.
- Placental products
- Dried feces in inhaled dust
- **Not by tick exposure**
- Occupational risk
  - Hunters
  - Farmers
  - Abattoir workers
  - Veterinarians
  - US military personnel recently deployed to Iraq and Afghanistan
- France and Australia cases outnumber those from the USA.

CLINICAL MANIFESTATIONS

- The incubation period is usually about 4 weeks. Many patients appear to be asymptomatically infected.
- **A self-limited, flu-like illness appears to be the most common infection**.
- A "chronic fatigue" syndrome has been reported in patients after infection with acute Q fever. This may have a genetic predisposition.
- Pulmonary
  - May present as an **atypical pneumonia**, often with fever, pleurisy, myalgias, diarrhea, and a **severe headache**

- Cough is nonproductive and may be absent despite the presence of pneumonia.
- Usually, Coxiella pneumonia is of mild-to-moderate severity, but it can be rapidly progressive and cause respiratory failure.
- Multiple rounded opacities may be seen.
- Pleural effusions in 1/3 of patients
- Hilar lymphadenopathy
- Thirty days is the average resolution time for the radiographs.
- If an lumbar puncture (LP) is performed for the headache, it is usually normal at this time.
- Liver
  - "Doughnut granulomas" on liver biopsy in patients with an fever of unknown origin (FUO)
  - Q fever hepatitis
    - Fever, abdominal pain, anorexia, nausea, vomiting, and diarrhea
    - Alkaline phosphatase, AST, and ALT levels are usually elevated to two to three times the normal level.
    - Autoantibodies are often present.
- Central nervous involvement
  - Meningoencephalitis occurs in 1% of cases.
  - Lumbar puncture will primarily show mononuclear cells, elevated protein, and normal glucose.
  - Patients with CNS involvement do not demonstrate differences in predisposing conditions but more frequently have occupational exposure to *goats* than patients with acute Q fever but no neurologic involvement.
  - **Headache is the most common symptom**, but Q fever can manifest in a variety of neurologic syndromes including aseptic meningitis and radiculitis.
- Pregnancy
  - Obstetric complications, such as spontaneous abortion, intrauterine growth retardation, intrauterine fetal death, and premature delivery, occur.
  - Pregnant women are at risk of developing of chronic Q fever.
  - A review suggested that the outcome was found to depend on the trimester.
    - **Abortions** occurred in 7 of 7 insufficiently treated patients infected during the **first trimester** as opposed to 1 of 5 patients infected later.
    - Co-trimoxazole given *until delivery* protected against abortion (0/4) but not against the development of chronic infections and did not significantly reduce the colonization of the placenta (2/4 vs. 4/4) in one study.
    - Endocarditis was not observed among any of the patients who received *long-term* co-trimoxazole therapy in another study.
- Heart
  - Myocarditis
    - One percent of Q fever cases
    - T-wave changes
    - Tachycardia, respiratory failure, and cardiac failure
    - May lead to death of the patient
    - Diagnosis by serology to phase II antigen, culture, and biopsy
  - Pericarditis
    - One percent of cases
    - Often associated with endocarditis or myocarditis
    - Effusions and T-wave changes are noted.
    - Chest pain

- Endocarditis
  - One of the causes of "culture-negative" endocarditis
  - Seventy percent of all chronic Q fever cases
  - More common in Europe than in the United States
  - **Abnormal native** valves (congenital, rheumatic, degenerative, or syphilitic)
  - Prosthetic valves can also be infected.
  - Mostly males
  - Age >40
    ○ Immunosuppression is a risk factor.
      - Organ transplant recipients
      - Cancer
      - Lymphoma
      - Rare in HIV patients
  - Symptoms are often related to heart failure.
  - Fever, often low-grade or remittent
  - Weight loss, chills, anorexia, and night sweats
  - Malaise
  - **Hepatosplenomegaly**
  - Marked clubbing
  - **Purpuric rash**
  - **Embolic phenomena in 20%**
  - Immune complex glomerulonephritis and microscopic hematuria
  - LVH on EKG can be seen.
  - Elevated erythrocyte sedimentation rate
  - Polyclonal increase in IgG, IgM, and IgA levels
  - Anemia and thrombocytopenia are often seen.
  - Most patients present with abnormal LFTs.
  - Lactate dehydrogenase and creatine phosphokinase levels may be abnormal.
  - Rheumatoid factor, circulating immune complexes, and cryoglobulin abnormalities can be found.
  - Anti–smooth muscle antibodies, circulating anticoagulant antibodies, antimitochondrial antibodies, antinuclear antibodies, and a positive Coombs test have also been reported.
  - Histologically, one may see significant fibrosis and calcifications, slight inflammation and vascularization, and small or absent vegetations.
    ○ These pathologic features might be confused with noninfectious valvular degenerative damage.
    ○ These histologic features are very similar to that observed with other blood culture–negative types of endocarditis, such as bartonellosis and Whipple disease. Meaning that the histologic features of Q fever endocarditis may be confused with degenerative damage.
- Usually, Q fever endocarditis is diagnosed serologically.
  ○ High levels of anti–phase I antibodies are found in chronic Q fever, **whereas anti–phase II antibodies predominate during acute Q fever**.
  ○ Note that the diagnosis of Q fever endocarditis can also be made by other means including *C. burnetii* isolation in cell *culture, polymerase chain reaction (PCR), or immunohistochemical examination.*
  ○ Patients should be serologically monitored for at least 5 years because of the risk of relapse.

- Vascular infections
  - Aortic aneurysms
  - Vascular grafts
  - Mortality (25%)
  - Surgery helpful

DIAGNOSIS

- Liver function tests are usually abnormal, the WBC count is normal to elevated, and the ESR may be high, but these findings are nonspecific.
- Lab workers must handle specimens by wearing gloves and masks **and only then in biosafety level 3 laboratories**.
- Tissue biopsy specimens
  - Can be tested either fresh, or following formalin fixation and paraffin embedding
  - Immunodetection may be performed by the immunoperoxidase technique, capture ELISA/ELIFA systems, or immunofluorescence with polyclonal or monoclonal antibodies.
  - Fibrin rings or "doughnut" granulomas can be seen.
- Human embryonic lung fibroblasts (HEL cells) grown in shell vials are often used to culture the organism.
  - Blood, cerebrospinal fluid, bone marrow, cardiac valve, vascular aneurysm or graft, bone biopsy, liver biopsy, milk, placenta, and fetal specimens after abortion are suitable for culture.
- *C. burnetii* DNA can be detected by PCR retrospectively in frozen samples and even in *paraffin-embedded* specimens.
- A nested PCR with primers targeted to the com1gene appeared to be a sensitive, specific, and useful method for the detection of *C. burnetii* in *serum* samples in one study.
- Serology
  - Antibodies are found only after 2 to 3 weeks from the onset of the disease.
  - Serology allows the differentiation of acute and chronic Q fever infections.
    ○ The IFA can be used for Q fever diagnosis.
    ○ Phase II antigen is obtained by growing *C. burnetii* in cell culture, while phase I antigen is obtained from spleens of infected mice.
    ○ Antibodies of the IgG, IgM, and IgA subclasses can be determined.
      – During **Acute Q fever**, seroconversion is usually detected from 7 to 15 days after the onset of clinical symptoms, and antibodies are detected by the third week in about 90% of cases.
  - **An IgG anti–phase II antibody titer of ≥200 and an IgM anti–phase II antibody titer of ≥50 are considered significant**.
  - The diagnosis of Q fever can definitely be ruled out if the serum sample was collected 1.5 months after the onset of symptoms or later and is found to be negative.
  - The presence of both an anti–phase II IgG titer of ≥1:200 and IgM titer of ≥1:50 is 100% predictive of acute Q fever.
  - However, such results are observed only in 10% of patients during the second week following the onset of symptoms, 50% during the third week, and 70% during the fourth week.

- **An IgG anti–phase I antibody titer of ≥800 is considered to be highly predictive of Q fever endocarditis, as seen with chronic Q fever**.
- Phase I IgG titers of ≥1:800 are highly indicative of chronic Q fever, with a 98% positive predictive value and 100% sensitivity, whereas titers of ≥1:1,600 are 100% predictive for chronic Q fever.
- Treatment of Q fever (see Table 26-2)
  - **Acute infections** are usually subclinical but should be treated when recognized because there is a risk of progression to endocarditis without therapy.
    - Studies suggest that the risk of endocarditis after acute infection in those patients with an *underlying valvular* abnormality approaches 40% to 75%.
    - Another study reported that *even minor* valvular abnormalities (i.e., mitral valve prolapse, bicuspid aortic valve, and minor valvular leak) could be associated with endocarditis. Patients who received doxycycline alone in one study (2 weeks to 6 months) had a >50% chance of developing endocarditis, whereas those treated with doxycycline and hydroxychloroquine (12 patients) for 1 to 15 months did not develop endocarditis.
    - The treatment of choice is 100 mg of oral doxycycline every 12 hours for 14 days.
    - Macrolides and ciprofloxacin might be useful as well.
- **Chronic infection/endocarditis**
  - Doxycycline (100 mg twice daily) plus hydroxychloroquine (200 mg 3 times daily)1 for at least 18 months; however, therapy may need to be prolonged.
  - **The rationale for hydroxychloroquine is that it will raise the pH within the phagolysosome vacuole of the monocyte. This will make the bacteria more susceptible to the effects of doxycycline**.
  - For patients unable to tolerate hydroxychloroquine, an alternative regimen of doxycycline plus an FQ for a minimum of 3 to 4 years has been proposed.
  - Doxycycline plus rifampin has also been suggested as an alternative therapy; however, drug interactions may limit the usefulness of this combination.
- Serologic follow-up for acute disease
  - Baseline TTE (*transthoracic*) echocardiography for all patients
  - Perform serology at *least twice over 6* months. Some would monitor for up to 2 years.
  - Phase I immunoglobulin (IgG) antibodies >1:800 or more require that a transesophageal echocardiography (TEE) be performed along with a serum PCR.
- Serologic follow-up for chronic disease
  - Monthly serology and clinical evaluation while on antimicrobial therapy
  - Then draw monthly serology for the first 6 months after you stop antibiotics, then every 6 months for 2 years, and possibly yearly thereafter
  - Phase I IgG titers of 1:200 or less are the best predictor of cure.
  - Perform *echocardiography* every 3 months while on antibiotics, and every 6 months for the first 2 years after you stop.

Table 26-1	Treatment Regimens for Q Fever		
Condition	Preferred Regimen	Alternative	Comments
Acute Q fever	Doxycycline	Quinolones, macrolides	Serologic follow-up
Endocarditis	Doxycycline plus hydroxychloroquine for a prolonged course		May need surgery for valve failure
			Monitor ratio of doxycycline to MIC. Keep ratio >1.
			Screen for glucose-6-phosphate dehydrogenase deficiency before receiving hydroxychloroquine and get annual eye exams.
			Perform frequent echocardiograms and get serial serology.
		Doxycycline plus quinolone or rifampin	
Pregnancy	Sulfamethoxazole		
Children (<8 yr)	Sulfamethoxazole	Macrolides?	
Bone	Doxycycline plus hydroxychloroquinolone Prolonged course	May add Rifampin to this regimen	Surgical debridement
Meningoencephalitis	Possibly, quinolones have an advantage here.		CSF penetration?

PREVENTION

- *C. burnetii* is a **category B bioterrorism** agent.
  - Postexposure prophylaxis for **5 days** by using doxycycline is effective if initiated **within 8 to 12** days of exposure.
  - Consider PEP with trimethoprim-sulfamethoxazole (160 mg/800 mg 2×/day) for the duration of the pregnancy for those at risk.
- Vaccines
  - Veterinarians
  - Abattoir workers
  - Farmers
  - Clinical trial (http://clinicaltrials.gov/ct2/show/NCT00584454).

SUGGESTED READING

Bernit E, Pouget J, et al. Neurological involvement in acute Q fever: a report of 29 cases and review of the literature. *Arch Intern Med* 2002;162(6):693–700.

Calza L, Attard L, et al. Doxycycline and chloroquine as treatment for chronic Q fever endocarditis. *J Infect* 2002;45(2):127–129.

Heart involvement is the most common clinical presentation of chronic Q fever, and it occurs almost invariably in patients with previous valvular disease or artificial valves and in the immunocompromised host.

Carcopino X, Raoult D, et al. Managing Q fever during pregnancy: the benefits of long-term cotrimoxazole therapy. *Clin Infect Dis* 2007;45(5):548–555.

Because of its ability to protect against placental infection, intrauterine fetal death, and maternal chronic Q fever, long-term co-trimoxazole treatment should be used to treat pregnant women with Q fever.

Fenollar F, Fournier PE, et al. Risks factors and prevention of Q fever endocarditis. *Clin Infect Dis* 2001;33(3):312–316.

Among patients with valvular defects, we estimate the risk of developing endocarditis to be 39%. A combination of doxycycline plus hydroxychloroquine was better at preventing the development of endocarditis than doxycycline alone (P = 0.009).

Fenollar F, Fournier PE, et al. Molecular detection of *Coxiella burnetii* in the sera of patients with Q fever endocarditis or vascular infection. *J Clin Microbiol* 2004;42(11):4919–4924.

LCN-PCR had a specificity of 100%. High IgG phase I titers decreased the sensitivity of LCN-PCR. In patient samples with titers below 1:25,600 tested prospectively, sensitivity was 100% (7 of 7). The LCN-PCR assay may be helpful in establishing an early diagnosis of chronic Q fever.

Fenollar F, Thuny F, et al. Endocarditis after acute Q fever in patients with previously undiagnosed valvulopathies. *Clin Infect Dis* 2006;42(6):818–821.

Authors concluded that, to prevent endocarditis, these minor valvulopathies must be actively searched for with echocardiography after diagnosis of acute Q fever. Previous studies have shown that the usual treatment regimen of doxycycline (200 mg/d for 3 weeks) for acute Q fever was not sufficient to prevent the occurrence of endocarditis in patients with acute Q fever and valvulopathy. A combination of doxycycline (200 mg/d) plus hydroxychloroquine (600 mg/d) for 12 months seemed to be more effective.

Gikas A, Kofteridis DP, et al. Newer macrolides as empiric treatment for acute Q fever infection. *Antimicrob Agents Chemother* 2001;45(12):3644–3646.

The effectiveness of newer macrolides in acute Q fever for 113 patients was recorded. The mean times to defervescence were 2.9 days for doxycycline and 3.3, 3.9, 3.9, and 6.4 days for clarithromycin, roxithromycin, erythromycin, and beta-lactams, respectively (P < 0.01 for macrolides vs. beta-lactams). We conclude that macrolides may be an adequate empirical antibiotic therapy for acute Q fever.

Hartzell JD, Wood-Morris RN, et al. Q fever: epidemiology, diagnosis, and treatment. *Mayo Clin Proc* 2008;83(5):574–579.

Excellent Review.

Healy B, van Woerden H, et al. Chronic Q fever: different serological results in three countries—results of a follow-up study 6 years after a point source outbreak. *Clin Infect Dis* 2011;52(8):1013–1019.

Authors recommend that all results are interpreted according to the clinical picture, and particular caution is applied in the interpretation of chronic serologic profiles. In order to further our understanding of Q fever infection, we propose that an international standard of Q fever serologic investigation be developed.

Helbig K, Harris R, et al. Immune response genes in the post-Q-fever fatigue syndrome, Q fever endocarditis and uncomplicated acute primary Q fever. *QJM* 2005;98(8):565–574.

There were significant differences between the three Q fever groups. QFS patients differed from both QFE and uncomplicated patients and controls in the frequency of carriage of HLA-DRB1*11 and of the 2/2 genotype of the interferon-gamma intron1 microsatellite. These immunogenetic differences support the concept of different immune states in chronic Q fever, determined by genetic variations in host immune responses, rather than by solely properties of C. burnetii.

Kampschreur LM, Oosterheert JJ, et al. Chronic Q fever-related dual pathogen endocarditis: a case series of three patients. *J Clin Microbiol* 2011;49(4):1692–1694.

Following C. burnetii infection, there is 1% to 5% risk of chronic Q fever. Endocarditis, mycotic aneurysm, and vascular prosthesis infection are common manifestations.

Karakousis PC, Trucksis M, et al. Chronic Q fever in the United States. *J Clin Microbiol* 2006;44(6):2283–2287.

Up to this point, the authors reviewed all cases of chronic Q fever reported in the United States and discussed important issues pertaining to epidemiology, diagnosis, and management of this disease.

Landais C, Fenollar F, et al. From acute Q fever to endocarditis: serological follow-up strategy. *Clin Infect Dis* 2007;44(10):1337–1340.

From these data, we propose a follow-up strategy of serologic testing at the third and sixth months after acute Q fever to obtain an early diagnosis of chronic infection.

*Figure A1 is an excellent tool to use to follow these patients.

Lecaillet A, Mallet MN, et al. Therapeutic impact of the correlation of doxycycline serum concentrations and the decline of phase I antibodies in Q fever endocarditis. *J Antimicrob Chemother* 2009;63(4):771–774.

During the treatment of Q fever endocarditis, serum concentrations of doxycycline should be monitored concomitantly with phase I antibodies in order to adjust the dose of doxycycline to achieve a higher concentration for patients with slow serologic evolution. Patients who had a rapid decline of antibody levels all have a serum doxycycline level >5 mg/L.

Lepidi H, Houpikian P, et al. Cardiac valves in patients with Q fever endocarditis: microbiological, molecular, and histologic studies. *J Infect Dis* 2003;187(7):1097–1106.

Histologically, Q fever endocarditis was characterized by significant fibrosis and calcifications, slight inflammation and vascularization, and small or absent vegetations. They found that the detection of C. burnetii in cardiac valves by immunohistochemical analysis, culture, and PCR decreased significantly only after 1 year of antibiotic treatment, which emphasizes the long persistence of this organism in valve tissues.

Madariaga MG, Pulvirenti J, et al. Q fever endocarditis in HIV-infected patient. *Emerg Infect Dis* 2004;10(3):501–504.

Authors describe a case of Q fever endocarditis in an HIV-infected patient. The case was treated successfully with valvular replacement and a combination of doxycycline and hydroxychloroquine. We review the current literature on Q fever endocarditis, with an emphasis on the coinfection of HIV and C. burnetii.

Marrie TJ. Q fever pneumonia. *Infect Dis Clin North Am* 2010;24(1):27–41.

The epidemiology of Q fever is that of the animal reservoirs of the infection including both direct and indirect contact and use of a variety of products from such animals as cattle, sheep, and goats. It is mild to moderate in severity, and mortality is unusual. It can occur as sporadic or outbreak cases.

Million M, Thuny F, et al. Long-term outcome of Q fever endocarditis: a 26-year personal survey. *Lancet Infect Dis* 2010;10(8):527–535.

The optimum duration of treatment with doxycycline and hydroxychloroquine in Q fever endocarditis is 18 months for native valves and 24 months for prosthetic valves. This duration should be extended only in the absence of favorable serologic outcomes. Patients should be serologically monitored for at least 5 years because of the risk of relapse.

Moodie CE, Thompson HA, et al. Prophylaxis after exposure to *Coxiella burnetii*. *Emerg Infect Dis* 2008;14(10):1558–1566.

On the basis of upper-bound probability estimates of PEP-related adverse events for doxycycline, they concluded that the risk for Q fever illness outweighs the risk for antimicrobial drug-related adverse events when the probability of C. burnetii exposure is >or=7% (pregnant women using trimethoprim-sulfamethoxazole = 16%).

Ong C, Ahmad O, et al. Optic neuritis associated with Q fever: case report and literature review. *Int J Infect Dis* 2010;14(suppl 3):e269–e273.

Reported the first case of ON associated with Q fever in Australia and review all previously reported cases in the medical literature. The impact of therapy with antibiotics and steroids on outcome is discussed.

Rafailidis PI, Dourakis SP, et al. Q fever endocarditis masquerading as mixed cryoglobulinemia type II. A case report and review of the literature. *BMC Infect Dis* 2006;6:32.
Entertain the diagnosis of Q fever endocarditis in cases of mixed type II cryoglobulinemia.

Raoult D, Fenollar F, et al. Q fever during pregnancy: diagnosis, treatment, and follow-up. *Arch Intern Med* 2002;162(6):701–704.
Their results show that C. burnetii infections cause abortion and that women who develop Q fever while pregnant should be treated with co-trimoxazole for the duration of pregnancy, specifically when infected during the first trimester.

Raoult D, Houpikian P, et al. Treatment of Q fever endocarditis: comparison of 2 regimens containing doxycycline and ofloxacin or hydroxychloroquine. *Arch Intern Med* 1999;159(2):167–173.

Raoult D, Tissot-Dupont H, et al. Q fever 1985-1998. Clinical and epidemiologic features of 1,383 infections. *Medicine (Baltimore)* 2000;79(2):109–123.

Reilly S, Northwood JL, et al. Q fever in Plymouth, 1972-88. A review with particular reference to neurological manifestations. *Epidemiol Infect* 1990;105(2):391–408.

Rolain JM, Boulos A, et al. Correlation between ratio of serum doxycycline concentration to MIC and rapid decline of antibody levels during treatment of Q fever endocarditis. *Antimicrob Agents Chemother* 2005;49(7):2673–2676.
The ratio of serum doxycycline concentration (shell vial assay, PCR) to MIC should be monitored during the course of therapy in patients with Q fever endocarditis. Keep ratio >1 if possible.

Scott JW, Baddour LM, et al. Q fever endocarditis: the Mayo Clinic experience. *Am J Med Sci* 2008;336(1):53–57.
Only three patients had valvular vegetations on TEE.

Tilburg JJ, Melchers WJ, et al. Interlaboratory evaluation of different extraction and real-time PCR methods for detection of *Coxiella burnetii* DNA in serum. *J Clin Microbiol* 2010;48(11):3923–3927.

Yeaman MR, Roman MJ, et al. Antibiotic susceptibilities of two *Coxiella burnetii* isolates implicated in distinct clinical syndromes. *Antimicrob Agents Chemother* 1989;33(7):1052–1057.

Zhang GQ, Nguyen SV, et al. Clinical evaluation of a new PCR assay for detection of *Coxiella burnetii* in human serum samples. *J Clin Microbiol* 1998;36(1):77–80.
A nested PCR method was developed for the detection of C. burnetii in human serum samples.

27 Tularemia

Dima Youssef and James W. Myers

INTRODUCTION

Tularemia is a zoonotic disease caused by *Francisella tularensis*.
- There are three subspecies of *F. tularensis*.
  - *Tularensis* (type A), which is the most common type in North America and is highly virulent in humans and animals
  - *Holarctica* (type B), a less virulent type, responsible for human tularemia infection in Europe, Asia, and North America
  - *Mediasiatica*, also less virulent and found in Asia
- *Francisella philomiragia* and *Francisella novicida* are closely related species that are found in immunocompromised patients.
- *F. tularensis* is a small, facultatively intracellular, gram-negative coccobacillus.

EPIDEMIOLOGY

- Small mammals such as voles, mice, squirrels, and rabbits that are reservoirs for *F. tularensis* acquire tularemia through bites from ticks, fleas, and mosquitoes and also through contact with contaminated environments.
- Survives for weeks in water, moist soil, or animal carcasses
- Human infection
  - Tick bites from hard tick species
    - Femoral-inguinal node involvement
    - Dog tick, *Dermacentor variabilis*
    - The lone star tick, *Amblyomma americanum*
    - Rocky Mountain wood tick, *Dermacentor andersoni*
  - Deer flies
  - Cat bites
  - Contact with infected animal tissues or fluids
  - Contact with or ingestion of contaminated water, food, or soil
  - Inhalation of bacteria
- Midwestern states usually have the highest incidence.
- The highest incidence is in 5- to 9-year-olds and 75- to 79-year-olds.
- Males
- Summer months
- Mortality rate around 10% overall

CLINICAL

- 2 to 5 days (up to 2 weeks) incubation period
- Fever, chills, cough, nausea, and other nonspecific symptoms predominate early.
- Symptoms can last for days to months without treatment.

TYPES OF TULAREMIA

- **Ulceroglandular (45% to 85% of cases. All others are 5% to 15%)**
  - Fever
  - The painful papule progresses to a vesicle, then a pustule and finally to an ulcer over several days in most patients
  - The ulcer is painful and may be associated with painful lymphadenitis. Make take several weeks to heal. May appear sporotrichoid.
  - Sinus tracts can form.
  - Scab formation
- **Glandular tularemia**
  - **Lymphadenopathy without a skin lesion**
  - Skin lesion may have been there but disappeared.
  - May persist for a long time and even suppurate
  - Often related to arthropod exposure
- **Oculoglandular tularemia** (Parinaud syndrome)
  - **Portal of injury is from the conjunctiva**, either from the patient's fingers or from splashes into the eye.
  - Usually but not always unilateral
  - Usually no loss of vision
  - Lid edema
  - A painful conjunctivitis, with occasional ulceration
  - Painful lymphadenopathy
    o Cervical
    o Preauricular
    o Submandibular
- **Oropharyngeal tularemia**
  - Eating poorly cooked game
  - **Ingestion of contaminated water or food**
  - Exudative pharyngitis or tonsillitis
  - Ulceration, stomatitis
  - Often, these patients have tender cervical lymph nodes that may suppurate and be complicated by fistula formation.
  - Previous, large outbreak in war-torn Kosovo reported
- **Pneumonic tularemia**
  - May be primary if the patient inhales infective dust. Often occupation related
  - **Usually arises weeks to months after other forms of tularemia, especially typhoidal and ulceroglandular**
    o Fever
    o Dry cough
    o Chest pain
    o Dyspnea
    o Hemoptysis
    o Abnormal radiographs
      - Subsegmental or lobar infiltrates
      - Hilar adenopathy
      - Less common manifestations are air space opacification of an entire lobe or segment, cavitation, oval opacities, pericardial effusion, linear opacities and septal lines,

apical and miliary disease resembling tuberculosis, a mediastinal mass, empyema with bronchopleural fistula, and residual cystic changes, calcification, and fibrosis.

- **Pleural effusions (30% of cases) mimic TB.**
  - High pleural fluid concentrations of adenosine deaminase, lysozyme, and beta 2-microglobulin occur in both diseases.
  - As is the case with tuberculous pleural effusions, pleural fluid in tularemia may show an abundance of lymphocytes, predominantly CD4-positive T lymphocytes.
- **Typhoidal tularemia**
  - Fever
  - **No predominant lymphadenopathy, or localizing signs**
  - May follow any form but probably from inapparent inhalation or ingestion
  - **The diagnosis can be made by isolation in blood cultures.**
  - Abdominal pain, **watery diarrhea**, and vomiting may be early symptoms.
  - Headache, myalgias, sore throat, and cough occur often.
  - Hepatomegaly, splenomegaly, cholangitis, and liver abscess have been described.
  - **Pulmonary infiltrates are common.**
  - **Can have a high mortality**
- **Complications of tularemia**
  - Septicemia, meningitis, endocarditis, hepatitis, skin rash, and renal failure

DIAGNOSIS

- The WBC and sedimentation rate may be normal or high.
- Thrombocytopenia, hyponatremia, and elevated serum transaminases are often seen.
- Culture
  - Biosafety level 3 needed for isolation
  - *F. tularensis* grows best on **cysteine-supplemented media** such as chocolate agar, cysteine heart agar, and buffered charcoal yeast extract (as for Legionella)
- PCR tests have been used for diagnosis.
  - Tissue, blood, or exudate may be used.
- Serology
  - Serologic methods include tube agglutination, microagglutination, hemagglutination, and enzyme-linked immunosorbent assays.
  - Fourfold increase between acute and convalescent serology or >1:160 on acute titer is suggestive.
  - Cross-reactivity may occur between *Brucella*, *Salmonella*, *Yersinia*, and *Legionella* antigens, but these reactions are usually lower in titers.

TREATMENT (SEE TABLE 27-1)

PREVENTION

- Currently, vaccination cannot be recommended for postexposure use.
- Use ciprofloxacin or doxycycline for mass casualty exposure.
- Not transmitted person-to-person. No isolation needed in the health care setting.

Table 27-1	Treatment of Tularemia	
	Dose	**Comments**
Streptomycin	7.5–10 mg/kg intramuscularly every 12 hours for 7–14 days	Historic drug of choice
Gentamicin	5 mg/kg/day in divided doses for 7–14 days	Equal to streptomycin Keep peak around 5. Once-daily dosing is probably effective as well.
Doxycycline	2 g/day in divided oral doses for at least 14 days	Higher relapse rate Postexposure prophylaxis for mass casualty?
Levofloxacin and ciprofloxacin	500 mg for 14 days 500 mg b.i.d. for 14 days	Effective. Some authors consider it to be a drug of choice but others disagree. Postexposure use?
Chloramphenicol	50–100 mg/kg/day intravenously in divided doses, may be added to streptomycin to treat meningitis	Consider combinations of streptomycin with chloramphenicol, or a combination of doxycycline with either streptomycin or gentamicin for meningitis.
Cephalosporins		Failures reported

SUGGESTED READING

Avashia SB, Petersen JM, et al. First reported prairie dog-to-human tularemia transmission, Texas, 2002. *Emerg Infect Dis* 2004;10(3):483–486.
  A tularemia outbreak, caused by F. tularensis type B, occurred among wild-caught, commercially traded prairie dogs.
Barry EM, Cole LE, et al. Vaccines against tularemia. *Hum Vaccin* 2009;5(12):832–838.
  This review summarizes the progress and promise of these various candidates.
Byington CL, Bender JM, et al. Tularemia with vesicular skin lesions may be mistaken for infection with herpes viruses. *Clin Infect Dis* 2008;47(1):e4–e6.
  Clinicians must recognize the cutaneous manifestations of tularemia and be able to distinguish these from lesions seen with herpes viruses.
Eliasson H, Broman T, et al. Tularemia: current epidemiology and disease management. *Infect Dis Clin North Am* 2006;20(2):289–311, ix.
Ellis J, Oyston PC, et al. Tularemia. *Clin Microbiol Rev* 2002;15(4):631–646.
  Review article.
Feldman KA, Enscore RE, et al. An outbreak of primary pneumonic tularemia on Martha's Vineyard. *N Engl J Med* 2001;345(22):1601–1606.
  Study of this outbreak of primary pneumonic tularemia implicates lawn mowing and brush cutting as risk factors for this infection.
Gangat N. Cerebral abscesses complicating tularemia meningitis. *Scand J Infect Dis* 2007;39(3):258–261.

Tularemia meningitis is a distinctly rare entity with only 14 cases reported in the literature, half of which occurred prior to 1950. In this case author provides the first description of cerebral microabscesses, which occurred as a complication of tularemia meningitis.

Hassoun A, Spera R, et al. Tularemia and once-daily gentamicin. *Antimicrob Agents Chemother* 2006;50(2):824.

Hepburn MJ, Purcell BK, et al. Live vaccine strain *Francisella tularensis* is detectable at the inoculation site but not in blood after vaccination against tularemia. *Clin Infect Dis* 2006;43(6):711–716.

Jensen WA, Kirsch CM. Tularemia. *Semin Respir Infect* 2003;18(3):146–158.
This article reviews the history, clinical features, diagnostic evaluation, and treatment of this organism with an emphasis placed on its potential role as an agent of biologic warfare.

Johansson A, Berglund L, et al. Comparative analysis of PCR versus culture for diagnosis of ulceroglandular tularemia. *J Clin Microbiol* 2000;38(1):22–26.
PCR was more sensitive than culture for demonstration of F. tularensis in wound specimens.

Johansson A, Berglund L, et al. Ciprofloxacin for treatment of tularemia. *Clin Infect Dis* 2001;33(2):267–268.

Khoury JA, Bohl DL, et al. Tularemia in a kidney transplant recipient: an unsuspected case and literature review. *Am J Kidney Dis* 2005;45(5):926–929.

Maurin M, Castan B, et al. Real-time PCR for diagnosis of oculoglandular tularemia. *Emerg Infect Dis* 2010;16(1):152–153.

Nigrovic LE, Wingerter SL. Tularemia. *Infect Dis Clin North Am* 2008;22(3):489–504, ix.

Petersen JM, Carlson JK, et al. Multiple *Francisella tularensis* subspecies and clades, tularemia outbreak, Utah. *Emerg Infect Dis* 2008;14(12):1928–1930.
In July 2007, a deer fly–associated outbreak of tularemia occurred in Utah.

Ruef C. Clinical and epidemiological features of tularemia. *Infection* 2009;37(6):477.

Splettstoesser W, Guglielmo-Viret V, et al. Evaluation of an immunochromatographic test for rapid and reliable serodiagnosis of human tularemia and detection of *Francisella tularensis*-specific antibodies in sera from different mammalian species. *J Clin Microbiol* 2010;48(5):1629–1634.
Developed a novel immunochromatographic test (ICT) to efficiently detect F. tularensis–specific antibodies in sera from humans and other mammalian species (nonhuman primate, pig, and rabbit).

Staples JE, Kubota KA, et al. Epidemiologic and molecular analysis of human tularemia, United States, 1964-2004. *Emerg Infect Dis* 2006;12(7):1113–1118.
Through a combined epidemiologic and molecular approach to human cases of tularemia, we provide new insights into the disease for future investigation.

Thomas LD, Schaffner W. Tularemia pneumonia. *Infect Dis Clin North Am* 2010;24(1):43–55.
This article describes the history of this infection, epidemiology, methods of diagnosis and treatment, and its potential as a bioterrorism weapon.

Tularemia—Missouri, 2000-2007. *MMWR Morb Mortal Wkly Rep* 2009;58(27):744–748.
Approximately 40% of all tularemia cases reported to CDC each year occur in Arkansas, Oklahoma, and Missouri.

VII Cardiovascular Infections

28 Infective Endocarditis: Diagnosis

Michael Davis and Jonathan P. Moorman

Infective endocarditis refers to the microbial infection of the valvular and nonvalvular endothelium of the heart. Classification of infective endocarditis has been based on clinical presentation, with both acute and subacute forms of disease. The annual incidence of endocarditis is estimated to be 2 to 7 per 100,000. Four components are characteristic: (i) cardiac involvement, (ii) systemic inflammation, (iii) embolic phenomena, and (iv) immune complex disease.

ETIOLOGY AND RISK FACTORS

- **Native valve endocarditis** (NVE) is primarily caused by streptococci and *Staphylococcus aureus* (>70% of cases), but less common bacterial causes include the HACEK group (*Haemophilus, Actinobacillus, Corynebacterium, Eikenella,* and *Kingella*), other gram-negative bacilli, community-acquired enterococci, and *Neisseria* species. Other organisms include *Chlamydia, Mycoplasma, Legionella, Bartonella, Brucella, Tropheryma, Rickettsia,* and fungi.
- *S. aureus* is the most common pathogen found in IV drug users, followed by streptococci and enterococci. The tricuspid valve is the most common site. Septic pulmonary emboli are common.
- **Prosthetic valve endocarditis** (PVE) is usually due to *Staphylococcus aureus* or *Staphylococcus epidermidis*. Early PVE occurs within 2 months of surgery, late PVE after 2 months.

Pathogen	Frequency (%)
S. aureus	32
Viridans streptococci	18
Enterococcus	11
Coagulase-negative Staphylococcus	11
Streptococcus bovis	7
Streptococcus (other)	5
HACEK	2
Gram-negative bacilli	2
Fungi	2
Culture-negative[a]	8

[a]May include *Coxiella, Legionella, Mycoplasma, Tropheryma whippelii, Brucella, Bartonella,* and *Chlamydia*.

CLINICAL PRESENTATION

Fever is found in the majority (>95%) of cases. Audible heart murmur is present in >85% of cases. Common findings include:

- Splenomegaly
- Petechiae
- Splinter hemorrhages
- Osler nodes
- Janeway lesions
- Major embolic phenomena
- Neurologic deficits
- Fatigue
- Weight loss
- Night sweats

DIAGNOSTIC FINDINGS

Diagnosis of infective endocarditis is based upon clinical, microbiologic, and echo-cardiographic criteria.

- Blood cultures (two to three sets) within 1 hour should be obtained.
- Echocardiogram is required to identify vegetations and evaluate valvular competence.
  - TTE: 98% specific, <60% sensitive
  - TEE: 76% to 100% sensitive, 94% specific
  - TEE the test of choice for PVE
- Other laboratory findings include elevated ESR, anemia, hematuria, and proteinuria.
- False-positive VDRL, elevated ANA, RF, and cryoglobulins can be seen.
- Modified Duke criteria:
  - Probable endocarditis: 2 major criteria or 1 major and 3 minor or 5 minor; possible endocarditis: 1 major and 1 minor or 3 minor

Clinical Manifestations (Minor Criteria)

- **Epidemiologic minor criteria**: predisposing heart conditions: rheumatic heart disease, valvular insufficiency, indwelling catheters, pacemakers, prosthetic heart valves, congenital heart disease, prior endocarditis, or IVDU
- **Fever**, temperature >38°C
- **Vascular phenomena**: major arterial emboli, septic pulmonary infarcts, mycotic aneurysm, intracranial hemorrhage, conjunctival hemorrhages, and Janeway lesions
- **Immunologic phenomena**: glomerulonephritis, Osler nodes, and Roth spots

Echocardiography (Major Criteria)

- **Major criteria**:
  - Echocardiographic evidence of vegetation, endocardial abscess, or new valvular regurgitation
- Echocardiography should be performed ASAP in all cases of suspected IE.
- TTE versus TEE depends on patient risk stratification. High-risk patients get initial TEE, and low initial risk patients get initial TTE.
- Repeat echocardiography and perform TEE if high clinical suspicion, for patients at high risk for complications, with worsening clinical status, and at the completion of therapy.
- Echocardiography may be used to suggest surgical intervention: unresolving infection or embolization, or valvular dysfunction causing heart failure.

Microbiology (Major and Minor Criteria)

- **Major criteria**:
  - Two *separate blood cultures with specific organisms* known to cause IE: Viridans streptococci, *S. bovis*, HACEK group, *S. aureus*, or community-acquired entero-cocci in the absence of a primary focus
  - *Persistently positive blood cultures*: 2 positive cultures drawn >12 hours apart, or all of 3 or a majority of >4 separate cultures of blood (with first and last sample drawn at least 1 hour apart)
  - Single positive blood culture for *Coxiella burnetii* or anti–phase 1 IgG antibody titer >1:800
- **Minor criteria**: positive blood culture not meeting major criteria or serologic evidence of active infection with organism consistent with IE

SUGGESTED READINGS

Baddour LM, et al. Infective endocarditis: diagnosis and management. *Circulation* 2005;111;e394–e434.
  This American Heart Association scientific statement thoroughly outlines the diagnosis, treatment, and management of complications in infective endocarditis using an evidence-based scoring system. This article also provides a reasonable approach to diagnosis of endocarditis (please see http://circ.ahajournals.org/content/111/23/e394/F1.large.jpg).

Cabell CH, Jollis JG, Peterson GE, et al. Changing patient characteristics and the effect on mortality in endocarditis. *Arch Intern Med* 2002;162:90–94.

Durack DT, Lukes AS, Bright DK. New criteria for diagnosis of infective endocarditis: utilization of specific echocardiographic findings. Duke Endocarditis Service. *Am J Med* 1994;96:200–209.

Fowler VG Jr, Sanders LL, Kong LK, et al. Infective endocarditis due to *Staphylococcus aureus*: 59 prospectively identified cases with follow-up. *Clin Infect Dis* 1999;28:106–114.

Fowler VG et al. *Staphylococcus aureus* endocarditis: a consequence of medical progress. *JAMA* 2005;293:3012–3021.

Fournier PE, et al. Comprehensive diagnostic strategy for blood culture-negative endocarditis: a prospective study of 819 new cases. *Clin Infect Dis* 2010;51(2):131–140.
  This study highlighted the role of zoonotic agents and noninfective diseases in blood culture–negative endocarditis. They propose a diagnostic approach for culture-negative endocarditis that includes serology and PCR (http://cid.oxfordjournals.org/content/51/2/131/F7.expansion.html).

Goldenberger D, Kunzli A, Vogt P, et al. Molecular diagnosis of bacterial endocarditis by broad-range PCR amplification and direct sequencing. *J Clin Microbiol* 1997;35:2733–2739.

Houpikian P, Raoult D. Diagnostic methods current best practices and guidelines for identification of difficult-to-culture pathogens in infective endocarditis. *Infect Dis Clin North Am* 2002;16(2):377–392.

Lindner JR, Case RA, Dent JM, et al. Diagnostic value of echocardiography in suspected endocarditis: an evaluation based on the pretest probability of disease. *Circulation* 1996;93:730–736.

Prendergast BD, Tornos P. Surgery for infective endocarditis: who and when? *Circulation* 2010;121:1141–1152.

Roder BL, Wandall DA, Frimodt-Moller N, et al. Clinical features of *Staphylococcus aureus* endocarditis. *Arch Intern Med* 1999;159:462–469.

29 Infective Endocarditis: Treatment and Prophylaxis

Hana Saleh and Jonathan P. Moorman

INTRODUCTION

- Empirical antibiotic treatment must be immediately started and targeted against the suspected organisms in patients with either native or prosthetic valve endocarditis.
- Antibiotic therapy would then be modified according to the specific organism growing in blood cultures, its susceptibility, and the antibiotic minimum inhibitory concentration (MIC).
- The antibiotic dose should be adjusted according to the patient's renal function, and patients should be monitored for development of medication side effects.
- Duration of antibiotic therapy starts from the time of first set of negative blood cultures.

ANTIBIOTIC THERAPY IN INFECTIVE ENDOCARDITIS:

I. Antibiotic regimens for treatment of infective endocarditis caused by streptococci and staphylococci species in patients with native valve and prosthetic valve are outlined in **Table 29-1** and **Table 29-2**. The use of initial, low-dose gentamicin in the setting of native valve *Staphylococcus aureus* endocarditis appears to add nephrotoxicity and is no longer recommended.

It is recommended to rule out colon cancer or other gastrointestinal lesions in patients with bacteremia or endocarditis caused by *Streptococcus bovis*.

II. Antibiotic regimens for treatment of infective endocarditis caused by *Streptococcus pneumoniae*, *Streptococcus pyogenes*, and groups B, C, and G streptococci:
- **S. pneumoniae** (highly susceptible to penicillin) or **S. pyogenes**: penicillin G IV, cefazolin, or ceftriaxone for 4 weeks. Vancomycin is considered as an alternative only in penicillin allergic patients.
- **S. pneumoniae** (intermediately or highly resistant to penicillin): High-dose penicillin or a third-generation cephalosporin.
- **Groups B, C, and G streptococci**: penicillin or cephalosporin for 4 to 6 weeks, plus gentamicin for 2 weeks

III. Antibiotic regimens for treatment of infective endocarditis caused by enterococci species in patients with native valve and prosthetic valve are outlined in Table 29-3.

Table 29-1	Treatment of Endocarditis Caused by Streptococci and Staphylococci Species in Patients with Native Valve		
Organism		**Antimicrobial Regimen**	**Alternative Regimen**[a]
Viridans group streptococci and S. bovis	**MIC ≤0.12 µg/mL** (highly susceptible to penicillin)	• Penicillin G 12–18 million U IV per day, in a continuous infusion, or given in four to six doses, for **4 weeks** • Penicillin G 12–18 million U IV per day, **plus** gentamicin 3 mg/kg IV/IM once daily, for **2 weeks** • Ceftriaxone 2 g IV once daily, **plus** gentamicin 3 mg/kg IV/IM once daily, for **2 weeks**	• Vancomycin 30 mg/kg divided in two IV doses per day (not more than 2 g/day), for **4 weeks**
	MIC >0.12 and ≤0.5 µg/mL (relative resistance to penicillin)	• Penicillin G 24 million U IV per day, for **4 weeks, plus** gentamicin 3 mg/kg IV/IM once daily, for **2 weeks** • Ceftriaxone 2 g IV once daily, for **4 weeks, plus** gentamicin 3 mg/kg IV/IM once daily, for **2 weeks**	• Vancomycin 30 mg/kg divided in two IV doses per day (not more than 2 g/day), for **4 weeks**
Staphylococci (S. aureus or coagulase-negative staphylococci)	Methicillin-sensitive	• Nafcillin or oxacillin[b] 12 g/day IV in four to six doses, for **6 weeks**	• Cefazolin[c] 6 g/day IV in three doses, for **6 weeks** • Daptomycin 6 mg/kg daily for **6 weeks**
	Methicillin-resistant	• Vancomycin 30 mg/kg divided in two IV doses per day, (not more than 2 g/day), for **6 weeks**[d]	• Daptomycin 6 mg/kg daily for **6 weeks**

Some experts believe vancomycin dose should be adjusted for a trough level of 10–20 µg/mL.

[a]Alternative therapy to be used in patients with penicillin intolerance

[b]In cases of uncomplicated right-sided endocarditis, **2-week** therapy with nafcillin/oxacillin **plus** gentamicin can be used.

[c]Substitute with vancomycin if history of anaphylaxis to penicillin is present.

[d]Daptomycin should be considered for treatment of methicillin-resistant S. aureus, if MIC to vancomycin is >1 µg/mL.

MIC, minimum inhibitory concentration.

Modified from Baddour LM, Taubert KA, et al. Infective endocarditis: diagnosis, antimicrobial therapy, and management of complications: a statement for healthcare professionals from the Committee on Rheumatic Fever, Endocarditis, and Kawasaki Disease, Council on Cardiovascular Disease in the Young, and the Councils on Clinical Cardiology, Stroke, and Cardiovascular Surgery and Anesthesia, American Heart Association. Circulation 2005;111(23):e394–e434.

Table 29-2   Treatment of Endocarditis Caused by Streptococci and Staphylococci Species in Patients with Prosthetic Valve

Organism		Antimicrobial Regimen	Alternative Regimen[a]
Viridans group streptococci and S. bovis	MIC ≤0.12 µg/mL (highly susceptible to penicillin)	• Penicillin G 24 million U IV per day, for **6 weeks**, ± gentamicin 3 mg/kg IV/IM once daily, for **2 weeks** • Ceftriaxone 2 g IV once daily, for **6 weeks**, ± gentamicin 3 mg/kg IV/IM once daily, for **2 weeks**	• Vancomycin 30 mg/kg divided in 2 IV doses per day, (not more than 2 g/day), for **6 weeks**
	MIC >0.12 (relative or complete resistance to penicillin)	• Penicillin G 24 million U IV per day, for **6 weeks**, **plus** gentamicin 3 mg/kg IV/IM once daily, for **6 weeks** • Ceftriaxone 2 g IV once daily, for **6 weeks**, **plus** gentamicin 3 mg/kg IV/IM once daily, for **6 weeks**	• Vancomycin 30 mg/kg divided in two IV doses per day, (not more than 2 g/day), for **6 weeks**
Staphylococci (S. aureus, or coagulase-negative staphylococci)	Methicillin-sensitive	• Nafcillin or oxacillin[b] 12 g/day IV in four to six doses, for **≥6 weeks, plus** rifampin 900 mg/day in 3 doses, for **≥6 weeks, plus** gentamicin 3 mg/kg IV/IM per day in two to three doses, for **2 weeks**	
	Methicillin-resistant	• Vancomycin 30 mg/kg divided in two IV doses per day, (not more than 2 g/day), for **≥6 weeks, plus** rifampin 900 mg/day in three doses, for **≥6 weeks, plus** gentamicin 3 mg/kg IV/IM per day in two to three doses, for **2 weeks**	

[a]Alternative therapy to be used in patients with penicillin intolerance
[b]Can substitute nafcillin or oxacillin with penicillin G 24 million U IV per day in four to six doses, if the staphylococcus strain is penicillin-sensitive (MIC ≤0.1 µg/mL)
Some experts believe vancomycin dose should be adjusted for a trough level of 10–20 µg/mL
MIC, minimum inhibitory concentration
Modified from Baddour LM, Taubert KA, et al. Infective endocarditis: diagnosis, antimicrobial therapy, and management of complications: a statement for healthcare professionals from the Committee on Rheumatic Fever, Endocarditis, and Kawasaki Disease, Council on Cardiovascular Disease in the Young, and the Councils on Clinical Cardiology, Stroke, and Cardiovascular Surgery and Anesthesia, American Heart Association. Circulation 2005;111:e394–e434.

Table 29-3 Treatment of Endocarditis Caused by Enterococci Species in Patients with Either Native or Prosthetic Valve

Organism	Antimicrobial Regimen	Alternative Regimen[a]
Enterococcal strains susceptible to penicillin, gentamicin, and vancomycin	• Ampicillin 12 g/day IV in six doses, for **4–6 weeks**,[b] **plus** gentamicin 3 mg/kg IV/IM per day in three doses, for **4–6 weeks**[b] • Penicillin G 18–30 million U IV per day, in a continuous infusion, or given in six doses, for **4–6 weeks**,[b] **plus** gentamicin 3 mg/kg IV/IM per day in three doses, for **4–6 weeks**[b]	Vancomycin 30 mg/kg divided in two IV doses per day, (not more than 2 g/day), for **6 weeks**, **plus** gentamicin 3 mg/kg IV/IM per day in three doses, for **6 weeks**
Enterococcal strains susceptible to penicillin, streptomycin, and vancomycin and resistant to gentamicin	• Ampicillin 12 g/day IV in six doses, for **4–6 weeks**,[b] **plus** streptomycin 15 mg/kg IV/IM per day in two doses, for **4–6 weeks**[b] • Penicillin G 24 million U IV per day, in a continuous infusion, or given in six doses, for **4–6 weeks**,[b] **plus** streptomycin 15 mg/kg IV/IM per day in two doses, for **4–6 weeks**[b]	Vancomycin 30 mg/kg divided in two IV doses per day, (not more than 2 g/day), for **6 weeks**, **plus** streptomycin 15 mg/kg IV/IM per day in two doses, for **6 weeks**
Enterococcal strains resistant to penicillin and susceptible to aminoglycoside and vancomycin	β-Lactamase producing	• Ampicillin–sulbactam 12 g/day IV in four doses, for **6 weeks**, **plus** gentamicin[c] 3 mg/kg IV/IM per day in three doses, for **6 weeks**	Vancomycin 30 mg/kg divided in two IV doses per day, (not more than 2 g/day), for **6 weeks**, **plus** gentamicin[c] 3 mg/kg IV/IM per day in three doses, for **6 weeks**

(Continued)

Table 29-3 Treatment of Endocarditis Caused by Enterococci Species in Patients with Either Native or Prosthetic Valve *(Continued)*

Organism		Antimicrobial Regimen	Alternative Regimen[a]
Enterococcal strains resistant to penicillin, aminoglycoside, and vancomycin	Intrinsic penicillin resistance	• Vancomycin 30 mg/kg divided in two IV doses per day, (not more than 2 g/day), **plus** gentamicin 3 mg/kg IV/IM per day in three doses, for **6 weeks**	
	Enterococcus faecium	• Linezolid 1,200 mg/day IV/PO in two doses, for **≥8 weeks** • Quinupristin–dalfopristin (Synercid) 22.5 mg/kg/day IV in three doses, for **≥8 weeks**	
	Enterococcus faecalis	• Imipenem/cilastatin 2 g/day IV in four doses, for **≥8 weeks**, **plus** ampicillin 12 g/day IV in six doses, for **≥8 weeks** • Ceftriaxone 4 g/day IV/IM in two doses, for **≥8 weeks**, **plus** ampicillin 12 g/day IV in six doses, for **≥8 weeks**	

[a]Alternative therapy to be used in patients with penicillin intolerance

Some experts believe vancomycin dose should be adjusted for a trough level of 10–20 μg/mL.

[b]For patients with **native valve** and with duration of symptoms <3 months, treat for 4 weeks. If symptomatic for >3 months, treat for 6 weeks. Patients with **prosthetic valve** should be treated for at least 6 weeks.

[c]If the enterococcal strain is resistant to gentamicin, the duration of therapy should be extended for more than 6 weeks.

Council on Cardiovascular Disease in the Young, and the Councils on Clinical Cardiology, Stroke, and Cardiovascular Surgery and Anesthesia, American Heart Association. *Circulation* 2005;111:e394–e434.

Modified from Baddour LM, Taubert KA, et al. Infective endocarditis: diagnosis, antimicrobial therapy, and management of complications: a statement for healthcare professionals from the Committee on Rheumatic Fever, Endocarditis, and Kawasaki Disease.

IV. Antibiotic regimens for treatment of infective endocarditis caused by the **HACEK microorganisms**:
- HACEK group includes *Haemophilus parainfluenzae, Haemophilus aphrophilus, Haemophilus paraphrophilus, Haemophilus influenzae, Actinobacillus actinomycetemcomitans, Cardiobacterium hominis, Eikenella corrodens, Kingella kingae,* and *Kingella denitrificans*.
- Drugs of choice are either ceftriaxone or ampicillin-sulbactam.
- In patients with β-lactam intolerance, fluoroquinolones can be used.
- Duration of therapy is 4 weeks in patients with native valve and 6 weeks in those with prosthetic valve.

V. Antibiotic regimens for treatment of infective endocarditis caused by **Enterobacteriaceae species**:
- Main therapy includes valvular surgery along with several weeks of antibiotics.
- Antibiotics should be chosen according to the gram-negative bacilli species and the antimicrobial susceptibility.
- Therapy for ***Escherichia coli*** *or **Proteus mirabilis*** endocarditis:
  - Ampicillin 2 g IV every 4 hours
  - Penicillin 20 million U IV daily
  - A broad-spectrum cephalosporin **plus** gentamicin 1.7 mg/kg every 8 hours
- Therapy for ***Salmonella*** endocarditis: third-generation cephalosporins
- Therapy for ***Klebsiella*** endocarditis: third-generation cephalosporins **plus** gentamicin or amikacin

VI. Antibiotic regimens for treatment of infective endocarditis caused by ***Pseudomonas*** **species**:
- For left- and right-sided endocarditis, antimicrobial therapy along with surgery is recommended in most cases.
- Antibiotic regimen: tobramycin 8 mg/kg IV/IM once daily, **plus** either penicillin (ticarcillin, piperacillin, azlocillin), **or** ceftazidime, or cefepime, for **6 weeks**

VII. Infective endocarditis caused by *Neisseria gonorrhoeae* species is uncommon and requires an infectious disease physician consult. Therapy is similar to that directed against *S. pneumoniae*.

VIII. Antibiotic regimens for treatment of infective endocarditis caused by ***Bartonella***:
- Culture-**negative** with suspected *Bartonella*:
  - Ceftriaxone 2 g IV once daily, for **6 weeks, plus** gentamicin 3 mg/kg IV/IM per day in three doses, for **2 weeks,** ± doxycycline 200 mg PO/IV daily in two doses, for **6 weeks**
- Culture-**positive** with confirmed *Bartonella*:
  - Doxycycline 200 mg PO/IV daily in two doses, for **6 weeks, plus** gentamicin 3 mg/kg IV/IM per day in three doses, for **2 weeks**
  - Can substitute gentamicin with rifampin 600 mg per day PO/IV in two doses

IX. Antibiotic regimens for treatment of **culture-negative** infective endocarditis are outlined in **Table 29-4**.

X. Antibiotic regimens for treatment of infective endocarditis caused by **fungi** (mainly ***Candida*** and ***Aspergillus*** species):
- Valve replacement **plus** 6 weeks of amphotericin, followed by lifelong suppressive therapy with an oral azole

Table 29-4	Treatment of Culture-Negative Endocarditis

Native Valve	Prosthetic Valve
• Ampicillin–sulbactam 12 g/day IV in four doses, for **4–6 weeks, plus** gentamicin 3 mg/kg IV/IM per day in three doses, for **4–6 weeks** • Vancomycin[a] 30 mg/kg divided in two IV doses per day, (not more than 2 g/day), for **4–6 weeks, plus** gentamicin 3 mg/kg IV/IM per day in three doses, for **4–6 weeks, plus** ciprofloxacin 1,000 mg PO daily, or 800 mg IV daily in two doses, for **4–6 weeks**	• If symptoms of endocarditis started **within 1 year** of valve replacement: • Vancomycin 30 mg/kg divided in two IV doses per day, (not more than 2 g/day), for **6 weeks, plus** gentamicin 3 mg/kg IV/IM per day in three doses, for **2 weeks, plus** cefepime 6 g/day IV in three doses, for **6 weeks, plus** rifampin 900 mg/day PO/IV in three doses for **6 weeks** • If symptoms of endocarditis started **after 1 year** of valve replacement: • Same treatment as for native valve, **plus** rifampin, for **6 weeks**

Some experts believe vancomycin dose should be adjusted for a trough level of 10–20 µg/mL.
[a]Use vancomycin in patients with penicillin allergy.
Modified from Baddour LM, Taubert KA, et al. Infective endocarditis: diagnosis, antimicrobial therapy, and management of complications: a statement for healthcare professionals from the Committee on Rheumatic Fever, Endocarditis, and Kawasaki Disease, Council on Cardiovascular Disease in the Young, and the Councils on Clinical Cardiology, Stroke, and Cardiovascular Surgery and Anesthesia, American Heart Association. *Circulation* 2005;111:e394–e434.

SURGERY IN INFECTIVE ENDOCARDITIS

• Consultation with a cardiac surgeon is indicated for patients with infective endocarditis with prosthetic valve.
• Indications of surgery in infective endocarditis are outlined in **Table 29-5**.

PROPHYLAXIS WITH INFECTIVE ENDOCARDITIS

• Dental procedures for which prophylaxis of endocarditis is reasonable include those that require manipulation of the gingiva or periapical area of the teeth or oral mucosa perforation.
• Prophylaxis is not recommended for patients receiving transesophageal echocardiogram, esophagogastroduodenoscopy, or colonoscopy.
• It is **reasonable** to provide prophylaxis to patients with:
  • Prosthetic valve or prosthetic material used in the valve repair
  • Previous episode of infective endocarditis
  • Congenital heart defect that is cyanotic with unrepaired defect, or with repaired defect using prosthetic material, within 6 months after the surgery, or with repaired defect with residual deformities at or close to the prosthetic material used
  • Heart transplant with regurgitation due to an abnormal valve structure
• Prophylaxis is **no longer required** in patients with: aortic stenosis, mitral stenosis, mitral valve prolapse, or native valve disease.
• Recommended antibiotic regimens to be given 30 to 60 minutes before the dental procedure:

Table 29-5	Indications of Surgery in Infective Endocarditis

Native Valve

Class I: surgery is **indicated** in the presence of:
- Heart failure due to valvular stenosis or regurgitation
- Hemodynamic evidence of elevated LV end-diastolic or left atrial pressures with aortic or mitral valve regurgitation
- Fungal endocarditis, or resistant microorganisms
- Heart block, annular or aortic abscess

Class IIa: surgery is **reasonable** in the presence of:
- Recurrent systemic emboli and persistent vegetations despite appropriate medical treatment

Class IIb: surgery **may be considered** in the presence of:
- More than 10-mm mobile vegetation regardless of the presence or absence of emboli

Prosthetic Valve

Class I: surgery is **indicated** in the presence of:
- Heart failure
- Prosthetic valve dehiscence
- Worsening obstruction or regurgitation
- Heart block, annular or aortic abscess

Class IIa: surgery is **reasonable** in the presence of:
- Recurrent systemic emboli and persistent vegetations despite appropriate medical treatment
- Relapsing infection

Class III: surgery is **not indicated** in the presence of:
- First time infection with a sensitive organism, with absence of complications

Modified from 2008 focused update incorporated into the ACC/AHA 2006 guidelines for the management of patients with valvular heart disease: a report of the American College of Cardiology/American Heart Association Task Force on Practice Guidelines (Writing Committee to Revise the 1998 Guidelines for the Management of Patients with Valvular Heart Disease): endorsed by the society of Cardiovascular Anesthesiologists, Society for Cardiovascular Angiography and Interventions, and Society of Thoracic Surgeons. *Circulation* 2008;118(15):e523–e661. 1

- Ampicillin 2 g PO/IV/IM **or** cefazolin or ceftriaxone 1 g IV/IM
- If patient is allergic to penicillin:
  - PO: cephalexin 2 g, clindamycin 600 mg, azithromycin 500 mg, or clarithromycin 500 mg
  - IV/IM: cefazolin or ceftriaxone 1 g, or clindamycin 600 mg

THE USE OF ANTICOAGULATION IN INFECTIVE ENDOCARDITIS

- There are no definite guidelines on the use of anticoagulation therapy in endocarditis.
- It is sometimes recommended to continue anticoagulation in the presence of mechanical prosthetic valve, but it should be stopped for a minimum of 2 weeks after starting antibiotic treatment in patients with *S. aureus* endocarditis who develop central nervous system emboli.
- It is not recommended to use aspirin in patients with endocarditis.

COMPLICATIONS OF INFECTIVE ENDOCARDITIS

- Congestive heart failure
  - It can occur in the presence of either native or prosthetic valve patients.
  - It is due to abnormality involving the valve (mainly aortic valve, then mitral, then tricuspid) rather than the myocardium.
  - Surgical intervention is recommended.
- Annular or aortic abscess
- Heart block
- Systemic embolic events
  - Mainly occurs early in the course of disease
  - Most common system involved is the central nervous system.

SUGGESTED READINGS

Baddour LM, et al. Infective endocarditis: diagnosis, antimicrobial therapy, and management of complications: a statement for healthcare professionals from the Committee on Rheumatic Fever, Endocarditis, and Kawasaki Disease, Council on Cardiovascular Disease in the Young, and the Councils on Clinical Cardiology, Stroke, and Cardiovascular Surgery and Anesthesia, American Heart Association. *Circulation* 2005;111(23):e394–e434.

This American Heart Association statement fully summarizes the antimicrobial treatment and management of patients with infective endocarditis. The role of daptomycin for S. aureus endocarditis had not yet been extensively discussed at the time of this guideline (http://circ.ahajournals.org/content/111/23/e394.full.pdf).

Bernard, et al. Valvular heart disease: changing concept in disease management. Surgery for infective endocarditis: who and when? *Circulation* 2010;121:1141–1152.

Bonow RO, et al. 2008 focused update incorporated into the ACC/AHA 2006 guidelines for the management of patients with valvular heart disease. *Circulation* 2008;118(15):e523–e661.

Cosgrove et al. Initial low-dose gentamicin for *Staphylococcus aureus* bacteremia and endocarditis is nephrotoxic. *Clin Infect Dis* 2009;48(6):713–721.

This study examined a prospective cohort with S. aureus endocarditis and found that any initial low-dose gentamicin as part of therapy for S. aureus bacteremia and native valve infective endocarditis was nephrotoxic and should not be used routinely, given the minimal existing data supporting its benefit.

Fowler VG Jr, et al. Daptomycin versus standard therapy for bacteremia and endocarditis caused by *Staphylococcus aureus*. *N Engl J Med* 2006;355(7):653–665.

This study found that daptomycin (6 mg/kg daily) is not inferior to standard therapy for S. aureus bacteremia and right-sided endocarditis.

Kullar R, et al. Effects of targeting higher vancomycin trough levels on clinical outcomes and costs in a matched patient cohort. *Pharmacotherapy* 2012;32(3):195–201.

Kim DH, et al. Impact of early surgery on embolic events in patients with infective endocarditis. *Circulation* 2010;122(11 suppl):S17–S22.

McDonald JR. Acute infective endocarditis. *Infect Dis Clin North Am* 2009;23(3):643–664.

Moore CL, et al. Daptomycin versus vancomycin for bloodstream infections due to methicillin-resistant *Staphylococcus aureus* with a high vancomycin minimum inhibitory concentration: a case-control study. *Clin Infect Dis* 2012;54(1):51–58.

The results of this retrospective, case-control study suggested that daptomycin was associated with a better outcome compared with vancomycin for the treatment of BSIs due to MRSA with higher vancomycin MICs (>1 mcg/mL).

Nishimura RA, et al. ACC/AHA 2008 guideline update on valvular heart disease: focused update on infective endocarditis. *Circulation* 2008;118(8):887–896.

Wilson W, et al. Prevention of infective endocarditis. *Circulation* 2007;116(15):1736–1754.

Cardiac Device Infections

Abdel Kareem Abu Malouh and Jonathan P. Moorman

EPIDEMIOLOGY

- The increased rate of cardiac device implantation in addition to an increased number of devices in older patients with more comorbid conditions has increased the rate of device infections.
- Recent studies suggest an infection rate of 0.9 to 2.1 per 1,000 devices with higher rates for automated implantable cardioverter-defibrillators (AICDs) than permanent pacemakers.

RISK FACTORS

Higher Risk	Lower Risk
Long-term corticosteroid use	Use of periprocedural antimicrobial prophylaxis
Heart failure	
History of generator replacement	Pectoral transvenous device placement
Renal dysfunction/hemodialysis	Higher physician experience
Oral anticoagulant use	
DM	
Presence of more than two pacing leads	
Fever within 24 hours before implantation	
History of preprocedural temporary pacing	
Immunomodulator use	

PATHOGENESIS

- Staphylococcal species cause the majority of infections.
- Other causes include *Corynebacterium* species, *Propionibacterium* acnes, gram-negative bacilli, *Candida* species, and atypical mycobacteria.
- Device contamination at the time of implantation appears to be the most common method of transmission.
- Hematogenous seeding during episodes of bacteremia also occurs: more likely with *Staphylococcus aureus* and rarely with gram-negative bacilli.
- Bacteria, particularly gram-positive cocci, adhere to hardware using biofilm production: difficult to sterilize.
- Pocket infection may track along the intravascular leads to cause lead infection and endocarditis.

CLINICAL PRESENTATION

- Local inflammatory changes at the generator site/pocket with or without cutaneous erosion of the generator or leads; abscess or sinus tract formation may occur.
- Pain or discomfort at the generator site
- Fever and other signs of systemic toxicity are often absent.
- Patients may present with positive blood cultures with no local inflammatory changes at pocket site.

DIAGNOSIS

- At least two sets of blood cultures should be obtained before the initiation of antimicrobial therapy in all patients with suspected cardiac device infection.
- Positive blood cultures, particularly due to staphylococcal species, provide a strong clue to device infection (especially in the first 3 months following device implantation).
- Transesophageal echocardiogram (TEE) is recommended in cases of bacteremia with underlying cardiac device and in cases of negative blood cultures with previous antibiotic use.
- TEE is more sensitive than transthoracic echo for the diagnosis of associated endocarditis or lead vegetations.
- Cultures of the generator pocket site may be useful in identifying the causative organism and guide future therapy.
- Percutaneous aspiration of the device pocket should be avoided because of risk of introducing microorganisms into the pocket and causing device infection.
- Lead tip culture at time of extraction can be misleading as it can be contaminated by organisms at the pocket site when extracted percutaneously.

MANAGEMENT

- Complete removal of all hardware is the recommended treatment for patients with definite cardiac device infection: includes patients with localized pocket infection with no systemic signs or positive blood cultures.
- Local pocket changes requiring device removal include device erosion, skin adherence, or chronic draining sinus.
- Device removal is not indicated for a superficial or incisional infection without involvement of the device and/or leads.
- Infection relapse rate is high with antimicrobial treatment and retention of hardware.
- Complete device removal should be done when patients undergo valve replacement for infective endocarditis because the device may be a nidus for future valve infection.
- Percutaneous lead extraction is the preferred method for hardware removal.
  - Risks include cardiac tamponade, hemothorax, pulmonary embolism, lead migration, and death.
- Surgical approach should be used after unsuccessful percutaneous attempts for removal or with lead vegetations more than 2 cm in diameter because of risk of PE with percutaneous extraction.

- Vancomycin should be given empirically until the causative organism is known.
- Blood cultures should be obtained from all patients after device removal.
- In cases of pocket site infection with inflammatory changes and negative blood cultures, antibiotics should be given for 10 to 14 days after device removal.
- If the presentation is device erosion without inflammatory changes and with negative blood cultures, antibiotics are given for 7 to 10 days after device removal.
  - Therapy can be switched to an oral agent if the organism is susceptible.
- Patients with positive blood culture and valvular vegetations should be treated like infective endocarditis.
- Patients with complicated lead vegetations should be treated with 4 to 6 weeks of antibiotics. Complications include:
  - Septic thrombophlebitis
  - Osteomyelitis
- Patients with *S. aureus* bacteremia with uncomplicated lead vegetations or negative TEE should be treated with 2 to 4 weeks of antibiotics.
- Patients with non–*S. aureus* bacteremia and uncomplicated lead vegetations or negative TEE can be treated with 2 weeks of antibiotics.
- Patients with sustained (>24 hours) bacteremia despite device removal and appropriate antibiotics should receive 4 weeks of IV antibiotics (even with a negative TEE).
- Adequate débridement and control of infection at all sites are important before any new device placement.
- Patients with *S. aureus* bacteremia and no localizing evidence of device infection will likely need device removal because of a high risk of seeding the leads during bacteremia. The following clues may indicate occult device infection:
  - Relapsing bacteremia after a course of appropriate antibiotic therapy
  - No other identifiable source of bacteremia
  - Bacteremia persisting more than 24 hours
  - If the device is an AICD
  - Presence of a prosthetic heart valve
  - Bacteremia within 3 months of device placement
- Secondary cardiac device infection is unlikely in patients with gram-negative bacteremia and no other evidence of device infection: TEE is not routinely recommended.
- Patients with bacteremia or fungemia due to other organisms (coagulase-negative staphylococci, streptococci, enterococci, and candida) and *no* evidence of device infection appear to have a low risk of infection.
- Long-term suppressive therapy is occasionally used in patients who are not candidates for device removal.

NEW DEVICE IMPLANTATION

- The need for new device should be evaluated in all patients with cardiac device infection.
  - One-third to one-half of patients will not need a new device.
- When implantation of a new device is necessary, it should be performed on the contralateral side if possible.
- Any new device can be placed after 72 hours of negative blood cultures following device removal or after 14 days when there is evidence of valvular vegetations.

PREVENTION

- Rule out active infection prior to device implantation
- Preoperative prophylaxis is generally with cefazolin given 1 hour prior to the procedure.
  - Shown to decrease the incidence of device infection significantly
  - Vancomycin can be substituted in patients who are allergic to penicillin or if the patient is at high risk for methicillin-resistant *Staphylococcus aureus* (MRSA) infection.
- Use antiseptic surgical technique including skin antiseptic preparation.
- Antibiotic prophylaxis is not recommended prior to dental or other invasive procedures.

SUGGESTED READINGS

Baddour LM, et al. Update on cardiovascular implantable electronic device infections and their management. *Circulation* 2010;121:458–477.

This American Heart Association scientific statement thoroughly summarizes the epidemiology, diagnosis, and treatment of cardiac device infections. They provide a useful approach to the patient with suspected infection (see http://circ.ahajournals.org/content/121/3/458/F3.expansion.html).

Dababneh AS, Sohail MR. Cardiovascular implantable electronic device infection: a stepwise approach to diagnosis and management. *Cleve Clin J Med* 2011;78:529–537.

Greenspon AJ, et al. Timing of the most recent device procedure influences the clinical outcome of lead-associated endocarditis: results of the MEDIC. *J Am Coll Cardiol* 2012;59:681–687.

Karchmer AW, Longworth DL. Infections of intracardiac devices. *Cardiol Clin* 2003;21:253–271.

Le KY, et al. Impact of timing of device removal on mortality in patients with cardiovascular implantable electronic device infections. *Heart Rhythm* 2011;11:1678–1685.

This study found that delay in device removal was associated with increased mortality. Early and complete device removal is advocated.

Le KY, et al. Clinical predictors of cardiovascular implantable electronic device-related infective endocarditis. *Pacing Clin Electrophysiol* 2011;34:450–459.

This study found pocket site infection was actually negatively associated with infective endocarditis, while comorbid conditions such as immunomodulator use, steroid use, hemodialysis, and remote infection were associated with an increased odds of infective endocarditis.

Uslan DZ. Infections of electrophysiologic cardiac devices. *Expert Rev Med Devices* 2008;5:183–195.

VIII Nosocomial Infections

31 Central Line–Associated Bloodstream Infections

David B. Banach, Michael J.Satlin, and
David P. Calfee

INTRODUCTION

- Central line–associated bloodstream infections (CLABSIs) are a major cause of morbidity and mortality among hospitalized patients and are associated with substantial costs to the health care system. A mortality rate of 12.3% and excess costs of $6,461 to $29,156 per infection have been reported.
- It has been estimated that 92,000 CLABSIs occurred in US hospitals in 2002.
- Although much attention toward CLABSI has focused on intensive care units (ICUs), there is an increasing awareness of these infections in non-ICU settings. In fact, in many US hospitals, the majority of patients with central venous catheters are outside the ICU, and many of these non-ICU areas have rates of CLABSI that are similar to or higher than those seen in ICUs.

PATHOGENESIS AND MICROBIOLOGY

- CLABSI is usually a complication of bacterial or fungal colonization of the extraluminal and/or intraluminal surfaces of the catheter. Contamination of the external surface of the catheter can occur during insertion or after insertion due to migration of bacteria present on the skin at the insertion site. Intraluminal colonization is typically the result of contamination of the catheter hub or tubing during use or manipulation of the catheter. More rarely, catheters can become colonized due to hematogenous seeding from a distant site of infection or by administration of contaminated medications or fluids.
- The organisms most commonly reported to the U.S. Centers for Disease Control and Prevention (CDC) in 2006 and 2007 as causes of CLABSI included, in descending order of frequency, coagulase-negative staphylococci (34.1%), *Enterococcus* species (16%), *Candida* species (11.8%), *Staphylococcus aureus* (9.9%), and *Klebsiella pneumoniae* (4.9%). Other gram-negative organisms make up the remainder of the ten most common causes of CLABSI.

SURVEILLANCE AND CLINICAL DEFINITIONS

- For surveillance and epidemiologic purposes, catheter-*associated* bloodstream infection is defined as a bloodstream infection in a patient with a central venous catheter in place at the time of or within 48 hours of collection of the blood sample, for which no other source of the bloodstream infection (e.g., pneumonia, surgical site infection) can be identified.
- Catheter-*related* bloodstream infection (CRBSI) is a term that is used when additional microbiologic testing has been done to provide more definitive evidence that

the bloodstream infection is truly related to and not just associated with a central venous catheter. (See section on Diagnosis.)

CLINICAL MANIFESTATIONS

- Patients with CLABSI often present with nonspecific signs and symptoms, such as fever and leukocytosis. Localized signs and symptoms of infection, such as erythema, tenderness, swelling, or purulent discharge at the catheter exit site or along the catheter tunnel, are seen in only a small minority of patients with CLABSI. Complications of CLABSI can include sepsis, endocarditis, septic thrombophlebitis, and metastatic infection (e.g., osteomyelitis, septic arthritis, epidural abscess).

DIAGNOSIS

- The diagnosis of CLABSI should be considered in any patient with a central venous catheter who develops a fever and/or other signs of systemic infection. Similarly, CLABSI should be considered in any patient with a central venous catheter who has a positive blood culture and no other obvious source of the bloodstream infection (e.g., pneumonia, urinary tract infection, surgical site infection).
- Inflammation and purulence at the catheter site are frequently absent in patients with CLABSI; however, the catheter exit site and tract should be thoroughly examined for signs of inflammation.
- In patients with suspected CLABSI, two sets of blood cultures should be obtained prior to the initiation of antibiotic therapy.
- Blood cultures should be drawn from two separate sites.
- Whenever possible, at least one set of blood cultures should be obtained by percutaneous venipuncture. Although blood cultures obtained by aspiration of blood through the central venous catheter are highly sensitive for the detection of CLABSI, they are of lower specificity than blood specimens obtained from peripheral veins.
- The sensitivity of a blood culture is dependent on the quantity of blood collected. Volumes of 30 to 40 mL provide optimal sensitivity. In clinical practice, however, 10 mL of blood per culture site are typically obtained.
- Several additional microbiologic tests can provide additional information that may help to determine if the catheter is the true source of a bloodstream infection and thus diagnose CRBSI.
  - Quantitative or semiquantitative cultures of the catheter tip: growth of $>10^2$ colony-forming units (CFU) per catheter segment of the same organism isolated from blood culture(s) by the quantitative method or >15 CFU by the semiquantitative method suggests that the catheter was the source of the bloodstream infection.
  - Paired quantitative blood cultures obtained from the catheter and from a peripheral vein: a microbial colony count from the catheter-aspirated blood specimen that is more than threefold greater than the colony count from a peripheral blood specimen is suggestive of CRBSI.
  - Differential time to positivity of paired blood cultures obtained from the catheter and from a peripheral vein: with the use of continuously monitored blood culture systems, detection of microbial growth from the blood specimen drawn through the catheter more than two hours before growth is detected in a simultaneously drawn peripheral blood sample is suggestive of CRBSI. Of the three mentioned methods, this is most likely to be readily available to most clinicians since most clinical microbiology laboratories use continuously monitored blood culture systems.

TREATMENT

- Guidelines published in 2009 by the Infectious Diseases Society of America (IDSA) provide evidence-based recommendations and a detailed review of the diagnosis and treatment of vascular catheter-related infections.
- The decision to initiate empiric antibiotic therapy and the selection of an empiric regimen are based on several factors, including severity of illness, underlying medical conditions, the suspected pathogens, and local antibiotic susceptibility patterns. Until culture results become available, it is reasonable to initiate empiric therapy with a broad-spectrum antibiotic regimen that provides coverage for the most likely bacterial pathogens. Antifungal agents are not typically included in an empiric regimen unless the patient has identified risk factors for candidemia. Empiric antibiotic therapy should be adjusted based on organism identification and susceptibility testing results, once available.
- Decisions regarding the duration of antibiotic therapy for the treatment of CLABSI are dependent upon the causative organism, the time until bacterial or fungal clearance, and the presence of secondary complications of infection (e.g., septic thrombophlebitis, endocarditis, septic arthritis, osteomyelitis).
- Figures 31-1 and 31-2 provide detailed guidance from IDSA regarding the selection of antimicrobial therapy, duration of therapy, and indications for catheter removal in the management of bloodstream infections associated with short-term and long-term catheters.
- The decision regarding catheter removal is an essential component of the management of CLABSI. The causative pathogen, catheter type (e.g., short-term or long-term), location of the catheter, and severity of illness should all be considered when making decisions regarding catheter removal.
- Long-term catheters should be removed in cases of severe illness (e.g., sepsis), persistent bloodstream infection despite appropriate antibiotic therapy, infection of the catheter tunnel tract, and complicated infections such as endocarditis, suppurative thrombophlebitis, or osteomyelitis. In addition, catheter removal is highly recommended in cases of CLABSI caused by *S. aureus* or *Candida* species. For uncomplicated infections due to other organisms, such as coagulase-negative staphylococci, *Enterococcus* species, and gram-negative bacilli, catheter salvage may be considered in conjunction with systemic antibiotic treatment and antibiotic lock therapy (ALT).
- In most cases of CLABSI associated with temporary, nontunneled catheters, the catheter should be removed. Catheter salvage may be considered in selected patients with infections due to coagulase-negative staphylococci.
- ALT refers to the introduction of a solution containing a high concentration (e.g., 1 to 5 mg/mL) of one or more antimicrobial agents with activity against the infecting organism into the lumen of a catheter where it is allowed to dwell while the catheter is not in use. The purpose of ALT is to provide an antibiotic at a concentration that is high enough and for a duration that is long enough to penetrate into the intraluminal biofilm and kill microorganisms living within the biofilm in order to increase the likelihood of successful catheter salvage. When used for the treatment of CLABSI, ALT should always be used in combination with systemic antimicrobial therapy. Agents other than antibiotics, such as ethanol, have also been used for catheter "lock" therapy. Prior to using such agents, it is important to determine that the catheter is compatible with the agent. For example, the use of an ethanol lock may damage a catheter that is made of polyurethane.

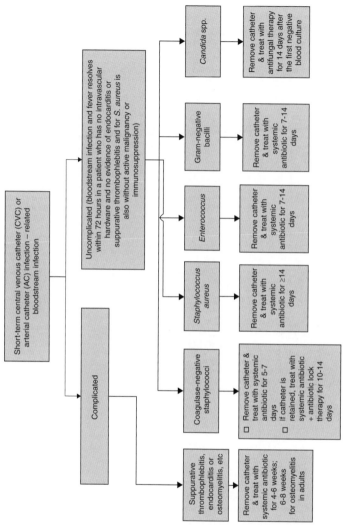

Figure 31-1. Approach to the management of patients with short-term central venous catheter-related bloodstream infection. CFU, colony-forming units. (From Mermel LA, Allon M, Bouza E, et al. Clinical practice guidelines for the diagnosis and management of intravascular catheter-related infection: 2009 update by the Infectious Diseases Society of America. *Clin Infect Dis* 2009;49:1–45. Used with permission from Oxford University Press and the Infectious Diseases Society of America.)

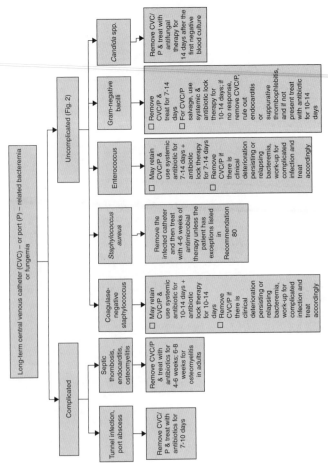

Figure 31-2. Approach to the management of patients with long-term central venous catheter–related bloodstream infection. Uncomplicated: bloodstream infection and fever resolve within 72 hours in a patient who has no intravascular hardware and no evidence of endocarditis or suppurative thrombophlebitis and for whom *S. aureus* is also without active malignancy or immunosuppression.

Recommendation 80: Patients can be considered for a shorter duration of antimicrobial therapy (i.e., a minimum of 14 days of therapy) if the patient is not diabetic; if the patient is not immunosuppressed; if the infected catheter is removed; if the patient has no prosthetic intravascular device; if there is no evidence of endocarditis or suppurative thrombophlebitis on transesophageal echocardiography and ultrasound, respectively; if fever and bacteremia resolve within 72 hours after initiation of appropriate antimicrobial therapy; and if there is no evidence of metastatic infection on physical examination and sign- or symptom-directed diagnostic tests. (From Mermel LA, Allon M, Bouza E, et al. Clinical practice guidelines for the diagnosis and management of intravascular catheter-related infection: 2009 update by the Infectious Diseases Society of America. *Clin Infect Dis* 2009;49:1–45. Used with permission from Oxford University Press and the Infectious Diseases Society of America.)

Table 31-1 Key Strategies for the Prevention of CLABSIs

	Catheter Insertion Procedure	Catheter Care and Maintenance	Catheter Use	Other
Strategies	Perform hand hygiene prior to beginning the catheter insertion procedure. Use maximal sterile barriers: sterile gown and gloves, surgical cap, and mask worn by all persons involved in the procedure, and cover the patient with a sterile full body drape. Avoid use of the femoral site in adult patients. Use a chlorhexidine and alcohol solution for skin antisepsis prior to catheter insertion. Use a checklist to ensure that all recommended infection prevention measures are implemented during catheter insertion. Consider use of antiseptic or antimicrobial-coated catheters if CLABSI rates are not decreasing with the use of standard preventive measures.	Assess the ongoing need for the catheter daily and remove the catheter as soon as it is no longer needed. Perform hand hygiene prior to performing catheter care activities. Use aseptic technique when performing catheter care. Keep the catheter insertion site covered with a sterile dressing at all times. Replace gauze dressings every 2 days. Replace transparent dressings at least every 7 days. Replace the dressing if it becomes loose, soiled, or damp. Use a 2% chlorhexidine solution for skin antisepsis during all dressing changes. Use a chlorhexidine-impregnated dressing at the catheter exit site if CLABSI rates are not decreasing with the use of standard preventive measures.	Perform hand hygiene prior to accessing or using the catheter. Clean the catheter injection port with chlorhexidine, 70% alcohol, or an iodophor prior to accessing the catheter.	Educate health care workers involved in catheter insertion, use, and/or maintenance about CLABSI prevention. Use 2% chlorhexidine for daily patient bathing.

PREVENTION

- It is important for clinicians to recognize that CLABSIs are not an inevitable complication of central venous catheter use. In fact, several recent studies have demonstrated that at least 65% to 70% of CLABSI can be prevented using current evidence-based preventive practices. Data from CDC indicate that there was a 58% decrease in the incidence of CLABSI in ICU patients in US hospitals between 2001 and 2009.
- Recommended practices and interventions for the prevention of CLABSI serve to reduce the risk of catheter contamination during catheter insertion, maintenance, and use (Table 31-1).
- Recently published guidelines provide additional evidence-based preventive strategies.

SUGGESTED READINGS

Berenholtz SM, Pronovost PJ, Lipsett PA, et al. Eliminating catheter-related bloodstream infections in the intensive care unit. *Crit Care Med* 2004;32:2014–2020.
One of the first published descriptions of a highly successful, multidisciplinary effort to prevent CLABSI in ICU patients. Describes the successful use of a "checklist" to ensure that all important infection prevention measures are implemented during central venous catheter insertion.

Bleasdale S, Trick W, Gonzalez I, et al. Effectiveness of chlorhexidine bathing to reduce catheter-associated bloodstream infections in medical intensive care unit patients. *Arch Intern Med* 2007;167(19):2073–2079.
One of the first published descriptions of the impact of daily bathing with chlorhexidine on the incidence of CLABSI.

Centers for Disease Control and Prevention. Vital signs: central line-associated blood stream infections-United States, 2001, 2008 and 2009. *MMWR Morb Mortal Wkly Rep* 2011;60:243–248.
Estimates of the number of and trends in CLABSI infections in ICU patients in US hospitals between 2001 and 2009.

Climo M, Diekema D, Warren D, et al. Prevalence of the use of central venous access devices within and outside of the intensive care unit: results of a survey among hospitals in the prevention epicenter program of the Centers for Disease Control and Prevention. *Infect Control Hosp Epidemiol* 2003;24(12):942–945.

Dudeck MA, Horan TC, Peterson KD, et al. National Healthcare Safety Network (NHSN) report, data summary for 2010, device-associated module. Centers for Disease Control and Prevention. http://www.cdc.gov/nhsn/PDFs/dataStat/NHSN-Report_2010-Data-Summary.pdf. Accessed February 19, 2012.
Summarizes data reported from US hospitals to the CDC's National Healthcare Safety Network and provides benchmarking data for rates of device-associated infections, including CLABSI.

Hidron AI, Edwards JR, Patel J, et al. NHSN annual update: antimicrobial resistant pathogens associated with healthcare-associated infections: annual summary of data reported to the National Healthcare Safety Network at the Centers for Disease Control and Prevention, 2006-2007. *Infect Control Hosp Epidemiol* 2008;29:996–1011.
Provides a summary of microbiologic data from cases of device- and procedure-associated infections reported to the CDC.

Horan T, Andrus M, Dudeck MA. CDC/NHSN surveillance definition of health care-associated infection and criteria for specific types of infections in the acute care setting. *Am J Infect Control* 2008;36(5):309–332.
Provides surveillance definitions for health care–associated infections, including CLABSI.

Klevens RM, Edwards JR, Richards CL, et al. Estimating health care-associated infections and deaths in U.S. hospitals, 2002. *Public Health Rep* 2007;122:160–166.

Provides estimates of the number of various types of health care–associated infections, including CLABSI, that occurred in US hospitals in 2002.

Mermel L, Allon M, Bouza E, et al.Clinical practice guidelines for the diagnosis and management of intravascular catheter-related infection: 2009 Update by the Infectious Diseases Society of America. *Clin Infect Dis* 2009;49:1–45.

Evidence-based recommendations for the diagnosis and treatment of CLABSI and other infectious complications of intravascular catheters.

O'Grady NP, Alexander M, Burns LA, et al. Guidelines for the prevention of intravascular catheter-related infections, 2011. *Clin Infect Dis* 2011;52:e1–e32.

Evidence-based recommendations for the prevention of CLABSI and other infectious complications of intravascular catheters.

Pronovost P, Needham D, Berenholtz S, et al. An intervention to decrease catheter-related bloodstream infections in the ICU. *N Engl J Med* 2006;355:2725–2732.

Description of a statewide initiative to prevent CLABSI that resulted in a 66% decrease in CLABSIs in ICU patients throughout the state of Michigan.

Scott RD. The direct medical costs of healthcare-associated infections in U.S. hospitals and the benefits of prevention. Centers for Disease Control and Prevention 2009. *http://www.cdc.gov/HAI/pdfs/hai/Scott_CostPaper.pdf* (Accessed February 15, 2012)

An economic analysis of the costs of health care–associated infections, including CLABSI, in the United States.

Umscheid CA, Mitchell MD, Doshi JA, et al. Estimating the proportion of healthcare-associated infections that are reasonably preventable and the related mortality and costs. *Infect Control Hosp Epidemiol* 2011;32:101–114.

Systematic review of the costs and preventability of the most common types of health care–associated infections, including CLABSI.

Health Care–Associated Urinary Tract Infection

Evgenia Kagan and Joseph F. John, Jr.

OVERVIEW

The genitourinary tract is a complex filtering and plumbing system. It can be attacked by microbial invasion at many intersections, creating diagnostic challenges and making localization of infections difficult. Much of the medical literature has concentrated on catheter-associated urinary tract infection (CA-UTI). While the threat of an indwelling catheter sets one backdrop of complexity, there are other conditions that predispose to complex UTI such as renal stones, ureteral diverticula, transplantation of the kidney and bladder, renal stents, chronic prostate disease, genital prosthesis, and ileal urinary drainage. The care team should discuss a method of collecting urine, transport to the clinical microbiology laboratory, and the meaning of bacterial (or fungal) quantitation that will be reported. Colony counts of bacteria and fungi in the setting of an abnormal or instrumented urinary tract are probably the greatest challenge to interpretation of infection. In this chapter, we discuss the current status of practical approaches to diagnosis and management of complex UTIs.

APPROACH TO THE PATIENT

Health care–associated urinary tract infection (HA-UTI) is a major cause of morbidity in hospitalized patients responsible for more than 40% of nosocomial infections. The most common bacterial specter of CA-UTI reflects the patients' own colonic flora. Other organisms are usually not found until the duration of catheterization exceeds 30 days.[1] Patients with long-term indwelling catheters tend to have polymicrobial bacteriuria, making laboratory interpretation difficult. Although *Escherichia coli* is the most common organism isolated, increasing use of broad-spectrum antimicrobials in health care has contributed to the emergence of multidrug-resistant pathogens. CA-UTI has served as an expanding reservoir for spread of such resistant pathogens as *Staphylococci* and *Enterococci* in health care settings. Other pathogens commonly found in HA-UTI include *Pseudomonas, Klebsiella, Enterobacter, Proteus, Citrobacter, Acinetobacter, Serratia*, Group B streptococci, yeast, and new fungal pathogens.[2] When HA-UTI is associated with bacteremia, *Enterococcus* and *Candida* are the most common pathogens.[3] The major predisposing factors to the development of nosocomial UTI are instrumentation of the genitourinary tract, most commonly presence of a urinary catheter, cystoscopy, underlying illness, diabetes, older age, and more advanced urologic procedures.

METHODS FOR LOCALIZATION

Criteria and definitions of UTI have changed in recent years.[4] Asymptomatic bacteriuria (ASB) (no clinical, histologic, or immunologic signs of infection) or candiduria are no longer considered "infection" and may better be described as "colonization." Under certain circumstances such as pregnancy, transurethral resection of the prostate, or traumatic genitourinary interventions associated with mucosal bleeding, ASB may be regarded as a precursor to development of symptomatic UTI and requires therapy to reduce the risk of associated complications such as bacteremia and sepsis.[5] Moreover, the recently modified CDC/NHSN surveillance guidelines introduce two new broad categories of symptomatic urinary tract infection and asymptomatic bacteremic urinary tract infection.[6]

A bacterial urinary tract infection is defined as the presence of bacteria in the urine in appropriate quantitative counts, pyuria, and symptoms or signs compatible with inflammation. A urine dipstick test is utilized as a screening tool for diagnosis of UTI. The dipstick nitrite test depends on the conversion of nitrate to nitrite by most bacteria in the urine (most often *Enterobacteriaceae*); normally, no detectable nitrite is present. Leukocyte esterase corresponds to pyuria. Clinical evaluation is always necessary because of the possibility of false-positive and false-negative test results.[7]

Urine samples for culture and sensitivity should be obtained prior to initiation of antibiotics. If ongoing catheterization is needed, ideally the catheter should be replaced prior to collecting a urine sample for culture in order to avoid culturing bacteria present in the microbial biofilm of the catheter and not within the bladder. In the absence of an indwelling urinary catheter, UTI is likely present when the level of bacteria in the urine is equal to or >10^5 CFU/mL in a "clean catch" specimen, or equal to or >10^2 CFU/mL in a catheterized specimen when there are symptoms attributable to the genitourinary tract. Diagnostic criteria of CA-UTI, catheter-associated asymptomatic bacteriuria (CA-ASB), and ASB in the absence of an indwelling catheter in adults are briefly summarized in Table 32-1.[8]

Clinical presentation may vary from severe obstructive acute pyelonephritis with imminent urosepsis to a catheter-associated postoperative UTI, with spontaneous resolution as soon as the catheter is removed. Diagnostic challenge arises when clinical symptoms of UTI are obscured by presence of the catheter[9] or when the patient is elderly, debilitated, or immunosuppressed. A patient's presentation with otherwise unexplained systemic manifestations compatible with infection (like fever, malaise, altered mental status, fall in blood pressure, leukocytosis, metabolic acidosis, respiratory alkalosis) should prompt evaluation for UTI.

HA-UTI is often associated with a urologic procedure such as placement of a ureteral stent. Bacterial stent colonization plays an essential role in the pathogenesis of stent-associated infections. Risk for stent colonization and UTI is significantly enhanced by the duration of stent retention (colonization is common if the indwelling time is more than 2 weeks), female sex, diabetes mellitus, chronic renal failure, and malignancies.[10] Proper culturing of stents can be challenging and is not needed when the same microorganisms grow repeatedly in routine urine cultures; however, difficulty may arise if significant biofilm formation has occurred as routine culture techniques do not accurately detect microorganisms embedded in these biofilms.

During manipulation or instrumentation, biofilm organisms could be shed into the urine and lead to ascending UTI and urosepsis. Novel developing technologies such as ureteral stents sonication offer a promising approach in the diagnosis of microbial ureteral stent colonization.[11] Real-time polymerase chain reaction (PCR) detection of pathogens has also been studied to supplement conventional culture methods for the diagnosis of UTI. The main advantage of PCR

Table 32-1	Diagnostic Criteria of CA-UTI, CA-ASB and ASB Without Indwelling Catheter in Adults	
Catheter Status	**Clinical Criteria**	**Laboratory Criteria**
CA-UTI[a] Indwelling urethral Indwelling suprapubic Intermittent catheterization	New onset or worsening of fever >38°C, rigors, altered mental status, malaise, or lethargy with no other identified cause; flank pain; costovertebral angle tenderness; acute hematuria; pelvic discomfort In those whose catheters have been removed: dysuria, urgent or frequent urination, or suprapubic pain or tenderness In patients with spinal cord injury: increased spasticity, autonomic dysreflexia, or sense of unease are also compatible with CA-UTI	10^3 units (CFU)/mL of more than one bacterial species in a single catheter urine specimen or in a midstream voided urine specimen from a patient whose urethral, suprapubic, or condom catheter has been removed within the previous 48 hours. *The absence of pyuria (urine specimen with >/=10 white blood cell mm³ or>/=3 WBC/high power field of unspun urine) in a symptomatic patient suggests a diagnosis other than CA-UTI.*
CA-ASB[b] Indwelling urethral Indwelling suprapubic Intermittent catheterization	Without symptoms	10^5 CFU/mL of more than bacterial species in a single catheter urine specimen. Man with a condom catheter is defined by the presence of 10^5 CFU/mL of one bacterial species in a single urine specimen from a freshly applied condom catheter. *Pyuria accompanying CA-ASB should not be interpreted as an indication for antimicrobial treatment.*
ASB[c] In the absence of indwelling urinary catheter	Asymptomatic women require two consecutive voided urine specimens. A single catheterized urine specimen in women or men A single, clean catch voided urine specimen in men	With isolation of the same bacterial strain in two consecutive voided urine specimens quantitative counts 10^5 CFU/mL. One bacterial species isolated in 10^2 CFU/mL quantitative count. One bacterial species isolated in a quantitative count 10^5 CFU/mL bacteriuria.

[a]CA-UTI, catheter-associated urinary tract infection.
[b]CA-ASB, catheter-associated asymptomatic bacteriuria.
[c]ASB, asymptomatic bacteriuria.
http://www.idsociety.org/uploadedFiles/IDSA/Guidelines-Patient_Care/PDF_Library/Comp%20UTI.pdf
http://www.idsociety.org/uploadedFiles/IDSA/Guidelines-Patient_Care/PDF_Library/Asymptomatic%20Bacteriuria.pdf

is time saved in pathogen identification.[12] The disadvantage of PCR is that they may have high sensitivity and thus lead to false-positive testing and cannot provide standardized susceptibility profiles.

The renal transplant patient looms as a special challenge. HA-UTI is the most common bacterial infection occurring in the renal transplant recipient with the highest rate within the first 3 months after surgery.[13,14] Renal transplant recipients with UTI are often clinically asymptomatic because of immunosuppression but may rapidly evolve to exhibit acute graft pyelonephritis, bacteremia, and sepsis. Risk factors for UTI in the renal transplant patient include urologic instrumentation during and after surgery, indwelling bladder catheters, anatomic abnormalities of the native or transplanted organ (such as vesicoureteral reflux, stones, or stents), neurogenic bladder especially in diabetic patients, microbial colonization of the ureteral stent, rejection, and intensified immunosuppression. The same criteria described above are used for diagnosis, but some experts suggest more sensitive definitions for quantification of bacteria in the renal transplant patient. Antimicrobial prophylaxis with TMP-SMX will reduce frequency of UTIs during the first months after kidney transplantation but leads to an increase in microbial resistance. Ureteral stents may be used to reduce urologic complications after renal transplantation; however, rapid colonization of the stent predisposes to infection, and thus, early removal of the stent (when possible) decreases risk of UTI.[14]

Imaging is largely unnecessary to manage lower UTI. Urgent diagnostic imaging or urologic investigation is indicated when patients have severe systemic symptoms or those who do not respond to appropriate antimicrobial therapy. The goal of early imaging is to identify obstruction or abscesses, for which immediate drainage may be necessary for source control. Even a plain radiograph of the abdomen may identify emphysematous infections and some stones. Computerized tomography (CT) is often the imaging modality of choice when confronted by a complex UTI as it identifies calculi, gas, hemorrhage, calcification, obstruction, renal enlargement, and inflammatory masses. Ultrasound examination is less sensitive and specific than other imaging modalities such as spiral CT and MRI, but it may be more accessible in some clinical settings.

Urinary diversion produces a very complex setting for development of HA-UTI. Discussion of this is beyond this chapter's scope, but the subject has been discussed in some detail.[15]

TREATMENT

Treatment of the majority of HA-UTI should be approached as treatment for complex UTI. These patients may be treated as outpatients but very often require hospitalization. Treatment constitutes management of the urologic abnormality, antimicrobial therapy, and supportive care. Antimicrobial selection should be based upon culture and sensitivity results (from the sample obtained prior to initiation of antibiotics). If empiric treatment is required prior to culture data, the antibacterial spectrum of the antibiotic agent should include the particular institution's most relevant pathogens based upon urine gram stain, previous culture results, or upon the antimicrobial sensitivity patterns of organisms in the hospital or nursing facility. Suspicion of bacteremia must influence empiric treatment. Once culture and susceptibility results are available, the antibiotic regimen should be tailored to the specific bacterial isolate to avoid the emergence of resistant strains. The optimal duration of therapy has not been rigorously studied, however, 10 to 14 days is generally appropriate. Shorter antimicrobial courses may be considered for patients who have prompt resolution of symptoms, without upper urinary tract symptoms, and if the indwelling catheter has been removed. Treatment should be individualized and often done under the guidance of an infectious disease specialist, particularly if immunosuppression is present. Intravenous antimicrobial therapy should be initiated in patients with signs of systemic toxicity and those who are unable to tolerate oral medications. Empiric therapy for the institutionalized or hospitalized patient with a serious UTI should include a parenteral antipseudomonal agent because of an increased risk of urosepsis with this organism.[16] In severe cases requiring hospitalization, empiric coverage for gram-negative bacilli such as a fluoroquinolone, an extended-spectrum cephalosporin, or an extended-spectrum penicillin, with or without an aminoglycoside or a carbapenem, should be considered. Gram-positive cocci may represent enterococci or staphylococci; empiric management with vancomycin is generally appropriate pending further susceptibility data. After a few days of parenteral therapy, organism identification and clinical improvement, a step-down to oral therapy may be considered. Recommendations for initial empiric antimicrobial treatment are summarized in Table 32-2. In patients with renal failure, appropriate dose adjustments are required.

European guidelines on antimicrobial therapy of UTI recently have been updated and reviewed.[16] The indwelling urinary catheter should be removed if the patient no longer requires it. In patients where long-term catheterization is needed and intermittent catheterization is not possible, the infected indwelling catheter should be replaced at the initiation of antibiotic therapy, as biofilm penetration of most antibiotics is poor[17] and catheter replacement has been associated with fewer relapses.[18] Whenever possible, ureteral stents or other urogenital prosthetic material should be removed as it could continue to shed biofilm organisms into the urine. If perirenal or intrarenal abscess is detected, acute percutaneous drainage after medical stabilization and antibiotic therapy is often indicated. *Staphylococcus aureus* causes a special syndrome of renal carbuncle, located in the cortex of the kidney, and as such can usually be treated with antibiotics alone.

PREVENTION AND FUTURE CONSIDERATIONS

Several recent guidelines elaborate on prevention of HA-UTI and are discussed in recently published reviews.[19,20] Disrupting the life cycle of the urinary catheter is the most important goal in preventing CA-UTI. Reduction of bladder colonization and biofilm formation may become possible with impregnated catheters, but their overall long-term efficacy is not known. Immunization for recurrent outpatient UTI may eventually have some impact on the risk of developing a nosocomial infection; however, the pathogen spectrum is different and there is little immunologic cross-reaction among the pathogenic genera. Technologic advances are needed in methods of urinary drainage, early detection of colonization and infection beyond culture techniques, and newer bladder and renal imaging concepts. Of late, third-party reimbursement for CA-UTI has been reduced producing a new economic incentive to eliminate and reduce the incidence of complex UTIs.[21]

Table 32-2	Recommended Initial Empirical Antimicrobial Therapy in Patient with Complex HA-UTI Without Bacteremia	
	Antimicrobial	**Comment**
Initial parenteral therapy	Ciprofloxacin 400 mg b.i.d. (for *Pseudomonas aeruginosa* 400 mg q8h) Levofloxacin 250–500 mg q.d. Levofloxacin 750 mg q.d. Cefotaxime 2 g t.i.d. Ceftriaxone 2 g q.d. Ceftazidime 2 g t.i.d. Cefepime 1–2 g b.i.d. Piperacillin/tazobactam 2.5–4.5 g t.i.d.	Use quinolone if resistance is not known to exceed 10%.
	Gentamicin 5–7 mg/kg q.d. Tobramycin 7 mg/kg q24h Amikacin 5 mg/kg q.d.	Use the nomogram to determine whether continued once-daily dosing is appropriate. VS adjust dosing based on peak/trough levels goal 10–12/<1.
	Ertapenem 1 g q.d. Imipenem/cilastatin 0.5/0.5 g t.i.d. Meropenem 1 g t.i.d.	
	Vancomycin 15 mg/kg q8–12h Fluconazole 200–400 mg (3–6 mg/kg) IV or PO daily Caspofungin 70 mg on day 1; subsequent dosing; 50 mg/day Micafungin 100 mg daily	Adjust dosing based on trough levels (goal 15–20 µg/mL).
Step-down oral therapy	Ciprofloxacin 500–750 mg b.i.d. Levofloxacin 250–500 mg q.d. Levofloxacin 750 mg q.d.	Consider giving an IV dose of the same or similar fluoroquinolone before starting oral dosing. If quinolone resistance is known to exceed 10%, give an IV dose of ceftriaxone or another long-acting agent.
	TMP-SMX b.i.d.	High rates of resistance. Give an IV dose of ceftriaxone or another long-acting agent
	Cefpodoxime 400 mg b.i.d. Amoxicillin/clavulanate 875 mg b.i.d.	
Not acceptable	Nitrofurantoin	Does not achieve acceptable levels in tissue or serum. Only used for uncomplicated cystitis

For patients with creatinine clearance (mL/min)>50. For dosing based on renal function see *http://kdpnet.louisville.edu/renalbook/adult*

REFERENCES

1. Sedor J, Mulholland SG. Hospital-acquired urinary tract infections associated with the indwelling catheter. *Urol Clin North Am* 1999;26(4):821–828.
2. Kang CI, Chung DR, Son JS, et al. Clinical significance of nosocomial acquisition in urinary tract-related bacteremia caused by gram-negative bacilli. *Am J Infect Control* 2011;39(2):135–140.
3. Chang R, Greene MT, Chenoweth CE, et al. Epidemiology of hospital-acquired urinary tract-related bloodstream infection at a university hospital. *Infect Control Hosp Epidemiol* 2011;32(11):1127–1129.
4. Johansen TE, Botto H, Cek M, et al. Critical review of current definitions of urinary tract infections and proposal of an EAU/ESIU classification system. *Int J Antimicrob Agents* 2011;38(suppl):64–70.
5. Nicolle LE, Bradley S, Colgan R, et al. Infectious Diseases Society of America guidelines for the diagnosis and treatment of asymptomatic bacteriuria in adults. *Clin Infect Dis* 2005;40(5):643–654.
6. Horan TC, Andrus M, Dudeck MA. CDC/NHSN surveillance definition of healthcare-associated infection and criteria for specific types of infections in the acute care setting. *Am J Infect Control.* 2008;36(5):309–332. Updated January 2012 http://www.cdc.gov/nhsn/pdfs/pscmanual/17pscnosinfdef_current.pdf
7. Lammers RL, Gibson S, Kovacs D, et al. Comparison of test characteristics of urine dipstick and urinalysis at various test cutoff points. *Ann Emerg Med* 2001;38(5):505–512.
8. Hooton TM, Bradley SF, Cardenas DD, et al. Diagnosis, prevention, and treatment of catheter-associated urinary tract infection in adults:2009 International Clinical Practice Guidelines from the Infectious Diseases Society of America. *Clin Infect Dis* 2010;50(5):625–663.
9. Tambyah PA, Maki DG. Catheter-associated urinary tract infection is rarely symptomatic: a prospective study of 1,497 catheterized patients. *Arch Intern Med* 2000;160(5):678–682.
10. Al-Ghazo MA, Ghalayini IF, Matani YS, et al. The risk of bacteriuria and ureteric stent colonization in immune-compromised patients with double J stent insertion. *Int Urol Nephrol* 2010;42(2):343–347.
11. Bonkat G, Rieken M, Rentsch CA, et al. Improved detection of microbial ureteral stent colonization by sonication. *World J Urol* 2011;29:133–138.
12. Lehmann LE, Hauser S, Malinka T, et al. Real-time polymerase chain-reaction detection of pathogens is feasible to supplement the diagnostic sequence for urinary tract infections. *BJU Int* 2010;106(1):114–120.
13. Ruth M. de Souza Jonathon Olsburgh. Urinary tract infection in the renal transplant patient. *Nat Clin Pract Nephrol* 2008;4(5):252–264.
14. Coskun AK, Harlak A, Ozer T. Is removal of the stent at the end of 2 weeks helpful to reduce infectious or urologic complications after renal transplantation? *Transplant Proc* 2011;43:813–815.
15. Falagas ME, Vergidis PI. Urinary tract infections in patients with urinary diversion. *Am J Kidney Dis* 2005;46(6)1030–1037.
16. Grabe M, Bjerklund-Johansen TE, Botto H, et al. International journal of antimicrobial agents 38S (2011) 1–2 antimicrobial therapy of urinary tract infections. http://www.uroweb.org/gls/pdf/Urological%20Infections%202010.pdf
17. Trautner BW, Darouiche RO. Role of biofilm in catheter-associated urinary tract infection. *Am J Infect Control* 2004;32(3):177.
18. Raz R, Schiller D, Nicolle LE. Chronic indwelling catheter replacement before antimicrobial therapy for symptomatic urinary tract infection. *J Urol* 2000;164(4):1254–1258.
19. Gould CV, Umscheid CA, Agarwal RK, et al. CDC Guideline for prevention of catheter-associated urinary tract infections 2009. *Infect Control Hosp Epidemiol* 2010;31(4):319–326.
20. Carol E, Chenoweth, Sanjay Saint. Urinary Tract Infections. *Infect Dis Clin North Am* 2011;25(1):103–115.
21. Fakih MG et al. Reducing inappropriate urinary Catheter use. *Arch Int Med* 2012;172: 255–260.

33 Pneumonia in Health Care

Curtis J. Coley, II and Melissa A. Miller

EPIDEMIOLOGY

As health care and associated technology have advanced, delivery of care has expanded to include not only the traditional hospital setting but also to long- and short-term acute and chronic care settings as well as to the home. As a consequence, the concept of the traditional nosocomial infection has changed. One example of this is nosocomial pneumonia, which is now largely classified according to recommendations from the American Thoracic Society and Infectious Diseases Society of America.[1]

- Hospital-acquired pneumonia (HAP) is defined as pneumonia identified 48 hours or more after admission to the hospital, which was not incubating at the time of admission.
- Ventilator-associated pneumonia (VAP) is defined as pneumonia in a patient who is currently intubated or who has been endotracheally intubated within the last 48 hours.
- Health care–associated pneumonia (HCAP) can occur in any patient who was hospitalized in an acute care hospital for two or more days within 90 days of the infection; resided in a nursing home or long-term care facility; received intravenous antibiotic therapy, chemotherapy, or wound care within the past 30 days of infection; or received hemodialysis in a clinic or hospital setting.

Pneumonia is the second most common nosocomial infection and associated with the highest potential morbidity and mortality.[2,3] HAP has been reported to occur at a rate between 5 and 10 cases per 1,000 hospital admissions, with the incidence increasing by 6- to 20-fold in mechanically ventilated patients. The incidence increases with duration of ventilation, and the risk is highest early in the hospital stay. It is estimated to be 3% per day during the first 5 days of mechanical ventilation, 2% per day during days 5 to 10, and 1% per day after this.[4] It has been estimated that pneumonia accounts for 25% or more of nosocomial infections in the intensive care unit (ICU) and for 50% or more of antibiotics prescribed there.[5] VAP is associated with longer length of stay in the ICU and an attributable cost of care ranging from $10,000 to over $40,000 per episode.[1] Also, VAP may lead to complications such as empyema, lung abscess, lengthy intubation times, and the need for additional procedures such as bronchoscopy and tracheostomy. Crude mortality associated with nosocomial pneumonia has been reported to be between 20% and 50% depending on the patient population under study and the infecting organism.[1–3] Increased mortality has been associated with cases complicated by bacteremia, especially with *Pseudomonas* and *Acinetobacter* species, medical (as opposed to surgical) illness, and ineffective empiric antibiotic therapy.[1]

Important risk factors for HAP are often presented as those which are modifiable and those which are not.[6]

- Modifiable risk factors include prolonged intubation and reintubation, oversedation, and continuous use of paralytic agents, which increase risk of aspiration. The use of H2 blockers and proton pump inhibitors for gastric acid suppression has also been suggested to increase risk.
- Nonmodifiable risk factors include advanced age, low functional status, underlying illness and lung disease, impaired immunity, and a diagnosis of acute respiratory distress syndrome (ARDS).

CLINICAL PRESENTATION

In order for pneumonia to occur, there must be a shift in the balance between host defense and a pathogen's ability to colonize and invade. Aspiration, which is common among seriously ill hospitalized patients, is the key pathogenic event, and depending on this balance, active infection may ensue. Clinical signs and symptoms may vary from patient to patient and include fever, tachypnea, increased oxygen requirement, cough, and increased production or a change in the character of sputum (including that suctioned from the endotracheal tube). In elderly patients, altered mental status may be a presenting symptom. Laboratory abnormalities may include an elevated white blood cell count with a neutrophil predominance.

Differential Diagnosis

The differential diagnosis for new pulmonary symptoms and fever in a hospitalized patient, including those receiving mechanical ventilation, is broad and includes pneumonia, aspiration pneumonitis, infectious tracheobronchitis, atelectasis, pulmonary embolism, and ARDS. Since the approach to management of each of these entities varies, it is important for the clinician to make the correct diagnosis and initiate appropriate therapy.

Microbiology

The microbiology of HCAP has been shown to be more similar to HAP and VAP compared to that of community-acquired pneumonia. Bacterial causes of HAP and VAP include gram-positive organisms, most notably *Staphylococcus aureus*, methicillin-resistant *S. aureus* (MRSA), and *Streptococcus spp.*, and gram-negative organisms, most notably *Escherichia coli*, *Klebsiella pneumoniae*, *Enterobacter spp.*, *Pseudomonas aeruginosa*, and *Acinetobacter spp.*, *S. aureus*, *P. aeruginosa*, *K. pneumoniae*, and *E. coli* account for more than half of cases. Patients who develop HAP or VAP within the first 4 days of hospitalization (early onset) tend to have infection due to more susceptible organisms and thus have a better prognosis, compared to those who develop infection after 5 days or more (late onset). However, if a patient develops early onset HAP or VAP and has risk factors for infection due to antibiotic-resistant organisms (Table 33-1), they should be treated similarly to patients with late onset disease.[1]

Clinicians should also be aware of other "atypical" causes of HAP including *Legionella pneumophila*, fungal pathogens (including Aspergillus species), and viruses such as influenza, parainfluenza, adenovirus, and respiratory syncytial virus. Patients who are immunosuppressed from disease, organ transplantation, or medications are at particular risk for HCAP due to these organisms. *Legionella* is more common in hospitals where the organism is present in the hospital water supply.

Table 33-1	Risk Factors for Multidrug-Resistant Pathogens Causing Hospital-Acquired Pneumonia, Healthcare-Associated Pneumonia, and Ventilator-Associated Pneumonia

- Antimicrobial therapy in preceding 90 days
- Current hospitalization of 5 days or more
- High frequency of antibiotic resistance in the community or in the specific hospital unit
- Presence of risk factors for HCAP:
    Hospitalization for 2 days or more in the preceding 90 days
    Residence in a nursing home or extended care facility
    Home infusion therapy (including antibiotics)
    Chronic dialysis within 30 days
    Home wound care
    Family member with multidrug-resistant pathogen
- Immunosuppressive disease and/or therapy

From ATS/IDSA. Guidelines for management of adults with hospital-acquired, ventilator associated, and healthcare-associated pneumonia. *Am J Respir Crit Care Med* 2005;171:388–416, with permission.

DIAGNOSIS

To diagnose HAP, the patient must have a new or worsening infiltrate on chest imaging as well as clinical characteristics mentioned above. Microbiologic criteria for diagnosis require clinical criteria in conjunction with a positive lower respiratory tract sample culture. In contrast, there has been no evidence suggesting a benefit in sampling the lower respiratory tract in the absence of clinical symptoms (surveillance sampling), and this practice may lead to unnecessary treatment, contribute to drug-resistant epidemiology, and expose patients to antibiotic side effects.

Approaches to sampling the lower airway are typically classified as bronchoscopic or nonbronchoscopic. Bronchoscopic sampling includes bronchoalveolar lavage (BAL) and protected brush sampling. Nonbronchoscopic sampling methods include tracheobronchial aspiration and mini-BAL. The advantages of bronchoscopic methods include visually directed sampling, higher specificity in culture results, and thus the potential of allowing for more rapid narrowing of antibiotic therapy. Conversely, nonbronchoscopic methods do not require a high level of clinical expertise and thus can be obtained quickly at a lower cost. Bronchoscopic sampling should be performed if possible. Quantitative culture thresholds have been recommended to aid in the diagnosis of VAP (Table 33-2), but their use has not been shown to improve clinical outcome compared to semiquantitative cultures (i.e., heavy, moderate, light, or no bacterial growth), where heavy to moderate growth are considered positive.

MANAGEMENT

ATS/IDSA guidelines have proposed four major principles to consider for management of HAP, VAP, and HCAP: (i) avoid untreated or inadequately treated HAP, VAP, or HCAP, which has been associated with increased mortality; (ii) recognize the variability of bacteriology from one hospital to another, specific sites within the hospital, and from one time period to another and use this information to alter the selection of an appropriate antibiotic regimen; (iii) avoid the overuse of antibiotics by focusing on accurate diagnosis, tailoring therapy to the results of lower respiratory tract cultures

Table 33-2	Bronchoscopic and Nonbronchoscopic Sampling Methods of the Lower Respiratory Tract

Protected Brush Sampling

A sheathed brush is guided through the bronchoscope until the sheath is adjacent to the desired airway wall location. A specimen is collected by brushing this area and a positive quantitative culture threshold is $>10^3$ CFU/mL.

Bronchoalveolar Lavage

Infusion and aspiration of sterile saline through the bronchoscope wedged into the desired bronchial segment. A positive quantitative culture threshold is $>10^4$ CFU/mL.

Tracheobronchial Aspiration

A catheter is advanced through the endotracheal tube until resistance is met, then suction is applied to the catheter to obtain the specimen. A positive quantitative culture threshold is $>10^5$ CFU/mL.

Mini-Bronchoalveolar Lavage

A catheter is advanced through the endotracheal tube until resistance is met and then sterile saline is infused through the catheter and aspirated to obtain the specimen. A positive quantitative culture threshold is $>10^5$ CFU/mL.

CFU/mL, colony forming units per milliliter.

and shortening duration of therapy to the minimal effective period; and (iv) apply prevention strategies aimed at modifiable risk factors.[1]

Recommendations for the management of patients with HAP, VAP, and HCAP are summarized in Figure 33-1. The presence and type of antibiotic-resistant pathogens are variable, including MRSA, extended spectrum β-lactamase–producing *Enterobacteriaceae*, beta-lactam–resistant *Pseudomonas* species, and multidrug-resistant *Acinetobacter* species. Thus, it is important for clinicians to be familiar with susceptibility patterns in their respective facilities. Coverage for resistant gram-positive organisms, specifically MRSA, should be considered in patients known to be colonized with the organism when a high prevalence of MRSA is present in the community, in critically ill patients, or in patients with risk factors for MRSA (previous use of antibiotics, HIV infection, hemodialysis, and residence in a long-term care facility). Vancomycin remains first-line therapy for MRSA in most institutions; however, linezolid has been shown in some trials to have a higher rate of treatment success for VAP. Additionally, MRSA strains with rising vancomycin minimum inhibitory concentration (MICS; >1) are more likely to be treated inadequately with vancomycin, even with higher doses. In patients with known colonization with these strains or in institutions where these strains are prevalent, linezolid should be more strongly considered.

Duration of antibiotics for VAP depends on the pathogen isolated and clinical response. If there is significant improvement in the first 48 to 72 hours of antibiotic administration, an organism is identified, and the empiric regimen was adequate, 7 to 8 total days of antibiotic therapy is sufficient. However, extended therapy (2 to 3 weeks) may be indicated for patients who failed to improve within the first 48 to 72 hours, for patients with infections due to *Pseudomonas*, and for patients with complicated infections due to MRSA.

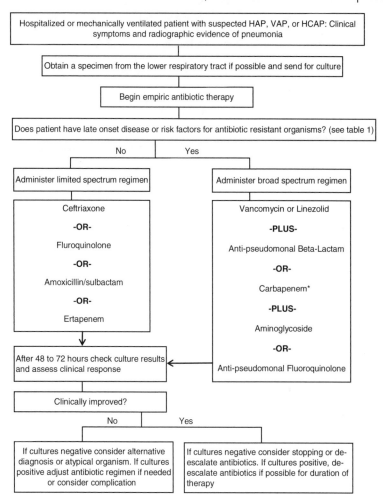

*Use of a carbapenem-based regimen is indicated in the setting of a high institutional prevalence of extended spectrum β-lactamase-producing *Enterobacteriaceae*, beta-lactam resistant *Pseudomonas* species, or multidrug-resistant *Acinetobacter* species.

Figure 33-1. Suggested management of patients with suspected HAP, VAP, or HCAP.[1]

PREVENTION

Since VAP is associated with a significant degree of morbidity and mortality, prevention is paramount. Recent guidelines have been proposed.[7,8] General strategies include adhering to hand hygiene guidelines, using noninvasive ventilation when possible, and minimizing the duration of ventilation by assessing daily for extubation readiness.

Strategies to prevent aspiration include placing the patient in a semirecumbent position (elevation of the head of the bed to >30 degrees), avoiding gastric overdistention, avoiding unplanned extubation and reintubation, use of a cuffed endotracheal tube with in-line and subglottic suctioning, and avoiding deep sedation and/or paralysis when possible. Measures to reduce colonization of the respiratory and digestive tract include providing a chlorhexidine oral rinse in combination with thorough mechanical cleaning of the oral cavity and avoiding H2-blocking agents and proton pump inhibitors among those not at high risk for stress ulcers.

REFERENCES

1. ATS/IDSA. Guidelines for management of adults with hospital-acquired, ventilator-associated, and healthcare-associated pneumonia. *Am J Respir Crit Care Med* 2005;171:388–416.
2. Chastre J, Fagon JY. Ventilator-associated pneumonia. *Am J Respir Crit Care Med* 2002;165:867–903.
3. Rello J, Ollendorf DA, Oster G, et al. Epidemiology and outcomes of ventilator-associated pneumonia in a large US database. *Chest* 2002;122:2115–2121.
4. Cook DJ, Walter SD, Cook RJ, et al. Incidence of and risk factors for ventilator-associated pneumonia in critically ill patients. *Ann Intern Med* 1998;129–440.
5. Richards MJ, Edwards JR, Culver DH, et al. Nosocomial infections in medical ICUs in the United States: National Nosocomial Infections Surveillance System. *Crit Care Med* 1999;27:887–892.
6. Tablan OC, Anderson LJ, Besser R, et al. Guidelines for preventing health-care–associated pneumonia, 2003: recommendations of CDC and the Healthcare Infection Control Practices Advisory Committee. *MMWR Morb Mortal Wkly Rep* 2004;53:1–36.
7. Lorente L, Blot S, Rello J. Evidence on measures for the prevention of ventilator-associated pneumonia. *Eur Respir J* 2007;30:1193–1207.
8. Coffin SE, Klompas M, Classen D, et al. Strategies to prevent healthcare-associated infections in acute care hospitals. *Infect Control Hosp Epidemiol* 2008;29:S31–S40.

34 Surgical Site Infections

Ioana Chirca and Camelia E. Marculescu

There are more than 25 million surgical procedures performed every year in the United States, and surgical site infections (SSI) complicate 1% to 5% of cases.[1] SSI increase the risk of death by 2- to 12-fold, length of hospitalization on average more than a week, and cost of treatment up to $60,000 depending on the type of SSI.[2,3]

DEFINITIONS

The clinical definition of an SSI in its simplest form is purulent drainage from a surgical incision site. This may or may not be accompanied by other local signs or symptoms of infection (swelling, redness, warmth) and may or may not be accompanied by a positive microbiologic culture. Because of this variation in clinical presentation and to better establish national benchmarks, the Centers for Disease Control and Prevention (CDC) has developed surveillance definitions for SSI. In general, a surgical site is monitored for 30 days for SSI if no implant is involved and for 12 months if an implant is utilized. SSIs are classified as superficial incisional, deep incisional, and organ/space.[4]

- Superficial incisional SSI involves only the skin and subcutaneous tissue of the incision. Additionally, the patient needs to have at least one of the following: (1) purulent drainage from the superficial site, (2) organisms aseptically isolated from fluid or tissue in the superficial incision, and (3) at least one sign/symptom of infection (pain, localized swelling, erythema, warmth) and the superficial incision is deliberately opened by the surgeon and is culture positive or not cultured; culture-negative does not meet the criterion.
- Deep incisional SSI involves deep soft tissues of the incision (fascia, muscles). Additionally, the patient needs to have at least one of the following: (1) purulent drainage from the incision but not from the organ/space component of the surgical site, (2) spontaneous dehiscence or deliberate opening of a deep incision with positive cultures or not cultured when the patient has fever or localized pain, and (3) abscess or other evidence of infection is found on examination, during reoperation, or by histopathologic or radiologic examination.
- Organ/space SSI is when the infection involves any part of the body but excludes categories mentioned above—skin, fascia, and muscles at the incision site. Additionally, the patient needs to have at least one of the following: (1) purulent drainage from a drain placed through a stab wound into the organ/space, (2) positive aseptically obtained cultures from tissue or fluid in the organ/space, and (3) abscess or evidence of infection of the organ/space on examination, reoperation, and histopathologic or radiologic examination. If an organ/space infection drains through the incision (often via a sinus tract), this is classified as a deep incisional SSI.

EPIDEMIOLOGY

The microbiology associated with SSI has not significantly changed over the previous few decades with the most common pathogens being *Staphylococcus aureus* and coagulase-negative staphylococci (Table 34-1).[5] Other important pathogens are *Enterococcus* spp., *Pseudomonas* spp., and other gram-negative bacteria. The site of surgery is generally the primary determinant of the organism responsible for the infection and depends on established colonizing organisms (e.g., staphylococcal predominance for orthopedic, cardiac, and vascular surgeries and gram negatives for abdominal surgeries). Antimicrobial resistance exhibited by some of these pathogens has been associated with poorer outcomes. Resistance also impacts antibiotic prophylaxis and empiric treatment of SSI. Surgeons and clinicians providing care for patients with SSI should be familiar with their local microbiology and resistance data. Recent CDC data report that approximately half of *S. aureus* SSI are methicillin resistant, 20% of enterococcal SSI are vancomycin resistant, and many gram-negative organisms causing SSI are resistant to fluoroquinolones and third-generation cephalosporins. Additionally, one needs to be aware of emerging SSI pathogens such as fungi, including invasive molds, and rapidly growing mycobacteria.

PATHOGENESIS AND RISK FACTORS

SSI is the result of complex interactions between multiple factors.

• *Microbial factors*: Bacteria can reach the surgical wound by endogenous and exogenous contamination. The most frequent mechanism is by endogenous contamination from organisms that reside on the skin and in skin appendages as antiseptic measures cannot completely eliminate bacteria.[6] Exogenous contamination is rare but has been reported such as colonization with *S. aureus* of operating room personnel and contamination of water sources or water-based solutions with organisms such as *Legionella*, *Pseudomonas*, or nontuberculous mycobacteria.[7-10] Bacterial virulence factors such as increased adhesion to wound matrix components by *S. aureus* and coagulase-negative staphylococci, biofilm production, exotoxin production by staphylococci and streptococci, and endotoxin production by gram-negative organisms may also be important for SSI risk and pathogenesis.[11-14] Also, it is intuitive that the higher the bacterial inoculum, the higher the risk of SSI and this served as the basis for classification of surgical wounds by the level of probable contamination (Table 34-2).[15]

Table 34-1	Major Pathogens Responsible for Surgical Site Infection[5]
Pathogen	**Percentage of SSI**
Staphylococcus aureus	30
Coagulase-negative staphylococci	13.7
Enterococcus spp.	11.2
Pseudomonas aeruginosa	5.6
Escherichia coli	9.6
Klebsiella pneumoniae	3
Acinetobacter, Serratia, Citrobacter	1 to 3
Candida spp.	2

Table 34-2	Wound Classification According to the Level of Contamination	
Class	**Type of Wound**	**Characteristics**
I	Clean	Uninfected, primarily closed, drained with closed drainage
II	Clean-contaminated	Respiratory, urinary, gastrointestinal (GI), and genital tract are entered under controlled conditions.
III	Contaminated	Open, fresh wounds; procedures with major breaks in sterile techniques, gross spillage from GI tract
IV	Dirty-infected	Old, traumatic wounds; perforated viscus; preexisting clinical infection.

Adapted from Mangram et al. Guideline for prevention of surgical site infection, 1999. Centers for Disease Control and Prevention (CDC) Hospital Infection Control Practices Advisory Committee. *Am J Infect Control* 1999;27:97–132, with permission.

- *Patient characteristics*: Age is not modifiable but has clearly been linked to the risk of developing an SSI, likely due to an increased incidence of other comorbid conditions.[16] Nutritional status has been considered to be important in determining risk for SSI; however, recent studies have not identified malnutrition as an independent risk factor. Conversely, obesity has been linked to increased risk for SSI due to mechanical issues of increased body mass as well as likely underdosing of prophylactic antimicrobials. Hyperglycemia increases the risk for SSI. Current recommendations suggest a goal serum glucose <180 mg/dL.[17] Smoking increases risk for SSI almost twofold, likely via vasoconstriction.[18] Smoking cessation is advised at least 4 weeks prior to surgery.[17] Nasal colonization with *S. aureus* has been reported as an independent risk factor for SSIs in some surgeries, including orthopedic procedures.[19,20] Nasal colonization has also been associated with colonization at other body sites, and thus, it is recommended to administer chlorhexidine bathing in close proximity to the surgical procedure.[17] Despite this recommendation, outcome data on SSI prevention have been mixed. Immunosuppressive medications have also been associated with increased risk of SSI, and if possible, they should be avoided in the perioperative period.[21]
- *Procedure-related factors*: Surgical technique is important. Limiting the degree of tissue injury and the introduction of a foreign body have been shown to reduce risk of SSI. Delayed primary closure and monofilament continuous sutures are preferred.[22,23] Proper ventilation in the operating room is achieved with high-efficiency particulate air (HEPA) filters or laminar flow systems. Minimizing traffic in and out of the OR may also be important.[24]

Hair removal should be done only if necessary and depilatory preparation or clipping are preferred over use of a razor.[17] Intraoperative hypothermia (34°C to 36°C) is associated with multiple adverse reactions, including increased SSI.[25] Perioperative oxygen supplementation has a theoretical benefit because of the oxygen-dependent bactericidal activity of the phagocytic system, but optimal concentration and duration of therapy remains unresolved.[26] Transfusion of blood products has also been associated with increased risk of SSI thought due to interaction with immune mechanisms.[27] Topical antibiotics are also used to reduce SSI, and multiple

Table 34-3	Elements of Systemic Antibiotic Prophylaxis[17]
Timing of administration	Within the first 30 minutes prior to incision, except vancomycin and fluorquinolones— 60 minutes prior to incision
	Should be discontinued within 24 hours of surgery completion (48 hours for cardiothoracic procedures)
Selection of antibiotic	According to the expected pathogens by surgical site, allergy status of the patient, and local resistance patterns
Dose adjustments	Renal impairment determines the dosing interval (except clindamycin and metronidazole) and obesity usually requires higher doses.
Redosing	For surgeries lasting longer than the half-life of the drug

techniques are utilized to deliver them to the surgical site, including irrigation with a syringe, sprinkling of powder, and antibiotic-impregnated implants for extended release.[28–30] The most commonly used antibiotics are aminoglycosides, vancomycin, cefazolin, and tetracyclines. Finally, systemic antibiotic prophylaxis has clearly been shown to reduce the risk of SSI, and the selection of antibiotic, timing of administration, and dosing recommendations are periodically updated and discussed in greater detail below (Table 34-3).[17,31]

PREVENTION AND CURRENT RECOMMENDATIONS

In order to identify individual patients at risk for developing SSI and for reporting purposes, surgery may be classified by level of wound contamination (Table 34-2) and by procedure (Table 34-4).[32,33] Historically, the risk for SSI has been estimated based

Table 34-4	Surgical Site Infection Rates by Procedure type and Nosocomial Infections Surveillance (NNIS) Risk Index (Pooled Mean, Per 100 Procedures)[33]			
Procedure Type	**SSI rates by NNIS Risk Index Category**			
	0	1	2	3
Cardiac		1.1	1.84	
CABG (chest & donor incision)	0.35	2.55	4.26	8.49
Colon	3.99	5.59	7.06	9.47
Bile duct/liver/pancreas		8.07	13.65	
Hip prosthesis	0.67	1.44	2.4	
Laminectomy	0.72	1.10	2.30	
Gallbladder	0.11	0.61	1.72	
Breast	0.95	2.95	6.36	
Cesarean section	1.46	2.43	3.82	

on a point system developed by CDC. A point is assigned at the time of perioperative assessment for each of the following: American Society of Anesthesiologists score of 3, 4, or 5; contaminated or dirty-infected wound; duration of surgery >75th percentile duration for that procedure; and a point subtracted for use of a laparoscope. Zero points has been associated with an overall risk of 1.5%, one point associated with a risk of 2.9%, two points a 6.8% risk, and three points a 13% risk of SSI.[32] Newer risk stratification systems are being developed and validated. These take additional variables into account such as patient comorbidities as well as whether or not the surgery is being performed in an academic setting. Summary measures to prevent SSI have recently been updated and are presented in Table 34-5.[15,17,21]

Table 34-5	Summary of Recommendations for Reduction of Surgical Site Infections [15,17]
Risk factor	**Risk reduction recommendation**
Hyperglycemia	Goal serum glucose <180 mg/dL, avoid hyperglycemia, close monitoring
Smoking	Smoking cessation 4 weeks prior to surgery
Obesity	Higher doses of antibiotics
Nutrition	Optimization, but not at the expense of delaying the surgery
Preoperative bathing	No formal recommendation; chlorhexidine baths if used should be in close proximity to the time of surgery
Hair removal	Only if necessary, immediately before surgery; use clippers; no shaving
Hypothermia	Maintain normothermia
Oxygenation, supplemental O_2	Should start with induction, at least 2 hours post procedure, but concentration and duration not established
Transfusions	Increase risk with increased number of transfusions; avoid large amount of crystalloid
Skin decontamination	Hand scrubs of 2–3 minutes for surgical team members with chlorhexidine/alcohol-based solutions
	Iodine/chlorhexidine—alcohol for the operative site
Operating room environment	HEPA filters and official ventilation recommendations, limitation of traffic, cleaning of environmental surfaces
Surgical technique	Limitation of tissue injury, introduction of foreign bodies, and use of electrocautery
	Obliteration of dead spaces by multilayered closures
	Delayed primary closure in highly contaminated wounds
Incise drapes usage	Proper technique recommended
Sutures	Monofilament, continuous sutures; antimicrobial-impregnated sutures may be beneficial (not enough evidence for formal recommendations)
Drains	Closed suction drains for large dead spaces not proved to prevent infection; conduit drains increase the risk for SSI
Topical antibiotic prophylaxis	Use throughout the procedure. Chlorhexidine/povidone not recommended
Systemic antibiotic prophylaxis	See Table 34-6.

Table 34-6	Select Recommendations for Prophylactic Antibiotics[17]		
Type of Procedure	Organisms	Routine Antibiotics	Penicillin Allergy
Cardiac and vascular with graft placement	*Staphylococcus aureus*, CoNS	cefazolin + vancomycin	vancomycin or clindamycin + gentamicin
Colorectal	Enteric gram negatives, anaerobes, enterococci	cefazolin + metronidazole or ertapenem[66]	clindamycin + gentamicin
Genitourinary	Gram negatives, anaerobes, group B streptococci	cefazolin	ciprofloxacin ± vancomycin
Orthopedic with implants	*Staphylococcus aureus*, CoNS	Cefazolin + vancomycin	vancomycin or clindamycin
Neurosurgery with craniotomy/device	*Staphylococcus aureus*, CoNS	cefazolin + vancomycin	vancomycin

CoNS, coagulase-negative *Staphylococcus*

Systemic antibiotic prophylaxis deserves additional discussion as one of the important risk reduction strategies for SSI. The goal is to ensure effective antibiotic levels in the serum and at the surgical site for the entire duration of the procedure (Table 34-3). The choice of antibiotic is sometimes challenging as the type of procedure as well as the local antibiogram need to be taken into consideration. First-generation cephalosporins are generally recommended either as monotherapy or in combination depending on surgery type and patient risks. Addition of vancomycin has been recommended for methicillin-resistant *Staphylococcus aureus* (MRSA) and coagulase-negative staphylococci coverage in procedures associated with a high prevalence of SSI due to these organisms (Table 34-6).[17]

Dosing of antibiotic prophylaxis should be weight-based. Cefazolin should be increased to 2 g for patients whose weight is 80 to 160 kg and 3 g for patients >160 kg. Vancomycin should be given at 20 mg/kg or a maximum of 3 g. Gentamicin is dosed at 4 mg/kg or a maximum of 540 mg. Clindamycin is dosed at 600 mg for <80 kg, 900 mg for 80 to 160 kg and 1,200 for >160 kg. Redosing should be done according to half-life for long surgeries and according to creatinine clearance; typically, cefazolin should be redosed at 4-hour intervals and vancomycin at 8 hours for patients with normal renal function.

Screening patients for *S. aureus* or MRSA colonization with the intention of providing decolonization prior to surgery has been successful in reducing SSI among certain surgical populations, namely, those undergoing orthopedic and cardiothoracic procedures; however, whether or not routine screening for all surgery patients remains unresolved.[21]

Institutions should monitor SSI rates and process measures for high-volume, high-impact procedures and provide feedback to individual surgeons regarding these rates in comparison with historic controls as well as national benchmarks. This feedback has been associated with increased awareness of SSI prevention as well as lower SSI rates.

REFERENCES

1. Gaynes RP, Culver DH, Horan TC, et al. Surgical site infection rates in the United States, 1992–1998: the national nosocomial infections surveillance system basic SSI risk index. *Clin Infect Dis* 2001;33(Suppl 2):S69–S77.

2. Anderson DJ, Kirkland KB, Kaye KS, et al. Underresourced hospital infection control and prevention programs: penny wise, pound foolish? *Infect Control Hosp Epidemiol* 2007;28:767–773.

3. Kirkland KB, Briggs JP, Trivette SL, et al. The impact of surgical-site infections in the 1990s: attributable mortality, excess length of hospitalization, and extra costs. *Infect Control Hosp Epidemiol* 1999;20:725–730.

4. Horan TC, Andrus M, Dudeck MA. CDC/NHSN surveillance definition of health care–associated infection and criteria for specific types of infections in the acute care setting. *Am J Infect Control* 2008;36:309–332.

5. National Healthcare Safety Network at the Centers for Disease Control and Prevention, 2006–2007. *Infect Control Hosp Epidemiol* 2008;29(11):996–1011.

6. Tuazon CU. Skin and skin structure infections in the patient at risk: carrier state of *Staphylococcus aureus*. *Am J Med* 1984;76:166–171.

7. Weber S, Herwaldt LA, McNutt LA, et al. An outbreak of *Staphylococcus aureus* in a pediatric cardiothoracic surgery unit. *Infect Control Hosp Epidemiol* 2002;23:77–81.

8. Lowry PW, Blankenship RJ, Gridley W, et al. A cluster of *Legionella* sternal-wound infections due to postoperative topical exposure to contaminated tap water. *N Engl J Med* 1991;324:109–113.

9. Mermel LA, McKay M, Dempsey J, et al. *Pseudomonas* surgical-site infections linked to a healthcare worker with onychomycosis. *Infect Control Hosp Epidemiol* 2003;24:749–752.

10. Furuya EY, Paez A, Srinivasan A, et al. Outbreak of mycobacterium abscessus wound infections among "lipotourists" from the United States who underwent abdominoplasty in the dominican republic. *Clin Infect Dis* 2008;46:1181–1188.

11. Paulsson M, Ljungh A, Wadstrom T. Rapid identification of fibronectin, vitronectin, laminin, and collagen cell surface binding proteins on coagulase-negative staphylococci by particle agglutination assays. *J Clin Microbiol* 1992;30:2006–2012.

12. Mack D, Becker P, Chatterjee I, et al. Mechanisms of biofilm formation in *Staphylococcus epidermidis* and *Staphylococcus aureus*: functional molecules, regulatory circuits, and adaptive responses. *Int J Med Microbiol* 2004;294:203–212.

13. Rogolsky M. Nonenteric toxins of *Staphylococcus aureus*. *Microbiol Rev* 1979;43:320–360.

14. Morrison DC, Ryan JL. Endotoxins and disease mechanisms. *Annu Rev Med* 1987;38:417–432.

15. Mangram AJ, Horan TC, Pearson ML, et al. Guideline for prevention of surgical site infection, 1999. Centers for disease control and prevention (CDC) hospital infection control practices advisory committee. *Am J Infect Control* 1999;27:97–132.

16. Kaye KS, Schmit K, Pieper C, et al. The effect of increasing age on the risk of surgical site infection. *J Infect Dis* 2005;191:1056–1062.

17. Alexander JW, Solomkin JS, Edwards MJ. Updated recommendations for control of surgical site infections. *Ann Surg*. 2011;253:1082–1093.

18. Myles PS, Iacono GA, Hunt JO, et al. Risk of respiratory complications and wound infection in patients undergoing ambulatory surgery: smokers versus nonsmokers. *Anesthesiology* 2002;97:842–847.

19. Perl TM, Cullen JJ, Wenzel RP, et al. Intranasal mupirocin to prevent postoperative *Staphylococcus aureus* infections. *N Engl J Med* 2002;346:1871–1877.

20. Kalmeijer MD, van Nieuwland-Bollen E, Bogaers-Hofman D, et al. Nasal carriage of *Staphylococcus aureus* is a major risk factor for surgical-site infections in orthopedic surgery. *Infect Control Hosp Epidemiol* 2000;21:319–323.

21. Anderson DJ, Kaye KS, Classen D, et al. Strategies to prevent surgical site infections in acute care hospitals. SHEA/IDSA Practice Recommendations. *Infect Control Hosp Epidemiol* 2008;29:S51–S61.

22. Duttaroy DD, Jitendra J, Duttaroy B, et al. Management strategy for dirty abdominal incisions: primary or delayed primary closure? A randomized trial. *Surg Infect (Larchmt)* 2009;10:129–136

23. Kathju S, Nistico L, Hall-Stoodley L, et al. Chronic surgical site infection due to suture-associated polymicrobial biofilm. *Surg Infect (Larchmt)* 2009;10:457–461.

24. Ayliffe GA. Role of the environment of the operating suite in surgical wound infection. *Rev Infect Dis* 1991;13(Suppl 10):S800–S804.

25. Beltramini AM, Salata RA, Ray AJ. Thermoregulation and risk of surgical site infection. *Infect Control Hosp Epidemiol* 2011;32:603–610.

26. Qadan M, Akca O, Mahid SS, et al. Perioperative supplemental oxygen therapy and surgical site infection: a meta-analysis of randomized controlled trials. *Arch Surg* 2009;144:359–366.

27. Hill GE, Frawley WH, Griffith KE, et al. Allogeneic blood transfusion increases the risk of postoperative bacterial infection: a meta-analysis. *J Trauma* 2003;54:908–914.

28. Calhoun JH, Mader JT. Antibiotic beads in the management of surgical infections. *Am J Surg* 1989;157:443–449.

29. Diefenbeck M, Muckley T, Hofmann GO. Prophylaxis and treatment of implant-related infections by local application of antibiotics. *Injury* 2006;37(Suppl 2):S95–S104.

30. Yamamoto K, Miyagawa N, Masaoka T, et al. Clinical effectiveness of antibiotic-impregnated cement spacers for the treatment of infected implants of the hip joint. *J Orthop Sci* 2003;8:823–828.

31. Bowater RJ, Stirling SA, Lilford RJ. Is antibiotic prophylaxis in surgery a generally effective intervention? Testing a generic hypothesis over a set of meta-analyses. *Ann Surg* 2009;249:551–556.

32. Culver DH, Horan TC, Gaynes RP, et al. Surgical wound infection rates by wound class, operative procedure, and patient risk index. national nosocomial infections surveillance system. *Am J Med* 1991;91:152S–157S.

33. Edwards JR, Peterson KD, Mu Y, et al. National healthcare safety network (NHSN) report: data summary for 2006 through 2008, issued december 2009. *Am J Infect Control* 2009;37:783–805.

Management of Occupational Blood-Borne Pathogen Exposure

Ivar L. Frithsen

INTRODUCTION

Blood-borne pathogen exposures (BBPE) among health care personnel (HCP) can occur in virtually all clinical settings with an estimated annual incidence of 650,000 in the United States.[1] Exposure to human immunodeficiency virus (HIV), hepatitis B virus (HBV), and hepatitis C virus (HCV) occurs when an infected patient's blood or other infectious material comes into contact with the blood of an exposed individual. Routes of exposure are percutaneous (sharp instrument), mucous membrane (eyes, nose, or mouth), or by contact with nonintact skin of the HCP.[2] Table 35-1 shows the risk of transmission after occupational BBPE by pathogen and route of exposure. Health care facilities should have policies in place to provide prompt response by someone familiar with current management guidelines in order to prevent transmission of pathogens and to reduce psychological trauma.[3,4] This chapter provides an outline for the management of occupational BBPE among HCP.

INITIAL MANAGEMENT

The first priority is immediate and thorough cleansing of the site of exposure. For percutaneous exposure or contact with nonintact skin, this should involve washing with soap and water with subsequent flushing for 5 minutes. In the case of mucous membrane exposure, the affected area should be flushed with water or saline solution for 5 to 10 minutes. Once the area has been cleaned or while this process is ongoing, the next step is to determine if there was penetration of the skin with a contaminated instrument, contact of blood/body fluids with mucous membranes, or contact of blood/body fluids with nonintact skin. Table 35-2 lists body fluids that are considered to be infectious versus those that are not considered infectious. Next, evaluate if the source patient is known to be infected with HIV, HBV, or HCV. Source patients whose HIV status is not known should have a rapid HIV test performed as soon as possible in accordance with state consent regulations. If the source patient's hepatitis status is not known, testing for HBV and HCV can be initiated at the same time.[2,5]

ONGOING MANAGEMENT

In the case of HIV exposure, baseline serologic testing of the HCP (HIV, complete blood count [CBC], and comprehensive metabolic panel [CMP]) should be performed, and postexposure prophylaxis (PEP) should be administered as described below.[5] If the source patient is known to be infected with HBV or HCV, baseline

Table 35-1	Risk of Transmission Following Occupational BBPE by Pathogen and Route of Exposure		
Pathogen	**Percutaneous**	**Mucous Membrane**	**Nonintact Skin**
HIV	0.9% (95% CI 0.2–0.5)	0.09% (95% CI 0.006–0.5)	Not quantified
HBV	22%–31% clinical disease 37%–62% seroconversion	Not quantified	Not quantified
HCV	1.8% (range 0%–7%)	Not quantified	Not quantified

From CDC. Updated U.S. Public Health Service guidelines for the management of occupational exposures to HBV, HCV, and HIV and recommendations for postexposure prophylaxis. *MMWR Morb Mortal Wkly Rep* 2001;50(RR-11):1–54; CDC. Updated U.S. Public Heath Service guidelines for the management of occupational exposures to HIV and recommendations for postexposure prophylaxis. *MMWR Morb Mortal Wkly Rep* 2005;54(RR-9):1–17.

testing on the exposed HCP should be performed as soon as feasible. When a hepatitis B exposure has occurred, determine both the vaccination and responder status of the exposed employee. Personnel who have not completed the three-shot HBV vaccination series are classified as unvaccinated; they should receive a single dose of hepatitis B immune globulin (HBIG; 0.06 mL/kg), and the vaccine series should be started. Those who have received the full vaccination series but have not been tested for antibody levels should undergo testing for anti-HBs antibody. For those with adequate antibody levels, no further treatment is indicated. For those with inadequate antibody levels, a single dose of HBIG should be administered with a vaccine booster. Immune globulin administered within 7 days of exposure has been shown to be effective in preventing transmission. HCP who have inadequate antibody response to two vaccine

Table 35-2	Body Fluids Considered to Be Infectious Versus Not Infectious Unless Containing Blood
Infectious	**Not Infectious (unless containing blood)**
Blood or any body fluid with visible blood Cerebrospinal fluid Synovial fluid Pericardial fluid Pleural fluid Amniotic fluid Peritoneal fluid Semen Vaginal secretions	Feces Nasal secretions Saliva Sputum Sweat Tears Urine Vomit

CDC. Updated U.S. Public Health Service guidelines for the management of occupational exposures to HBV, HCV, and HIV and recommendations for postexposure prophylaxis. *MMWR Morb Mortal Wkly Rep* 2001;50(RR-11):1–54.

series should receive two doses of HBIG. Health care workers who have completed the three-shot HBV series and are known responders will require no further treatment or evaluation. Since there is no recommendation for PEP in the case of HCV exposure, the next step is to obtain baseline serologic testing for HCV as soon as feasible. When the HBV/HCV status of the source patient is not known initially, follow-up should be arranged to discuss the results of hepatitis testing when that information is available. PEP for HBV may be considered if the source patient is at high risk for having HBV. HCP should be advised to refrain from unprotected sexual activity and breast-feeding until hepatitis test results have been determined.[2]

HIV POSTEXPOSURE PROPHYLAXIS

If the source patient is found to be HIV positive by either known history or rapid HIV testing, PEP should be started without delay. Consultation with an infectious disease expert is preferred but not if initiation of treatment will be delayed.[5] If the patient is known to be HIV positive, it will be helpful to obtain the patient's HIV treatment history, viral load, CD4 count, and any resistance testing performed in addition to details about the nature of the exposure when contacting a consultant. This information will be used to determine the optimal PEP regimen. If local consultation is not readily available, the National Clinicians' Post-Exposure Prophylaxis Hotline (PEPline 1-888-448-4911) can provide assistance in evaluating exposures and determining PEP regimens. Centers for Disease Control and Prevention (CDC) describes methodology for determining optimal PEP regimens in the updated 2005 guidelines; Table 35-3 summarizes those recommendations and Table 35-4 describes HIV PEP regimens with dosing.[5]

Prior to starting PEP therapy, HCP of child-bearing age should have their pregnancy status determined. Prescription or over-the-counter medications, supplements, and herbal remedies should be reviewed prior to initiating PEP therapy. Prescribers should be familiar with HIV medication interactions and side effects; HCP should be advised to refrain from unprotected sexual activity and breastfeeding while on PEP. When PEP is initiated based on the results of a rapid HIV test, a confirmatory test should be performed, and if that test is negative, PEP can be discontinued.[5]

FOLLOW-UP

All HCP with BBPE should be seen by someone familiar with the management of exposures either at the time of the event or on the next business day in order to receive counseling and further testing as indicated. For HCP who are taking PEP, this should occur within 72 hours postexposure in order to asses for side effects/toxicity and to provide further information about the source patient that may not have been available at the time of exposure. HIV PEP is continued for 4 weeks following exposure; a CBC and CMP should be done after 2 weeks to assess for drug toxicity. HIV tests should be done at 6 weeks, 12 weeks, and 6 months after exposure. HIV testing should be offered to all HCP exposed to HIV regardless of whether they are taking PEP. Further HIV testing at 1 year is only indicated for HCP who develop HCV after exposure to a patient coinfected with HIV and HCV.[5] No follow-up testing is indicated in cases of exposure to HBV unless the HBV immunization series was initiated at the time of exposure in which case anti-HBs antibody testing should be performed 1 to 2 months following completion of the vaccination series. If HBIG was administered,

Table 35-3 Methods for Determining Appropriate PEP Regimens by Exposure Type and Degree of Exposure

Exposure Type	HIV-Positive Class 1	HIV-Positive Class 2	Source Unknown HIV Status	Unknown Source
	Asymptomatic or known low viral load (< 1,500 RNA copies/mL)	Symptomatic, AIDS, acute seroconversion, known high viral load	Source not available for testing or refuses testing	Needle in sharps container—do not perform HIV testing on needles or other instruments
Percutaneous				
Less severe	Recommend basic two-drug regimen	Recommend expanded three-drug regimen	Generally no PEP warranted; consider basic two-drug regimen for source with HIV risk factors	Generally no PEP warranted; consider basic two-drug regimen in settings where HIV exposure likely
• Solid needle				
• Superficial injury				
More severe	Recommend expanded three-drug regimen	Recommend expanded three-drug regimen	Generally no PEP warranted; consider basic three-drug regimen for source with HIV risk factors[a]	Generally no PEP warranted; consider basic two-drug regimen in settings where HIV exposure likely[a]
• Large-bore hollow needle				
• Deep puncture				
• Visible blood on device				
• Needle from artery or vein				
Mucous membrane/nonintact skin				
Small volume	Consider basic two-drug regimen[a]	Recommend basic two-drug regimen	Generally no PEP warranted	Generally no PEP warranted
• A few drops				
Large volume	Recommend basic two-drug regimen	Recommend expanded three-drug regimen	Generally no PEP warranted; consider basic two-drug regimen for source with HIV risk factors[a]	Generally no PEP warranted; consider basic two-drug regimen in settings where HIV exposure likely[a]
• Large splash				

[a]The recommendation to "consider" PEP indicates that PEP is optional. The decision to treat is based on a discussion between the exposed HCP and treating physician where the risks versus benefits of PEP are described.

Adapted from CDC Updated U.S. Public Heath Service guidelines for the management of occupational exposures to HIV and recommendations for postexposure prophylaxis. *MMWR Morb Mortal Wkly Rep* 2005;54(RR-9):1–17.

Table 35-4	HIV Postexposure Prophylaxis Regimens	
	Preferred	**Alternatives**[a]
Basic two-drug regimen	• Tenofovir (TDF) 300 mg once daily + emtricitabine (FTC) 200 mg once daily (Truvada)[b] • Zidovudine (AZT) 300 mg twice daily + lamivudine (3TC) 150 mg twice daily (Combivir)[c]	• Stavudine (d4T) 40 mg twice daily or 30 mg twice daily if body weight is <60 kg + lamivudine (3TC) or emtricitabine (FTC) • Didanosine (ddI) 200 mg twice daily or 400 mg once daily for patients weighing >60 kg and 125 mg twice daily or 250 mg once daily for patients weighing >60 kg. + lamivudine (3TC) or emtricitabine (FTC)
Expanded three-drug regimens	Basic regimen + • lopinavir–ritonavir (LPV/r) 400/100 mg twice daily (Kaletra)	Basic regimen + • atazanavir +/- ritonavir (ATV/RTV) • fosamprenavir +/- ritonavir (FPV/RTV) • indinavir +/-ritonavir (IDV/RTC) • saquinavir + ritonavir (SQV/RTV) • nelfinavir (NFV) • efavirenz (EFV)

[a]Dosing same as for preferred regimen when not indicated, dosing for alternative expanded regimens described in CDC-Updated U.S. Public Heath Service guidelines for the management of occupational exposures to HIV and recommendations for postexposure prophylaxis. *MMWR Morb Mortal Wkly Rep.*. 2005;54(RR-9):1–17.
[b]Fewer side effects, contraindicated in pregnancy.
[c]More side effects, considered safe in pregnancy.

anti-HBs antibody testing should be delayed for 3 to 4 months. For exposure to HCV, follow-up testing for alanine aminotransferase (ALT) and anti-HCV should be performed after 4 to 6 months. HCV RNA can be performed at 4 to 6 weeks for earlier diagnosis.[2] HCP who demonstrate evidence of acute HCV infection clinically or through HCV RNA detection may wish to be referred to hepatology for follow-up. Some institutions would repeat HCV RNA levels at monthly intervals to determine if the HCP is going to clear the virus and if not would consider therapy for HCV.

REGULATIONS

The United States Occupational Health and Safety Administration (OSHA) standard number 1910.1030 pertains to blood-borne pathogens. Health care workers responsible for managing BBPE should review this document in detail and be familiar with any relevant state regulations. This OSHA standard requires that all health care facilities develop a written exposure control plan that is available to all employees;

engineering and work practice controls should be utilized to avoid exposures; personal protective equipment shall be provided to employees at no cost when appropriate; immunization for HBV shall be provided; and postexposure management shall include PEP if indicated, follow-up testing, counseling, and a written report.[3]

PREVENTION

Engineering controls such as safety needles, sharps disposal boxes, needleless systems, and other safety devices should be utilized by health care organizations to prevent BBPE. Hepatitis B vaccination should be provided at no cost to all HCP. Hand washing should be performed on a regular basis. Gloves should be worn for all procedures involving potential contact with blood or infectious materials, and face shields should be used when there is a potential for body fluids to splash.[2,3,5] Double gloving, use of a neutral zone, and blunt instruments are effective methods to reduce blood-borne exposures.[6-8]

RESOURCES

Exposure to Blood: What HCP Need to Know:
   http://www.cdc.gov/HAI/pdfs/bbp/Exp_to_Blood.pdf
PEP steps:
   http://www.mpaetc.org/downloads/PEP%20final%20(2006).pdf
Rapid HIV test comparison chart:
   http://www.cdc.gov/hiv/topics/testing/rapid/rt-comparison.htm
AIDS *info* (service of the United States Department of Health and Human Services that includes detailed medication information):
   http://aidsinfo.nih.gov/

REFERENCES

1. Perry J, Jagger J. Healthcare worker blood exposure risks: correcting some outdated statistics. *Adv Expo Prev* 2003;6(3):28–31.
2. CDC. Updated U.S. Public Health Service guidelines for the management of occupational exposures to HBV, HCV, and HIV and recommendations for postexposure prophylaxis. *MMWR Morb Mortal Wkly Rep* 2001;50(RR-11):1–54.
3. OSHA. Bloodborne pathogens. *Occupational Safety and Health Standards* http://www.osha.gov/pls/oshaweb/owadisp.show_document?p_table=STANDARDS&p_id=10051. Accessed January 5, 2012.
4. Wald J. The psychological consequences of occupational blood and body fluid exposure injuries. *Disabil Rehabil* 2009;31(23):1963–1969.
5. CDC. Updated U.S. Public Heath Service guidelines for the management of occupational exposures to HIV and recommendations for postexposure prophylaxis. *MMWRMorb Mortal Wkly Rep* 2005;54(RR-9):1–17.
6. Catanzarite V, Byrd K, McNamara M, et al. Preventing needlestick injuries in obstetrics and gynecology: how can we improve the use of blunt tip needles in practice? *Obstet Gynecol* 2007;110(6):1399–1403.
7. Cicconi L, Claypool M, Stevens W. Prevention of transmissible infections in the perioperative setting. *AORN J* 2010;92(5):519–527.
8. Tanner J, Parkinson H. Double gloving to reduce surgical cross-infection. *Cochrane Database Syst Rev* 2006;3:1–38.

36 Health Care–Associated *Clostridium difficile* Infection

Carlene A. Muto

INTRODUCTION

- *Clostridium difficile* is a spore-forming, obligate anaerobic, gram-positive rod. It derives its name from observations in the laboratory. The organism was "difficult" to isolate because of its slow growth compared to other species of *Clostridium* and its aerointolerant nature when in the vegetative form.
- *C. difficile* is a ubiquitous organism found in the environment; however, its major reservoir is within health care facilities.
- *C. difficile* spores are the transmissible form of the organism and contribute to its survival in the environment and in the host. Spores can survive for months and have been recovered from many common hospital surfaces (toilets, bedpans, bedrails, floors, and thermometers). *C. difficile* spores are problematic in health care because typical hospital cleaning products have no activity against them.
- After exposure to *C. difficile*, the patient may develop either asymptomatic colonization or *Clostridium difficile* infection (CDI). Approximately 3% to 5% of healthy adults are colonized with *C. difficile*, and up to 25% of hospitalized patients are found to be colonized at some point during their hospital stay.
- CDI is an inflammatory condition of the colon with clinical illness ranging from mild diarrhea to life-threatening conditions such as toxic megacolon, perforation, or sepsis.
- The colonic inflammatory response is a result of toxin-induced cytokines (toxins A and B). Only strains of toxin-producing *C. difficile* are able to cause disease, and the pathopneumonic condition associated with CDI is pseudomembranous colitis.
- Toxigenic strains of *C. difficile* contain a pathogenicity locus (PaLoc) that harbors the genes *tcdA*, *tcdB*, *tcdC*, *tcdR*, and *tcdE* responsible for encoding and regulating toxins A and B. Nontoxigenic strains do not contain PaLoc.
- CDI is the most common cause of health care–associated infectious diarrhea.
- Recent data suggest that the incidence of health care–associated *C. difficile* colonization and infection is 29.5 and 28.1 cases per 10,000 patient days, respectively.
- Recently, CDI has been associated with increased mortality. This has been attributed to an emerging strain of *C. difficile*, which has a mutation of the toxin regulatory gene *tcdC*. This strain (referred to as BI/NAP1/027) produces severalfold more toxin A and B as well as a binary toxin, which may contribute to more severe disease.
- Recent data report that among patients colonized or infected with *C. difficile*, 36% and 63% have the NAP1 strain, respectively.
- Acquisition of *C. difficile* generally occurs after exposure to broad-spectrum antibiotics. Clindamycin, cephalosporins, and beta-lactams have been repeatedly associated with *C. difficile*. Fluoroquinolones have emerged as a significant risk as well,

particularly with the NAP1 strain. Even short-term exposure to antibiotics, such as that with prophylactic perioperative courses, increases risk for *C. difficile*.

- Traditional risks beyond antibiotic use include advanced age, increased severity of illness, prior hospitalization, use of feeding tubes, gastrointestinal surgery, and the use of proton pump inhibitors; however, risk factors may differ between those merely colonized with the organism and those who develop CDI. These risks appear to be associated with defined host as well as pathogen variables.
  - Risks for *C. difficile* colonization include recent (within 60 days) hospitalization, use of chemotherapy, proton pump inhibitors, H2 blockers, and the presence of antibodies against toxin B.
  - Risks for CDI include older age, antibiotics, and use of proton pump inhibitors.

CLINICAL PRESENTATION

- A number of clinical features have been described for CDI including malaise, anorexia, abdominal cramping, diarrhea (frequently watery and up to 20 times per day), and fever. Severe disease may cause paralytic ileus or toxic megacolon resulting in no diarrhea.
- Physical exam may reveal tenderness (especially in the lower quadrants) and distension. Absence of bowel sounds may indicate severe disease complicated by toxic megacolon. Fever and altered mental status also suggest moderate or severe disease.
- Systemic findings, such as fever and leukocytosis, are usually absent in mild disease but are common in moderate or severe disease. Renal failure and shock have also been described.
- Laboratory findings consistent with CDI include leukocytosis with bandemia, fecal leukocytes, renal insufficiency, hypoalbuminemia, and elevated lactate.
- Visual exam by endoscopy may reveal extensive pseudomembranes or raised yellow-white plaques overlying an erythematous and edematous mucosa. Microscopic evaluation demonstrates an inflammatory exudate composed of mucinous fibrinous material with polymorphonuclear cells.
- CT scan may reveal colonic wall thickening and/or pericolonic stranding.
- Many facilities employ a scoring criteria to determine severity of disease. Older age (>60), WBC >15,000 or bandemia >10%, elevated serum creatinine (≥1.5 times baseline), low albumin, and altered mental status may be markers for severe or complicated disease.

DIAGNOSIS

- Definitive diagnosis requires laboratory identification of *C. difficile* toxin in a stool sample and/or visualization of pseudomembranes during endoscopy.
- Several laboratory testing methods are available to aid in the diagnosis of CDI, each with described advantages and disadvantages (Table 36-1).

MANAGEMENT

- Historically, metronidazole and oral vancomycin were viewed as equivalent with regard to efficacy and relapse rates, and thus, given the higher cost of oral vancomycin and the concern for development of vancomycin-resistant enterococci, metronidazole (orally or intravenously) was the preferred initial agent of choice.

Table 36-1	Various Stool Testing Methods for Diagnosis of *Clostridium difficile* Infection[a]		
Method	**Identifies**	**Advantages**	**Disadvantages**
Cell culture cytotoxin assay	Observes toxin-induced cytopathic effect of a cell line inoculated with stool infiltrate	Good sensitivity (67%–86%) but less than newer methods of detection	Requires tissue culture facility, labor intense, takes 24–48 hours, no longer the gold standard
Toxin enzyme immunoassay (EIA)	Toxin A or A and B. Best to use a test that detects both toxins	Fast (2–6 hours), easy to perform, high specificity (84%–100%), most common method used in US hospitals	EIAs generally have variable sensitivity (often <90%). Practice guidelines consider EIA suboptimal for diagnosis of CDI
Glutamate dehydrogenase (GDH) EIA	Common enzyme (GDH) expressed at high levels by all (toxigenic and nontoxigenic) strains of *C. difficile*	Fast (<1 hour), easy to perform, high negative predictive value (98.5%–99.7%)	Must be combined with another method that detects toxin to verify diagnosis if GDH test is positive
Anaerobic culture	Toxigenic and nontoxigenic *C. difficile*	High sensitivity, permits strain typing and antibiotic resistance testing during epidemics, useful for comparing new diagnostics	Labor intense (not practical), cannot distinguish between toxin-producing strains, typically takes 2–5 days
Nucleic acid amplification assays	Some assays target conserved regions of *tcdB*. Some assays detect the PaLoc at a conserved region of *tcdA*.	Rapid (<1 hour); high sensitivity (77%–100%) and specificity (93%–100%). Gaining popularity for use in hospital clinical microbiology laboratories	Assays vary in methodology, ease of use, instrumentation, and cost

[a]Specimen should be watery, loose, or unformed and promptly submitted to the hospital laboratory.

Table 36-2	Treatment for *Clostridium difficile* Infection[a]

Initial Episode

*Mild to moderate disease:*oral metronidazole 500 mg three times a day for 10–14 days

*Severe disease without ileus:*oral vancomycin 125 mg enterally four times a day for 10–14 days. Colectomy may be necessary if no response to medical management.

*Severe disease with ileus:*IV metronidazole 500 mg every 8 hours for 10–14 days and oral vancomycin 500 mg enterally four times a day for 10–14 days. Colectomy may be necessary if no response to medical management.

Recurrent Disease

First Recurrence	**Subsequent (≥2) Recurrences**
Treat with the same drug used to treat the initial episode	Oral vancomycin 125 mg enterally four times a day for 10–14 days followed by vancomycin taper or pulse dose over 4–6 weeks[b]
	Sequential oral vancomycin followed by rifaximin (resistance already described)
	Concomitant oral vancomycin with rifampin (resistance already described)
	Passive antibody
	Infuse donor stool

[a]In patients who are unable to tolerate oral medications, intracolonic vancomycin could be utilized.
[b]Vancomycin rather than with metronidazole, in part because of the adverse effects (e.g., peripheral neuropathy) resulting from long-term exposure to metronidazole.

- Vancomycin was reserved for patients with severe disease, intolerance, or contraindication (pregnancy) to metronidazole, or to those who failed to respond to metronidazole.
- Recent observational studies have reported increased failure and recurrence rates with metronidazole, and prospective trials have reported vancomycin to be superior to metronidazole in the setting of severe disease. Thus, treatment recommendations are based on severity of illness (Table 36-2).

Management of Severe CDI

- Metronidazole should be given in combination with oral vancomycin. In the absence of ileus, metronidazole should be administered orally. With ileus, vancomycin should be administered via nasogastric tube or via rectal instillation.
- Although higher doses of oral vancomycin are recommended for severe CDI, no data have demonstrated a difference in outcome with these higher dosage regimens.
- Patients with severe CDI should have surgical consultation without delay. In the event that there is limited response to medical treatment, surgery (colectomy) can be lifesaving.

- Ileus, marked leukocytosis (>20,000/μL), serum lactate >5 mmol/L, and rising serum creatinine are all poor prognostic indicators and are considerations for surgical intervention.
- Intravenous immunoglobulin (IVIG) use has been considered, but outcomes data are limited.

Management of Recurrent CDI

- It has been estimated that 20% to 25% of patients with CDI will experience at least one episode of recurrence, and among those who have experienced one recurrence, 45% will have another. Unfortunately, some patients have multiple relapses.
- Recurrent CDI has not been associated with antibiotic resistance.
- A first recurrence should be treated in the same manner as the initial episode (according to disease severity); however, metronidazole should not be utilized beyond treatment of the first recurrence and for durations exceeding 14 days due to the potential for hepatic and neuropathic toxicity.
- For further recurrences, tapered or pulse dosing of vancomycin has been the most widely used regimen (Table 36-2).
- Adjunctive treatment with various therapies has been trialed. Probiotics, such as *Saccharomyces boulardii* or *Lactobacillus* GG, have been used with hopes of repopulating the colonic microflora and restricting the growth of toxigenic *C. difficile*. Most studies are limited to a small number of patients.
- *Saccharomyces* has been associated with a beneficial effect on recurrence rates when added to and continued after treatment with metronidazole or vancomycin; however, fungemia has been reported.
- Probiotics are generally safe and easy to administer in most patient populations; however, most studies have failed to demonstrate a consistent benefit of probiotics for the prevention of CDI.
- Anecdotal reports of treatment success for patients with multiple relapses with the use of rifampin in combination with oral vancomycin exist. Similarly, rifamycin and rifaximin may have a potential role for treatment in this setting. Of note however, widespread rifampin resistance has already been described among *C. difficile* isolates.
- Nitazoxanide, a nitrothiazolide compound, and fidaxomicin, a macrolide antibiotic, both have activity against *C. difficile* and have been compared to oral vancomycin with similar efficacy results. Fidaxomicin use has been associated with lower recurrence rates with infection due to non-NAP1 strains.
- Finally, fecal transplantation (restoration of bacterial homeostasis) may be considered as an alternative therapy for recurrent CDI. The donor specimen must be fresh and homogenized using normal saline. After filtration, the preparation is delivered by nasogastric tube. This treatment has been associated with a 94% cure rate (no recurrence) in survivors.

CONTROL MEASURES IN HEALTH CARE

- In order to control *C. difficile* in the health care setting, it is important to follow recommendations designed to prevent emergence of the organism as well as prevent transmission from the environment, the transiently contaminated health care worker, and affected patients.
- The use of a comprehensive bundle, which includes education, early case finding methodologies, expanded infection control measures, a *C. difficile* management

team, and targeted antimicrobial management (restricting the use of agents known to be associated with *C. difficile*), has been associated with rapid and sustainable control.

Limiting Environmental Contamination

• Environmental surface contamination with *C. difficile* spores is common. Importantly, both asymptomatic colonized patients and patients with active disease contribute to this contamination.

• Environmental cleaning and enhanced disinfection measures are necessary to kill *C. difficile* spores.

• Although a variety of approved hospital cleaners are effective in killing vegetative forms of *C. difficile*, only chlorine-based disinfectants, high-concentration vaporized hydrogen peroxide, or select liquid hydrogen peroxides are sporicidal.

Limiting Health Care Worker Contamination

• Contamination of the health care worker (hands, clothing, and equipment) can lead to and result from contamination of the environment, particularly in the setting of poor compliance with hand hygiene.

• Alcohol-based hand rubs, now commonly used for hand hygiene, do not kill *C. difficile* spores and are not effective at removing them from hands.

• When caring for patients with suspected or confirmed *C. difficile*, hand washing (30 seconds to 2 minutes with soap and water) followed by proper hand drying with a disposable paper towel is effective for spore removal.

• Barrier precautions (gloves and gown) and dedicated equipment should also be used when caring for any *C. difficile* patient and when contact with their environment is anticipated.

Limiting Patient Contamination

• Recent data suggests that patients with active CDI or asymptomatic carriage have high rates of skin contamination (61% to 78%) and even noncarriers have skin contamination rates of 19%. Spores on the skin of patients are easily transferred to their environment as well as to the hands of care providers.

• Cleansing patients with chlorhexidine-saturated cloths has been shown to reduce contamination of patient's skin and subsequently contamination of health care workers' hands.

SUGGESTED READINGS

Bartlett JG, G. DN. Clinical recognition and diagnosis of *Clostridium difficile* infection. *Clin Infect Dis* 2008;46:S12–S18.

Carroll KC, Bartlett JG. Biology of *Clostridium difficile*: implications for epidemiology and diagnosis. *Annu Rev Microbiol* 2011;65:501–521.

Cohen S, et al. Clinical practice guidelines for *Clostridium difficile* infection in adults: 2010 update by the Society for Healthcare Epidemiology of America (SHEA) and the infectious diseases society of America (IDSA). *Infect Control Hosp Epidemiol* 2010;31(5):431–455.

Loo VG, Bourgault AM, Poirier L, et al. Host and pathogen factors for *Clostridium difficile* infection and colonization. *N Engl J Med* 2011;365:1693–1703.

Loo VG, et al. A predominantly clonal multi-institutional outbreak of *Clostridium difficile*-associated diarrhea with high morbidity and mortality. *N Engl J Med* 2005;353(23): 2442–2449.

Louie TJ, Miller MA, Mullane KM, et al. Fidaxomicin versus vancomycin for *Clostridium difficile* infection. *N Engl J Med* 2011;364:422–431.

McFarland LV. Alternative treatments for *Clostridium difficile* disease: what really works? *J Med Microbiol* 2005;54(2):101–111.

Musher D, et al. Relatively poor outcome after treatment of *Clostridium difficile* colitis with metronidazole. *Clin Infect Dis* 2005;40:1586–1590.

Muto CA, et al. Control of an outbreak of infection with the hypervirulent *Clostridium difficile* BI strain in a university hospital using a comprehensive "bundle" approach. *Clin Infect Dis* 2007;45(10):1266–1273.

Parkes GC, Sanderson JD, Whelan K. The mechanisms and efficacy of probiotics in the prevention of *Clostridium difficile*-associated diarrhoea. *Lancet Infect Dis* 2009;9:237–244.

Sunenshine RH, McDonald LC. *Clostridium difficile*-associated disease: new challenges from an established pathogen. *Cleve Clin J Med* 2006;73:187–197.

Zar FA, et al. A comparison of vancomycin and metronidazole for the treatment of *Clostridium difficile*-associated diarrhea, stratified by disease severity. *Clin Infect Dis* 2007;45(3): 302–307.

37

Epidemiologically Important Resistant Gram-Positive Bacteria in Health Care

Cassandra D. Salgado

The incidence of clinically relevant antimicrobial resistance among gram-positive organisms has significantly increased. This has resulted in important changes in the way clinicians approach treatment of infections caused by these pathogens as well as fostered increased awareness for prevention and control, particularly in health care. This chapter focuses on three epidemiologically important gram-positive bacteria, *Streptococcus pneumoniae, Staphylococcus aureus* (including methicillin-resistant *Staphylococcus aureus* (MRSA) and *S. aureus* with reduced susceptibility to vancomycin), and *Enterococcus* species. Common infections due to these organisms, common resistance mechanisms, treatment options, and prevention measures are discussed.

STREPTOCOCCUS PNEUMONIAE

- *S. pneumoniae* replicates in chains when grown in liquid medium.
- In the laboratory, pneumococci have been identified by (1) α-hemolysis when grown on blood agar media, (2) a negative catalase reaction, (3) susceptibility to optochin, and (4) solubility in bile salts.
- In a susceptible host, several characteristics of *S. pneumoniae* likely contribute to infection; however, it is the outer polysaccharide capsule that is largely responsible for virulence of the organism.
- The polysaccharide capsule protects the organism against phagocytosis from the cells it invades. The hosts' specific immune response to capsular antigen (anticapsular antibodies) has served as the basis for serotype identification. There are currently more than 90 different serotypes, but serotypes 6, 14, 18, 19, and 23 are most prevalent and are responsible for the majority of disease.[1]
- The cell wall, primarily composed of glycopeptides, covalently binds to the capsule. Antigens within the cell wall result in a profound inflammatory reaction, and most clinically relevant pneumococcal isolates produce an important virulence factor, pneumolysin, a cytotoxin, responsible for injuring neutrophils, endothelial cells, and alveolar epithelium.
- *S. pneumoniae* colonizes the nasopharynx in 5% to 10% of adults and 20% to 40% of children.[2] The rate of invasive disease has been reported as 15 per 100,000 persons per year worldwide. US data suggest that the incidence of pneumococcal disease has decreased, likely as a result of the administration of the protein-conjugate vaccine in children.[3]
- *S. pneumoniae* is a common cause of pneumonia, sinusitis, and otitis media, likely resulting from direct spread and invasion. *S. pneumoniae* also causes meningitis, endocarditis, peritonitis, or bone and joint infections; however, these infections are more likely from hematogenous spread.

- *S. pneumoniae* has developed resistance to many classes of antibiotics, including β-lactams, macrolides, tetracyclines, trimethoprim-sulfamethoxazole, and fluoroquinolones. Previous exposure to antibiotics, day care or preschool, nursing home, or other long-term care facility residence and a history of a recent respiratory infection (including viral infections) are risk factors for resistance. The most clinically relevant antibiotic resistance is that toward penicillin.
- Penicillin inhibits *S. pneumoniae* by binding to penicillin binding proteins (PBPs); however, in resistant strains, the PBPs are altered and have much less affinity for penicillin (and often other β-lactams).
- Resistance to penicillin is considered to be concentration dependent and the definition based upon achievable drug concentration in the cerebral spinal fluid (CSF); however, achievable drug concentration in CSF is often lower than what is achieved in plasma, inner ear fluid, or alveolar fluid.
- In a nonmeningeal infection, *S. pneumoniae* is susceptible to penicillin when the minimum inhibitory concentration (MIC) is $2\,\mu g/mL$, intermediately resistant to penicillin when the MIC is $4\,\mu g/mL$, and resistant to penicillin when the MIC is $\geq 8\,\mu g/mL$. In meningeal infection, *S. pneumoniae* is considered susceptible to penicillin when the MIC $0.06\,\mu g/mL$ and resistant when $\geq 0.12\,\mu g/mL$.[4] Rates of penicillin resistance vary by geographic location and patient population. The clinician should be aware of the local and regional epidemiology corresponding to their patient cohort.
- In the United States, use of the 7-valent protein conjugate pneumococcal vaccine has resulted in an 80% reduction in invasive disease and a >95% decrease in invasive *S. pneumoniae* isolates covered by the vaccine.[3] However, there has been an increase among strains not included in the vaccine (type 6 (non-B), 19 (non-F), 35, 11, and 15), and many of these strains have demonstrated antimicrobial resistance.
- Susceptibility to ceftriaxone, a common third-generation cephalosporin used for treatment of *S. pneumoniae* infections, is defined as susceptible if the MIC is $<1.0\,\mu g/mL$, intermediately resistant if the MIC is $= 2.0\,\mu g/mL$, and resistant if the MIC $>4.0\,\mu g/mL$.
- Up to one-third of *S. pneumoniae* isolates are resistant to macrolides, 20% to tetracyclines, 30% to trimethoprim-sulfamethoxazole, up to 10% resistant to clindamycin, and 5% to fluoroquinolones (higher among long-term care residents).[5]
- Because of differing achievable drug concentrations, treatment decisions depend on the site of infection. First-line therapy for otitis media and sinusitis is high-dose amoxicillin (90 mg/kg/day divided into twice or three time daily doses). In the case of treatment failure or in the presence of a penicillin allergy, a macrolide may be used. If cross-resistance to penicillin as well as the macrolide class of antibiotics is common in the region, alternatives such as a third-generation cephalosporin should be considered.
- For treatment of bacteremia in a normal host, most experts would recommend cefuroxime, cefotaxime, or ceftriaxone at standard doses as achievable plasma levels typically exceed the desired MIC.
- For meningitis suspected to be due to *S. pneumoniae* in a patient who has risk factors for resistance or in a geographic area where isolates exist with intermediate or high resistance to penicillin or ceftriaxone, higher doses of third-generation cephalosporins (cefotaxime 2 g IV every 4 hours or ceftriaxone 2 g IV every 12 hours) plus vancomycin should be utilized. Vancomycin does not readily penetrate the blood-brain barrier; thus, once susceptibilities return, if possible, treatment should be continued with a β-lactam.

STREPTOCOCCUS PNEUMONIAE PREVENTION

- Limiting the use of unnecessary antibiotics in both the inpatient and outpatient setting, combined with continued vaccination of susceptible hosts are important measures to control the emergence of resistant *S. pneumoniae*.
- The pneumococcal conjugate vaccine, PCV13, is routinely given to infants as a series of four doses (ages 2 months, 4 months, 6 months, and 12 through 15 months). The 23-valent pneumococcal polysaccharide vaccine, PPSV, is given for prevention of disease among older children and adults. These vaccines are currently recommended for use in all adults who are older than 65 years of age and for persons who are 2 years and older and at high risk for disease (e.g., sickle cell disease, asthma, smoking, HIV infection, or other immunocompromising condition.)

STAPHYLOCOCCUS AUREUS

- *S. aureus* are named for their ability to grow in grape-like clusters in solid media. They are characterized by a positive catalase test and identified as *S. aureus* by a positive coagulase test.
- Several virulence factors have been described including exotoxins (such as toxic shock syndrome toxin) and enterotoxins; leukocidin, which causes destruction of phagocytes; and catalases, coagulases, and hyaluronidases, which promote invasion and survival in tissue. Presence of the Panton Valentine leukocidin (PVL) gene encodes for release of a cytotoxin, which causes tissue necrosis and leukocyte destruction and has been associated with infections of greater severity.[6]
- *S. aureus* colonizes the skin and mucosa, preferably the anterior nares. Ten percent to forty percent of the population are transiently colonized, and less commonly, some may become chronically colonized and as such may be at increased risk for clinical disease.
- Synthetic penicillins (such as methicillin, oxacillin, and nafcillin) have been recommended as first-line therapy for *S. aureus* infections for decades; however, methicillin resistance among *S. aureus* has been a continuously emerging problem.
- Methicillin resistance results when *S. aureus* acquires the staphylococcal cassette chromosome *mec* (SCC*mec*). Within this large mobile genetic element, the *mec*A gene mediates β-lactam resistance. Specifically, *mec*A encodes for an altered PBP, PBP2a, which has little affinity for β-lactam antibiotics conferring resistance to the entire class. Additionally, *mec*A is often flanked by IS431, an insertion sequence that acts as a "collector" for additional antibiotic-resistance genes for other classes of agents.
- At least eight SCC*mec* cassettes have been described (types I through VIII) based largely on the *mec*A genes; however, types I through V have been the most studied. Types I, II, and III are large and are more likely to have multiple antibiotic-resistance encoding genes. Types IV and V are smaller, more mobile, and contain fewer antibiotic-resistance encoding genes.
- MRSA is defined as having an MIC of >16 mg/L to methicillin or an MIC of >4 mg/L to oxacillin; however, rapid methods, which detect the presence of the *mec*A gene or its product, PBP2a, for identification of methicillin-resistance, are commonly utilized in health care.[7]
- The epidemiology of MRSA continues to develop, but most continue to rely on whether or not the organism is considered health care associated or community associated, as the prevalence, resistance patterns, and clinical syndromes depend on this classification.

Health Care–Associated MRSA

- Health care–associated MRSA (HA-MRSA) has traditionally been defined as being isolated from a patient 72 hours or more after admission to a health care facility. These strains often harbor the SCC*mec* types I, II, or III and may be multidrug resistant.
- HA-MRSA infections include pneumonia, central line–associated bloodstream infections (CLABSI), and surgical site infections (SSI). In 2008, the National Healthcare Safety Network (NHSN) of the Centers for Disease Control (CDC) released a report of antimicrobial-resistant pathogens associated with hospital infections in the United States. The pooled mean proportion of all device-related infections due to MRSA was 8%; however, this varied by type of infection and by patient care area.[8] In 2009, a report by the International Nosocomial Infection Control Consortium (INICC) described hospital infections in 173 ICUs from 25 countries in Latin America, Asia, Africa, and Europe.[9] Rates of MRSA infections in these international ICUs were generally higher than rates reported from NHSN ICUs. For example, the proportion of *S. aureus* CLABSI resistant to methicillin among INICC ICUs was 84.1% versus 56.8% reported among NHSN ICUs.
- Risk factors for HA-MRSA include prolonged hospital stay, receipt of care in the ICU, exposure to broad spectrum antibiotics, receipt of invasive procedures or foreign bodies and being in close proximity to other MRSA colonized or infected patients.
- Patient-to-patient spread from the contaminated hands, clothing, and medical equipment of health care providers is the predominant way the organism is transmitted in health care.
- Compared to patients who acquire infections due to susceptible strains of *S. aureus*, those who acquire infections due to MRSA suffer increased morbidity (longer hospital and ICU stays), mortality (nearly twofold increase for those with BSI and nearly threefold for those with SSI), and greater hospital costs (nearly threefold increase).[10,11]

Community-Associated MRSA

- Community-associated MRSA (CA-MRSA) has traditionally been defined as that identified in a patient at the time of or within 48 to 72 hours of admission into health care. Also, MRSA may be considered CA if it has been isolated from a patient presenting as an outpatient or to an emergency department.
- CA-MRSA typically harbor SCC*mec* IV and less often SCC*mec* V and often are more susceptible to other classes of antibiotics. Also, CA-MRSA isolates are more likely to possess the gene responsible for encoding PVL and are often identified as the USA 300 clone when subjected to pulsed-field gel electrophoresis.
- Data from the CDC's Active Bacterial Core surveillance and Emerging Infections Program Network indicate that 13.7% of invasive MRSA disease in the United States occurred in persons without established health care–associated risks.[12] This emerging epidemiology of MRSA is the result of clonal dissemination of novel strains of MRSA that are genetically and epidemiologically distinct from typical HA strains.
- A landmark study from 2006 documented that MRSA was the single most common identifiable cause of skin and soft tissue infections among patients presenting to emergency departments in 11 US cities. The overall prevalence of MRSA was 59%, and among those, 97% were the USA 300 clone and 98% harbored SCC*mec* IV and were PVL positive.[13]

- Even though the majority of infections due to CA-MRSA have involved skin and soft tissue, the organism may also cause more invasive infections such as necrotizing fasciitis, bacteremia, or necrotizing pneumonia.
- A 2005 US population–based active case finding study reported that more than 94,000 invasive MRSA infections occurred for an estimated incidence rate of 31.8 per 100,000 persons. These infections were associated with more than 18,000 deaths for an estimated mortality rate of 6.3 per 100,000 persons.[12] Most were HA, 58.4% were HA community onset and 26.6% were HA hospital onset. Only 13.7% of invasive MRSA infections were CA.
- Further study and molecular analysis has provided evidence that community strains of MRSA (USA 300) comprise a measurable amount of hospital onset disease ranging from 16% to 25%.[12,14] Additionally, recent studies have demonstrated that some community strains of MRSA are becoming more resistant to non-beta-lactam antibiotic classes.[15]
- Historically, treatment for serious MRSA infections has been somewhat limited to agents such as vancomycin; however, newer agents are now available. Vancomycin is given intravenously, and blood levels, as well as renal function, need to be monitored while on therapy. Daptomycin is indicated for MRSA skin and soft tissue infections (at 4 mg/kg IV daily dose) and bacteremia, including right-sided endocarditis (at 6 mg/kg IV daily dose). Patients receiving daptomycin should be followed for the onset of muscle pain or weakness and have weekly creatine phosphokinase (CPK) levels measured. Tigecycline, another intravenous drug is also approved for treatment of complicated MRSA skin and skin structure infections at an initial dose of 100 mg, followed by 50 mg every 12 hours. Linezolid, which can be given orally, has clinical efficacy comparable to that of vancomycin for common infections, including skin and soft tissue infections, and may be associated with more favorable outcomes when used for treatment of MRSA nosocomial pneumonia.[16,17] Ceftaroline (600 mg IV every 12 hours) is also indicated for treatment of acute MRSA skin and skin structure infections. Trimethoprim-sulfamethoxazole, clindamycin, and tetracyclines may also have activity against MRSA, and these agents are used predominantly for outpatient management of skin and soft tissue infections.

S. aureus with Elevated MICs to Vancomycin, Vancomycin-Intermediate S. aureus, and Vancomycin-Resistant S. aureus

- *S. aureus* infections with MICs to vancomycin in the 1.5 to 2.0 μg/mL range present clinicians with treatment dilemmas. Studies have shown poorer outcomes for patients with these infections, mostly bacteremias[18,19]; however, it still remains unclear what treatment options are best. Guidelines would recommend treatment with an agent other than vancomycin (such as daptomycin, tigecycline, ceftaroline, or linezolid) and consultation with an expert in treating resistant organisms.[20]
- Vancomycin-intermediate *Staphylococcus aureus* (VISA) is defined as having an MIC toward vancomycin of 8 to 16 μg/mL. Infections have occurred primarily among those receiving long courses of vancomycin.[21] The mechanism of resistance has been described as due to cell wall thickening, which causes the large vancomycin molecule to become trapped and unable to reach its functional targets. Vancomycin-resistant *Staphylococcus aureus* (VRSA) is defined as having an MIC toward vancomycin of ≥64 μg/mL. The mechanism of resistance for this worrisome pathogen is acquisition of the *vanA* gene from vancomycin-resistant *Enterococcus* (VRE). Emergence of this organism has originated in areas where MRSA and VRE have coexisted. Fortunately, these VISA and VRSA strains have retained susceptibility to many alternative

antibiotic agents, but their mere existence highlights the importance of controlling their spread in health care facilities.[22]

ENTEROCOCCUS SPECIES

- Enterococci are facultative anaerobic organisms that grow at extreme temperatures and hydrolyze esculin in the presence of bile. They are resident normal flora of the gastrointestinal and genitourinary tract.
- *Enterococcus* is a common cause of nosocomial infections including CLABSI, endocarditis, wound infections, and catheter-associated urinary tract infections. Two species, *Enterococcus faecalis and Enterococcus faecium*, cause 90% of these infections.[23]
- Enterococci exhibit intrinsic resistance to many antibiotics traditionally used to treat gram-positive infections, particularly the cephalosporins. Also, *E. faecalis'* MIC toward ampicillin is 1 μg/mL, and its MIC toward penicillin and piperacillin is 2 μg/mL. Resistance to β-lactams results from reduced affinity of the PBP. Even if enterococci are initially susceptible to penicillins, if they are exposed to this class, they may develop tolerance.
- Acquired resistance toward the aminoglycosides (streptomycin and gentamicin) and toward the glycopeptide, vancomycin, is also of concern as these infections have limited treatment options.
- Enterococci become resistant to vancomycin by acquisition of vancomycin-resistance gene clusters, most commonly the vanA, vanB, or vanD genes. The product of these genes leads to the substitution of D-Ala-D-Ala-ending peptidoglycan precursors within the cell wall with D-alanyl-D-lactate termini. This altered terminus has markedly decreased affinity for binding with vancomycin, rendering the drug inactive.
- Similar to other antibiotic-resistant organisms, data from US hospitals suggest that the prevalence of VRE nosocomial infections has continued to increase over the past decade and now has surpassed 30% among ICU patients.[8]
- Like MRSA, emergence of VRE has resulted from overuse of broad-spectrum antibiotics and spread from patient to patient occurs almost always by contaminated hands and equipment of health care workers.
- Risk factors for VRE include serious underlying illness, prolonged stay in the hospital, receipt of broad-spectrum antibiotics, the presence of indwelling devices, and being in close proximity to another VRE colonized or infected patient.
- Compared to patients who develop infections due to susceptible enterococci, those who develop infection with VRE suffer increased morbidity (longer hospital stay, need for ICU care, more bacteremic days and need for surgery), mortality (increased two to threefold for those with BSI), and greater hospital costs.[24,25]
- Treatment of infections due to VRE is challenging because there are a limited number of agents available with activity against the organism and even fewer that have been studied in clinical trials.
- Quinupristin-dalfopristin has activity against *E. faecium*, but not most strains of *E. faecalis*. It also has a significant side effect profile and must be given through a central venous catheter. Linezolid has activity against VRE, but this drug is bacteriostatic and should be used with caution among patients with bacteremia or endocarditis (bactericidal therapy preferred). Linezolid is also associated with myelosuppression and thus may not be optimal for long-term therapy or for patient populations where this side effect is less tolerated (patients on chemotherapy). Daptomycin is

bactericidal against VRE and may be considered for invasive infections; however, there are no comparative clinical studies specifically directed toward its use against VRE. Tigecycline also has *in vitro* activity against VRE and has been studied among patients with complicated skin and soft tissue infections and intra-abdominal infections where VRE was isolated.

- Occasionally, ampicillin may have some activity against strains of VRE. For isolates with MICs to ampicillin ranging from 16 to 64 μg/mL, high doses of the drug may be used (24 g a day divided every 4 hours). For deep-seated infections or endocarditis, ampicillin in combination with gentamicin or streptomycin is recommended. Invasive disease due to ampicillin-resistant VRE should prompt consultation with an expert in treating these infections. Daptomycin or tigecycline may be considered, again often in combination with an aminoglycoside or other agent that has demonstrated susceptibility *in vitro*.

- Given these difficulties in treating VRE infections, every attempt should be made to remove unnecessary foreign bodies or drain areas of infection, as well as improving underlying host factors.

PREVENTION OF MRSA AND VRE

- Extensively referenced guidelines have been published regarding prevention and control of antibiotic-resistant organisms, such as MRSA and VRE. Generally, measures include reducing emergence of the organism by limiting unnecessary use of broad-spectrum agents through effective stewardship, reducing patient-to-patient spread by identifying the reservoir (surveillance culturing or screening) and utilizing measures that reduce contamination of the environment (disinfection, terminal cleaning, dedicated patient equipment) and contamination of the health care worker (hand hygiene, gowns, and gloves).[26,27]

- Additionally, health care–acquired infections can be effectively controlled by instituting best practices outlined in the prevention guidelines for CLABSI and ventilator-associated pneumonia.[28,29]

REFERENCES

1. Lee C, Banks SD, Li JP. Virulence, immunity and vaccine related *Streptococcus pneumoniae*. *Crit Rev Microbiol* 1991;18:89–114.
2. Ekdahl K, Ahlinder I, Hansson HB, et al. Duration of nasopharyngeal carriage of penicillin-resistant *Streptococcus pneumoniae*: experiences from South Swedish Pneumococcal Intervention Project. *Clin Infect Dis* 1997;25:1113–1117.
3. Whitney CG, Farley MM, Hadler J, et al. Decline in invasive pneumococcal disease after the introduction of protein-polysaccharide conjugate vaccine. *N Engl J Med* 2003;348:1737–1746.
4. Clinical and Laboratory Standards Institute. *Performance standards for antimicrobial susceptibility testing; eighteenth informational supplement. CLSI Document M100–S18.* Wayne, PA: CLSI; 2008.
5. Doern GV, Richter SS, Miller A, et al. Antimicrobial resistance among *Streptococcus pneumoniae* in the United States; have we begun to turn the corner on resistance to certain antimicrobial classes? *Clin Infect Dis* 2005;41:139–148.
6. Francis JS, Doherty MC, Lopatin U, et al. Severe community-onset pneumonia in healthy adults caused by methicillin-resistant *Staphylococcus aureus* carrying the Panton Valentine leukocidin genes. *Clin Infect Dis* 2005;40:100–107.

7. CLSI, *Surveillance for methicillin-resistant Staphylococcus aureus: principles, practices, and challenges; a report. CLSI document X07-R.* Wayne, PA: Clinical and Laboratory Standards Institute; 2010.

8. Hidron AI, Edwards JR, Patel J, et al. NHSN annual update: antimicrobial-resistant pathogens associated with healthcare-associated infections: annual summary of data reported to the National Healthcare Safety Network at the Centers for Disease Control and Prevention, 2006-2007. *Infect Control Hosp Epidemiol* 2008;29(11):996–1011.

9. Rosenthal VD, Maki DG, Jamulitrat S, et al. International Nosocomial Infection Control Consortium (INICC) report, data summary for 2003-2008, issued June 2009. *Am J Infect Control* 2010;38(2):95–104 e2.

10. Cosgrove SE, Sakoulas G, Perencevich EN, et al. Comparison of mortality associated with methicillin-resistant and methicillin-susceptible *Staphylococcus aureus* bacteremia: a meta-analysis. *Clin Infect Dis* 2003;36:53–59.

11. Engemann JJ, Carmeli Y, Cosgrove SE, et al. Adverse clinical and economic outcomes attributable to methicillin resistance among patients with *Staphylococcus aureus* surgical site infection. *Clin Infect Dis* 2003;36:592–598.

12. Klevens RM, Morrison, MA, Nadle J, et al. Invasive methicillin-resistant *Staphylococcus aureus* infections in the United States. *JAMA* 2007;298:1763–1771.

13. Moran GJ, Krishnadasan A, Gorwitz RJ, et al. Methicillin-resistant *S. Aureus* infections among patients in the emergency department. *N Engl J Med* 2006;355:666–674.

14. Freitas EA, Harris RM, Blake RK, et al. Prevalence of USA300 strain type of methicillin-resistant *Staphylococcus aureus* among patients with nasal colonization identified with active surveillance. *Infect Control Hosp Epidemiol* 2010;31(5):469–475.

15. McDougal LK, Fosheim GE, Nicholson A, et al. Emergence of resistance among USA300 methicillin-resistant *Staphylococcus aureus* isolates causing invasive disease in the United States. *Antimicrob Agents Chemother* 2010;54(9):3804–3811.

16. Sharpe JN, Shively EH, Polk HC Jr. Clinical and economic outcomes of oral linezolid versus intravenous vancomycin in the treatment of MRSA-complicated, lower-extremity skin and soft-tissue infections caused by methicillin-resistant *Staphylococcus aureus. Am J Surg* 2005;189(4):425–428.

17. Kollef MH, Rello J, Cammarata SK, et al. Clinical cure and survival in gram-positive ventilator-associated pneumonia: retrospective analysis of two double-blind studies comparing linezolid with vancomycin. *Intensive Care Med* 2004;30(3):388–394.

18. Van Hal SJ, Lodise TP, Paterson DL. The clinical significance of vancomycin minimum inhibitory concentration in *Staphylococcus aureus* infections: a systematic review and meta-analysis. *Clin Infect Dis* 2012;54:755–771.

19. Moore CL, Osaki-Kiyan P, Hague NZ, et al. Daptomycin versus vancomycin for bloodstream infections due to methicillin-resistant *Staphylococcus aureus* with a high vancomycin minimum inhibitory concentration: a case control study. *Clin Infect Dis* 2010;54: 51–58.

20. Liu C, Bayer A, Cosgrove SE, et al. Clinical practice guidelines by the infectious diseases society of America for the treatment of methicillin-resistant *Staphylococcus aureus* infections in adults and children: executive summary. *Clin Infect Dis* 2011;52:285–292.

21. Rice LB. Antimicrobial resistance in gram-positive bacteria. *Am J Med* 2006;119:S11–S19.

22. Sievert DM, Rudrik JT, Patel JB, et al. Vancomycin-resistant *Staphylococcus aureus* in the United States, 2002-2006. *Clin Infect Dis* 2008;46:668–674.

23. Murray BE. Vancomycin-resistant enterococcal infections. *N Engl J Med* 2000;342: 710–721.

24. Carmeli Y, et al. Health and economic outcomes of vancomycin-resistant enterococci. *Arch Intern Med* 2002;162:2223–2238.

25. Salgado CD, Farr BM. Outcomes associated with vancomycin-resistant enterococci: a meta-analysis. *Infect Control Hosp Epidemiol* 2003;24:690–698.

26. Siegel JD, Rhinehart E, Jackson M, et al; Healthcare Infection Control Practices Advisory Committee. Management of multidrug-resistant organisms in healthcare setting 2006. *Am J Infect Control* 2007;35(10 suppl 2):S165–S193.

27. Calfee DP, Salgado CD, Classen D, et al. Strategies to prevent transmission of methicillin—resistant *Staphylococcus aureus* in acute care hospitals. *Infect Control Hosp Epidemiol* 2008;29(S1):S62–S80.

28. Marschall J, Mermel LA, Classen D, et al. Strategies to prevent central line–associated bloodstream infections in acute care hospitals. *Infect Control Hosp Epidemiol* 2008;29(S1): S22–S30.

29. Coffin SE, Klompas M, Classen D, et al. Strategies to prevent ventilator—associated pneumonia in acute care hospitals. *Infect Control Hosp Epidemiol* 2008;29(S1):S31–S40.

38 Multidrug-Resistant Gram-Negative Bacteria

Ramzy H. Rimawi and Paul Cook

INTRODUCTION

Health care–associated infections are the leading cause of mortality in acute care hospitals, with over 50% of them due to infections caused by multidrug-resistant (MDR) bacteria. These resistant pathogens result in a number of disturbing sequelae including increased morbidity, increased mortality, prolonged hospitalizations, and increased medical cost. Common nosocomial gram-negative organisms (e.g., *Pseudomonas aeruginosa, Klebsiella pneumoniae, Acinetobacter baumannii*, and *Enterobacter* species) are adept at acquiring genes that confer resistance to a variety of classes of antimicrobial agents. Moreover, there has been a dramatic decline in the discovery and development of antimicrobial agents active against gram-negative microorganisms in the past two decades. We are now in the presence of gram-negative bacilli (GNB) that are resistant not only to first-line antimicrobials (amikacin, tobramycin, cefepime, ceftazidime, imipenem, meropenem, piperacillin-tazobactam, ciprofloxacin, moxifloxacin, and levofloxacin) but also to second-line agents such as tigecycline and polymyxins.[1,2]

EPIDEMIOLOGY

The Infectious Diseases Society of America has identified six top-priority perilous pathogens for which there are few effective drugs surfacing in the near future. These pathogens are termed ESKAPE (extended-spectrum beta-lactamase [ESBL]-producing Enterobacteriaceae, methicillin-resistant *Staphylococcus aureus*, *K. pneumoniae*, *A. baumannii*, *P. aeruginosa*, and vancomycin-resistant *Enterococcus faecium*), four of which are GNB.

The principle cause of antimicrobial resistance is inappropriate antimicrobial use, though other factors play a part as well, including population demographics, patient compliance, comorbidities, poor infection control, increased travel, and alcohol and drug abuse. Doctors prescribe over 133 million courses of antibiotics in an outpatient setting and over 190 million courses in a hospital setting.[3] Risk factors for developing MDR GNB include age over 65 years, hospitalization in the preceding 90 days, recent antibiotic use, residence in a nursing home or long-term treatment facility, fecal incontinence, chronic indwelling catheter or feeding tube, mechanic ventilation, and/or long-term hemodialysis.[4]

COMMON MICROORGANISMS AND MECHANISMS OF RESISTANCE

Table 38-1 demonstrates the four major types of MDR GNB resistance mechanisms: (1) production of enzymes that destroy the integrity of the antibiotic (e.g., ESBL-producing and carbapenemase-producing Enterobacteriaceae), (2) mutations in the

| Table 38-1 | Multidrug-Resistant Gram-Negative Bacilli Resistance Mechanisms |

Organism	Mechanism of Resistance					
	ESBL/ Metallo-β- lactamase	OMP Changes	AME	Efflux Pumps	Porin Channels	Membrane Changes to Polymyxin
Enterobacteria- ceae	+	−	−	−	−	−
P.aeruginosa	+	+	+	+	+	−
Acinetobacter spp.	+	+	+	+	+	+
Stenotrophamo- nas malto- philia	+	+	+	+	+	−

ESBL, extended-spectrum β-lactamases; OMP, outer membrane protein; AME, aminoglycoside-modifying enzymes.
Enterobacteriaceae includes *Citrobacter, Enterobacter, E. Coli, Klebsiella* and *Serratia*.

antimicrobial binding site (e.g., DNA gyrase and topoisomerase mutations causing resistance to fluoroquinolones), (3) down-regulation of outer membrane proteins (e.g., imipenem-resistant *P. aeruginosa*), and (4) efflux pumps that efficiently remove an antibiotic from the cell.

ESBL enzymes are perhaps the most common clinically significant mechanism of resistance demonstrated by all gram-negative bacteria. ESBLs are beta-lactamases that are able to hydrolyze the penicillins, cephalosporins, and monobactams but not the cephamycins or carbapenems. The plasmids carrying the ESBLs frequently also carry resistant genes for other antimicrobial agents, so that resistance to fluroquinolones and aminoglycosides frequently coexist with resistance to penicillins and cephalosporins. Suspicion for ESBLs should be high in elderly patients with comorbid conditions, recent hospitalization(s), invasive devices, and/or recent use of broad-spectrum antibiotics (quinolones, cephalosporins).[5] Carbapenemases are the beta-lactamases with the broadest gamut of activity. The plasmid-borne *Klebsiella pneumoniae* carbapenemases (KPCs) are among the most widely recognized and prevalent. The recommended method for detecting carbapenemases is the modified Hodge test, which is labor intensive and requires an additional day to perform, making the detection of carbapenemases rather difficult. The Clinical and Laboratory Standards Institute (CLSI) has recently lowered the breakpoints that define susceptibility of Enterobacteriaceae in an effort to improve the screening process for detection of carbapenemases. The recent discovery of the New Dehli metallo-beta-lactamase (NDM-1) in Enterobacteriaceae is concerning as this class of beta-lactamase confers resistance to all beta-lactam drugs, including carbapenems. NDM-1 is transmitted on plasmids that frequently cotransmit resistance genes to fluoroquinolones and aminoglycosides. Other metallo-beta-lactamases are prevalent in *P. aeruginosa, A. baumannii,* and *Stenotrophomonas maltophilia* (Table 38-1).

Following *S. aureus, P. aeruginosa* is the second most frequent cause of infectious health care–associated pneumonia and skin and soft tissue infections. *Pseudomonas* exhibits additional resistance mechanisms, including aminoglycoside-modifying enzymes, efflux pumps, porin loss, and metallo-beta-lactamases (primarily VIM-2)

(Table 38-1). A porin is the outer membrane channel through which an antibiotic must pass in order to gain entry into the organism. Loss or changes of these porins in conjunction with efflux pumps allows for antibiotic resistance. For example, the loss of 54-kD outer membrane protein, known as OprD, is the most common mechanism of imipenem resistance in *P. aeruginosa*.[6]

Acinetobacter is a gram-negative coccobacillus of the family Moraxellaceae. The most common species is *A. baumannii*, which has been a common wound isolate in military personnel returning from the Middle East. The organism has become increasingly resistant to nearly all antimicrobial therapies via multiple resistance mechanisms similar to those of *P. aeruginosa*. Like *P. aeruginosa*, *A. baumannii* is primarily a nosocomial pathogen causing ventilator-associated pneumonia, as well as infections of central lines, the urinary tract, and surgical wounds.

TREATMENT

Empiric therapy for suspected MDR gram-negative infections should include broad-spectrum agent(s) that cover(s) the suspected organisms[7] (Table 38-2). Universal antimicrobial recommendations are of limited value. Rather, individual institutional and unit-specific antibiograms are crucial factors in determining appropriate empiric therapy. For example, if your hospital has a low incidence of infections with ESBLs or KPCs, there may be no reason to use carbapenems or polymyxins, respectively, as first-line therapy while awaiting culture and susceptibility results. On the other hand, if the patient has come from a long-term care facility that is experiencing an outbreak of MDR Acinetobacter infections, then empiric therapy needs to include polymyxins and/or tigecycline, depending on local antibiograms.

Empiric therapy in suspected or proven *Pseudomonas* species infections with an antipseudomonal carbapenem (doripenem, meropenem, or imipenem) or piperacillin-tazobactam plus either tobramycin or ciprofloxacin is recommended pending final culture and susceptibility results. Again, unit-specific and/or institutional antibiograms should guide choices of drugs for combination therapy. For example, if more *Pseudomonas* are susceptible to tobramycin than to ciprofloxacin on your hospital's antibiogram, then tobramycin should be the empiric combination drug of choice. Once the susceptibilities are available, monotherapy is adequate in most cases.

The increase in rates of carbapenem-resistant *P. aeruginosa* and *A. baumannii* has led to the resurgence in the use of polymyxins, which had fallen out of favor due to

Table 38-2	Empirical Multidrug-Resistant Gram-Negative Bacteria Suggested Antimicrobial Approach	
Infection Type	**First-Line Therapy**	**Second-Line Therapy**
Monomicro-bial	Carbapenem Tigecycline +/– antipseudomonal agent	Piperacillin-tazobactam Colistin
Polymicrobial	Anti-MRSA agent + Carbapenem Tigecycline +/– antipseudomonal agent	Anti-MRSA agent + Piperacillin-tazobactam Anti-MRSA agent + Colistin

Table 38-3	Suggested Directed Therapy for Multidrug-Resistant Gram-Negative Bacteria	

Organism	Recommended Therapy	Other Recommendations
ESBL-producing Enterobacteriaceae	Doripenem 500 mg IV q 8 hours; meropenem 1 g IV q 8 hours; or imipenem 1 g IV q 8 hours	Extended infusions of carbapenems over 4 hours to maximize time above MIC. Adjust dose for renal insufficiency.
Carbapenemase-producing Enterobacteriaceae	Tigecycline 100 mg IV loading dose followed by 50 mg IV q 12 hours Colistin 1.25–2.5 mg/kg IV q 12 hours	For pneumonia: Nebulized colistimethate sodium, 1 million to 3 million IU/day in divided doses (diluted in sterile normal saline), administered with a conventional nebulizer; or nebulized aminoglycosides
Carbapenem-resistant A. baumannii	Colistin 1.25–2.5 mg/kg IV q 12 hours or tigecycline, 100 mg given intravenously as a loading dose, then 50 mg given intravenously every 12 hours	For pneumonia: Nebulized colistimethate sodium, 1 million to 3 million IU/day in divided doses (diluted in sterile normal saline), administered with a conventional nebulizer; or nebulized aminoglycosides
Carbapenem-resistant P. aeruginosa	Colistin 1.25–2.5 mg/kg IV q 12 hours	For pneumonia: Nebulized colistimethate sodium, 1 million to 3 million IU/day in divided doses (diluted in sterile normal saline), administered with a conventional nebulizer; or nebulized aminoglycosides

ESBL, extended-spectrum β-lactamases; MRSA, methicillin-resistant *Staphylococcus aureus*; MDR, multidrug resistant.

their adverse effects, mainly nephrotoxicity. These drugs have been used both intravenously and as nebulizer therapy for patients with ventilator-associated pneumonia (Tables 38-2 and 38-3). Treatment of MDR gram-negative infections frequently involves use of extended infusion of drugs such as piperacillin-tazobactam and doripenem to maximize the time of drug above the minimal inhibitory concentration (MIC) for the organism (Tables 38-2 and 38-3). Dosing of drugs such as aminoglycosides, on the other hand, are frequently dosed once daily to maximize the concentration-dependent killing of this class of drugs.

Many options exist to help tackle the tribulations of gram-negative bacterial resistance. Limiting the spread and impact of antimicrobial resistance requires a multifaceted approach, including infection control and antimicrobial stewardship. Antibiotic use can be effectively controlled through reliance on clinical scoring tools, adherence to evidence-based national and international treatment guidelines and/or pharmacy controlled monitoring. Though some antimicrobial drugs are currently in phase 1 and phase 2 trials, it will be several years before new agents are available for clinical use.

REFERENCES

1. Kollef MH, Golan Y, Micek ST, et al. Appraising contemporary strategies to combat multidrug resistant gram-negative bacterial infections-proceedings and data from the gram-negative resistance summit. *Clin Infect Dis* 2011:53(suppl 2):S33–S55.
2. Lee JH, Jeong SH, Cha SS, et al. New disturbing trend in antimicrobial resistance of gram-negative pathogens. *PLoS Pathog* 2009;5(3): e1000221.
3. Engel LS. The dilemma of multidrug-resistant gram-negative bacteria. *Am J Med Sci* 2010:340(3):232–237.
4. Kasper DL, Fauci AS. *Harrison's Infectious Diseases*. New York: McGraw-Hill Medical; 2010:188–200.
5. Bonomo R, Szabo D. Mechanisms of multidrug resistance in *Acinetobacter* Species and *Pseudomonas aeruginosa*. *Clin Infect Dis* 2006;43:S49–S56.
6. Nicasio A, Kuti J, Nicolau D. The current state of multidrug-resistant gram negative bacilli in North America: common mechanisms of resistance within gram negative bacilli. *Pharmacotherapy* 2008;20(2):235–249.
7. Kanj SS, Kanafani ZA. Current concepts in antimicrobial therapy against resistant gram-negative organisms: extended-spectrum β-lactamase-producing Enterobacteriaceae, Carbapenem-Resistant Enterobacteriaceae, and multidrug-resistant *Pseudomonas aeruginosa*. *Mayo Clin Proc* 2011;86(3):250–259.

39 Candidemia

Keith W. Hamilton and Ebbing Lautenbach

INTRODUCTION

- The incidence of invasive fungal infections has increased as an unintended consequence of increased use of immunosuppression to treat certain medical conditions and the improved ability of medical technology to treat critically ill patients.
- *Candida* species are the most common cause of health care–acquired invasive fungal infections and represent 5% to 10% of all central line–associated bloodstream infections (CLABSIs).
- A blood culture positive for yeast should never be considered a contaminant and should be treated promptly with appropriate empiric antifungal therapy.
- Delayed treatment has been associated with increased morbidity and mortality.
- Possible sources of candidemia and presence of complications and focal organ involvement should also be investigated as these factors will impact the type and duration of therapy.
- In critically ill patients, the most common sources of infection are indwelling catheters and gastrointestinal pathology.
- Risk factors associated with candidemia include (i) presence of a central venous catheter, (ii) total parenteral nutrition, (iii) recent gastrointestinal surgery or perforation, (iv) receipt of broad-spectrum antibiotics, (v) acute renal failure, (vi) receipt of hemodialysis, (vii) mechanical ventilation, (viii) ICU admission, (ix) older age, (x) number of red blood cell transfusions, (xi) immunosuppression (including neutropenia), (xii) known fungal colonization, and (xiii) increased severity of illness.
- Despite developments in the diagnosis and treatment of candidemia, mortality rates remain substantial, with an overall mortality of 30% to over 50% and attributable mortality of 19% to 38%.

CLINICAL PRESENTATION

- Clinical manifestations of candidemia are variable and depend on host immune factors and the extent of infection. Symptoms range from a low-grade fever to sepsis. Skin lesions may also occur and often appear as small pustules or nodules with surrounding erythema, but appearance can be variable, and patients may even develop large, necrotic lesions.
- Candidemia can also be associated with metastatic foci of infection through hematogenous seeding. Commonly involved sites include heart valves, spleen, liver, central nervous system, joints, and bones.
- Candidemia can also result in endovascular seeding of the highly vascular choroid plexus in the eye, causing chorioretinitis or endophthalmitis. The possibility of *Candida* chorioretinitis should be evaluated in all patients with candidemia regardless of symptoms because many patients lack visual symptoms early in the course of illness.

Failure to identify *Candida* chorioretinitis may result in loss of vision due to inappropriate or inadequate duration of treatment, which should be a minimum of 4 to 6 weeks.

DIAGNOSIS

- Blood cultures have been the standard diagnostic tool for candidemia, but the sensitivity of traditional blood culture methods has been only about 50%. However, newer automated culture modalities likely have significantly better performance characteristics.
- Fungal culture and direct microscopic examination of a biopsy or drainage sample from possible focal sources of infection, including skin lesions and abscesses, provide important additive diagnostic ability.
- Growth in specialized chromogenic media can expedite identification of certain *Candida* species.
- More rapid identification methodologies, such as the antigen-based assay β-D-glucan, have been used as an adjunct for diagnosis in some invasive fungal infections.
- The β-D-glucan test detects a cell wall antigen present in most fungi. However, its presence in multiple types of fungi also makes the test less specific for use in the diagnosis of candidemia. Pooled sensitivity and specificity for all invasive fungal infections are 76.8% and 85.3%, respectively. The β-D-glucan test should be approached with the caveat that it cannot distinguish *Candida* infections from those caused by other fungi. Identification and isolation of the particular organism by other means is still necessary to make a definitive diagnosis and to tailor appropriate therapy.
- Consultation with an institution's clinical microbiology department or an expert in the diagnosis and management of patients with fungal disease should be initiated to discuss performance characteristics of diagnostic tests available at the institution and to aid in the interpretation of the results. These individuals are also knowledgeable of institutional protocols to optimize chances of isolating *Candida* species.
- Historically, *Candida albicans* was the most common species involved in nosocomial candidemia, but over the past decade, there has been a progressive shift toward non-albicans *Candida* species. These non-albicans species now outnumber *C. albicans* in many health care institutions. This increase is generally thought to be the consequence of increased use of broader-spectrum antifungal agents.
- Identification of the species responsible for infection is important, as each species has a different antifungal susceptibility pattern (Table 39-1). Within their own institutions, clinicians should be aware of the most common species of *Candida* and the susceptibility profiles.

MANAGEMENT

- The selection of empiric therapy for any patient with candidemia, pending identification of the species, should take into consideration the severity of illness, comorbidities, previous history of *Candida* infection, exposure to or intolerance to certain antifungal agents, and available susceptibility reports. Consultation with an expert familiar with the management of patients with serious fungal infections is advised.
- Candidemia in the neutropenic patient has been associated with a higher incidence of multifocal disease, higher rates of sepsis, multiorgan system failure and death.
- Recommendations for the treatment of candidemia in both the neutropenic and nonneutropenic host have been published by the Infectious Diseases Society of America and are presented in Table 39-2.

Table 39-1	Common *Candida* Species Susceptibility Patterns

	Candida albicans	Candida glabrata	Candida parapsilosis	Candida tropicalis	Candida krusei	Candida lusitaniae
Fluconazole	S	S-DD to R	S	S	R	S
Voriconazole	S	S-DD to R	S	S	S	S
Posaconazole	S	S-DD to R	S	S	S	S
Echinocandins	S	S	S to R	S	S	S
Amphotericin B products	S	S-DD to I	S to R	S	S to I	S to R

S, susceptible; S-DD, susceptible dose-dependent; I, intermediately susceptible; R, resistant.

Table 39-2	Summary of Treatment Recommendations for Candidemia

	Primary	Alternative	Comments
Nonneutropenic patients	Fluconazole 800 mg loading dose, then 400 mg daily; or an echinocandin	LFAmB 3–5 mg/kg daily; or voriconazole 400 mg b.i.d. for two doses, then 200 mg b.i.d.	Choose an echino-candin for moder-ate to severe illness and for patients with recent azole exposure. Transi-tion to fluconazole after initial echino-candin is appropri-ate in many cases.
Neutropenic patients	An echinocandin or LFAmB 3–5 mg/kg daily	Fluconazole 800 mg load-ing dose, then 400 mg daily; or voriconazole 400 mg b.i.d. for two doses, then 200 mg b.i.d.	An echinocandin or LFAmB is preferred for most patients. Fluconazole is recommended for patients without recent exposure to azoles and who are not critically ill. Voriconazole is rec-ommended when additional coverage for molds is desired.

Echinocandin dosing in adults is as follows: anidulafungin, 200 mg loading dose, then 100 mg daily; caspofungin, 70 mg loading dose, then 50 mg daily, and micafungin, 100 mg daily.

For patients with endocarditis or other cardiovascular infections, higher daily doses of an echinocan-din may be appropriate.

LFAmB, lipid formulation of amphotericin B.

Adapted from Clinical practice guidelines for the management of candidiasis: 2009 update by the Infectious Diseases Society of America. *Clin Infect Dis* 2009;48:503–535, Table 2.

- Due to the increasing prevalence of *Candida glabrata* resistance toward fluconazole, the preferred empiric agent for this species in many institutions is an echinocandin.
- Fluconazole should not be used for empiric therapy against *C. glabrata* or other species with high endemic rates of resistance unless the isolate is confirmed to be susceptible.
- If possible, for all cases of candidemia, metastatic foci should be drained or debrided and gastrointestinal pathology should be repaired.
- Prompt removal of existing central venous catheters is paramount, as failure to do so results in prolonged illness and higher mortality rates.
- The duration of therapy for uncomplicated candidemia has not been well studied, but experts suggest a minimum of 2 weeks of appropriate antifungal therapy from the day of documented clearance of blood cultures and resolution of symptoms.
- Longer durations of 4 to 6 weeks should be used if blood cultures are persistently positive, if there have been metastatic foci identified, if there are persistent abscesses, if there is focal involvement of deep tissues or organs, or if there is an endovascular focus such as endocarditis. Surgical intervention often plays a critical role in effectively treating these complications of candidemia.
- When clusters of candidemia develop in a hospital or an area of a hospital, cross-contamination from health care workers should be considered. Some outbreaks have also been linked to clonal isolates of various *Candida* species, indicating a common source or horizontal transmission.
- Any increase in candidemia rates in a hospital can be a sign of general lapses in infection control measures, and appropriate consultation with the Infection Prevention and Control Department is encouraged to ensure that infection control procedures, including line care, hand hygiene, and universal precautions, are reinforced.
- Antifungal prophylaxis has been considered for use in certain high-risk patients in order to decrease rates of candidemia, but on the basis of current evidence, there are no data to support routine use of this practice in the immunocompetent host, except in certain compelling situations such as necrotizing pancreatitis or gastrointestinal perforation.

SUGGESTED READINGS

Blumberg HM, Jarvis WR, Soucie JM, et al. Risk factors for candidal bloodstream infections in surgical intensive care unit patients: the NEMIS prospective multicenter study. The national epidemiology of mycosis survey. *Clin Infect Dis* 2001;33:177–186.

Chow JK, Golan Y, Ruthazer R, et al. Risk factors for albicans and non-albicans candidemia in the intensive care unit. *Crit Care Med* 2008;36:1993–1998.

Falagas ME, Roussos N, Vardakas KZ. Relative frequency of albicansand the various non-albicans *Candida spp* among candidemia isolates from inpatients in various parts of the world: a systematic review. *Int J Infect Dis* 2010;14:e954–e966.

Garey KW, Rege M, Pai MP, et al. Time to initiation of fluconazole therapy impacts mortality in patients with candidemia: a multi-institutional study. *Clin Infect Dis* 2006;43:25–31.

Hernández-Castro R, Arroyo-Escalante S, Carrillo-Casas EM, et al. Outbreak of *Candida parapsilosis* in a neonatal intensive care unit: a health care workers source. *Eur J Pediatr* 2010;169:783–787.

Karageorgopoulos DE, Vouloumanou EK, Ntziora F, et al. β-D-glucan assay for the diagnosis of invasive fungal infections: a meta-analysis. *Clin Infect Dis* 2011;52:750–770.

Kuhn DM, Mikherjee PK, Clark TA, et al. *Candida parapsilosis* characterization in an outbreak setting. *Emerg Infect Dis* 2004;1074–1081.

Méan M, Marchetti O, Calandra T. Bench-to-bedside review: *Candida* infections in the intensive care unit. *Crit Care* 2008;12:204.

Montagna MT, Caggiano G, Borghi E, et al. The role of the laboratory in the diagnosis of invasive candidiasis. *Drugs* 2009;69(Suppl 1):59–63.

Morgan J, Meltzer MI, Plikaytis BD, et al. Excess mortality, hospital stay, and cost due to candidemia: a case-control study using data from population-based candidemia surveillance. *Infect Control Hosp Epidemiol* 2005;26:540–547.

Ortega M, Marco F, Soriano A, et al. Candida species bloodstream infection: epidemiology and outcome in a single institution fro 1991 to 2008. *J Hosp Infect* 2011;77:157–161.

Pappas PG, Kauffman CA, Andes D, et al. Clinical practice guidelines for the management of candidiasis: 2009 update by the Infectious Diseases Society of America. *Clin Infect Dis* 2009;48:503–535.

Playford EG, Lipman J, Sorrell TC, et al. Prophylaxis, empirical and preemptive treatment of invasive candidiasis. *Curr Opin Crit Care* 2010;16:470–474.

Wisplinghoff H, Bischoff T, Tallent SM, et al. Nosocomial bloodstream infections in US hospitals: analysis of 24,179 cases from a prospective nationwide surveillance study. *Clin Infect Dis* 2004;39:309–317.

Scabies

Stephan Albrecht and Helmut Albrecht

Scabies (ICD-9 133.0) from Latin scabere, "to scratch," is a disease caused by infestation with the mite *Sarcoptes scabiei* variety hominis (Fig.40-1) resulting in a characteristic and intensely pruritic skin eruption. Adult scabies mites are whitish-brown microscopic parasites with eight legs that belong to the phylogenetic class Arachnida, as do spiders and ticks. Related mite species cause mange in animals.

The mite is an obligate human parasite that completes its entire life cycle on humans. Larvae emerge 2 to 5 days after eggs are laid, and maturation, which involves molting into nymphal stages, takes approximately 2 weeks. Only female mites burrow into the skin, and they survive 3 to 4 weeks on humans, which is longer than their smaller male counterparts. Classical scabies is usually associated with infestation of 5 to 15 female mites, but the number can reach thousands or even millions in cases of crusted scabies.

EPIDEMIOLOGY/TRANSMISSION

The worldwide prevalence has been estimated at about 300 million cases annually.[1] Mites cannot fly or jump, but crawl at the rate of 2.5 cm/min on warm skin. Transmission of scabies therefore usually requires spread via direct contact from person to person. Transmission from parents to children, and especially from mother to infant, is common. In adolescents, infection is often associated with sexual encounters. Institutional transmission from patient to patient or patient to caregiver is common. Spread via fomites (bedding, clothing) is less frequent, but well documented and is facilitated by the fact that mites can survive off a host for 24 to 36 hours at room temperature and average humidity, but longer in colder, more humid conditions. Probability of transmission is determined by parasite density and the duration of close contact.

CLINICAL COURSE

The skin eruption of classic scabies is considered a consequence of both infestation and a type IV hypersensitivity reaction to the mite. The prominent clinical feature of scabies is itching. It is often severe and usually worse at night. Incubation period between infection and development of symptoms is 3 to 6 weeks for primary infestation, but may be as short as 1 to 3 days in cases of reinfestation. Scabies is generally a nuisance on account of itching, rash, and its ability to spread among people, but bacterial superinfection or severe infestation may occur. The risk of severe outbreaks and complicated scabies is particularly high in institutions (including nursing homes and hospitals) and among socially disadvantaged populations and immunocompromised hosts.

The initial lesion is a small, nondescript erythematous papule, which is often excoriated through manipulation by the patient before presentation. Not always present, but essentially pathognomonic is the burrow, a thin, grayish, reddish, or brownish line that is 2 to 15 mm long. Burrowing is facilitated by secretion of proteolytic enzymes, which can trigger allergic reactions. Allergic miniature wheals, vesicles, pustules, and rarely urticaria or bullae may also be present. All of these are more common in recurrent infection.

Predilection sites for scabies include the sides and webs of the fingers, the flexor aspects of the wrists, elbows, axilla, breast, the periumbilical areas, waist, male genitalia, the lower buttocks and upper thighs, the extensor surface of the knees, and the lateral and posterior aspects of the feet. Head and back are usually spared except in very young children or in crusted scabies. Nonspecific secondary lesions, including eczematization and impetiginization, may occur.

CRUSTED SCABIES

Patients with an impaired immune system, such as patients with HIV, with cancer, or on immunosuppressive medications may develop widespread infestation, usually referred to as crusted scabies (formerly "Norwegian scabies"). Affected patients experience only mild itching, but exhibit thick crusts of skin that contain thousands of mites resulting in high infectivity.

DIAGNOSIS

The diagnosis of scabies is generally made from the history and the distribution of lesions. Scabies should be suspected in patients with

Widespread itching sparing the head (except in infants and young children), which is worse at night and out of proportion to the visible changes in the skin
Pruritic papular lesions with typical distribution
Other household members with similar symptoms

Definitive diagnosis relies on the identification of mites, eggs, eggshell fragments, or mite pellets in skin scrapings or biopsy specimens or invivo, using dermoscopy. For skin scrapings, multiple superficial skin samples should be obtained from characteristic lesions—specifically, burrows or papules and vesicles in vicinity of burrows—by scraping laterally across the skin with a blade without causing bleeding. Alternatively, adhesive tape can be applied to a skin lesion and pulled off. Obtained specimens can be examined with a light microscope under low power. Since the number of mites is low in cases of classic scabies, failure to find mites is common and does not rule out scabies. When direct examination is not possible, a skin biopsy may confirm the diagnosis. However, mites or other diagnostic findings are frequently absent, and the histologic examination shows a nonspecific, delayed hypersensitivity reaction, requiring clinical correlation.

DIFFERENTIAL DIAGNOSIS

The differential diagnosis is broad and includes eczema, tinea, atopic dermatitis, Langerhans cell histiocytosis, systemic or cutaneous lupus, syphilis, various urticaria-related syndromes, allergic reactions, other ectoparasites such as lice and fleas, bullous pemphigoid, papular urticaria, seborrheic dermatitis, and acropustulosis of infancy.

TREATMENT

Despite the relatively low sensitivity of diagnostic testing, empirical treatment is not recommended for patients with generalized pruritus, but should be reserved for patients with a history of exposure, a typical eruption, or both. Infested persons and their close physical contacts should be treated at the same time, regardless of whether symptoms are present. Topical or oral products may be used, although there are few rigorous studies to guide their use. Patients should be advised that itching can persist for up to 4 weeks after the end of correctly administered and successful scabicide therapy. Symptomatic treatment includes antihistamines for the, at times, intense prurigo.

Permethrin

Topical permethrin (5%) is highly effective for the treatment of classical scabies. It is applied from the neck down to the bottom of the feet, including areas under the fingernails and toenails, usually before bedtime and left on for about 8 to 14 hours, then showered off in the morning. The hairline, neck, temples, and forehead may be infested in infants and geriatric patients. In such patients, permethrin should also be applied to the scalp and face, sparing the eyes and mouth. One application of around 30 g is sufficient for mild infections but moderate to severe cases may require another application 1 to 2 weeks later. There are other cheaper topical products including lindane, benzyl benzoate, crotamiton, malathion, and sulfur preparations, but permethrin is considered the standard of care because of its unparalleled efficacy and excellent tolerability, with side effects being rare except for a generally mild irritation of the skin. Five percent cream appears to be safe and effective even when applied to infants <1 month of age with neonatal scabies, and it is classified as category B for use in pregnancy.

Ivermectin

Ivermectin is an oral medication shown by many clinical studies to be effective in eradicating scabies, often in a single dose of 0.2 mg/kg. Human tablets are available at 3 mg and are significantly more costly than veterinary preparations. Ivermectin is thought to interrupt glutamate-induced and γ-aminobutyric acid–induced neurotransmission in parasites causing paralysis and death. In one randomized trial compared with an overnight application of 5% permethrin, a single dose of ivermectin cured 70% of patients, as compared with a 98% cure rate with permethrin ($p < 0.003$), but a second ivermectin dose taken 2 weeks later increased the cure rate to 95%.[2] The lower efficacy of single-dose ivermectin was thought to be due the lack of an ovicidal action of the drug. Randomized trials and clinical experience have suggested that ivermectin is safe. Encephalopathy has rarely been reported in patients who are treated with repeated dosing of ivermectin. The CDC recommends not using ivermectin in pregnant or lactating women and states that safety has not been determined in children who weigh <15 kg.[3]

Crusted Scabies

Topical 5% permethrin applied daily for 7 days, then twice weekly until cure and oral ivermectin (0.2 mg/kg/dose) given on days 1, 2, 8, 9, and 15 is recommended by the CDC.[3] Patients with severe infestations may require even longer courses of oral ivermectin, with two additional doses given after 3 and 4 weeks.

PREVENTION

There is no preventative vaccine. Because scabies is transmitted by close or skin-to-skin contact, usual recommendations are that all members of the family and close contacts be treated at the same time to avoid an endless chain of cross contamination and reinfestation.

As mites can survive in the environment for only a few days, options for items used within several days before treatment (clothing, bedding, stuffed animals, etc.) include placing in a plastic bag for at least 3 days, machine washing with hot water and then ironing or drying in a hot dryer, or dry cleaning. Fumigation is not indicated. Affected individuals can return to work, child care, or school the day after treatment.

Patients with crusted scabies, however, should be isolated immediately and strict barrier procedures instituted if transmission to others is to be avoided. Serious institutional epidemics of scabies have resulted from failure to recognize the disease and take proper precautions. Rooms previously used by patients with crusted scabies should be vacuumed and cleaned thoroughly and bedding should be washed and dried utilizing high heat cycles.

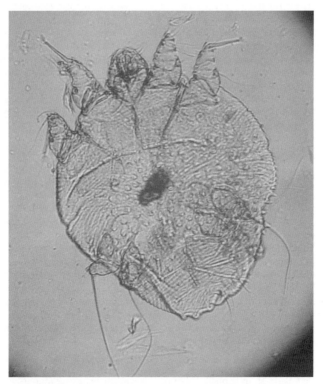

Figure 40-1. Adult *Sarcoptes scabiei*. (From http://upload.wikimedia.org/wikipedia/commons/c/c0/Sarcoptes_scabei_2.jpg?uselang=de; For public use including for publication. For details, see http://en.wikipedia.org/wiki/File:Sarcoptes_scabei_2.jpg)

REFERENCES

1. Chosidow O. Clinical practice: scabies. *N Engl J Med* 2006;354:1718–1727.
2. Usha V, Gopalakrishnan Nair TV. A comparative study of oral ivermectin and topical permethrin cream in the treatment of scabies. *J Am Acad Dermatol* 2000;42:236–40
3. Workowski KA, Berman S; Centers for Disease Control and Prevention. Sexually transmitted diseases treatment guidelines, 2010. *MMWR Recomm Rep* 2010;59(RR-12):1–110.

IX Zoonoses

Animal Bites

Paras Patel and James W. Myers

INTRODUCTION

- Animal bites account for 1% of all visits to emergency rooms in the United States.
- Two to five million animal bites occur every year.
- More than 1 million victims of animal bites visit their physician at a total cost of approximately $30 million per year.
- Animal bites result in 10 to 20 deaths every year in the United States, mainly among infants and small children.

EPIDEMIOLOGY

Dog bites account *for 85% to 90% of all animal bites*, with the remainder caused by cats (5% to 10%), rodents (2% to 3%), and rarely, other animals such as monkeys, ferrets, raccoons, foxes, livestock, bats, minks, kinkajous, and other wild animals.

- Animal bites involving joints or bones are more likely to get complicated by septic arthritis, tenosynovitis, or local abscesses.
- Bites to the hand require careful radiographic and surgical evaluation if a puncture or a severe laceration has been noticed.
- *Most casualties from animal bites are due to dog bites.*
- Note that human bites and cat bites account for the majority of infected wounds by clinicians.

INITIAL EVALUATION AND MANAGEMENT OF BITE WOUNDS

- Initial steps include the use of ice, elevation, and control of any bleeding.
- Washing the wound with soap and water as soon as possible will help decrease the risk of rabies infection if done within 3 hours.
- Note the circumstances of the bite attack, focusing on the behavior of the biting animal and whether the animal is in captivity and has been immunized against rabies.
- Assess tetanus immunization status and allergies to antibiotics.
- Provide good wound care in the form of adequate irrigation and debridement of nonviable tissue as needed.
- General wound management measures such as rabies vaccine, tetanus toxoid administration, and wound closure should also be employed (see Table 41-1).
- Specific inquiry should be made about risks for poor wound healing (see Table 41-2):
  - Diabetes
  - Peripheral vascular disease
  - Steroid use, splenectomy, or alcoholism

Table 41-1 Initial Evaluation and Management of Animal Bites

History	Physical Examination	Wound Care	Imaging	Indication for Hospitalization	Reporting
An exact history should be elicited and should include the type of animal that attacked the patient, whether the bite was provoked or unprovoked, and the circumstances in which the bite occurred.	Record a diagram of the wound with the location, type, and depth of injury; range of motion; possibility of joint penetration; presence of edema or crush injury; nerve and tendon function; signs of infection; and odor of exudate.	Obtain Gram stain, and wound cultures should be done in the presence of abscesses, sepsis, serious cellulitis, devitalized tissue, or foul odor of the exudate.	X-rays should be obtained if fracture bone penetration or foreign bodies are suspected	Fever, sepsis, spreading cellulitis, significant edema or crush injury, loss of function, compromised host, and patient noncompliance.	Require the reporting of bites by any animals known to be potential carriers of rabies, such as bats, raccoons, skunks, foxes, and cattle, to prevent cases of human rabies and control the spread of rabies within the animal community.
If animal can be rabid, locate the animal for 10 days' observation or sacrifice.	Photo documentation may be useful in case that may involve litigation such as unleashed dog bite.	Animal bite wounds should be irrigated with copious amounts of normal saline.			
Obtain general health and immunization status of animal.		Puncture wounds should be irrigated with a "high-pressure jet" from a 20–50 mL syringe and an 18–20 gauge needle.			
Document the time and location of the attack.		Irrigation with either normal saline or Ringer's lactate can decreased infection rate by 20-fold.			
		Debridement			
Obtain patient's medical history such as splenectomy, steroid use, lung disease, peripheral vascular disease, diabetes, mastectomy, liver disease, and immunosuppression.		Necrotic skin tags or devitalized tissues should be debrided and any foreign bodies should be removed			
		Wound closure: may be necessary for selected, fresh, uninfected wounds, especially facial wounds, but primary wound closure is not usually indicated.			
		Wound edges should be approximated with adhesive strips in selected cases			

Table 41-2	Risk Factors in Bite Wound Infections	
Factor	**High Risk**	**Low Risk**
Animal	Cat	Dog
	Human	Rodent
	Pig	
Site of wound	Hand	Face
	Leg	Scalp
	Oral through and through	Mucosa
	Joint	
Type of wound	Puncture wound	Large
	Contaminated	Superficial
	Crush	Clean
	Old	Recent
Co-morbidity	Diabetes mellitus	
	History of splenectomy	
	Peripheral vascular disease	
	Prosthetic heart valve	
	Use of corticosteroids and Cytotoxic drugs.	
	Alcoholism	

ASSESSMENT OF RISK FACTORS FOR INFECTION

- Wounds inflicted on the *hands and below the knee* are the highest sites for infection risk. A *dog bite to the hand* may lead to infection 30% of the time as opposed to only 9% if bitten elsewhere. Hand injuries from cat bites have a nearly 20% infection rate.
- In contrast, dog bites of the face and neck have an infection rate of only 0% to 5% even when sutured, unless they are severe and require hospitalization.
- Patients with underlying medical conditions such as diabetes, peripheral vascular disease, splenectomy, liver disease, use of steroids, and an immunocompromised status have increased risk of infection and poor outcomes (Table 41-2).

ANTIBIOTIC THERAPY FOR COMMON ANIMAL BITE WOUNDS

- Antibiotic prophylaxis is considered reasonable if the risk of infection is 5% to 10%.
- Prophylactic antibiotics are *not indicated for most routine* dog bite wounds, except for hand wounds.
- Because *cat bites* have been reported to have a high likelihood of infection, and infected cat bites often require hospitalization, it is not unwise to consider prophylactic antibiotics for cat bites, especially hand wounds (Table 41-3).
- For dog bite wound infections, coverage of *Pasteurella multocida* must be used.
  - A second- or third-generation cephalosporin or *amoxicillin-clavulanate* is an excellent first-line agent.
  - Clindamycin plus sulfamethoxazole can be used for the patient having history of *penicillin allergy*.

Table 41-3	Antimicrobial Therapy: Indications for Prophylactic Antibiotics

Presentation more than 8 hours after bites?
Moderate or severe injury?
Cat bites (most)
Diabetes mellitus
Asplenic patient
Immunocompromised patient (mastectomy, liver disease, or steroid therapy)
Hand or facial involvement
Deep puncture wounds with possible bone or joint penetration

- Doxycycline and fluoroquinolones are also effective but should *not be routinely used in children.*
- For penicillin-allergic **children**, clindamycin plus trimethoprim-sulfamethoxazole (TMP-SMX) is used as an alternate (Table 41-4).
- The species of the animal will help to determine the bacteria that might be present in the wound (see Table 41-5 to 41-7).
- Sulfonamides should not be given to pregnant women or newborns.
- Fluoroquinolones are not approved for children

RABIES

- Most human cases occur in the *developing areas following dog* bites, while most human cases of rabies occur following exposure to rabid wild animals *in regions where dogs are immunized.*

TABLE 41-4	Rabies Postexposure Prophylaxis guide—United States, 2008	
Animal Type	**Evaluation and Disposition of Animal**	**Postexposure Prophylaxis Recommendations**
Dogs, cats, and ferrets	Animal is healthy and available for 10 days observation.	Do not initiate prophylaxis unless animal develops clinical signs of rabies.
	Rabid or suspected rabid	Initiate immediate antirabies prophylaxis.
	Unknown (e.g., escaped)	Consult public health officials.
Skunks, raccoons, foxes and coyotes, bats	Considered as rabid unless animal was proven negative by laboratory tests	Initiate immediate prophylaxis.
Squirrels, rats, mice, hamsters, guinea pigs, gerbils, chipmunks, rabbits, and hares	No antirabies postexposure prophylaxis	

| Table 41-5 | Microbiology and Choice of Prophylactic Antibiotics | | | |

Animal	Microbiology	Prophylactic Antibiotics	Alternative Antibiotic	Others
Dog	*Pasteurella* species. *Staphylococcus aureus*, *Streptococcus viridans*, *Capnocytophaga canimorsus*, and *Bacteroides* and *Fusobacterium*	Amoxycillin-clavulinic acid 875 mg bid or 500 mg t.i.d. for 3–5 days	Clindamycin 300 mg q.i.d. and a fluoroquinolone or TMP-SMX	Capnocytophaga in splenectomized patient may cause sepsis
Cat bites	*Pasteurella* spp., *Staphylococcus*, and *S. viridans*	Amoxycillin-clavulinic acid 875 mg b.i.d. or 500 mg t.i.d. for 3–5 days	Cefuroxime 500 mg b.i.d. or doxycycline 100 mg b.i.d.	Increased risk of infection after cat bite without prophylactic antibiotics. *P. multocida* is resistant to dicloxacillin, clindamycin, erythromycin and cephalexin
Human bite	Streptococci, *S. aureus*, *Eikenella corrodens*, and *Bacteroides* and *Peptostreptococcus*	Amoxycillin-clavulinic acid 875 mg b.i.d. or 500 mg t.i.d. for 3–5 days	Clindamycin 300 mg q.i.d. and a fluoroquinolone or TMP-SMX Azithromycin Moxifloxacin	

| Table 41-6 | Duration of Antimicrobial Prophylaxis |

Type of Wound	Duration of Treatment
<8 hours after animal bite	Prophylaxis for 3–5 days
Cellulitis	7–14 days
Bone/joint	For 3–8 weeks

Considerations for antibiotic prophylaxis should include:
  Wounds seen <8 hours after animal bites
  Those that might involve hands, joints and bones
  Punctures wounds especially close to joint
  Wounds in those with comorbid conditions such as
  immunosuppression and DM

Table 41-7	Less Common Animal Bites
Species	**Microbiology**
Monkey bites	B virus (also known as herpesvirus simiae or cercopithecine herpes virus 1)
Horse bites	*S. aureus, Streptococcus* species., *Neisseria* spp., *Escherichia coli, Actinobacillus lignieresii, Pasteurella* species, *Bacteroides ureolyticus, Bacteroides fragilis*, other anaerobic gram-negative bacilli, *Prevotella melaninogenica*, and *Prevotella heparinolytica*
Pig bites	*Staphylococcus* spp., *Streptococcus* spp. (including *Streptococcus sanguis, Streptococcus suis* and *Streptococcus milleri*), diphtheroids, *P. multocida*, other *Pasteurella* spp., *Haemophilus influenzae, Actinobacillus suis, Flavobacterium* IIb–like organisms, *B. fragilis*, and other anaerobic gram-negative bacilli
Bird pecking and bites	*Streptococcus bovis, Clostridium tertium*, and *Aspergillus niger, Bacteroides* species, *Pseudomonas aeruginosa*
Ferrets	*S. aureus*
Rat	*S. moniliformis, Spirillum minus*
Shark bites	*Vibrio carchariae*
Piranha and alligator bites	*Aeromonas hydrophila*

- In low-prevalence regions, an increasing percentage of cases *are imported* and occur after long incubation periods or lack a known source of exposure.
- Reported incubation period for rabies varies from a *few days to more than 19 years*, although 75% of patients become ill in the first *90 days* after exposure.
- The initial symptoms of rabies resemble those of other systemic viral infections, but the first neurologic symptoms involve *personality changes and cognition* deficits. The prodromal phase will usually last from 4 to 10 days. *Paresthesias or pain* near the exposure site may occur early as well.
- Human rabies infections are divided into two forms:
  1. The *furious form* or encephalitic type presents with the hydrophobia, delirium, and agitation that form the common picture of rabies.
  2. About a fifth of patients present with the *paralytic form* and have very little clinical evidence of cerebral involvement until late in the course.
- Diagnosis
  - Direct fluorescent antibody (DFA) staining of a skin biopsy obtained from the **nape of the neck**, above the hairline
  - The reverse transcriptase–polymerase chain reaction (RT-PCR)
  - The rapid fluorescent focus inhibition test (RFFIT)
  - MRI images reveal areas of **increased T_2 signal** in the hippocampi, hypothalamus, and brain stem.

- *Preexposure prophylaxis* is used for people with a *relatively high risk o*f rabies exposure, such as veterinarians, laboratory workers, spelunkers, and travelers who plan to visit countries with a significant risk of dog rabies.
  - A series of **three** intramuscular or intradermal injections (days 0, 7, and 21 or 28) is given.
  - **Booster doses** every 2 to 3 years are usually recommended for individuals frequently at risk of exposure.
- It is cost saving to administer postexposure prophylaxis (PEP) if a patient is bitten by a rabid animal that has tested positive for rabies or if a patient is bitten by a reservoir vector species, *even if the animal is not available* for testing (Table 41-8).
- **Proper wound care** with a 20% soap solution or povidone-iodine reduces the risk of rabies by 90%.
- In low-prevalence regions, a *healthy dog or cat* should be observed for 10 days. If infection is suspected and confirmed by a pathologic exam, there is still adequate time to institute PEP.
- *Wild mammal exposure*, especially if the animal exhibits uncharacteristic behavior, warrants PEP in almost all circumstances.

Table 41-8	Postexposure Prophylaxis		
	Wound Care	**Intramuscular Vaccines**	**RIG**
Nonimmunized person	Immediate thorough cleansing of all wounds with soap and water. If available, a virucidal agent such as povidone-iodine solution should be used to irrigate the wounds.	HDCV or PCECV 1.0 mL, IM (deltoid area), one dose on 0, 3, 7, 14	If possible, the **full dose** should be infiltrated around any wound(s) and any remaining volume should be administered IM at an anatomical site distant from vaccine site
Previously immunized individuals	Immediate thorough cleansing of all wounds with soap and water. If available, a virucidal agent such as povidone-iodine solution should be used to irrigate the wounds	HDCV or PCECV 1.0 mL, IM (deltoid area), one dose on 0, 3	No need.

- If the animal **is available** for pathologic examination, and if pathologic examination of the brain does not indicate the presence of rabies virus, PET may be discontinued.
  - Discovery of a bat in a room with an infant or a child who cannot report the occurrence of a bite reliably, and on whom no bite is found, raises the issue of PEP. If the bat is captured and tests positive for rabies, PEP is indicated.
  - If the bat is not captured, the decision about PEP must be individualized but should probably be given by many physicians.
- PEP appears to be safe in **pregnant women** and should not be withheld when an indication exists.
- Postexposure treatment should always include two types of immunizing agents:
  - **Rabies immune globulin** is available in human (HRIG) and equine forms, which provide immediate passive immunity that can persist for a short period of time.
  - **Rabies vaccines are available** in human diploid cell vaccine (HDCV; Imovax) and purified chick embryo cell vaccine (PCECV; RabAvert). Both are inactivated virus vaccines that are remarkably safe and induce immunogenic response.
- Both immunizing agents are used simultaneously for postexposure prophylaxis, unless person *immunized previously* (Table 41-8).
- For adults, the vaccination should always be administered in **the deltoid area** rather than the gluteal area in adults and older children, while vaccines should be given in the lateral thigh in small children.
- The vaccine must not be given in the same region as the immunoglobulin.
- Patients who have received preexposure prophylaxis or prior postexposure prophylaxis with rabies vaccines should receive 1.0 mL IM on **days 0 and 3 only without any** immune globulin.

SUGGESTED READINGS

Blanton JD, Palmer D, et al. Rabies surveillance in the United States during 2009. *J Am Vet Med Assoc* 2010;237(6):646–657.
  Relative contributions by the major animal groups were as follows: 2,327 (34.8%) raccoons, 1,625 (24.3%) bats, 1,603 (24.0%) skunks, 504 (75%) foxes, 300 (4.5%) cats, 81 (1.2%) dogs, and 74 (1.1%) cattle.
Brook I. Microbiology and management of human and animal bite wound infections. *Prim Care* 2003;30(1):25–39, v.
  This article describes the microbiology, diagnosis, and management of human and animal bite wound infections.
Chutivongse S, Wilde H, et al. Postexposure rabies vaccination during pregnancy: effect on 202 women and their infants. *Clin Infect Dis* 1995;20(4):818–820.
  Tissue culture–derived rabies vaccines as well as immune globulins are safe to use for postexposure prophylaxis during pregnancy. Such treatment should never be withheld or delayed if the patient possibly was exposed to rabies.
Cummings P. Antibiotics to prevent infection in patients with dog bite wounds: a meta-analysis of randomized trials. *Ann Emerg Med* 1994;23(3):535–540.
  Meta-analysis of published studies. Prophylactic antibiotics reduce the incidence of infection in patients with dog bite wounds. The full costs and benefits of antibiotics in this situation are not known. It may be reasonable to limit prophylactic antibiotics to patients with wounds that are at high risk for infection.
De Serres G, Skowronski DM, et al. Bats in the bedroom, bats in the belfry: reanalysis of the rationale for rabies postexposure prophylaxis. *Clin Infect Dis* 2009;48(11):1493–1499.

These authors feel that current RPEP recommendations related to occult bat contact should be reconsidered. A controversial but interesting position in my opinion.

Dire DJ, Hogan DE, et al. Prophylactic oral antibiotics for low-risk dog bite wounds. *Pediatr Emerg Care* 1992;8(4):194–199.
This study suggests that prophylactic oral antibiotics in low-risk dog bite wounds are not indicated.

Elliott S. Rat bite fever and *Streptobacillus moniliformis*. *Clin Microbiol Rev* 2007;20(1):13–22.
The clinical and biologic features of rat bite fever and Streptobacillus moniliformis are reviewed, providing some distinguishing features to assist the clinician and microbiologist in diagnosis.

Goldstein EJ. Bite wounds and infection. *Clin Infect Dis* 1992;14(3):633–638.
One of every two Americans will be bitten by an animal or by another person at some point. The principles of management of bite wounds are discussed.

Jackson AC. Update on rabies diagnosis and treatment. *Curr Infect Dis Rep* 2009;11(4): 296–301.
The Milwaukee protocol involves induction of therapeutic coma; however, there is no clear rationale for a neuroprotective role of this therapy, many reports exist of its failures, and its use should be abandoned. Basic research is needed on the mechanisms of rabies pathogenesis. This may allow the development of new therapeutic approaches for this ancient disease.

Jackson AC. Therapy of human rabies. *Adv Virus Res* 2011;79:365–375.
More basic research is needed on the mechanisms involved in rabies pathogenesis, which will hopefully facilitate the development of new therapeutic approaches in the future for this ancient disease.

Kristinsson G. *Pasteurella* multocida infections. *Pediatr Rev* 2007;28(12):472–473.

Laothamatas J, Hemachudha T, et al. MR imaging in human rabies. *AJNR Am J Neuroradiol* 2003;24(6):1102–1109.
Both forms of human rabies share a similar MR imaging pattern. Such pattern and the lack of enhancement in a noncomatose patient with suspected encephalitis may differentiate rabies from other viral encephalitides.

Manning SE, Rupprecht CE, et al. Human rabies prevention—United States, 2008: recommendations of the Advisory Committee on Immunization Practices. *MMWR Recomm Rep* 2008;57(RR-3):1–28.

Medeiros I, Saconato H. Antibiotic prophylaxis for mammalian bites. *Cochrane Database Syst Rev* 2001;(2):CD001738.
There is evidence from one trial that prophylactic antibiotics reduce the risk of infection after human bites, but confirmatory research is required. There is no evidence that the use of prophylactic antibiotics is effective for cat or dog bites. There is evidence that the use of antibiotic prophylactic after bites of the hand reduces infection, but confirmatory research is required.

Rupprecht CE, Briggs D, et al. Evidence for a 4-dose vaccine schedule for human rabies post-exposure prophylaxis in previously non-vaccinated individuals. *Vaccine* 2009;27(51):7141–7148.
Based upon the available evidence, a reduced schedule of cell-culture rabies vaccine, administered on days 0, 3, 7, and 14, given in conjunction with rabies immune globulin, was supported and recommended by the United States Advisory Committee on Immunization Practices.

42 Bartonella

James W. Myers

INTRODUCTION

Bartonella

- Gram-negative
- Intracellular
- Grow on solid media (shell vial tissue cultures, blood enriched)

CLINICAL FEATURES

1. Classic *Bartonella*, Carrion Disease.
- Epidemiology/Pathology
  - ***Bartonella bacilliformis***
  - Human reservoir
  - Found between altitudes 800 and 3,000 m on the western slopes of the Andes Mountains in the countries of Columbia, Peru, and Ecuador
  - Sandfly transmission (*Lutzomyia verrucarum*)
  - The bacteria destroy red cells and invade cells of the reticuloendothelial system (RES).
  - Nucleated RBCs and reticulocytes, intravascular hemolysis
- Clinical
  - ***Bacteremic phase, Oroya Fever***
    - Primary bacteremia
    - ≥3-week incubation period
    - Fever
    - Malaise
    - Anemia
    - Head, abdominal, and joint and long bone pain
    - The liver, spleen, and lymph nodes are enlarged and often tender.
    - ≥30% death rate by 3 weeks
    - Superinfection with salmonella is common, up to 50%
    - Salmonellosis is the most frequent complication, occurring in 40% to 50% of cases of Oroya fever. Toxoplasmosis has been reported as well.
    - Parotitis, thromboses, pleurisy, and meningoencephalitis may complicate the infection in some patients.
  - ***Eruptive phase, verruga peruana***
    - Crops of skin lesions occur *several weeks to-months* after resolution of the initial infection.
    - Miliary or nodular lesions
    - Face and legs > trunk
    - May also occur with visceral involvement, especially dysphagia and vaginal bleeding

Table 42-1	Diagnostic Tests for *Bartonella*				
	Warthin-Starry Silver Stain	Culture	Serology	Giemsa Stain of Blood	PCR
Oroya Fever	+	+	+ (travelers)	++	+
Typical CSD	+	+ (20%)	++		+ tissue
CNS					+
Endocarditis	+	+			++
BA	+	+			+
PH	+	+			+
Neuroretinitis			+		+
Trench Fever		+	+		+

- ○ Recurring crops over several months is not uncommon.
- ○ As seen in yaws, the constitutional symptoms disappear with the appearance of the skin lesions.
- Diagnosis (see Table 42-1)
  - The organism can be seen in the red cells during Oroya fever and in smears from verruga lesions.
  - Can be cultured from the blood on special media
  - Serology is usually not helpful
- Treatment (see Table 42-2)
  - *Chloramphenicol* (2 to 4 gm daily in divided doses) for 1 to 2 weeks is the traditional antibiotic of choice in South America.
  - Other effective antibiotics include tetracycline, streptomycin, rifampin, ciprofloxacin, ampicillin, and cotrimoxazole.
2. *Bartonella Quintana*
  - Epidemiology
    - *Pediculus humanus*, **the human body louse**, is the vector.
    - *B. quintana* has historically caused worldwide outbreaks of *trench fever*.
    - 1 million people infected during WWI
    - *B. quintana* presentations commonly seen today:
      - ○ Asymptomatic infections
      - ○ A relapsing febrile illness with headache *and leg* pain
      - ○ A cause of "culture-negative" endocarditis
      - ○ May cause bacillary angiomatosis (BA), chronic lymphadenopathy, bacteremia, and endocarditis *in HIV-infected patients*
      - ○ Outbreaks in homeless patients, most notably in Seattle and France. Associated with poverty and alcoholism
  - Clinical Features
    - Classic trench fever
      - ○ Transmission occurs primarily by the *rubbing of louse feces* into broken skin. Less often by actual biting by the lice
      - ○ Incubation period was usually 7 days but ranged from 3 to 38 days
      - ○ Onset of fever and chills was usually sudden, resembling influenza

Table 42-2	Treatment Options for *Bartonella*		
	Drugs of Choice	**Alternates**	**Comments**
CSD	None, as the course is self-limited in most patients.	Azithromycin is dosed 500 mg PO on day 1, then 250 mg PO on days 2–5 as a single daily dose.	Only treat for bulky or extensive lymph-adenopathy. No evidence it will prevent complications.
Oroya Fever	Chloramphenicol at 500 mg PO or IV q.i.d. for 14 days plus a beta-lactam.	Ciprofloxacin 500 mg PO b.i.d. for 10 days. Perhaps trimethoprim-sulfamethoxazole.	
Verruca	Rifampin 10 mg/kg/day PO for 14 days	Streptomycin at 15–20 mg/kg/day IM for 10 days.	
Suspected *Bartonella* endocarditis	Gentamicin at 3 mg/kg/day.IV for 14 days and ceftriaxone at 2 g IV or IM q.d. for 6 weeks with or without doxycycline at 100 mg PO or IV b.i.d. for 6 weeks		
Documented *Bartonella* endocarditis	Doxycycline at 100 mg PO b.i.d. for 6 weeks and Gentamicin at 3 mg/kg/day IV for 14 days.		
Retinitis	Doxycycline at 100 mg PO b.i.d. for 4–6 weeks and rifampin at 300 mg PO b.i.d. for 4–6 weeks		Steroids are of unproven benefit but may be recommended by ophthalmology.
Trench Fever and *B. quintana* bacteremia.	Doxycycline at 200 mg PO q.d. for 4 weeks plus gentamicin 3 mg/kg IV q.d. for 2 weeks		
BA	Erythromycin at 500 mg PO q.i.d. for 3 months	Or doxycycline at 100 mg PO b.i.d. for 3–4 months.	
PH	Erythromycin at 500 mg PO q.i.d. for 4 months.	Or doxycycline at 100 mg PO b.i.d. for 3–4 months.	

- º Military physicians previously described four distinct patterns of illness:
  - A single febrile episode, a short febrile period lasting roughly 5 days, a relapsing febrile illness occurring at 5-day intervals with asymptomatic intervening periods, and a debilitating and persistent typhoidal illness, often lasting many months
- º Retroorbital headache
- º Anterior tibial pain or *shin bone fever* was a characteristic feature.
- º Splenomegaly and rash occurred.
- º Vertigo, conjunctivitis, and arthralgias were also seen.
- Urban homeless patients
  - º Seattle cluster
    - Had fever, weight loss, and endocarditis
    - Typical features of trench fever were missing.
  - º Marseille
    - One patient had shin pain.
    - Several with endocarditis
    - Less likely to be febrile compared to Seattle patients
    - Five of ten patients were bacteremic for several weeks but did not develop endocarditis.
  - º Raoult reported on 22 patients with endocarditis, 5 with quintana shared several common features.
    - Aortic valve
    - Preexisting damage
    - Valve replacement
- HIV-infected patients
  - º Fever
  - º Cutaneous lesions
  - º Bone
  - º Less likely to cause peliosis hepatitis than *Bartonella henselae*
  - º Endocarditis
3. Other species of *Bartonella*
   - One isolate of *Bartonella elizabethae* has been reported as a cause of bacteremia and endocarditis. One case of neuroretinitis with this organism was also reported.
   - *Bartonella vinsonii* was associated with bacteremia in a healthy rancher from the western United States.
   - *Bartonella koehlerae* and *Bartonella alsatica* have been reported to cause endocarditis as well.
   - A *Bartonella clarridgeiae*–like isolate was found to cause fever and bacteremia in a patient with arthropod bites returning from Peru.
   - *Bartonella tamiae* bacteremia has been described in Thailand with rat exposure.
   - *Bartonella grahamii* has been reported to cause retinitis.
   - *Bartonella washoensis* has been associated with myocarditis.
4. Cat scratch disease (CSD), caused by *B. henselae*
   - Epidemiology
     - *B. henselae* has been recovered from the blood of healthy cats and from cat fleas (*Ctenocephalides*)
     - *B. henselae* >> *B. clarridgeiae*> *vinsonii* subsp. *berkhoffii* in terms of frequency.
     - Antibodies are more common in kittens and feral cats.
     - Domestic cats, fleas, ruminants, ticks, and dogs have all been implicated as sources of disease. Most infections in cats are asymptomatic and can last for several months.
     - Usually affects patients under 21, especially children.

- Clinical
  - Typical CSD.
    - Enlargement of lymph nodes after being *bitten, licked, or scratched* by a kitten or feral cat is the typical presentation.
      - A small papule usually occurs within about a week of the event. It may persist for a while and be found on exam later. A more diffuse rash may occur rarely.
      - Involvement of the lymph nodes (most commonly head, neck, axilla) that drain the site of the bite may be delayed for a few weeks.
      - Usually, this is a single node, but 1/3 may have multiple nodes.
      - Low-grade fever and malaise may be present in 1/3 to 2/3 of patients.
      - Rash, headache, and sore throat may rarely occur.
      - The lymph nodes resolve spontaneously over several months. Ten percent to fifteen percent may suppurate.
      - This typical course is more common in children than adults.
- Other features of CSD.
  - *Parinaud oculoglandular syndrome* occurs in 10% of cases.
    - A granulomatous, ipsilateral conjunctivitis
    - Preauricular, lymph node involvement
    - The granulomas may occur in bulbar or palpebral conjunctiva, upper or lower.
    - Fever and other systemic signs may or may not be present.
    - The conjunctivitis and the regional lymph node abnormalities usually resolve over 1 month.
    - May rarely suppurate
    - Tularemia and sporotrichosis may mimic this as well
  - Other syndromes reported to be associated with CSD include FUO, atypical pneumonia, osteomyelitis, erythema nodosum, arthralgia, nephritis, endocarditis, arthritis, and thrombocytopenic purpura, and splenitis.
  - CNS changes
    - Around 2% of patients with CSD develop encephalopathy or other neurologic manifestations.
    - Possible explanations for disease include toxin- or immune-mediated processes, vasculitis, and direct bacterial invasion of the brain.
    - Encephalopathy and seizures are common.
    - Long-term intellectual changes are rare.
    - Death is rare.
    - Transient findings include nuchal rigidity, aphasia, ataxia, cranial nerve palsy, hemiplegia, and sphincter dysfunction.
    - Patients typically recover fully. Most recover within 12 months of presentation; however, complete recovery does not always occur.
  - Ocular
    - Neuroretinitis usually follows the onset of lymphadenopathy.
    - Choroiditis
    - Eye exam can show hemorrhages, cotton-wool spots, multiple discrete lesions in the deep retina, *and stellate macular exudates.*
- HIV-infected patients
  - *B. henselae* or *B. quintana* have been reported to cause meningoencephalitis, and encephalopathy.
  - *B. henselae* and *B. quintana* cause BA and peliosis hepatis (PH).

- BA
  - Red skin papules or vascular nodules
  - Fever, headache, weight loss
  - Respiratory and gastrointestinal mucosa involvement may be seen.
  - Occasional heart, liver, spleen, and bone lesions as well
  - Bone marrow
  - May resemble KS
- PH
  - Nausea, vomiting, diarrhea, and abdominal distension are features of PH
  - Cystic, blood-filled spaces
  - *B. henselae* >> quintana

DIAGNOSIS

- *Bartonella* syndromes are often made clinically, but useful diagnostic tests are found in Table 42-1.
- If blood cultures are drawn, EDTA or Isolator systems can be used. Blood or choco-late agar can be used. The organism may take a while to grow, at least 7 days, and acridine orange staining can be useful.
- Consider cocultivation with eukaryotic cells, in addition to plating onto rabbit blood and chocolate agars.
- Acute and convalescent serum specimens are positive for antibody testing (70% to 90% positive in immunocompetent patients) in patients with CSD.
- Cerebrospinal fluid (CSF) analysis may show elevated lymphocytes and protein. Culture is typically negative and glucose levels are usually normal in cases with encephalopathy.

TREATMENT

- MICs from antibiotic susceptibility testing may correlate poorly with clinical out-comes.
  - The lack of a bactericidal effect for monotherapy gentamicin, for example, may in part due to sequestration in erythrocytes.
  - CSD typically does not respond to nor need antibiotic therapy. The clinical mani-festations of the disease may be due to an immunologic reaction in the lymph nodes, and there are probably few or no viable *Bartonella* bacilli by the time that a biopsy is performed.
  - See Table 42-2 for treatment of specific disease states.

SUGGESTED READINGS

Agan BK, Dolan MJ. Laboratory diagnosis of *Bartonella* infections. *Clin Lab Med* 2002;22(4):937–962.

Avidor B, Graidy M, et al. *Bartonella koehlerae*, a new cat-associated agent of culture-negative human endocarditis. *J Clin Microbiol* 2004;42(8):3462–3468.
  B. koehlerae is reported for the first time to be a human pathogen that causes culture-negative endocarditis.

Bass JW, Freitas BC, et al. Prospective randomized double blind placebo-controlled evaluation of azithromycin for treatment of cat-scratch disease. *Pediatr Infect Dis J* 1998;17(6):447–452.
  Treatment of patients with typical CSD with oral azithromycin for 5 days affords significant clini-cal benefit as measured by total decrease in lymph node volume within the first month of treatment.

Breitschwerdt EB, Maggi RG, et al. PCR amplification of *Bartonella koehlerae* from human blood and enrichment blood cultures. *Parasit Vectors* 2010;3:76.

Future studies should more thoroughly define modes of transmission and risk factors for acquiring infection with B. koehlerae. In addition, studies are needed to determine if B. koehlerae is a cause or cofactor in the development of arthritis, peripheral neuropathies, or tachyarrhythmias in patients.

Brouqui P, Lascola B, et al. Chronic *Bartonella quintana* bacteremia in homeless patients. *N Engl J Med* 1999;340(3):184–189.

In an outbreak of urban trench fever among homeless people in Marseilles, B. quintana infections were associated with body lice in patients with nonspecific symptoms or no symptoms.

Cadenas MB, Maggi RG, et al. Identification of bacteria from clinical samples using *Bartonella* alpha-Proteobacteria growth medium. *J Microbiol Methods* 2007;71(2):147–155.

In an effort to overcome historical problems associated with the isolation of Bartonella species from animal and human blood samples, our laboratory developed a novel, chemically modified, insect-based, liquid culture medium (Bartonella alpha-Proteobacteria growth medium, BAPGM).

Carithers HA. Cat-scratch disease. An overview based on a study of 1,200 patients. *Am J Dis Child* 1985;139(11):1124–1133.

1,200 patients with CSD are reviewed.

Chomel BB, Boulouis HJ, et al. *Bartonella* spp. in pets and effect on human health. *Emerg Infect Dis* 2006;12(3):389–394.

Transmission of B. henselae by cat fleas is better understood, although new potential vectors (ticks and biting flies) have been identified. We review current knowledge on the etiologic agents, clinical features, and epidemiologic characteristics of these emerging zoonoses.

Chomel BB, Kasten RW. Bartonellosis, an increasingly recognized zoonosis. *J Appl Microbiol* 2010;109(3):743–750.

Daly JS, Worthington MG, et al. Rochalimaea elizabethae sp. nov. isolated from a patient with endocarditis. *J Clin Microbiol* 1993;31(4):872–881.

Dreier J, Vollmer T, et al. Culture-negative infectious endocarditis caused by *Bartonella* spp.: 2 case reports and a review of the literature. *Diagn Microbiol Infect Dis* 2008;61(4):476–483.

Foucault C, Brouqui P, et al. *Bartonella quintana* characteristics and clinical management. *Emerg Infect Dis* 2006;12(2):217–223.

Fouch B, Coventry S. A case of fatal disseminated *Bartonella henselae* infection (cat-scratch disease) with encephalitis. *Arch Pathol Lab Med* 2007;131(10):1591–1594.

This case illustrates the extreme severity of the spectrum with which CSD can present and provides evidence of brain histopathology that may be representative of the disease.

Lamas C, Curi A, et al. Human bartonellosis: seroepidemiological and clinical features with an emphasis on data from Brazil—a review. *Mem Inst Oswaldo Cruz* 2008;103(3):221–235.

This review provides updated information on clinical manifestations and seroepidemiologic studies with an emphasis on data available from Brazil.

Larson AM, Dougherty MJ, et al. Detection of *Bartonella (Rochalimaea) quintana* by routine acridine orange staining of broth blood cultures. *J Clin Microbiol* 1994;32(6):1492–1496.

*B. quintana was isolated from 34 BACTEC nonradiometric aerobic resin blood cultures for 10 adults. Nine patients were initially diagnosed by routine **acridine orange staining** of routine cultures that had been incubated for 8 days. All subcultures grew on chocolate agar within 3 to 12 days (median, 6 days). The PLUS 26 high-volume aerobic resin medium, combined with acridine orange stain and subculture, is an effective system for detection and isolation of B. quintana from blood.*

Lepidi H, Fournier PE, et al. Quantitative analysis of valvular lesions during *Bartonella* endocarditis. *Am J Clin Pathol* 2000;114(6):880–889.

Lynch T, Iverson J, et al. Combining culture techniques for *Bartonella*: the best of both worlds. *J Clin Microbiol* 2011;49(4):1363–1368.

In this study, they were able to overcome these temperature- and cell-dependent limitations and accommodate all of the strains tested by combining mammalian cell culture–based medium with insect cell culture–based medium.

Maguina C, Garcia PJ, et al. Bartonellosis (Carrion's disease) in the modern era. *Clin Infect Dis* 2001;33(6):772–779.

Maguina C, Guerra H, et al. Bartonellosis. *Clin Dermatol* 2009;27(3):271–280.
The clinical manifestations, differential diagnosis, laboratory diagnosis, and treatment of these conditions are discussed.

Minnick MF, Battisti JM. Pestilence, persistence and pathogenicity: infection strategies of *Bartonella. Future Microbiol* 2009;4(6):743–758.

O'Halloran HS, Draud K, et al. Leber's neuroretinitis in a patient with serologic evidence of *Bartonella elizabethae. Retina* 1998;18(3):276–278.

Pérez GJ, Munita SJ, et al. Cat scratch disease associated neuroretinitis: clinical report and review of the literature. *Rev Chilena Infectol* 2010;27(5):417–422.

Raoult D, Roblot F, et al. First isolation of *Bartonella alsatica* from a valve of a patient with endocarditis. *J Clin Microbiol* 2006;44(1):278–279.
B. alsatica was identified by serology and culture and by PCR of an aortic valve specimen. B. alsatica should be added to the list of zoonotic agents of blood culture-negative endocarditis.

Reed JB, Scales DK, et al. *Bartonella henselae* neuroretinitis in cat scratch disease. Diagnosis, management, and sequelae. *Ophthalmology* 1998;105(3):459–466.
*B. henselae is a cause of neuroretinitis in CSD. Compared to historic cases, doxycycline and rifampin appeared to shorten the course of disease and hasten visual recovery. **Long-term prognosis is good**, but some individuals may acquire a mild postinfectious optic neuropathy.*

Riess T, Dietrich F, et al. Analysis of a novel insect cell culture medium-based growth medium for *Bartonella* species. *Appl Environ Microbiol* 2008;74(16):5224–5227.
Human- and animal-pathogenic Bartonella species are fastidious and slow-growing bacteria difficult to isolate and cultivate. We describe a novel, easy-to-prepare liquid medium for the fast and reliable growth of several Bartonella spp. that does not affect bacterial protein expression patterns or interactions with host cells.

Rolain JM, Brouqui P, et al. Recommendations for treatment of human infections caused by *Bartonella* species. *Antimicrob Agents Chemother* 2004;48(6):1921–1933.
Excellent review. Several good tables in this article.

43 Rabies

Abdel Kareem Abu-Malouh and Jonathan P. Moorman

INTRODUCTION

- Rabies is an acute CNS disease caused by rabies virus infection.
- Rabies virus is a bullet-shaped virus with a single-stranded RNA, a member of the genus Lassa virus and the family rhabdoviridae.
- The virus is highly neurotropic and replicates slowly within muscle cells.
- It causes more than 50,000 deaths each year worldwide, mostly in developing countries.
- The infection is invariably fatal if prophylactic measures are not applied.

EPIDEMIOLOGY

- All mammals can transmit rabies virus.
  - Infection is usually caused by dog bites in Asia and Africa and by bat bites in North America.
  - Transmission from cats, cattle, raccoons, skunks, and foxes have been reported.
- Infection can be transmitted by salivary contact with nonintact skin or mucus membranes.
- Transmission can occur without awareness of the bite or exposure (sleeping adult or child).
- Transmission by transplanted cornea and other solid organs has been reported.
- No known person-to-person transmission
  - Infected patients still need to be in contact and respiratory isolation.
- Forty percent of cases occur in children under 15 years of age.
- >Fifteen million people worldwide receive rabies postexposure prophylaxis (PEP) yearly (Table 43-1).

PATHOGENESIS

- Incubation period is 1 to 3 months in human but can be up to more than 1 year.
- After inoculation into muscle cells, the virus is transmitted from the peripheral nerves to dorsal root ganglia and then to the brain.
- PEP is *ineffective* once the virus enters into the peripheral nerve.
- The virus spreads rapidly throughout the CNS, undergoing massive replication.
  - Induces neuronal dysfunction rather than neuronal death
  - Causes Negri bodies, the most characteristic pathologic change in the CNS
  - Mainly in Purkinje cells of the cerebellum and pyramidal cells of the hippocampus
- The virus then spreads from the CNS through peripheral nerves to salivary glands, liver, muscle, skin, adrenals, and heart.
  - Excreted abundantly in saliva

Table 43-1	Postexposure Prophylaxis of Rabies	

Vaccination Status	Intervention	Regimen
Not previously vaccinated	Wound cleansing	All PEP should begin with immediate thorough cleansing of all wounds with soap and water. If available, a virucidal agent (e.g., povidine-iodine solution) should be used to irrigate the wounds.
	Human rabies immune globulin (HRIG)	Administer 20 IU/kg body weight. If anatomically feasible, the full dose should be infiltrated around and into the wound(s), and any remaining volume should be administered at an anatomical site (intramuscular) distant from vaccine administration. Also, HRIG should not be administered in the same syringe as vaccine. Because RIG might partially suppress active production of rabies virus antibody, no more than the recommended dose should be administered.
	Vaccine	Human diploid cell vaccine (HDCV) or purified chick embryo cell vaccine (PCECV) 1.0 mL, IM (deltoid area), one each on days 0, 3, 7, and 14.
Previously vaccinated	Wound cleansing	All PEP should begin with immediate thorough cleansing of all wounds with soap and water. If available, a virucidal agent such as povidine-iodine solution should be used to irrigate the wounds.
	HRIG	HRIG should not be administered.
	Vaccine	HDCV or PCECV 1.0 mL, IM (deltoid area), one each on days 0 and 3.

Adapted from Rupprecht CE, et al; CDC. Use of a reduced (4 dose) vaccine schedule for postexposure prophylaxis to prevent human rabies. *MMWR Morb Mortal Wkly Rep* 2010;59(RR-2):1–9.

CLINICAL MANIFESTATIONS

- The disease is divided into three main stages: the prodrome, the acute neurologic phase, and coma/death.
- Prodrome: Usually lasts for 1 to 7 days; symptoms are nonspecific including fever, headache, nausea, vomiting, anxiety, and agitation
- Paresthesia, pain, or itching may occur at the site of exposure.
  - Reflects infection of the dorsal roots or cranial sensory ganglia

- There are two clinical forms of the disease: encephalitic (80%) and paralytic (20%).
- Encephalitic form is characterized by fever, confusion, hallucinations, muscle spasms, seizures, and hyperexcitability separated by intervals of lucidity.
  - Autonomic dysfunction may occur and results in hypersalivation, excessive sweating, pupillary dilatation, and priapism.
  - The brain stem is usually involved early in the encephalitic form, resulting in hydrophobia and aerophobia.
  - Other manifestations of the encephalitic form include SIADH, noncardiogenic pulmonary edema, and cardiac arrhythmias.
- Paralytic form is manifested by muscle weakness, which begins in the bitten extremity and spreads to produce quadriparesis and bilateral facial weakness and respiratory paralysis.
  - Sphincter involvement is common, and sensory involvement is not prominent.
  - The paralytic form has a higher survival rate than encephalitic form.
- The clinical course is usually followed by coma and death within 5 days in the encephalitic form and within a few weeks in the paralytic form.

DIAGNOSIS

- Rabies is usually misdiagnosed in developed countries due to lack of experience.
- Diagnosis should be considered in any case of progressive encephalitis or ascending paralysis as an exposure may be not recognized.
- Diagnosis requires multiple testing modalities and several specimens (saliva, skin, serum, CSF) as the sensitivity of any single test is low.
- All samples should be considered potentially infectious and should be shipped immediately to a state lab or CDC.
- Rabies serum antibodies are diagnostic in previously unimmunized patients and usually appear within a few days after the onset of symptoms but may be undetectable until later in the course.
- CSF exam shows minimal lymphocytic pleocytosis (5 to 30 WBCs/μL) and mildly elevated protein.
- Rabies antibodies in CSF are diagnostic regardless of immunization status.
- Viral shedding can be intermittent so serial samples should be collected.
- Testing of viral DNA by reverse transcription PCR can detect the virus in saliva, CSF, and tissue
- Skin biopsies from the nape of the neck can detect the virus by direct fluorescent antibody testing.
  - Biopsy should include at least 10 hair follicles with their cutaneous nerves.
- Studies showed that PCR of skin biopsy has the highest sensitivity and specificity, followed by saliva specimens.
- Postmortem testing can be done by using immunofluorescence staining for viral antigens and looking for Negri bodies in the brain stem and other neural tissues.
- If possible, the suspected rabid animal should be captured.
  - If it is not overtly rabid, it should be quarantined for 10 days and observed for signs of rabies.
  - If the animal shows signs of rabies during the observation period, it should be euthanized and its brain tissue examined with PCR or immunofluorescence.

TREATMENT/POSTEXPOSURE PROPHYLAXIS

- No established treatment is available for rabies, and it is almost always a fatal disease.
- Treatment is mainly supportive, with supplemental oxygen, mechanical ventilation, sedation, and anticonvulsants.
- Treatment relies mostly on PEP with rabies immunoglobulin and rabies vaccine before the development of symptoms.
- The wound should be washed thoroughly with soap and water and debrided if needed. Tetanus prophylaxis should be given as well as antibiotics if bacterial infection is suspected. This will decrease the risk of rabies by as much as 90%.
- An unprovoked bite by an animal is more likely to indicate that the animal is rabid.
- If dogs, cats, and ferrets are healthy and available for 10 days observation, persons should not receive prophylaxis unless the animal develops clinical signs of rabies.
- Any animal other than a dog, a cat, or ferret should be euthanized immediately and the brain submitted for examination
- Skunks, raccoons, foxes, and bats are regarded as rabid unless the animal is proven negative by lab tests.
  - Bitten persons should receive PEP immediately unless the animal is available for testing and public health authorities are facilitating expedite lab testing.
  - In rabies endemic areas, prophylaxis should be started without waiting for lab results.
- If the lab results are negative, prophylaxis can be discontinued.
- PEP should be started when a sleeping adult or a small child is present in the same space with a bat even without evidence of a bite.
- The administration of PEP to a clinically rabid human is ineffective.
- Rabies human immunoglobulin (RIG) should be given to previously unvaccinated patients as soon as possible, no later than 7 days after the first vaccine dose.
- The entire dose of RIG (20 IU/kg) should be infused at the site of the bite if feasible and the remaining dose should be given intramuscularly (IM) at a distant site.
- RIG and rabies vaccine should not be given at the same site or in the same syringe.
- Cell culture rabies vaccine should be given in four 1-mL doses, starting at the day of presentation at days 0, 3, 7, and 14.
- The deltoid area is the preferred site of giving the vaccine in adults, and the anterolateral thigh is used in children.
- Immunosuppressant medications should be held during PEP if possible as they interfere with antibody production.
- The antibody response develops after 7 to 10 days and generally persists for several years.
- Antibody titer measurement is not required unless the patient is immunocompromised, in which case the titer should be checked after 2 to 4 weeks
- Local or mild systemic reactions to the vaccine can be treated with anti-inflammatory medications and the vaccination should not be discontinued.

PREVENTION

- Preexposure prophylaxis should be considered for people at risk of exposure by travel to endemic areas or occupation.
- Three doses of rabies vaccine are given at days 0, 7, and 21 or 28 for preexposure prophylaxis.

- Previously immunized patients exposed to rabies should receive two booster doses of rabies vaccine at days 0 and 3 without the need for RIG.
- Periodic measuring of antibody titer should be done based on a person's risk of exposure.
- Persons at continuous risk, including rabies researchers and vaccine producers, should check their titer every 6 months.
- The frequent risk category includes animal control and wildlife workers, bat handlers, rabies diagnostic lab workers, veterinarians and their staff working in endemic areas, and cave explorers.
  - Individuals in this category should have their titer checked every 2 years.
- The infrequent risk category includes veterinarians, veterinary students, and animal control workers in nonendemic areas.
  - This group should not have their titer checked routinely.
- A booster dose of rabies vaccine should be given to persons in the continuous and frequent risk groups if their titers fail to completely neutralize the virus at a 1:5 serum dilution.
- Animal rabies can be controlled by proper induction of herd immunity through vaccination of domestic animals.

SUGGESTED READINGS

Fooks AR, et al. Emerging technologies for the detection of rabies virus: challenges and hopes in the 21st century. *PLoS Negl Trop Dis* 2009;3(9):e530.
   This article discusses the current and emerging techniques available for diagnosis of rabies infection.
Jackson AC. Rabies. *Neurol Clin* 2008;26:717–726.
Jackson AC. Therapy of human rabies. *Adv Virus Res* 2011;79:365–375.
Leung AK, Davies HD, Hon KL. Rabies: epidemiology, pathogenesis and prophylaxis. *Adv Ther* 2007;24:1340–1347.
Laothamatas J, et al. Neuroimaging in rabies. *Adv Virus Res* 2011;79:309–327.
   This article discusses the radiographic findings in rabies infection, with a focus on MRI and potential new neuroimaging techniques for assessing rabies.
Manning SE, et al. Human rabies prevention, recommendations of the advisory committee on immunization practices. *MMWR Recomm Rep* 2008;57(RR-3):1–28.
   This consensus document provides clear guidance on immunization in the setting of rabies exposure. An update to the schedule, reducing the number of doses to four, was published in 2010 (see Rupprecht et al. 2010 MMWR).
Nigg AJ, Walker PL. Overview: prevention and treatment of rabies. *Pharmacotherapy* 2009;29:1182–1195.
Rupprecht CE, Gibbons RV. Prophylaxis against rabies. *N Engl J Med* 2004;351:2626–2635.
Rupprecht CE, et al; CDC. Use of a reduced (4 dose) vaccine schedule for post-exposure prophylaxis to prevent human rabies. *MMWR Recomm Rep* 2010;59(RR-2):1–9.
   This article provides the most recent guidance for immunization after rabies exposure, including the dosing schedule and routes of administration.
Willoughby RE, et al. Survival after treatment of rabies with induction of coma. *N Engl J Med* 2005;16:2508–2514.

44 Brucellosis

Waseem Ahmad and James W. Myers

ORGANISM

Brucellosis is a zoonotic disease, reported for the first time in 1859 by Marston, in Malta.

Brucellae are intracellular pathogens that can survive and multiply within phagocytic cells. The inhibition of tumor necrosis factor α (TNF-α) by brucella affects natural killer cells and macrophages. *Brucella* are taken up by local tissue lymphocytes, then travel through lymphatics to lymph nodes, and then reach the bloodstream to disseminate to all organs of the body. Caseation and granuloma formation can be seen on pathology.

Patients can be reinfected or relapse with brucellosis.

- Four species of *Brucella*:
  1. ***Brucella melitensis* (goats, sheep, camel). Most common cause in the world**
  2. *Brucella abortus* (cattle, buffalo, yaks)
  3. *Brucella suis* (pigs, reindeer)
  4. *Brucella canis* (dogs, foxes)
- *Brucella* are nonmotile, nonsporulating, noncapsulated gram-negative coccobacilli.
  - Growth on culture media is increased by the adding serum or blood.
  - Serum enhances growth.
  - Grows slowly, up to 4 weeks
  - Aerobic but may require carbon dioxide
- Able to survive in unpasteurized cheese for long periods of time
- Resists freezing but **not pasteurization** or boiling
- Shed in animal urine, stool, and after birth
- *Remains viable in soil for over a month*

EPIDEMIOLOGY

- Worldwide
- Highest prevalence
  - Mediterranean
  - India
  - Mexico and Central and South America

TRANSMISSION

- Gastrointestinal tract is the usual route.
  - Untreated dairy, raw meat, liver
- Inhalation
  - Occupational hazard of herdsmen and dairy farmers

- Lab personnel
  - Brucellosis is the number one laboratory-associated bacterial infection.
  - Biosafety level 3 precautions.
  - PEP recommendations are doxycycline 100 mg orally twice a day plus rifampin 600 mg orally once a day for 21 days.
- Penetration by pieces of bone affects abattoir workers.
- Accidents related to animal vaccination by veterinarians.
- Transplacental transmission, transmission via breast milk feeding, and possibly even sexual transmission.
- Blood transfusion or marrow or organ transplantation.

CLINICAL FEATURES

- Incubation period is usually several weeks.
- Nonspecific symptoms
  - An **undulant fever pattern** (rising and falling like a wave) is sometimes observed.
  - Fever is accompanied by nonspecific complaints of fatigue, back pain, weight loss, poor appetite, body aches, and **depression**.
  - Peculiar taste sensations
  - Twenty percent to thirty percent have lymphadenopathy, hepatosplenomegaly.
- Organ localization
  - Gastrointestinal
    - Nausea, vomiting, diarrhea, or constipation in up to 70%
    - Tonsillitis, hepatitis, ileitis, cholecystitis, and pancreatitis
    - Mild changes in liver function tests
    - No cirrhosis
    - Abscesses; granulomas occasionally
  - Genitourinary
    - Fifty percent may have a positive urine culture.
    - **Epididymo-orchitis in 20% of men**
    - Prostatitis, cystitis
    - Cervicitis, tubo-ovarian abscesses, changes in menses
    - Found in semen
    - Interstitial nephritis, pyelonephritis, renal calcifications
    - Granulomatous lesions with abscesses in the kidneys
  - Ocular
    - Endophthalmitis. Cultures may be positive.
    - Uveitis. Usually a later complication
    - Conjunctivitis
    - Keratitis
    - Retinal detachment
  - Skeletal
    - Knees
    - Hips
    - Sternoclavicular joint
    - **Sacroiliitis in younger patients**
    - **Lumbar spondylitis in older patients**
    - Vertebral osteomyelitis
    - Psoas abscesses are common.
    - *Lymphocytes* are seen in synovial fluid.

- Pregnancy
  - Abortion
  - Premature delivery
  - Transmission via breast milk
- Cardiovascular
  - Endocarditis is rare but fatal if untreated. **Overall mortality from brucellosis is low (<1%) and almost exclusively occurs from cardiac complications**.
  - The median duration of symptoms prior to diagnosis is around 3 months.
  - Forty-five percent have underlying valvular damage, and in 55% of cases, it involved a normal valve.
  - Aortic involvement is found in 82% of cases.
  - Blood cultures were positive in 63% of the patients.
  - Surgical treatment was undertaken in eight patients (72%).
  - Pericarditis occasionally
- Respiratory
  - Pneumonia
  - Lung nodules
  - Abscess
  - Empyema
- Neurologic
  - Meningitis, encephalitis, brain and epidural abscesses
  - Guillain-Barré syndrome, a multiple sclerosis–like illness, paraplegia, and rhabdomyolysis
  - Acute or chronic meningitis syndromes are most common.
    - **Lymphocytic pleocytosis**, high protein, and normal or low glucose
    - Results of an agglutination test for *Brucella* in serum were positive for all patients in one review.
- Six of sixteen patients had positive blood cultures, and four of 14 had positive CSF cultures.
    - Gram stains and cultures of cerebrospinal fluid are usually negative.
    - Specific antibodies or real-time polymerase chain tests can help make the diagnosis.
- Skin
  - Purpura; maculopapular lesions
  - Stevens-Johnson syndrome
- Relapses are common.
- Ten percento
- Usually occur in the first year
- Retreat with the same antibiotics
- Milder than the initial infectiono

DIAGNOSIS

CDC Classification

Probable: A clinically compatible illness with at least one of the following:

- Epidemiologically linked to a confirmed human or animal brucellosis case
- Presumptive laboratory evidence, but without definitive laboratory evidence, of *Brucella* infection

Confirmed: A clinically compatible illness with *definitive laboratory* evidence of *Brucella* infection.

- Gram-negative coccobacillus
- The white blood cell count is usually not elevated.
- Liver function tests might be abnormal.
- Culture of brucellae from blood or bone marrow occurs more often than from other tissues.
  - Forty percent to ninety percent in acute cases
  - Five percent to twenty percent in chronic cases
    - Bone marrow is the most sensitive site and remains positive for the longest time after treatment begins.
    - **Blood** cultures are positive in 45% to 70%.
    - The time-to-detection of *Brucella* can take up to 30 days using the Castaneda blood culture method.
    - Automated blood culture systems have reduced the potential growth time of *Brucella* to less than a week, but in the absence of this, weekly subcultures might be useful for 4 weeks.
    - Biohazard risk to laboratory personnel
- Serology
  - If Rose Bengal or rapid dipstick tests are used for screening, they should be confirmed by running a serum agglutination test (SAT).
  - **The SAT measures both IgG and IgM antibodies**.
    - *Tularemia and Yersinia enterocolitica can give false-positive reactions.*
    - *SAT to detects antibodies to B. abortus, melitensis, and suis. Special tests must be run for canis.*
    - IgG is measured by using 2-mercaptoethanol to inactivate IgM. Acutely infected patients may develop both IgM and IgG antibodies.
    - **A bacterial agglutination titer of>160 suggests past or recent infection; a fourfold rise in titer between acute and convalescent samples is evidence of recent infection**.
    - Blocking antibodies can lead to false-negative results at low dilutions of serum. Dilute to >1:640
    - **Elevated levels of specific antibodies may remain present in some patients treated for brucellosis for a long time, limiting the usefulness of the SAT as a follow-up test**.
      - IgG antibody titers slowly decline over a period of months, but IgM antibodies may persist at a low level in the serum for several years.
      - **However, persistently high IgG antibody titers or a second rise in IgG antibody levels are seen in chronic infection or relapse**.
  - The **ELISA test** appears to *be more sensitive* than and *at least as specific* as the SAT.
    - Use cytoplasmic proteins as antigens.
    - ELISA measures class M, G, and A.
    - **Better for patients with neurobrucellosis**
    - In patients with **chronic brucellosis**, IgG and IgA were consistently positive (100%), while IgM was only positive in 33% of their sera.
    - In the CSF of patients with CNS brucellosis, ELISA was positive in 100%, 20%, and 85% for IgG, IgM, and IgA.

- ○ ELISA **was negative in the CSF specimens from patients with brucellosis without CNS** involvement or meningitis other than *Brucella*.
- ○ Other serologic tests used in endemic areas include *rapid point-of-care tests*, and immunochromatographic *Brucella* IgM/IgG *lateral flow* assays, which are highly sensitive and specific in some studies.
- Polymerase chain reaction (PCR)
  - ○ Can confirm the identity and species
  - ○ Both sensitive and specific
  - ○ Useful for initial diagnosis, follow-up, and relapse diagnosis.
  - ○ Many patients, however, maintain a low-level positive PCR for an indefinite period despite an initial decline after therapy.

THERAPY

- **Single drug therapy is ineffective (See Tables 44–1 and 44–2).**
- Doxycycline has increased activity in the *acidic environment* in macrophages. Conversely the activities of quinolones are decreased in the acidic environment of phagolysosomes.
- Pregnancy, meningitis, spondylitis, endocarditis, and the treatment of children pose additional challenges.

Table 44-1	Treatment Regimens
Drug Regimen	**Comments**
Tetracycline	Monotherapy ineffective. Use only in combinations.
Doxycycline (200 mg/d PO for 6 wk) plus gentamicin (5 mg/kg/d IM for 7 days).	**Essentially replaces tetracycline and streptomycin as the most effective regimen.** Duration is for uncomplicated disease. "Oral only" regimen can be an advantage.
The combination of doxy-cycline (200 mg/d PO for 6 weeks) plus rifampin (600–900 mg/d PO for 6 wk)	Not advised in cases of spondylitis, or other complicated cases. WHO endorsed. Higher relapse rate.
Trimethoprim-sulfamethoxazole	Must be used in combination with either rifampin, an aminoglycoside, or a quinolone. Useful in treating children.
Trimethoprim-sulfamethoxa-zole and rifampin.	Safer for pregnancy.
Quinolones	Use only in combinations. Monotherapy ineffective.
Doxycycline has been used successfully with trime-thoprim-sulfamethoxazole and rifampin for compli-cated disease.	Meningitis and Endocarditis. ? Third-generation cephalosporins for meningitis. Consider steroids for neurologic complications. Surgical consultation for valvular involvement. Treat for several (~6) months in some cases.

Table 44-2	Useful Web Resources
Map of *Brucella*	http://www.thelancet.com/journals/laninf/article/ PIIS1473-3099(06)70382-6/fulltext
CDC	http://www.cdc.gov/ncidod/dbmd/diseaseinfo/ brucellosis_t.htm

- Relapse
  - Defined by symptom recurrence within a year after completion of treatment but usually occurs in <6 months
  - SAT rises, with or without positive blood culture in most patients.
  - PCR may be helpful but can remain positive at a low level for a long time.
  - Aminoglycosides associated with lower relapse rates. Rifampin can lower doxycycline levels, so relapse might be higher with this combination.

PREVENTION

- No human vaccine
- Avoid unpasteurized milk products.
- There are veterinary vaccines available for *B. abortus* and *B. melitensis*.
- There is no vaccine available for *B. suis*.

SUGGESTED READINGS

Amirghofran AA, Karimi A, et al. Brucellosis relapse causing prosthetic valve endocarditis and aortic root infective pseudoaneurysm. *Ann Thorac Surg* 2011;92(4):e77–e79.

Araj GF. Update on laboratory diagnosis of human brucellosis. *Int J Antimicrob Agents* 2010;36(suppl 1):S12–S17.

Baysallar M, Aydogan H, et al. Evaluation of the BacT/ALERT and BACTEC 9240 automated blood culture systems for growth time of *Brucella* species in a Turkish tertiary hospital. *Med Sci Monit* 2006;12(7):BR235–BR238.
  Authors concluded that the mean time-to-detection could be ≤3 days, which is considered rapid enough for starting appropriate evidence-based treatment in an endemic setting.

Celik AK, Aypak A, et al. Comparative analysis of tuberculous and brucellar spondylodiscitis. *Trop Doct* 2011;41(3):172–174.
  A prolonged clinical course of the disease, constitutional symptoms, lymphocytosis, increased erythrocyte sedimentation rate (ESR), presence of posterior vertebrae lesions and psoas abscesses were significantly more frequent in the TB group.

Del Arco A, De La Torre-Lima J, et al. Splenic abscess due to *Brucella* infection: is the splenectomy necessary? Case report and literature review. *Scand J Infect Dis* 2007;39(4):379–381.
  On the basis of this case and the literature review, one should consider that surgical treatment must be considered in patients with splenic abscess due to Brucella infection.

Dhand A, Ross JJ. Implantable cardioverter-defibrillator infection due to *Brucella* melitensis: case report and review of brucellosis of cardiac devices. *Clin Infect Dis* 2007;44(4):e37–e39.
  Device removal, followed by antibiotic therapy for 6 weeks, is probably required for cure. Table one in this article describes six cases.

Fedakar A, Cakalagaoglu C, et al. Treatment protocol and relapses of brucella endocarditis; cotrimoxazole in combination with the treatment of brucella endocarditis. *Trop Doct* 2011;41(4):227–229.

This treatment should be continued for at least 6 months after surgery in order to prevent relapses.

Franco MP, Mulder M, et al. Human brucellosis. *Lancet Infect Dis* 2007;7(12):775–786.

This review summarizes current knowledge of the pathogenic mechanisms, new diagnostic advances, therapeutic options, and the situation of developing countries in regard to human brucellosis.

Gulsun S, Aslan S, et al. Brucellosis in pregnancy. *Trop Doct* 2011;41(2):82–84.

Appropriate antimicrobial therapy of brucellosis in pregnancy will reduce morbidity and prevent complications.

Hasanjani Roushan MR, Mohraz M, et al. Efficacy of gentamicin plus doxycycline versus streptomycin plus doxycycline in the treatment of brucellosis in humans. *Clin Infect Dis* 2006;42(8):1075–1080.

The combination of oral doxycycline for 45 days plus intramuscular gentamicin for 7 days is equally as effective as traditional therapy using doxycycline for 45 days plus streptomycin for 14 days.

Kasim RA, Araj GF, et al. *Brucella* infection in total hip replacement: case report and review of the literature. *Scand J Infect Dis* 2004;36(1):65–67.

A 47-year-old female underwent revision of a left total hip replacement because of a loose prosthesis.

Mantur B, Parande A, et al. ELISA versus conventional methods of diagnosing endemic brucellosis. *Am J Trop Med Hyg* 2010;83(2):314–318.

For accurate diagnosis in suspected brucellosis cases detection, authors recommend both ELISA IgM and IgG tests.

McLean DR, Russell N, et al. Neurobrucellosis: clinical and therapeutic features. *Clin Infect Dis* 1992;15(4):582–590.

Eighteen patients with neurobrucellosis are described.

Navarro E, Segura JC, et al. Use of real-time quantitative polymerase chain reaction to monitor the evolution of *Brucella* melitensis DNA load during therapy and post-therapy follow-up in patients with brucellosis. *Clin Infect Dis* 2006;42(9):1266–1273.

Using Q-PCR techniques, we consistently detected B. melitensis DNA in the blood samples of patients with brucellosis throughout treatment and follow-up, despite apparent recovery from infection. These findings may have diagnostic, pathogenic, and therapeutic implications.

Obiako OR, Ogoina D, et al. Neurobrucellosis-a case report and review of literature. *Niger J Clin Pract* 2010;13(3):347–350.

Ozdemir M, Feyzioglu B, et al. A comparison of immuncapture agglutination and ELISA methods in serological diagnosis of brucellosis. *Int J Med Sci* 2011;8(5):428–432.

Pappas G, Akritidis N, et al. Brucellosis. *N Engl J Med* 2005;352(22):2325–2336.

Excellent review article. Table 4 summarizes treatment data.

Reguera JM, Alarcon A, et al. *Brucella* endocarditis: clinical, diagnostic, and therapeutic approach. *Eur J Clin Microbiol Infect Dis* 2003;22(11):647–650.

Presented here are 11 cases of Brucella endocarditis, all managed uniformly. The median duration of symptoms prior to diagnosis was 3 months. Five patients (45%) had underlying valvular damage, and in six (55%), endocarditis involved a normal valve. There was a predominance of aortic involvement (82%) and a high incidence of left ventricular failure (91%). All the other patients received antibiotic therapy for 3 months, with no signs of relapse of the infection or malfunction of the prosthesis during a minimum follow-up period of 24 months.

Sasmazel A, Baysal A, et al. Treatment of *Brucella* endocarditis: 15 years of clinical and surgical experience. *Ann Thorac Surg* 2010;89(5):1432–1436.

For Brucella endocarditis, perioperative antibiotic therapy combined with surgical treatment (prosthetic valve replacement) has satisfactory results and increases the quality of life in the long-term follow-up.

Skalsky K, Yahav D, et al. Treatment of human brucellosis: systematic review and meta-analysis of randomised controlled trials. *BMJ* 2008;336(7646):701–704.

There are significant differences in effectiveness between currently recommended treatment regimens for brucellosis. The preferred treatment should be with dual or triple regimens including an aminoglycoside.

Theegarten D, Albrecht S, et al. Brucellosis of the lung: case report and review of the literature. *Virchows Arch* 2008;452(1):97–101.

In the right setting, granulomatous inflammation negative for Ziehl-Neelsen and Grocott stains presenting together with other localized lesions should lead to specific investigations on brucellosis.

Ustun I, Ozcakar L, et al. *Brucella* glomerulonephritis: case report and review of the literature. *South Med J* 2005;98(12):1216–1217.

The pathogenesis and the mechanism of renal involvement in brucellosis is discussed in light of the pertinent literature.

Weil Y, Mattan Y, et al. *Brucella* prosthetic joint infection: a report of 3 cases and a review of the literature. *Clin Infect Dis* 2003;36(7):e81–e86.

They reviewed several cases of B. melitensis infection of prosthetic hips and knees. Tables 1 and 2 summarize the data.

Wortmann G. Pulmonary manifestations of other agents: brucella, Q fever, tularemia and smallpox. *Respir Care Clin N Am* 2004;10(1):99–109.

Brucella, Q fever, tularemia, and smallpox are all rare infections in the United States but are potential agents of biologic terrorism.

X Infections in Transplantation

Immunosuppression in Transplantation

Holly B. Meadows and Michael S. Boger

INTRODUCTION

Maintenance immunosuppression for solid organ transplant recipients has been utilized for over 50 years. Initially, azathioprine and corticosteroids were the mainstay of immunosuppression until the approval of calcineurin inhibitors in the 1980s and 1990s. Since the mid-1990s, several immunosuppressants have been approved, including mycophenolic acid, the mammalian target of rapamycin inhibitors, sirolimus and everolimus, and the newly approved belatacept. While immunosuppression is vital to allograft survival, all available agents are associated with significant adverse effects, including infection and malignancy. Transplant health care providers struggle to find the balance between efficacy and tolerability regarding immunosuppression.[1–5]

CALCINEURIN INHIBITORS: INHIBIT INTERLEUKIN-2 PRODUCTION

Mechanism of Action
• Prevent interleukin-2 production and therefore cytotoxic T-cell activation[1–3]

Efficacy
• Tacrolimus is considered a more potent immunosuppressant than cyclosporine.[3,6]
• Efficacy trials between the two agents have shown that tacrolimus decreases rates of acute rejection at 1 year after transplant. However, long-term outcome data between cyclosporine and tacrolimus have not shown a clear benefit of one over the other in regard to patient and allograft survival.[6–8]

Dosing and Monitoring
• Dosing is transplant center–specific. Guidelines are displayed in Table 45-1.[2,9]
• Calcineurin inhibitors are usually monitored by 12-hour trough levels. Target trough levels are transplant center–specific and dependent on a variety of factors, including time since transplant, organ transplanted, renal function, and concomitant immunosuppression.[2,3,9]

Drug Interactions and Adverse Effects
• Calcineurin inhibitors are metabolized in the liver and are substrates for the cytochrome P450 3A4 isoenzyme and P-glycoprotein.
• Significant drug interactions are displayed in Table 45-2.
• Adverse effects are displayed in Table 45-3 and include nephrotoxicity, infection, and malignancy.[1–3,9]

Table 45-1	Immunosuppression Dosing and Monitoring		

Immunosuppressant	Standard Dosing	IV:PO	Typical Target Trough Levels
Cyclosporine	1.5–2.5 mg/kg P.O. b.i.d.	~1:3	50–200 ng/mL
Tacrolimus	1 mg P.O. b.i.d. 0.02–0.05 mg/kg b.i.d.	~1:4	5–12 ng/mL
Azathioprine	1–4 mg/kg/day	~1:1	N/A
Mycophenolate mofetil[a]	1,000–1,500 mg P.O. b.i.d.	~1:1	Therapeutic drug monitoring is controversial.
Sirolimus	2–5 mg daily (May give loading dose)	N/A	5–15 ng/mL
Everolimus	0.5–0.75 mg P.O. b.i.d.	N/A	3–8 ng/mL
Belatacept	10 mg/kg days 1[b] and 5[c] 10 mg/kg after 2 and 4 wk 10 mg/kg after 8 and 12 wk 5 mg/kg after 16 wk and every 4 wk thereafter	N/A	N/A

[a]Mycophenolate sodium 720 mg is equivalent to mycophenolate mofetil 1,000 mg. (There is no IV formulation of mycophenolate sodium)
[b]To be given prior to organ reperfusion
[c]~96 hours after dose 1

Table 45-2	Common Drug Interactions with Calcineurin Inhibitors and mTOR Inhibitors

Increase Concentrations (CYP3A4 Inhibitor)	Decrease Concentrations (CYP3A4 Inducer)
"Azole" antifungals, including voriconazole, fluconazole, itraconazole, and ketoconazole	Phenytoin
Diltiazem	Carbamazepine
Verapamil	Phenobarbital
Amiodarone	Rifampin
Clarithromycin	Rifabutin
Erythromycin	St. John's wort
Danazol	
Protease Inhibitors	
Grapefruit Juice	

Table 45-3	Common and Serious Adverse Effects of Immunosuppressants
Immunosuppressant	**Adverse Effects**
Cyclosporine	Nephrotoxicity, neurotoxicity, hyperglycemia, hyperkalemia, hypomagnesemia, hyperuricemia, hyperlipidemia, hypertension, **hirsutism, gingival hyperplasia**, infection, malignancy
Tacrolimus	Nephrotoxicity, neurotoxicity, hyperglycemia, hyperkalemia, hypomagnesemia, hyperuricemia, hyperlipidemia, hypertension, **alopecia**, infection, malignancy
Azathioprine	Leukopenia, anemia, thrombocytopenia, gastrointestinal disturbances, pancreatitis, liver toxicity, alopecia, skin cancers (likely related to overall level of immunosuppression)
Mycophenolate mofetil/sodium	Nausea, vomiting, **diarrhea**, abdominal pain, leukopenia, anemia, thrombocytopenia, malignancy, increased tissue-invasive cytomegalovirus (CMV) infection, increased risk of progressive multifocal leukoencephalopathy (PML)
Sirolimus/Everolimus	**Hyperlipidemia, delayed would healing**, proteinuria, anemia, thrombocytopenia, gastrointestinal disturbances, **pneumonitis**, infections
Corticosteroids	Hyperglycemia, osteoporosis, infection, mood disturbances, psychosis, fluid retention, weight gain, hypertension, cataracts, peptic ulcers
Belatacept	Posttransplant lymphoproliferative disorder (increased in EBV seronegative recipients), infusion reactions (rare), infection

CYCLOSPORINE (SANDIMMUNE, NEORAL, GENGRAF)

Cyclosporine products are not bioequivalent. Practitioners should always confirm cyclosporine products with patients and continue them on the same formulation. If this is not possible, cyclosporine concentrations should be monitored closely.[3,9]

- Sandimmune, the original cyclosporine formulation, is dependent on bile for absorption and associated with erratic pharmacokinetics. Bioequivalent generic products are available.[3,9]
- Neoral, cyclosporine modified, is less dependent on bile for absorption and has more predictable pharmacokinetics than the original formulation.[3,9]
  - Gengraf is a branded generic product of Neoral and is bioequivalent.[3,9]

Cyclosporine has also been monitored using levels 2 hours after dose (C_2 levels), which have been shown to more closely correlate with area under the concentration-time curve (AUC).[10]

The following adverse effects are more common with cyclosporine than tacrolimus:[2,11]

- Hyperlipidemia, hypertension, hirsutism, and gingival hyperplasia

TACROLIMUS (PROGRAF)

Most transplant centers utilize tacrolimus as their calcineurin inhibitor of choice due to the decrease in both acute rejection rates and cosmetic side effects.[2,6,11] The following adverse effects are more common with tacrolimus than cyclosporine:[2,11]

- Hyperglycemia, neurotoxicity, and alopecia

ANTIMETABOLITES: INHIBIT PURINE SYNTHESIS AND LYMPHOCYTE PROLIFERATION

Mechanism of Action

- Most cell lines use both the salvage and de novo pathways for purine synthesis, but lymphocytes rely almost exclusively on the de novo pathway. These agents block de novo purine synthesis necessary for lymphocyte proliferation.[12]

Efficacy

- Mycophenolate mofetil is considered a more potent and selective immunosuppressant than azathioprine.
- In kidney transplantation, mycophenolate mofetil has improved graft survival[13] and long-term patient survival[14] compared with azathioprine.

AZATHIOPRINE (IMURAN)

Mechanism of Action

- Converted to a purine analog that is incorporated into DNA, inhibiting DNA synthesis, and inhibits enzymes involved in the de novo pathway. It blocks both the salvage and de novo pathways. Because it is nonspecific and affects all hematopoietic cell lines, it has more myelosuppressive effects than mycophenolate mofetil.[12]
- Typically used in conjunction with cyclosporine or tacrolimus

Dosing and monitoring are displayed in Table 45-1.[3,9,15]
Noteworthy drug interactions:[15]

- Allopurinol
  - Inhibits xanthine oxidase (responsible for azathioprine metabolism) and concomitant use may cause azathioprine toxicity[15]
  - Reduce azathioprine dose by 1/3 to 1/4 of usual dose
  - Contraindicated with febuxostat (may cause azathioprine toxicity)

Adverse effects (Table 45.3) include:[15,16]

- Bone marrow suppression: dose dependent, intensified in renal insufficiency
  - Reduce dose or hold further doses if white blood cell count (WBC) <3000 or if 50% reduction in WBC compared to prior level
  - Usually resolves within 7 to 10 days after dose reduction[17]
- Black box warning: posttransplant lymphoma and hepatosplenic T-cell lymphoma reported in patients with inflammatory bowel disease[15]

MYCOPHENOLATE MOFETIL (MMF, CELLCEPT)

Mechanism of Action

- Inhibits inosine monophosphate dehydrogenase (IMDPH), an enzyme crucial in the de novo pathway. It is lymphocyte-selective as it only inhibits the de novo pathway, on which lymphocytes are dependent, resulting in a more potent and specific inhibition of lymphocyte proliferation than azathioprine, with less myelosuppressive effects.[12]
- The antiproliferative agent of choice due to decreased acute rejection and improved patient and graft survival[2]
- Used in conjunction with cyclosporine or tacrolimus[2]

Dosing and monitoring are displayed in Table 45-1.[3,9,18]
Noteworthy drug interactions:[18]

- Enterohepatic recirculation of MMF is inhibited by cyclosporine, which may lower mycophenolic acid exposure.

Key adverse effects are displayed in Table 45-3.[2,3,18–20]

- Birth defects (must use reliable form of contraception)
- Gastrointestinal
  - Dosage reduction may decrease symptoms.[17]
  - Mycophenolate sodium (EC-MPS, Myfortic): enteric coated, delayed release formulation developed to reduce gastrointestinal side effects[21]
- Myelosuppression[20]

mTOR INHIBITORS: CELL CYCLE INHIBITORS, RENAL SPARING

Mechanism of Action

- Bind to FK binding protein (FKBP12) and the resultant complex binds to mammalian target of rapamycin (mTOR), a serine-threonine kinase, arresting cell division by preventing progression from G_1 to S phase of the cell cycle. The net effect is blocking IL-2 postreceptor signaling and, thus, T-cell proliferation.[12,22]

Efficacy

- Changing from a calcineurin inhibitor- to sirolimus-based immunosuppressive regimen 3 months after kidney transplantation was associated with improved renal function with no significant difference in patient and graft survival.[23]
- Dosing and monitoring are displayed in Table 45-1.[1,3,9,11,24,25]

SIROLIMUS (RAPAMUNE)

- If used with calcineurin inhibitors may increase risk of nephrotoxicity but when used without calcineurin inhibitors does not appear to cause renal impairment
- Sirolimus has inhibitory effects on vascular smooth muscle proliferation and has been shown to attenuate cardiac allograft vasculopathy.[26]

Noteworthy drug interactions are listed in Table 45-2.[1,2,24]
Adverse effects (Table 45-3) include[24]

- Hyperlipidemia (monitor serum lipids)—may respond to dose reduction[17,27]
- Impaired wound healing[28]

- Hold prior to planned surgery (usually 3 to 4 weeks), then restart 2 to 3 months postoperatively
- Noninfectious pneumonitis[29]
  - Risk factors: age, late switch to sirolimus, and elevated serum creatinine
  - Treatment: withdrawal of sirolimus or dose reduction
- Myelosuppression
- Hepatic artery thrombosis (black box warning) after liver transplantation[30]
  - Should not be used for the first 30 days after liver transplantation

EVEROLIMUS (ZORTRESS)

- Analog of sirolimus with shorter half-life compared to sirolimus (30 hours vs. 60 hours)
- Similar side effect profile and drug interactions as sirolimus[25]

CORTICOSTEROIDS

Mechanism of Action

- Decrease serum lymphocytes, down-regulate proinflammatory cytokines, and prevent cytotoxic T-cell activation.[2,11]
- Many transplant centers withdraw steroids posttransplant to decrease long-term complications associated with their use.[2,3,11]
  - Timing of steroid withdrawal may be days, months, or years posttransplant depending on organ transplanted and transplant center protocol.
  - Adverse effects (displayed in Table 45-3) are notable for hyperglycemia, psychosis, fluid retention, peptic ulcers, and osteoporosis.[3,11]

BELATACEPT (NULOJIX)[3,31]

Mechanism of Action

- Blocks CD28 stimulation by antagonizing CD80 and CD86, inhibiting T-cell activation
- First intravenous *maintenance* immunosuppressant approved for use in solid organ transplantation. FDA-approved for prevention of acute rejection in renal transplant recipients.
- Contraindicated in Epstein-Barr virus (EBV)–seronegative patients
- Used in place of calcineurin inhibitor
- Most clinical data have studied belatacept versus cyclosporine. Immunosuppression protocols consisted of basiliximab induction therapy followed by mycophenolate mofetil, corticosteroids, and either cyclosporine or belatacept.

Advantages: increased glomerular filtration rate at 1 and 2 years posttransplant, more controlled environment to assess medication compliance, no required drug monitoring, and limited drug-drug interactions. Belatacept is an attractive option in renal transplant recipients unable to tolerate conventional immunosuppression regimens.

Disadvantages: increased rates of acute cellular rejection compared to cyclosporine

Adverse Effects

- Malignancy, specifically posttransplant lymphoproliferative disorder, especially in EBV–seronegative recipients

REFERENCES

1. Gaston RS. Current and evolving immunosuppressive regimens in kidney transplantation. *Am J Kidney Dis* 2006;47:S3–S21.
2. Halloran PF. Immunosuppressive drugs for kidney transplantation. *N Engl J Med* 2004;351:2715–2729.
3. Hardinger KL, Koch MJ, Brennan DC. Current and future immunosuppressive strategies in renal transplantation. *Pharmacotherapy* 2004;24:1159–1176.
4. Martin ST, Tichy EM, Gabardi S. Belatacept: a novel biologic for maintenance immuno-suppression after renal transplantation. *Pharmacotherapy* 2011;31:394–407.
5. Patel PS. Overcoming the force and power of immunity: a history of immunosuppression in kidney transplantation. *J Nephrol* 2006;19:137–143.
6. First MR. Improving long-term renal transplant outcomes with tacrolimus: speculation vs evidence. *Nephrol Dial Transplant* 2004;19(suppl 6):vi17–vi22.
7. Kaplan B, Schold JD, Meier-Kriesche HU. Long-term graft survival with Neoral and tacro-limus: a paired kidney analysis. *J Am Soc Nephrol* 2003;14:2980–2984.
8. Kramer BK, Montagnino G, Del Castillo D, et al. Efficacy and safety of tacrolimus com-pared with cyclosporine A microemulsion in renal transplantation: 2-year follow-up results. *Nephrol Dial Transplant* 2005;20:968–973.
9. Ensor CR, Trofe-Clark J, Gabardi S, et al. Generic maintenance immunosuppression in solid organ transplant recipients. Pharmacotherapy 2011;31:1111–1129.
10. Levy G, Thervet E, Lake J, et al. Patient management by Neoral C(2) monitoring: an international consensus statement. *Transplantation* 2002;73(9 suppl):S12–S18.
11. Yang H. Maintenance immunosuppression regimens: conversion, minimization, with-drawal, and avoidance. *Am J Kidney Dis* 2006;47:S37–S51.
12. Duncan MD, Wilkes DS. Transplant-related immunosuppression: a review of immunosup-pression and pulmonary infections. *Proc Am Thorac Soc* 2005;2:449–455.
13. Sollinger HW. Mycophenolate mofetil for prevention of acute rejection in primary cadav-eric renal allograft recipients. US Renal Transplant Mycophenolate Mofetil Study Group. *Transplantation* 1995;60:225–232.
14. Wang K, Zang H, Li Y, et al. Efficacy of mycophenolate mofetil versus azathioprine after renal transplantation: a systematic review. *Transplant Proc* 2004;36:2071–2072.
15. Imuran [package insert]. San Diego, CA: Prometheus Laboratories Inc; 2011.
16. Romagnuolo J, Sadowski DC, Lalor E, et al. Cholestatic hepatocellular injury with azathio-prine: a case report and review of the mechanisms of hepatotoxicity. *Can J Gastroenterol* 1998;12:479–483.
17. Lindenfeld J, Miller GG, Shakar SF, et al. Drug therapy in the heart transplant recipient: Part II: immunosuppressive drugs. *Circulation* 2004;110:3858–3865.
18. CellCept [package insert]. San Francisco, CA: Genentech USA, Inc.; 2010.
19. Berger JR. Progressive multifocal leukoencephalopathy and newer biological agents. *Drug Saf* 2010;33:969–983.
20. Ritter ML and Pirofski L. Mycophenolate mofetil: effects on cellular immune subsets, infec-tious complications, and antimicrobial activity. *Transplant Infect Dis* 2009;11:290–297.
21. Myfortic [package insert]. New Hanover, NJ: Novartis Pharmaceutical Corp; 2010.
22. Benjamin D, Colombi M, Moroni C, et al. Rapamycin passes the torch: a new generation of mTOR inhibitors. *Nat Rev Drug Discov* 2011;10:868–880.
23. Lebranchu Y, Thierry A, Toupance O, et al. Efficacy on renal function of early conver-sion of cyclosporine to sirolimus 3 months after renal transplantation: concept study. *Am J Transplant* 2009;9:1115–1123.
24. Rapamune [package insert]. Philadelphia, PA: Wyeth Pharmaceuticals Inc; 2010.
25. Zortress [package insert]. East Hanover, NJ: Novartis Pharmaceuticals Corp; 2010.
26. Topilsky Y, Hasin T, Raichlin E, et al. Sirolimus as primary immunosuppression attenuates allograft vasculopathy with improved survival and delayed cardiac events following cardiac transplantation. *Circulation* 2012;125(5):708–720.

27. Dummer JS. Risk factors and approaches to infections in transplant patients. In: Mandell GL, Bennett JE, Dolin R, eds. *Mandell, Douglas, and Bennett's Principles and Practice of Infectious Diseases*. 6th Ed. Philadelphia, PA: Elsevier; 2005.

28. Zuckermann A, Barten MJ. Surgical wound complications after heart transplantation. *Transplant Int* 2011;24:627–636.

29. Weiner SM, Sellin L, Vonend O, et al. Pneumonitis associated with sirolimus: clinical characteristics, risk factors and outcome—a single center experience and review of the literature. *Nephrol Dial Transplant* 2007;22:3631–3637.

30. Trotter JF. Sirolimus in liver transplantation. *Transplant Proc* 2003;35:193S–200S.

31. Nulojix [package insert]. Princeton, NJ: Bristol-Myers Squibb; 2011.

46 Donor-Derived Infections in the Transplant Patient

Claire E. Magauran

Donor-derived infections are those that are transmitted from a donor to one or more recipients.

BACKGROUND

- Twenty-one thousand three hundred and fifty-four solid organ transplants were performed in the United States from January–September 2011 utilizing 10,556 donors.[1] Seven thousand and twelve allogeneic and 9,778 autologous hematopoietic stem cell transplants (HSCTs) were performed in the United States in 2009.
- Up to eight lives can be saved with a single organ donor. Eighteen people die daily awaiting an organ.[2]
- Sixteen percent of unrelated donor recipients died due to infection compared to 12% of human leukocyte antigen (HLA)–identical sibling recipients between 2008 to 2009.[3]
- Despite a large number of transplants performed, the rate of donor-derived infection is reported to be <1%.[4] Any transmission of infection can have devastating consequences for the recipient, leading to significant morbidity and mortality.

DONOR SCREENING FOR SOLID ORGAN TRANSPLANT AND HEMATOPOIETIC STEM CELL TRANSPLANT

- A thorough history and physical examination including exposures, travel history, and history of prior transfusions is required.
- In HSCT, donor screening is performed within 8 weeks of donation; serologic testing is done within 30 days or less and followed by repeat testing within a week prior to transplant.[5] The purpose of such screening is to rule out active infection in donors and assess risk for possible infection.

Lab Testing

SOT	HSCT
FDA-licensed HIV 1 and 2 antibody	FDA-licensed HIV 1 and 2 antibody[a]
Hepatitis B surface antigen (HBsAg), Hepatitis B core antibody (HBcAb)	Hepatitis B surface antigen (HBsAg), Hepatitis B surface antibody (HBcAb)
Hepatitis C antibody (anti-HCV)	Hepatitis C antibody (anti-HCV)[a]
CMV antibody (CMV IgG)	CMV antibody (CMV IgG)

SOT	HSCT
EBV antibody (EBV IgG)	EBV antibody (EBV IgG)
Rapid plasma reagin (RPR) or VDRL	Rapid plasma reagin (RPR) or VDRL
Purified protein derivative (PPD) or interferon-gamma release assay (IGRA) in potential living donors	
	Herpes simplex virus (HSV IgG) antibody[b]
	HTLV-I/II antibodies[b]

[a]Nucleic acid testing (NAT) used for HIV and HCV.
[b]Tested in HSCT not SOT.

• Other specific tests depending on organ or exposure history may be performed (e.g., Toxoplasma or Strongyloides antibody testing if the donor is from an endemic area).

Deceased Donors

• Blood cultures, urine cultures, and sputum or bronchoalveolar lavage cultures from hospitalized patients should be obtained in addition.[6]

Deceased Donor Screening Problems

• Limited information about deceased donors
• Short time frame to accept or reject donor organ from deceased donors
• Lack of rapid, sensitive, specific, and cost-effective testing

High-Risk Donor (CDC Classification)[7]

Donors that are considered high risk for possible HIV transmission include:
(1) Men who have sex with men in the last 5 years; (2) nonmedical intravenous, intramuscular, or subcutaneous injection of drugs in the last 5 years; (3) persons with hemophilia or other clotting disorders who have received human-derived clotting factor concentrates; (4) men and women engaging in sex in exchange for money or drugs in the last 5 years; (5) sexual exposure in the last 12 months with any person described above or with known or suspected HIV; (6) exposure in the last 12 months to known or suspected HIV-positive blood through percutaneous inoculation or through contact with an open wound, nonintact skin, or mucus membrane; (7) inmates of a correctional facility

• The risks of rejecting a donor need to be weighed against those of possibly transmitting an infection, and informed consent from the potential recipient is required.

TIMELINE OF INFECTION AFTER SOLID ORGAN TRANSPLANTATION

0- to 1-Month Posttransplant

• Infections related to surgery or indwelling devices are common. This includes wound infection, anastomotic leak, urinary tract infection (UTI), catheter-related bloodstream infection, ventilator-associated pneumonia, and *Clostridium difficile* colitis.
• Nosocomial or health care–related infections including multidrug-resistant organisms (MDRO) such as methicillin-resistant *Staphylococcus aureus*, vancomycin-resistant *Enterococcus*, MDR gram-negative bacilli, and *Candida species* also occur.

- **Donor-derived infections**: Any febrile illness early after transplant should be considered to be possibly donor-derived. These include known or unknown infections prior to transplant such as donor CMV IgG (+) in CMV IgG (–) recipient; donor with UTI, bacteremia, or meningoencephalitis (e.g., lymphocytic choriomeningitis virus [LCMV], West Nile virus [WNV], rabies).
- **Recipient infections**: previously undiagnosed or insufficiently treated colonization or infection

1- to 6-Months Posttransplant

- Antimicrobial prophylaxis has led to decreases in infections due to *Pneumocystis*, *Nocardia*, *Toxoplasma*, and *Listeria*; however, these opportunistic infections are still possible.
- Prior to antiviral prophylaxis human herpes virus infections (CMV, EBV, HSV, VZV, HHV 6 and 7) were frequently seen during this time frame.
- Infection due to BK virus, recurrent HCV, *Cryptococcus*, *tuberculosis*, adenovirus, influenza, and HBV (without prophylaxis) are possible.
- Complications related to anastomosis are common in this time period.
- **Reactivation of latent donor or recipient infections may occur among patients who received prophylaxis**.

>6-Months Posttransplant

- Community-acquired infections such as respiratory viruses, pneumonia, and UTI are common.
- Late viral infections may occur such as HBV, HCV, or CMV after the prophylaxis period (e.g., colitis).
- Infections due to atypical pathogens such as *Nocardia* and *Rhodococcus species* may occur as well as fungal infections due to *Aspergillus*, *Mucor*, or other molds.
- Posttransplant lymphoproliferative disorder (PTLD) which may be EBV related may occur.
- Reactivation of latent infections when treating for acute graft dysfunction may surface during this time period.

TIMELINE OF INFECTION AFTER HEMATOPOIETIC STEM CELL TRANSPLANTATION

Pre-Engraftment (Days 0 to 45)

- Starts from infusion of stem cells to end of engraftment (about 30 days for allogeneic HSCTs, shorter for autologous and longer for cord-blood stem cell transplants)
- Engraftment = absolute neutrophil count (ANC) >500 for 3 consecutive days and platelets 20,000 to 50,000 per mL/blood
- Patients with neutropenia, mucocutaneous barrier breakdown, and the presence of central venous catheters are at risk for bacterial or fungal infections. Septicemia, pneumonia, catheter-related infections, invasive fungal infections, and skin infections are examples. Patients are at risk for infection due to enteric gram negative organisms and gram positive skin flora.
- Antifungal and antimicrobial prophylaxis are utilized to decrease risk of gram-negative infections and invasive fungal infections.
- Reactivation of HSV is common without prophylaxis.

Post-Engraftment (Days 30 to 100)

- Humoral and cellular immunity are impaired and affected by the presence of graft versus host disease (GVHD) and its treatment.
- See CMV disease or reactivation.
- *Pneumocystis* and *Aspergillus* infections may occur as well as reactivation of *Toxoplasma*, adenovirus, and HHV-6.

Late Phase (>100 Days Posttransplantation)

- Impaired humoral and cellular immunity persists, particularly in the presence of chronic GVHD (cGVHD) and its treatment.
- Patients are at risk for opportunistic and community-acquired infections including CMV, VZV, and encapsulated bacteria such as *Streptococcus pneumonia*.

DONOR-DERIVED INFECTIONS

"Expected" Infections Transmitted[8]

Expected infections such as HCV, HBV, CMV, EBV, and toxoplasmosis may be detected by screening tests, can be monitored closely for early infection, or may be universally prophylaxed.

"Unexpected" Infections Transmitted

- Unrecognized infections prior to transplant or not screened for in the donor include HIV,[9] HCV,[10,11] WNV,[12] rabies,[13] Chagas disease,[14] Mycobacterium tuberculosis (MTB),[15] LCMV,[16,17] Balamuthia,[18] aspergillosis,[19] human T-cell leukemia virus type I (HTLV-I),[20] and endemic fungi. Unrecognized infections or infections not screened for prior to transplant can have devastating consequences for the recipient.

"Expected" Infections Transmitted

HCV

- HCV Ab(+) donors have been used for HCV Ab(+) recipients. In exceptional cases, HCV Ab(+) donors have been used for HCV Ab(−) recipients when transplant is urgent with stringent informed consent.
- Need to monitor the recipient for HCV RNA and immunosuppression should be modulated carefully. The decision to start or need for treatment is based on multiple factors and should be done under the guidance of an expert.

HBV

Donor is HBcAb(+)[21]

Liver Transplant Recipient
- High risk of primary infection regardless of recipient serology. Prophylaxis with lamivudine 100 mg daily (add) indefinitely. Entecavir 0.5 mg daily or tenofovir 300 mg daily may be used by some centers.
- If recipient is HBsAg(−), HBsAb(+) but <100 mIU/mL, vaccinate.
- If recipient is HBsAg(−), while on prophylaxis check HBsAg every 3 months for 1 year, then every 6 months afterwards (for breakthrough infection).

Nonliver Transplant Recipient

- If recipient is HBsAb(+) then no prophylaxis is needed. Follow HBcAb, HBsAg, HBsAb, and liver function tests every 3 months for 1 year.
- If recipient is HBsAb(–), check donor serum HBV-DNA. If donor serum (+) HBV-DNA, prophylaxis with lamivudine 100 mg daily ≥12 months or give HBIG 10,000 IU daily for 7 days, then monthly for 3 to 6 months. Start prophylaxis while awaiting donor serum HBV-DNA results if not immediately available. If donor serum (–) HBV-DNA, no need for continued prophylaxis. Follow HBcAb, HBsAg, HBsAb, and liver function tests every 3 months for 1 year.[22,23]

CMV

Highest Risk for Disease

- CMV (D+/R-) status in SOT = donor is CMV IgG(+) and recipient is CMV IgG(–)
- CMV (D-/R+) status in allogeneic HSCT = donor is CMV IgG(–) and recipient is CMV IgG(+)

Prevention Strategies

Two Approaches:
- Universal prophylaxis, antivirals given to all "at risk" patients after transplant, for a defined period of time. This is rarely used in allogeneic HSCT.
- Preemptive prophylaxis, antivirals given to patients with evidence of CMV replication prior to onset of clinical disease. This approach is often utilized in HSCT.

Clinical Manifestations

- Classically seen 1 to 4 months posttransplant but can see late-onset disease with prophylaxis. May have **asymptomatic viremia**, **CMV syndrome** (fever, malaise, myalgias, and bone marrow suppression—particularly leukopenia, thrombocytopenia), or **tissue invasive disease** (i.e., colitis, pneumonitis, hepatitis, retinitis, meningoencephalitis)

Diagnosis

- Serum CMV PCR or antigenemia. Criteria varies for treatment threshold.
- Rapid shell-vial culture, histopathology of specimens from bronchoscopy with biopsy, endoscopy with biopsy, funduscopic examination, and lumbar puncture

Treatment

- For **asymptomatic viremia or CMV syndrome**, consider decreasing immunosuppression and initiating valganciclovir 900 mg PO b.i.d. or ganciclovir 5 mg/kg q12h IV (renally dosed).
- For **tissue invasive disease**, reduce immunosuppression and initiate ganciclovir 5 mg/kg q12h IV. Consider valganciclovir 900 mg PO b.i.d. if NOT severe disease and no malabsorption issues. If concern for resistance or intolerance to ganciclovir, consider other options such as foscarnet 60 mg/kg q8h or 90 mg/kg q12h or cidofovir 5 mg/kg weekly for 2 weeks and every 2 weeks thereafter. All medications should be renally dosed. For CMV retinitis intravitreal ganciclovir or fomivirsen may also be needed (consult Ophthalmology) Intravitreal ganciclovir or fomivirsen (consult Ophthalmology) may also be needed. Consider CMV IgG (Cytogam) if very ill with CMV pneumonitis.[24]
- If viremia persists despite adequate treatment, viral load increases after 2 weeks of treatment, or if the patient is still clinically symptomatic, consider the possibility of ganciclovir resistance.

EBV

High Risk for Disease

- EBV D(+)/R(−) status in SOT = donor is EBV IgG(+) and recipient is EBV IgG(−)
- Monitor quantitative EBV PCR every 2 weeks for 3 months, then monthly for the rest of year 1, then every 2 to 3 months in year 2. May consider prophylaxis with valganciclovir, ganciclovir, acyclovir, or valacyclovir for 3 months.
- EBV D(−)/R(−) = donor EBV IgG(−) and recipient is EBV IgG(−)—at risk of community-acquired disease. If detectable EBV PCR, look for signs or symptoms of PTLD (fever, weight loss, pharyngitis, GI symptoms, enlarged liver or spleen, lymphadenopathy, leukopenia, anemia, atypical lymphocytosis) and repeat EBV PCR.
- If only viremia found, monitor closely.
- If viremia and signs/symptoms of PTLD are found, reduce immunosuppression, consider antiviral treatment, follow EBV PCR every 2 weeks, monitor for rejection, and consider Rituxan if persistent high-grade viremia.[25]
- Be aware there is significant variation between different assays at different institutions so hard to compare different lab testing facility results.

TOXOPLASMOSIS

High Risk for Disease

- Toxoplasma D(+)/R(−) status in heart or heart-lung recipient = donor toxoplasma IgG(+) and recipient toxoplasma IgG(−). Recommended screening at time of transplant (donor and recipient). Trimethoprim-sulfamethoxazole prophylaxis should be given (DS 1 tab PO daily or three times weekly) or pyrimethamine if allergy or intolerance is a concern.
- Clinically may present with meningitis, meningoencephalitis, focal brain abscess, or pneumonia without prophylaxis
- For CNS disease, pneumonitis or disseminated disease, treat with pyrimethamine (200 mg PO loading dose, then 75 mg/day) + sulfadiazine (1 to 1.5 g q6h PO)+ folinic acid (10 to 25 mg/day PO).

SUMMARY

- Donor-derived infections are rare but cause significant morbidity and mortality.
- Always consider donor-derived infection in ill posttransplant recipients.
- Good communication is essential between transplant centers and organ procurement organizations.
- We will never completely eliminate the risk of transmission of infection from donor to recipient, but hopefully with careful screening and assessment, we can significantly mitigate risk.

REFERENCES

1. OPTN: Organ Procurement and Transplantation Network, http://optn.transplant.hrsa.gov/data. Accessed December 13, 2011.
2. U.S. Department of Health and Human Services, http://www.organdonor.gov. Accessed December 13, 2011.

3. Pasquini MC, Wang Z. Current use and outcome of hematopoietic stem cell transplantation: CIBMTR Summary Slides, 2011. Available at: http://www.cibmtr.org. Accessed January 14, 2012.

4. Ison MG, Hager J, Blumberg E, et al. Donor-derived transmission events in the United States: data reviewed by the OPTN/UNOS Disease Transmission Advisory Committee. *Am J Transplant* 2009;9(8):1929–1935.

5. Centers for Disease Control and Prevention (CDC). Guidelines for preventing opportunistic infections among hematopoietic stem cell transplant recipients. *MMWR Recomm Rep* 2000;49(RR-10);1–125, CE1–CE7.

6. Organ Procurement and Transplantation Network—OPTN Policy 2.0 http://optn.transplant.hrsa.gov/PoliciesandBylaws2/policies/pdfs/policy_2.pdf. Accessed January 16, 2012.

7. Rogers MF, Simonds RJ, Lawton KE, et al. National Center for Infectious Diseases. Guidelines for preventing transmission of human immunodeficiency virus through transplantation of human tissue and organs. *MMWR Recomm Rep* 1994;43:1–17. Accessed January 14, 2012, http://www.cdc.gov/mmwr/preview/mmwrhtml/00031670.htm.

8. Ison MG. The epidemiology and prevention of donor-derived infections. *Adv Chronic Kidney Dis* 2009;16(4):234–41.

9. Bowen PA II, Lobel SA, Cuarana RJ, et al. Transmission of human immunodeficiency virus (HIV) by transplantation: clinical aspects and time course analysis of viral antigenemia and antibody production. *Ann Intern Med* 1998;108(1);46–48.

10. Ahn J, Cohen SM. Transmission of human immunodeficiency virus and hepatitis C virus through liver transplantation. *Liver Transpl* 2008;14(11);1603–1608.

11. Shuhart MC, Myerson D, Childs BH, et al. Marrow transplantation from hepatitis C virus seropositive donors: transmission rate and clinical course. *Blood* 1994;84(9);3229–3235.

12. Centers for Disease Control and Prevention (CDC). West Nile virus transmission via organ transplantation and blood transfusion—Louisiana, 2008. *MMWR Morb Mortal Wkly Rep* 200920;58(45):1263–1267.

13. Srinivasan A, Burton EC, Kuehnert MJ, et al. Transmission of rabies virus from an organ donor to four transplant recipients. *N Engl J Med* 2003;348:2196–2203.

14. Chagas' disease after organ transplantation—United States, 2001. *MMWR Morb Mortal Wkly Rep* 2002;51:210–212.

15. Transplantation-transmitted tuberculosis—Oklahoma and Texas, 2007. *MMWR Morb Mortal Wkly Rep* 2008;57(13):333–336.

16. Palacios G, Druce J, Du L, et al. A new arenavirus in a cluster of fatal transplant-associated diseases. *N Engl J Med* 2008;358:991–998.

17. Fischer SA, Graham MB, Kuehnert MJ, et al. Transmission of lymphocytic choriomeningitis virus by organ transplantation. *N Engl J Med* 2006;354:2235–2249.

18. Centers for Disease Control and Prevention (CDC). *MMWR Morb Mortal Wkly Rep* 2010;59(36):1165–1170.

19. Mueller NJ, Weisser M, Fehr T, et al. Donor-derived aspergillosis from use of a solid organ recipient as a multiorgan donor. *Transpl Infect Dis* 2010;12(1):54–59.

20. Kikuchi H, Ohtsuka E, Nakayam T, et al. Allogeneic bone marrow transplantation-related transmission of human T lymphotropic virus type I (HTLV-1). *Bone Marrow Transplant* 2000;26:1685–1690.

21. Doucette KE. Management of Recipients of Hepatitis B Core Antibody-Positive Donar Organ. In: Kumar D, ed. *The AST handbook of transplant infections.* Wiley-Blackwell; 2011;99.

22. Chung RT, Feng S, Delmonico FL. Approach to the management of allograft recipients following the detection of hepatitis B virus in the prospective donor. *Am J Transplant* 2001;1(2):185–191.

23. Cholongitas E, Papatheodoridis GV, Burroughs AK. Liver grafts from anti-hepatitis B core positive donors: a systematic review. *J Hepatol* 2010;52(2):272–279.

24. Razonable RR, Humar A. Cytomegalovirus. In: Kumar D, ed. *The AST handbook of transplant infections.* Wiley-Blackwell Hoboken, NJ; 2011;35–41.

25. Madan R, Herold B. Epstein-Barr Virus and Post-transplant Lymphoproliferative Disoders. In: Kumar D, ed. The AST handbook of transplant infections. Wiley-Blackwell; 2011;42.

47

Reactivation Infections in Solid Organ Transplant Recipients

Ellie S. Walker and Michael G. Ison

INTRODUCTION

Infection is one of the leading causes of morbidity and mortality in solid organ transplant recipients despite advances in preoperative screening, infection prophylaxis, and immunosuppressive regimens.[1] Posttransplant infection may be the result of an infection acquired from the organ donor, of de novo acquisition of a typical or opportunistic pathogen posttransplant, or of reactivation of infection latently infecting the recipient at the time of transplantation.[1] Pretransplant screening of transplant candidates is directed at identifying patients at risk of such reactivation infections posttransplant.[2] When latent infection is identified, patients may be managed through application of pretransplant treatment, posttransplant prophylaxis, or careful monitoring for reactivation coupled with early therapy posttransplant.[2] Although a range of pathogens may lie dormant in a patient and reactivate posttransplant to cause infection, viruses and mycobacteria are associated with the most frequent morbidity and mortality.[1,3] Herpes viruses, hepatitis viruses, and polyoma viruses are the most common viral infections that may reactivate in the recipient posttransplant.[1] Extensive reviews of the epidemiology and prevention of hepatitis and BK virus infection have been published recently.[4,5] Here, we focus on the current state-of-the-art of screening for and preventing cytomegalovirus (CMV) and tuberculosis in the posttransplant period.

CASE PRESENTATION: PART A

The patient is a 60-year-old Hispanic man who was originally born in rural Mexico with end-stage renal disease on hemodialysis. He had a history of hyperlipidemia, type II diabetes, heart failure, pulmonary hypertension, and anemia. During pretransplant screening for renal transplant, he was found to have a positive interferon-γ release assay (IGRA) (QuantiFERON-TB Gold) and was diagnosed with latent TB infection (LTBI). Isoniazid (INH) and vitamin B_6 were initiated to complete a 9-month course. The patient followed up regularly and reported compliance with INH and completed treatment.

Latent *Mycobacterium tuberculosis* Infection

The incidence of reactivation of latent *M. tuberculosis* is 20- to 74-fold higher among transplant recipients than in the general population.[6] In the United States, the majority of posttransplant tuberculosis occurs as the result of reactivation of latent TB, and screening of candidates is associated with a reduction in the rate of posttransplant infection.[7,8] As a result, current guidelines recommend the screening of all transplant candidates for tuberculosis.[2] The American Society of Transplantation Infectious Diseases Community of Practice guidelines recommend screening for LTBI and treatment of LTBI in all transplant candidates.[2,9] Screening consists of a detailed patient history, chest x-ray, and either tuberculin skin testing (TST) or an IGRA. The three currently approved IGRAs in the United States are the QuantiFERON-TB gold, QuantiF-ERON-TB Gold In-Tube, and TB. Studies comparing TST with the approved IGRA assays have shown similar sensitivity and specificity, and the Centers for Disease Control (CDC) and American Society of Transplantation (AST) recommend that the tests may be used interchangeably.[10] Studies comparing pretransplant screening with TST and the QuantiFERON-TB gold IGRA show comparable, low rates of posttransplant TB infections.[11] However, IGRAs have benefits over TST, in some settings. IGRAs may increase the proportion of patients who complete pretransplant LTBI screening as patients do not need to return for TST reading.[10] IGRAs also have a lower rate of false-positive results, have less cross-reactivity with other *Mycobacteria*, and may be used for patients who have previously received bacillus calmette-guerin (BCG) vaccination.[11] In addition, IGRAs may yield fewer false-negative results than TST in patients with immunosuppression as these patients may have cutaneous anergy.[9,10]

Current recommendations state that patients diagnosed with LTBI should be treated with either 9 months of isoniazid with supplemental vitamin B_6 or 4 months of rifampin.[12] An alternative regimen of 3 months of directly observed once-weekly therapy with rifapentine (900 mg) plus isoniazid (900 mg) was recently found to be equally effective but with a higher treatment completion rate than 9 months of isoniazid.[13] Ideally, LTBI treatment is initiated prior to organ transplantation. Typically, isoniazid/B_6 regimens are utilized in the pretransplant period since rifampin may induce cytochrome P450 enzymes and effect posttransplant immunosuppressive levels; if rifampin is utilized (typically because of isoniazid intolerance), the patient should be placed on medical hold until approximately 1 month after completing therapy. Although there is a concern about hepatotoxicity, particularly with isoniazid-containing regimens, isoniazid is generally well tolerated by patients with end-organ failure awaiting transplant as long as liver function testing is performed regularly.[14] Patients with end-stage liver disease and baseline liver function test abnormalities greater than three to five times the upper limits of normal should typically have LTBI delayed until posttransplant.[15]

CASE PRESENTATION: PART B

The patient underwent cadaveric renal transplant approximately 2 months prior to admission when he presented with fever, cough, nausea, and peripheral edema as well as evidence of allograft rejection on imaging. His immunosuppressive medications were mycophenolic acid and tacrolimus. He initially presented to another hospital with similar symptoms and was felt to be in acute heart failure exacerbation and was treated with diuretics. He was transferred to a tertiary care center because of findings consistent with acute allograft rejection on imaging. On transfer, he was noted to have fever, leukocytosis, and worsening cough. He was started on empiric antimicrobials for pneumonia. Admission blood and urine cultures were negative. He later developed altered mental status, severe hypotension, and worsening thrombocytopenia on top of baseline anemia. A nonbronchoscopic bronchoalveolar lavage was performed and acid fast bacillus (AFB) smear was positive. Disseminated tuberculosis was then suspected given pulmonary disease, altered mental status possibly due to TB meningoencephalitis, new pancytopenia possibly due to bone marrow involvement, and severe hypotension due to adrenal involvement. His immunosuppressive medications were discontinued, and he was started on four-drug TB therapy and moxifloxacin for treatment of disseminated TB.

Posttransplant *M. tuberculosis* Infection

Tuberculosis is a significant opportunistic infection that typically results from reactivation of latent infection in 1.2% to 6.4% of solid organ transplant (SOT) recipients in developed countries; less commonly, TB can be transmitted from the donor (~4% of all cases) or from posttransplant de novo exposure to the pathogen.[6] Primary infection is uncommon in developed countries. Tuberculosis infection typically develops within the first year after transplant and is associated with significant morbidity, including graft loss, and high mortality (up to 30%).[6,7] About half of patients affected will develop pulmonary disease followed by disseminated disease and extrapulmonary infection. Diagnosis may be delayed due to atypical or nonspecific clinical presentation. The American Thoracic Society (ATS) and CDC recommend starting with a three or more typically four-drug treatment for the first 2 months for active TB and then completion of an additional 4 months of two-drug therapy, for susceptible strains.[9] Six months of treatment is generally sufficient with some important exceptions: central nervous system (CNS) disease should be treated for 9 to 12 months total; bone and joint disease should be treated for 6 to 9 months total; patients with cavitary pulmonary tuberculosis who continue to have positive *M. tuberculosis* cultures after 2 months of treatment should be treated for 9 months. Patients who receive second-line agents, typically for resistant mycobacteria or intolerance, should also have prolonged treatment.[9] In cases where prolonged treatment is necessary, it is the maintenance phase that is lengthened. Some transplant infectious diseases experts have also advocated for longer treatment courses if disease is particularly severe or if there is enhanced immunosuppression (such as recent lymphodepletion). Consideration should be given to reducing immune suppression, particularly early during the treatment of tuberculosis in transplant patients; immune reconstitution syndrome (IRIS) has been described in some such patients. Since rifampin is associated with significant induction of the cytochrome P450 system, patients receiving calcineurin (cyclosporine or tacrolimus) or mTOR inhibitors (everolimus or sirolimus) should have rifabutin used instead of rifampin because of lesser impact on drug levels. Nonetheless, all transplant patients require very close monitoring of immunosuppressive levels when starting, changing, or stopping antituberculosis therapy because of drug interactions by isoniazid and the rifamycins. Transplant patients are at risk for allograft rejection if doses are not adjusted appropriately.[8,9,16] There is evidence that even with close monitoring, rejection and graft loss increase in frequency with rifamycin use.[6,7,17] Fluoroquinolones may be used as an alternative in patients who experience drug-induced hepatotoxicity.[9,18]

CYTOMEGALOVIRUS

CMV is one of the most common causes of posttransplant infections among SOT recipients. It is estimated that in the United States, up to 70% of adults have been exposed to CMV.[19] Because of the high prevalence of infection and the scarcity of organs, CMV seromatching of donor and recipients is generally not performed.[20] This is important in that the highest risk of CMV occurs in CMV seronegative recipients of seropositive donor organs (D+/R-); without prophylaxis, the majority of such patients would experience viral replication. Intermediate risk groups include seropositive recipients (D±/R+). The risk of CMV in D-/R- patients is approximately 2%, with acquisition of infection through exposure to infected individuals, hemodialysis or blood transfusion, and false-negative test results.[20] Since cellular immunity plays a central role in the control of CMV, lymphocyte depletion, as part of induction or

TABLE 47-1	Pros and Cons for Available CMV Preventative Strategies	
	Prophylaxis	**Preemptive**
Pros	• Improved graft survival • Low rate of rejection • Less monitoring required by center	• Lower medication costs • Less potential for development of resistance
Cons	• Potential for development of CMV resistance • Late onset infections more prevalent • Greater drug toxicity • Greater cost of medication	• Increased graft loss due to rejection • Need for frequent follow-up • High monitoring cost (direct testing costs and need for staff to follow up and intervene when missed labs)

for the treatment of rejection, is also a significant risk factor for CMV infection.[21] Further, lung, intestine, and pancreatic transplants are the highest risk followed by heart transplants. Liver and renal transplants result in the lowest risk of CMV infection.[20,21] This is likely due to the differing levels of immunosuppression required and the potential CMV load in the transplanted organ. In the absence of prophylaxis, CMV infection typically occurs during the first 6 months posttransplant, with the peak incidence 2 to 4 months posttransplant. In the presence of prophylaxis, CMV typically occurs 2 to 4 months after stopping prophylaxis.[22] Prevention of CMV is typically achieved either by use of universal prophylaxis, in which all at risk recipients receive antiviral agents (typically oral valganciclovir, oral ganciclovir, or valacyclovir) for a fixed period of time, or by preemptive monitoring, in which patients have assessments for CMV replication (typically plasma or whole blood PCR) at regular intervals coupled with therapy with evidence of replication.[21] Although there are relative pros and cons to using either preventative strategy (see Table 47-1), most guidelines favor universal prophylaxis.[20,21] Recent studies of universal valganciclovir prophylaxis in high-risk kidney transplant patients have demonstrated that 200 days of prophylaxis is associated with fewer patients developing CMV disease by 12 months than those who receive 100 days of prophylaxis (16.1% vs. 36.8%); similar benefit was found with less CMV viremia with 200 days of prophylaxis (37.4% vs. 50.9%).[23]

CMV infection is known to have direct and indirect effects. Direct effects of CMV reactivation may result in symptoms ranging from mild, self-limited mononucleosis-like syndrome to tissue invasive disease including hepatitis, pneumonia, or gastrointestinal illness to disseminated disease causing critical illness.[20] Indirect effects include increased levels of immunosuppression with resultant superinfection with fungal pathogens and epstein-barr virus (EBV) reactivation potentially leading to post-transplant lymphoproliferative disorder (PTLD).[21] Data also suggest that CMV replication may contribute to acute and chronic rejection; this is one of the strongest drivers to recommendation of universal prophylaxis.[20,21,24,25]

REFERENCES

1. Fishman JA. Infection in solid-organ transplant recipients. *N Engl J Med* 2007;357(25): 2601–2614.
2. Fischer SA, Avery RK. Screening of donor and recipient prior to solid organ transplantation. *Am J Transplant* 2009;9(suppl 4):S7–S18.

3. Holty JE, Sista RR. Mycobacterium tuberculosis infection in transplant recipients: early diagnosis and treatment of resistant tuberculosis. *Curr Opin Organ Transplant* 2009;14(6): 613–618.

4. Hirsch HH, Randhawa P. BK virus in solid organ transplant recipients. *Am J Transplant* 2009;9(suppl 4):S136–S146.

5. Levitsky J, Doucette K. Viral hepatitis in solid organ. *Am* transplant recipients. *J Transplant* 2009;9(suppl 4):S116–S130.

6. Singh N, Paterson DL. Mycobacterium tuberculosis infection in solid-organ transplant recipients: impact and implications for management. *Clin Infect Dis* 1998;27(5): 1266–1277.

7. Munoz P, Rodriguez C, et al. Mycobacterium tuberculosis infection in recipients of solid organ transplants. *Clin Infect Dis* 2005;40(4):581–587.

8. Aguado JM, Torre-Cisneros J, et al. Tuberculosis in solid-organ transplant recipients: consensus statement of the group for the study of infection in transplant recipients (GESITRA) of the Spanish Society of Infectious Diseases and Clinical Microbiology. *Clin Infect Dis* 2009;48(9):1276–1284.

9. Subramanian A, Dorman S. Mycobacterium tuberculosis in solid organ transplant recipients. *Am J Transplant* 2009;9(suppl 4):S57–S62.

10. Mazurek GH, Jereb J, et al. Updated guidelines for using Interferon Gamma Release Assays to detect Mycobacterium tuberculosis infection—United States, 2010. *MMWR Recomm Rep* 2010;59(RR-5):1–25.

11. Theodoropoulos N, Lanternier F, et al. Use of the QuantiFERON-TB Gold interferon-gamma release assay for screening transplant candidates: a single-center retrospective study. *Transpl Infect Dis* 2012;14(1):1–8.

12. CDC. Treatment Options for Latent Tuberculosis Infection. Retrieved January 18, 2012, from http://www.cdc.gov/tb/publications/factsheets/treatment/LTBItreatmentoptions.htm.

13. Sterling TR, Villarino ME, et al. Three months of rifapentine and isoniazid for latent tuberculosis infection. *N Engl J Med* 2011;365(23):2155–2166.

14. Antony SJ, Ynares C, et al. Isoniazid hepatotoxicity in renal transplant recipients. *Clin Transplant* 1997;11(1):34–37.

15. Yee D,Valiquette C, et al. Incidence of serious side effects from first-line antituberculosis drugs among patients treated for active tuberculosis. *Am J Respir Crit Care Med* 2003;167(11):1472–1477.

16. Dromer C, Nashef SA, et al. Tuberculosis in transplanted lungs. *J Heart Lung Transplant* 1993;12(6 Pt 1):924–927.

17. Aguado JM, Herrero JA, et al. Clinical presentation and outcome of tuberculosis in kidney, liver, and heart transplant recipients in Spain. Spanish Transplantation Infection Study Group, GESITRA. *Transplantation* 1997;63(9):1278–1286.

18. Ho CC, Chen YC, et al. Safety of fluoroquinolone use in patients with hepatotoxicity induced by anti-tuberculosis regimens. *Clin Infect Dis* 2009;48(11):1526–1533.

19. Mandell GL, Bennett JE, et al. *Mandell, Douglas, and Bennett's principles and practice of infectious diseases.* Philadelphia, PA: Churchill Livingstone/Elsevier; 2010.

20. Humar A, Snydman D. Cytomegalovirus in solid organ transplant recipients. *Am J Transplant* 2009;9(suppl 4):S78–S86.

21. Kotton CN, Kumar D, et al. International consensus guidelines on the management of cytomegalovirus in solid organ transplantation. *Transplantation* 2010;89(7):779–795.

22. Fishman JA, Rubin RH. Infection in organ-transplant recipients. *N Engl J Med* 1998;338(24):1741–1751.

23. Humar A, Lebranchu Y, et al. The efficacy and safety of 200 days valganciclovir cytomegalovirus prophylaxis in high-risk kidney transplant recipients. *Am J Transplant* 2010;10(5):1228–1237.

24. Toupance O, Bouedjoro-Camus MC, et al. Cytomegalovirus-related disease and risk of acute rejection in renal transplant recipients: a cohort study with case-control analyses. *Transpl Int* 2000;13(6):413–419.

25. Cainelli F, Vento S. Infections and solid organ transplant rejection: a cause-and-effect relationship? *Lancet Infect Dis* 2002;2(9):539–549.

48 Community-Acquired Infections in Solid Organ Transplant Recipients

Tue H. Ngo

The risk of infection in solid organ transplant (SOT) recipients changes over time. More than 6 months after transplantation, the intensity of immunosuppression is decreased in recipients who have a good functioning allograft.[1] Their risk for most opportunistic infections declines in this late posttransplant period, and thus, other typical community-acquired infections predominate. SOT recipients may have manifestations from reactivated or chronic viral infections, such as varicella-zoster virus (VZV), hepatitis C virus (HCV), and hepatitis B virus (HBV).[1-3] A small group of patients who experience recurrent episodes of acute or chronic rejection, and thus require higher doses of immunosuppression, remain at high risk for opportunistic infections.[3]

Patients in the late posttransplant period usually reside in their home and are predisposed to community-acquired infections found in the general population, such as community-acquired bacterial pneumonia, urinary tract infection, and community respiratory viral infection. These infections may be more severe in the transplant population due to immunosuppression.[1-3] Organisms commonly identified in community-acquired bacterial pneumonia include *Streptococcus pneumoniae*, *Haemophilus influenzae*, and *Legionella* species. However, microorganisms may not be isolated from cultures in bacterial pneumonia.[2,4] The incidence of invasive pneumococcal disease is 12.8-fold greater among SOT recipients compared to the general population with 90% of infections associated with bacteremia.[5]

SOT recipients are at risk for illnesses due to community-acquired respiratory viruses such as rhinovirus, coronavirus, respiratory syncytial virus, influenza, parainfluenza, human metapneumovirus, and adenovirus. Common presenting symptoms include coryza, cough, sore throat, dyspnea, and fever.[6,7] A high rate of progression to lower respiratory tract infection has been reported, with 26% of patients with influenza and parainfluenza infection progressed to viral pneumonia in one study.[7] Community respiratory viruses can also have an indirect effect on the graft as well, possibly leading to increased risk for graft rejection.[6-8] Among 21 SOT recipients with influenza at the University of Pittsburgh who had a biopsy performed on their transplanted organs, 62% showed acute rejection in their lung or kidney grafts.[8]

Reactivation of latent infections can also occur during this period. *Mycobacterium tuberculosis* infection after transplantation is typically due to reactivation of a latent infection, although donor transmission, community acquisition, and nosocomial acquisition have been described. The incidence of tuberculosis (TB) varies from 0.35% to 15% among SOT recipients worldwide[9] and occurs at a median of 6 to 9 months posttransplant, with the majority (63% to 95%) of cases diagnosed within the first year after transplantation.[9,10] TB most commonly involves the lungs (>70%)[9,10];

however, extrapulmonary TB (16%) and disseminated infection (33%) have been described. Radiographic pulmonary presentation is variable, ranging from focal infiltrate to a miliary pattern, nodules, pleural effusions, diffuse interstitial infiltrates, and cavitary disease.[9] TB-attributable mortality remains high with a reported incidence of 9.5%.[10] The recommended initial phase of treatment for active TB includes isoniazid (INH), rifampin (RIF), pyrazinamide (PZA), and ethambutol (EMB) for the first 2 months. If the TB isolate is sensitive to INH, RIF, and PZA, then EMB can be discontinued. Then, treatment is tapered generally to INH and RIF in the continuation phase. Treatment regimen and duration should be guided by an expert in treating these patients.[11] Drug-drug interactions occur between RIF and the immunosuppressant medications with RIF significantly reducing the serum concentrations of cyclosporine, tacrolimus, sirolimus, and everolimus. Graft rejection has been reported with subtherapeutic immunosuppressant levels due to interactions with RIF, and thus, close monitoring of drug levels is warranted. Rifabutin, a weaker inducer of cytochrome P3A4, may have less drug interactions and result in more manageable immunosuppressant levels and thus, provides an alternative to RIF.[11] Hepatotoxicity due to INH is a concern in particular among liver transplant recipients, and hepatotoxicity can be increased in conjunction with RIF. Close monitoring of liver function tests is needed.[9,11]

Infections in the late posttransplant period usually occur as a result of reactivated or chronic viral infections.[1-3] VZV in SOT recipients typically manifests as herpes zoster (HZ), representing predominantly reactivation disease, but cases of primary community-acquired infection have been reported.[12] HZ is characterized by a painful, vesicular rash in a dermatomal distribution, which can involve one or two adjacent dermatomes, and can be associated with risk for cutaneous and visceral dissemination. Patients may experience pain and paresthesia a few days prior to the development of rash.[12] The overall incidence of HZ is 8.6% among SOT recipients, and the median time to development of disease is 9 months, with 63% of recipients experiencing HZ by 12 months after transplantation. Postherpetic neuralgia developed in 43% of patients in one study.[13]

Primary infection with JC virus (JCV), a polyomavirus, typically occurs at a young age with establishment of a latent infection. Reactivation of JCV can induce progressive multifocal leukoencephalopathy (PML), which is a demyelinating disease of the central nervous system. Neurologic deficit is the hallmark of PML, characterized by motor, sensory, visual deficit, ataxia, cognitive, or behavioral changes.[14] Disease develops at a median of 17 months posttransplantation with 71% of cases diagnosed within 24 months after transplantation.[15] MRI of the brain demonstrates T1 hypointense, T2 hyperintense lesions in the subcortical areas, cerebellum, and brain stem without enhancement or mass effect.[16] Brain biopsy is needed for definitive diagnosis. If a tissue sample cannot be obtained, then the diagnosis can be suggested by the constellation of compatible clinical history, characteristic MRI findings, and JCV DNA in the cerebrospinal fluid.[14] Treatment for PML in transplant recipients involves decreasing immunosuppression. There is no effective antiviral agent for treatment of PML.[14,15]

Posttransplantation lymphoproliferative disorder (PTLD) is the most important disease associated with Epstein-Barr virus (EBV) infection in SOT recipients. PTLD results from abnormal lymphoid proliferation.[17,18] The spectrum of disease can range from an infectious mononucleosis-like syndrome to B cell lymphoma, T cell lymphoma, or Hodgkin lymphoma. The disease can be nodal or extranodal involving the gastrointestinal tract, thorax, brain, or other parts of the body; localized or

Table 48-1	Risk Factors for Posttransplantation Lymphoproliferative Disorders
Early PTLD	Primary Epstein-Barr virus infection
	Cytomegalovirus mismatch or cytomegalovirus disease
	Young recipient age
	Type of organ transplanted
	OKT3 and polyclonal antilymphocyte antibodies
Late PTLD	Older recipient age
	Type of organ transplanted
	Duration of immunosuppression

From Cockfield SM. Identifying the patient at risk for posttransplant lymphoproliferative disorder. *Transpl Infect Dis* 2001;3:70–78, with permission from John Wiley & Sons.

disseminated; and with the allograft often affected.[2,17,18] EBV has been etiologically associated with the development of most cases of PTLD in particular with disease occurring within the first year after transplantation. Late PTLD commonly occurs at >3 to 5 years posttransplantation and tends to have EBV negative lesions.[17,18] The incidence of PTLD varies for the type of organ transplanted: 1% for kidneys, 2.2% for liver, 3.4% for heart, 1.8% to 7.9% for lung, 9.4% for heart-lung, 7% to 11% for intestine, and 13% to 33% for multivisceral organs.[19] The risk factors for PTLD are shown in Table 48-1.

PTLD diagnosis is made by pathologic examination of tissue. High EBV viral load in the blood has been observed in SOT recipients with PTLD. However, the clinical utility of EBV viral load testing to predict PTLD needs to be further evaluated.[18] The initial treatment for PTLD involves reduction or cessation of immunosuppression, if possible. Surgical resection or local irradiation can be used as adjunctive therapy for localized PTLD lesions. Antiviral agents, such as acyclovir and ganciclovir, have been employed in the treatment of PTLD, but there have been no prospective studies that provide evidence to support their effectiveness in treating PTLD alone. Additional strategies used in the treatment of PTLD include anti–CD20 monoclonal antibody and cytotoxic chemotherapy, and adoptive immunotherapy is being investigated.[17,18]

Without a preventive treatment strategy, cytomegalovirus (CMV) infection has been reported to occur in 36% to 100% of SOT recipients with symptomatic CMV disease occurring in 11% to 72% of recipients usually during the first 3 months after transplantation. Currently, antiviral prophylaxis is routinely administered, resulting in reduced incidence of early CMV disease.[20] However, after discontinuation of antiviral prophylaxis, late-onset CMV disease can occur, usually 3 to 6 months after transplantation or sometimes later following a standard 3-month course of antiviral prophylaxis.[21] Clinical manifestations of CMV infection range from asymptomatic infection to CMV disease, with the latter classified as CMV syndrome or tissue invasive disease. CMV syndrome is characterized by fever, malaise, elevated liver function tests, leukopenia, or thrombocytopenia. Tissue invasive disease can present as pneumonitis, hepatitis, gastrointestinal tract disease, retinitis, nephritis, or other end-organ involvement.[2,21] The incidence of late-onset CMV disease varies from 7% to 29% in SOT recipients, with CMV syndrome observed in 5% to 14% and invasive tissue disease in 3% to 15%. Late-onset CMV disease occurs at a median of 1.5 to 2 months after completing 3 months of antiviral prophylaxis.[22–24] Extending the duration of antiviral prophylaxis beyond the standard 3 months may reduce the incidence of late-onset CMV disease.[25] Very late-onset CMV disease occurring more than 1 year after transplantation has been described. In one study, 8.5% of liver transplant recipients developed very late-onset CMV disease at a mean of 5.9 years posttransplant. Patients commonly presented with fever and hepatitis, with pneumonitis and retinitis observed less frequently.[26] Atypical very late-onset CMV disease at a median of 25 months after transplantation (range, 6 months to 22 years) has been described occurring in the absence of recent rejection. Many patients had atypical presentation reflected by leukocytosis, normal platelet count, normal liver function tests, and lack of fever.[27]

CMV infection has been implicated in chronic allograft injury. CMV has been associated with bronchiolitis obliterans syndrome (BOS), a form of chronic allograft rejection in lung transplant recipients.[28] Recipients with BOS are susceptible to recurrent bronchitis and pneumonia.[2,4] Among heart transplant recipients, CMV has been implicated in the pathogenesis of accelerated cardiac allograft vasculopathy, characterized by graft arteriosclerosis.[29] Among liver transplant recipients, CMV has been associated with vanishing bile duct syndrome, a manifestation of chronic liver rejection.[30]

Prior to the routine use of posttransplant antiviral prophylaxis, HBV recurrence in the liver allograft was high and associated with graft loss. The use of hepatitis B immune globulin (HBIG) and antiviral agents is effective in preventing recurrent HBV infection in the liver graft. The risk of HBV recurrence has decreased to ≤10% 1 to 2 years after transplantation with combined HBIG and lamivudine prophylaxis.[31] A high rate of HBV recurrence of 35% to 40% in the first 2 to 3 years after transplantation has been observed with lamivudine monotherapy prophylaxis, and it is not recommended. For patients with lamivudine resistance, alternative anti–HBV agents are available, including adefovir, entecavir, tenofovir, emtricitabine, and telbivudine.[31] The efficacy of using only antiviral prophylaxis following discontinuation of HBIG after a defined period posttransplantation is being investigated and has been demonstrated to be effective in preventing recurrent HBV infection in the liver graft.[32] Surveillance for HBV recurrence with viral load monitoring is necessary posttransplantation to detect for recurrence of infection. HBV treatment should be changed if HBV viral load >3 log copies/mL is persistently detected.[31]

Reinfection of the allograft with HCV is universal for liver transplant recipients with HCV viremia prior to transplantation.[33] Histologic recurrence of HCV hepatitis in the liver allograft has been reported to occur in 40% to 88% of patients posttransplant.[34,35] The proportion of recipients with HCV-induced graft cirrhosis varies from 6% to 18% occurring at a median of 25.6 to 44.4 months posttransplantation.[35,36] After the onset of graft cirrhosis, progression of recurrent HCV infection is accelerated. The cumulative probability of developing liver decompensation is 30% at 1 year from diagnosis of cirrhosis, and the probability of survival at 1 year is 46% following onset of decompensation.[36] Current antiviral treatment for recurrent HCV infection posttransplantation includes ribavirin and pegylated interferon. Combination therapy with (pegylated) interferon and ribavirin results in sustained virologic response (SVR) rates of 37% to 42%. Clinical benefits are observed in patients who have SVR. Patients with SVR have a histologic response with decreased or stable fibrosis and improved inflammatory activity, are less likely to progress to graft cirrhosis, and have a higher 5-year survival rate compared to nonresponders.[37,38] Two protease inhibitors, Boceprevir and Telaprevir, have recently been approved for the treatment of HCV genotype 1 infection in conjunction with peginterferon and ribavirin. However, the use of protease inhibitors in treating recurrent HCV infection posttransplantation needs to be evaluated.

SOT recipients who have recurrent episodes of acute and chronic rejection require higher doses of immunosuppression and thus have continued risk for community-acquired opportunistic infections.[3] Some of the opportunistic pathogens causing infections include CMV (discussed above), *Cryptococcus neoformans*, *Pneumocystis carinii*, *Listeria monocytogenes*, and *Nocardia* species. These patients are also at risk for invasive fungal infections due to *Aspergillus* species, dematiaceous molds, and mucormycosis. Infection due to unusual organisms such as *Rhodococcus* has also been reported.[1,3]

REFERENCES

1. Fishman JA. Infection in solid-organ transplant recipients. *N Engl J Med* 2007;357: 2601–2614.
2. Dummer JS, Singh N. Infections in solid organ transplant recipients. In: Mandell GL, Bennett JE, Dolin R, eds. *Mandell, Douglas, and Bennett's principles and practice of infectious diseases*. 7th ed. Philadelphia, PA: Churchill Livingstone Elsevier; 2010:3839–3850.
3. Patel R, Paya CV. Infections in solid-organ transplant recipients. *Clin Microbiol Rev* 1997;10:86–124.
4. Kotloff RM, Ahya VN, Crawford SW. Pulmonary complications of solid organ and hematopoietic stem cell transplantation. *Am J Respir Crit Care Med* 2004;170:22–48.
5. Kumar D, Humar A, Plevneshi A, et al. Invasive pneumococcal disease in solid organ transplant recipients-10 year prospective population surveillance. *Am J Transplant* 2007;7:1209–1214.
6. Kumar D, Erdman D, Keshavjee S, et al. Clinical impact of community-acquired respiratory viruses on bronchiolitis obliterans after lung transplant. *Am J Transplant* 2005;5: 2031–2036.
7. Vilchez R, McCurry K, Dauber J, et al. Influenza and parainfluenza respiratory viral infection requiring admission in adult lung transplant recipients. *Transplantation* 2002;73:1075–1078.
8. Vilchez RA, McCurry K, Dauber J, et al. Influenza virus infection in adult solid organ transplant recipients. *Am J Transplant* 2002;2:287–291.
9. Singh N, Paterson DL. *Mycobacterium tuberculosis* infection in solid-organ transplant recipients: impact and implications for management. *Clin Infect Dis* 1998;27:1266–1277.
10. Torre-Cisneros J, Doblas A, Aguado JM, et al. Tuberculosis after solid-organ transplant: incidence, risk factors, and clinical characteristics in the RESITRA cohort. *Clin Infect Dis* 2009;48:1657–1665.
11. Subramanian A, Dorman S. *Mycobacterium tuberculosis* in solid organ transplant recipients. *Am J Transplant* 2009;9(suppl 4):S57–S62.
12. Miller GG, Dummer JS. Herpes simplex and varicella zoster viruses: forgotten but not gone. *Am J Transplant* 2007;7:741–747.
13. Gourishankar S, McDermid JC, Jhangri GS, et al. Herpes zoster infection following solid organ transplantation: incidence, risk factors and outcomes in the current immunosuppressive era. *Am J Transplant* 2004;4:108–115.
14. Kwak EJ, Vilchez RA, Randhawa P, et al. Pathogenesis and management of polyomavirus infection in transplant recipients. *Clin Infect Dis* 2002;35:1081–1087.
15. Shitrit D, Lev N, Bar-Gil-Shitrit A, et al. Progressive multifocal leukoencephalopathy in transplant recipients. *Transpl Int* 2005;17:658–665.
16. Hirsch HH. Polyoma and papilloma virus infections after hematopoietic cell or solid organ transplantation. In: Bowden RA, Ljungman P, Snydman D, eds. *Transplant infections*. 3rd ed. Philadelphia, PA: Lippincott Williams & Wilkins; 2010:465–482.
17. Evens AM, Roy R, Sterrenbert D, et al. Post-transplantation lymphoproliferative disorders: diagnosis, prognosis, and current approaches to therapy. *Curr Oncol Rep* 2010;12:383–394.
18. Allen U, Preiksaitis J.Epstein-Barr virus and posttransplant lymphoproliferative disorder in solid organ transplant recipients. *Am J Transplant* 2009;9(suppl 4):S87–S96.

19. Cockfield SM. Identifying the patient at risk for post-transplant lymphoproliferative disorder. *Transpl Infect Dis* 2001;3:70–78.

20. Sun H, Wagener MM, Singh N. Prevention of posttransplant cytomegalovirus disease and related outcomes with valganciclovir: a systematic review. *Am J Transplant* 2008;8: 2111–2118.

21. Humar A, Snydman D. Cytomegalovirus in solid organ transplant recipients. *Am J Transplant* 2009;9(suppl 4):S78–S86.

22. Arthurs SK, Eid AJ, Pedersen RA, et al. Delayed-onset primary cytomegalovirus disease and the risk of allograft failure and mortality after kidney transplantation. *Clin Infect Dis* 2008;46:840–846.

23. Akalin E, Sehgal V, Ames S, et al. Cytomegalovirus disease in high-risk transplant recipients despite ganciclovir or valganciclovir prophylaxis. *Am J Transplant* 2003;3:731–735

24. Limaye AP, Bakthavatsalam R, Kim HW, et al. Late-onset cytomegalovirus disease in liver transplant recipients despite antiviral prophylaxis. *Transplantation* 2004;78:1390–1396.

25. Humar A, Lebranchu Y, Vincenti F, et al. The efficacy and safety of 200 days of valganciclovir cytomegalovirus prophylaxis in high-risk kidney transplant recipients. *Am J Transplant* 2010;10:1228–1237.

26. Shibolet O, Ilan Y, Kalish Y, et al. Late cytomegalovirus disease following liver transplantation. *Transpl Int* 2003;16:861–865.

27. Slifkin M, Tempesti P, Poutsiaka DD, et al. Late and atypical cytomegalovirus disease in solid-organ transplant recipients. *Clin Infect Dis* 2001;33:e62–e68.

28. Westall GP, Michaelides A, Williams TJ, et al. Bronchiolitis obliterans syndrome and early human cytomegalovirus DNAaemia dynamics after lung transplantation. *Transplantation* 2003;75:2064–2068

29. Fateh-Moghadam S, Bocksch W, Wessely R, et al. Cytomegalovirus infection status predicts progression of heart-transplant vasculopathy. *Transplantation* 2003;76:1470–1474.

30. Lautenschlager I, Hockerstedt K, Jalanko H, et al. Persistent cytomegalovirus in liver allografts with chronic rejection. *Hepatology* 1997;25:190–194.

31. Coffin CS, Terrault, NA. Management of hepatitis B in liver transplant recipients. *J Viral Hepat* 2007;14(suppl 1):37–44.

32. Saab S, Desai S, Tsaoi D, et al. Posttransplantation hepatitis B prophylaxis with combination oral nucleoside and nucleotide analog therapy. *Am J Transplant* 2011;11:511–517.

33. Gane E. The natural history and outcome of liver transplantation in hepatitis C virus-infected recipients. *Liver Transpl* 2003;9(suppl 3):S28–S34.

34. Gane EJ, Portmann BC, Naoumov NV, et al. Long-term outcome of hepatitis C infection after liver transplantation. *N Engl J Med* 1996;334:815–820.

35. Testa G, Crippin JS, Netto GJ, et al. Liver transplantation for hepatitis C: recurrence and disease progression in 300 patients. *Liver Transpl* 2000;6:553–561.

36. Firpi RJ, Clark V, Soldevila-Pico C, et al. The natural history of hepatitis C cirrhosis after liver transplantation. *Liver Transpl* 2009;15:1063–1071.

37. Bizollon T, Pradat P, Mabrut JY, et al. Benefit of sustained virological response to combination therapy on graft survival of liver transplanted patients with recurrent chronic hepatitis C. *Am J Transplant* 2005;5:1909–1913.

38. Berenguer M, Palau A, Aguilera V, et al. Clinical benefits of antiviral therapy in patients with recurrent hepatitis C following liver transplantation. *Am J Transplant* 2008;8:679–687.

XI Foodborne Infections

Foodborne Illness

Paras Patel and James W. Myers

INTRODUCTION

According to a report from the Centers of Disease Control and Prevention, foodborne illnesses account for approximately 76 million illnesses, leading to 325,000 hospitalizations and 5,000 deaths each year in the United States.

Diarrheal diseases represent one of the five leading causes of death worldwide. Morbidity and mortality are significant even in the United States, where diarrhea is more often than not a "nuisance disease" in the normally healthy individual.

DEFINITIONS

- Clinically, *diarrhea* is defined as stool weight in excess of 200 g/day or more than or equal to three loose or watery stools per day, or a definite decrease in consistency and increase in frequency based upon an individual baseline.
- Diarrhea reflects increased water content of the stool, whether due to impaired water absorption and/or active water secretion by the bowel.
- In *severe infectious diarrhea*, the number of stools may reach 20 or more per day, with defecation occurring every 20 or 30 minutes. In this situation, the total daily volume of stool may exceed 2 L, with resultant volume depletion and hypokalemia.
- Most patients with acute diarrhea have three to seven movements per day with total stool volume <1 L/day.
- When diarrhea lasts for 14 days, it can be considered *persistent*; the term *chronic* generally refers to diarrhea that lasts for at least 1 month.

The following definitions have been suggested according to the duration of diarrhea (Table 49-1).

PATHOGENIC MECHANISMS IN FOODBORNE ILLNESS

- The following divides foodborne diseases into a variety of syndromes, mostly based on signs and symptoms and time of onset after consumption of contaminated food, and indicates the agents most likely responsible for the illness (Table 49-2).
- If the pathogen makes the toxin before the food is eaten, the onset of symptoms will be sooner, around 6 hours, and primarily be vomiting or other upper intestinal in nature.
- On the other hand, if the toxin is made after ingestion, the symptoms will take longer, around 24 hours, and be more of a watery diarrhea illness.
- Pathogens that damage or invade tissue are often associated with fever and systemic illness, but a variety of symptoms are possible.

Table 49-1	Definitions of Diarrhea	
Entity	**Days**	**Comment**
Diarrhea		Diarrhea is defined as stool weight in excess of 200 g/day
Acute	<14	
Persistent	>14	
Chronic	>30	
Severe		The number of stools may reach 20 or more per day, with defecation occurring every 20 or 30 minutes. In this situation, the total daily volume of stool may exceed 2 L, with resultant volume depletion and hypokalemia.

FOODBORNE DISEASE SYNDROMES

• Most cases of acute diarrhea are due to infections with viruses and bacteria and are self-limited.
• Noninfectious etiologies become more common as the course of the diarrhea persists and becomes chronic.
• The evaluation of patients for a noninfectious etiology should be considered in those patients in whom evaluation fails to identify a pathogen (e.g., bacterial, viral, or protozoal) and the diarrhea worsens or becomes chronic.

TABLE 49-2	Major Pathogenic Mechanisms in Some Foodborne Illness		
Preformed Bacterial Toxin	**Toxin Production In Vivo**	**Tissue Invasion**	**Seafood Toxins**
Staphylococcus aureus	Clostridium perfringens	Campylobacter jejuni	Ciguatera
Bacillus cereus[a]	Shiga toxin–producing E. coli	Salmonella	Paralytic shellfish poisoning
Clostridium botulinum	C. botulinum	Shigella	Scombroid
	Enterotoxigenic E. coli	Invasive E. coli	Poisonous mushrooms
	Vibrio cholerae O1 or O139	Listeria monocytogenes	
	Clostridium difficile	Yersinia enterocolitica?	
	V. cholerae non-O1	Norovirus?	
		Cryptosporidium, Cyclospora, Giardia?	

[a]Also has a long incubation form with toxin production in vivo.

- Foodborne disease can appear as an isolated sporadic case or, less frequently, as an outbreak of illnesses affecting a group of people after a common food exposure.
  - The diagnosis of foodborne disease should be considered when an acute illness, especially one with gastrointestinal or neurologic manifestations, affects two or more people who had shared a common meal.
  - Important clues to the etiologic agent are provided by the signs and symptoms of affected persons and the incubation period.
  - The incubation period in an individual illness is usually unknown, but it is often apparent in the focal outbreak setting.
- Tables 49-3 and 49-4 divide foodborne diseases into a variety of syndromes, mostly based on signs and symptoms and time of onset after consumption of contaminated food, and indicate the agents most likely responsible for the illness see Table 49-5 for a comparison of common foodborne illnesses.

TREATMENT

- Often, the most important measures are general ones such as hydration and alteration of diet.
- Antibiotic therapy is **not required** in most cases.
- The treatment of specific infections is listed in Tables 49-6 and 49-7.
- Antimotility agents can occasionally be helpful:
  - Loperamide is useful in those patients in whom **fever is absent** or low grade and the **stools are not bloody**.
  - **In two randomized controlled studies, loperamide compared with placebo significantly decreased the number of liquid bowel movements or diarrhea when given with ciprofloxacin. The dose of loperamide is two tablets (4 mg) initially, then 2 mg after each unformed stool, not to exceed 16 mg/day for ≤2 days**.
  - Diphenoxylate (Lomotil) is an alternative agent, but it has not been studied in randomized controlled studies.
  - The dose of diphenoxylate is two tablets (4 mg) four times daily for ≤2 days. Diphenoxylate has central opiate effects and may cause cholinergic side effects.
  - Note that both drugs can precipitate the development of the hemolytic uremic syndrome (HUS) in patients infected with Enterohemorrhagic E. coli (EHEC).
- Bismuth subsalicylate (Pepto-Bismol) has also been used for symptomatic treatment of acute diarrhea.
  - When compared with placebo, bismuth subsalicylate significantly reduced the number of unformed stools and increased the proportion of patients free of symptoms at the end of treatment trials.
  - **However, in studies that compared bismuth subsalicylate with loperamide, loperamide brought significantly faster relief**.
  - A role for bismuth subsalicylate may be in patients with significant fever and dysentery, **conditions in which loperamide should be avoided**.
  - The dose of bismuth subsalicylate is 30 mL or two tablets every 30 minutes for eight doses.
- Probiotics, including bacteria that assist in recolonizing the intestine with non-pathogenic flora, can also be used as alternative therapy.
- Probiotics have been shown to be useful in treating traveler's diarrhea and acute nonspecific diarrhea in children.

Table 49-3	Infectious Syndromes			

Syndrome	Etiology	Pathogenesis	Clinical Features	Associated Foods
Nausea and vomiting within 1–6 hours	*S. aureus, B. cereus*[a]	Preformed enterotoxins, heat-resistant toxins; food may not smell or look bad.	Severe nausea and vomiting, very little fever with *Staph*, short duration of illness (12–24 hours); patients with this illness are not contagious. Toxins are not transmitted from one person to another. Supportive care	*S. aureus:* unrefrigerated meats, potato, or egg salad, cream-filled pastries *B. cereus:* fried rice, meats, vegetables
Abdominal cramps and diarrhea within 8–16 hours	*C. perfringens* and *B. cereus*	Enterotoxin mediated; toxin is not preformed.	Watery diarrhea, nausea, abdominal cramps. Vomiting is NOT a major feature in these illnesses.	Meats, poultry, gravy, time- or temperature-abused food
Fever, abdominal cramps, and diarrhea within 6–48 hours	*C. jejuni, E. coli, Salmonella, Shigella,* and *Vibrio parahaemolyticus.*	Tissue invasion	Diarrhea, **fever,** abdominal cramps, vomiting	Contaminated eggs, poultry, unpasteurized milk or juice, contaminated water
Abdominal cramps and watery diarrhea within 16–72 hours	Enterotoxigenic strains of *E. coli* (ETEC), *V. parahaemolyticus, V. cholerae* non-O1, and, in endemic areas, *V. cholerae* O1 and O139; *C. jejuni, Salmonella,* and *Shigella*	Enterotoxins	Watery diarrhea, abdominal cramps, nausea, and vomiting	Water or food contaminated with human feces, undercooked or raw seafood such as fish, shellfish
Vomiting and nonbloody diarrhea within 24–48 hours	Noroviruses[b]	Tissue invasion	Vomiting, diarrhea, abdominal pain, and nausea; **fever occurs in one-third** to one-half of patients, is usually low grade, and lasts for <24 hours. Cruise ships; aerosol transmission is possible. Very contagious, low infectious dose, no lasting immunity	Salads, shellfish

Fever and abdominal cramps within 16–48 hours, without diarrhea	*Y. enterocolitica*	Tissue invasion	May closely resemble acute appendicitis in older children and adults. Nausea and vomiting are relatively uncommon, occurring in <25%–40% of the cases. Illness can last up to 4 weeks.	Milk, pork, chitterlings
Bloody diarrhea without fever within 72–120 hours	*E. coli* most often serotype O157:H7	Shiga toxin or verotoxins	Severe diarrhea, often bloody, abdominal pain, and vomiting, little or no fever	Undercooked beef, especially hamburger; unpasteurized milk and juice; raw fruits and vegetables
Nausea, vomiting, diarrhea, and paralysis within 18–36 hours	*C. botulinum*	Heat-labile protein neurotoxins	Vomiting, diarrhea, blurred vision, diplopia, dysphagia, and descending muscle weakness	Home-canned foods with low acid content, improperly canned commercial foods
Persistent diarrhea within 1–3 weeks	Cyclosporiasis, cryptosporidiosis, giardiasis, and Brainerd diarrhea	Tissue invasion	Watery diarrhea, anorexia, weight loss, abdominal cramps, nausea, and body aches; vomiting and low-grade fever may be noted.	Contaminated water and food, milk

[a]Food handler contaminates it and leaves the food at room temperature. Vomitus or food can be tested for toxin if necessary for *Bacillus* or *Staphylococcus*.
[b]RT-PCR useful for diagnosis.

Table 49-4	Foodborne Disease Syndromes Caused by Nonbacterial Toxins		
Syndromes	**Etiology**	**Signs and Symptoms**	**Associated Foods**
Nausea, vomiting, and abdominal cramps within 1 hour	Heavy metals such as copper, zinc, tin, and cadmium	Nausea, vomiting, and abdominal cramps result from direct irritation of the gastric and intestinal mucosa and usually resolve with 2–3 hours if minor amounts are ingested.May result to serious illness and even death if larger amounts are ingested.	Acidic beverages
Paresthesias within 1 hour	Histamine fish poisoning (scombroid)[a]	**Flushing**, rash, burning sensation of skin, mouth and throat, dizziness, **urticaria**, paresthesias	Fish: bluefin, **tuna**, mackerel, **marlin**, mahi mahi, contaminated dark meat fish; decarboxylated histidine is responsible, self-limited, but responds to antihistamines.
	Paralytic shellfish poisoning[b]	Diarrhea, nausea, vomiting leading to paresthesias of the mouth and lips, weakness, respiratory paralysis, death in 10%; shellfish taste normal. Heating or freezing does not affect the toxin.	Scallops, mussels, clams, often seen during a red tide along the northwest or northeast coasts; toxin is from Alexandrium dinoflagellates, blocks sodium channels.
Paresthesias within 1–6 hours	Ciguatera[c]	Supportive care Gastrointestinal: abdominal pain, nausea, vomiting, diarrhea Neurologic: paresthesias, **reversal of hot and cold**, pain, weakness, **painful teeth** Cardiovascular: bradycardia, hypotension, heart block	A variety of large reef fish, grouper, **red snapper**, **amberjack**, and barracuda tastes normal. Dinoflagellates of the genus Gambierdiscus produce the toxin.

Abdominal cramps and diarrhea within 6–24 hours, followed by hepatorenal failure	Poisonous mushrooms	The illness is typically biphasic; the abdominal cramps and diarrhea, which may be severe, usually resolve within 24 hours. The patient then remains well for 1–2 days before evidence of hepatic and renal failure supervenes. A mortality rate of 20%–50% has been reported.	
Puffer fish syndrome	Tetrodotoxin-containing fish	Deadly toxin binds to sodium channels. Weakness, paralysis due to saxitoxin. Supportive care, edrophonium?	Japan: Fugu, blowfish
PEAS	Estuary syndrome from a neurotoxin-mediated Pfiesteria dinoflagellate illness	Eye irritation, cramps, vomiting, neurocognitive changes, visual contrast sensitivity may improve with cholestyramine.	Fish kills and ulcers along Maryland's eastern shore

[a]Histamine levels are >50 to 100mg per 100g fish if measured. Usually a clinical diagnosis.

[b]Neurotoxic shellfish poisoning is found in the southeast and causes an aerosolized red tide syndrome from inhaled sea spray resulting in rhinorrhea and asthmatic symptoms. It also causes a gastrointestinal/paresthesia syndrome after eating shellfish contaminated with Gymnodinium breve dinoflagellate toxins. Diarrhetic shellfish poisoning is found worldwide and causes diarrhea secondary to okadaic acid toxins. Amnestic shellfish poisoning results from ingestion of the heat-stable domoic acid toxin found in mussels eaten in Canada. Glutamate analogue causes anterograde memory loss in survivors.

[c]No commercially available tests. Mannitol if often used but no good evidence to suggest that it is better than saline.

Table 49-5 Domestically Acquired Common Foodborne Illness

Species	Clinical Features	Most Common Route of Transmission	Stool Findings	Complications	Outbreaks[a]	Case Per 100,000 Person According to Fed Net Data in 2007
Norovirus	Vomiting, diarrhea, and abdominal pain	Noroviruses spread from person to person, through contaminated food or water and by touching contaminated surfaces.	Nonbloody, lack mucous, and may be loose to watery; fecal leukocytes are not seen.	NA	The epidemic form of family and community-wide outbreaks	NA
Salmonella, nontyphoidal	Abdominal cramps, headache myalgia, fever	Ingestion of poultry, eggs, and milk products; nontyphoidal Salmonellae have been associated with fresh produce, meats, milk, and other foodstuff.	Watery, may have WBC	NA	Most recent outbreak was associated with eating food from a Mexican-style fast food restaurant chain in 2012 linked to ground beef.	13.9
E. coli (STEC) O157	Abdominal pain, often bloody diarrhea, fever	Ingestion of undercooked ground beef	Stool sample cultures	Hemolytic uremic syndrome	Most recent multistate outbreak in 2011 reported due to romaine lettuce.	0.99

Campylobacter spp.	Abdominal cramp, bloody diarrhea, fever, myalgia	Ingestion of poultry	Stool cultures	Guillain-Barre syndrome	Most recent outbreak in February 2012 from consumption of raw dairy milk.	13.02
Shigella	Abdominal cramp, fever, diarrhea	Direct person-to-person spread as well as from contaminated food and water	Stool culture	Reiter syndrome	NA	3.99
L. monocytogenes	Fever, abdominal pain, diarrhea	Acquired by humans primarily through consumption of contaminated food	Stool culture, blood culture	Fetal loss in pregnant patient, cause invasive disease, including sepsis and meningo-encephalitis	Most recent outbreak in September 2011 associated with cantaloupe	NA

[a]http://www.cdc.gov/outbreaknet/outbreaks.html#201.

Table 49-6   Antimicrobial Therapy in Bacterial Diarrhea

Diarrheal Disease	Treatment	Dose	Comment
Shigellosis, Aeromonas species diarrhea, Plesiomonas shigelloides diarrhea, enteroinvasive E. coli infection	FQ or azithromycin	Ciprofloxacin, 750 mg once a day for 3 days; or azithromycin, 500 mg once a day for 3 days	Immunocompromised patients for 10–14 days
Enterotoxigenic E. coli diarrhea, enteroaggregative E. coli diarrhea, or traveler's diarrhea	FQ or azithromycin or rifaximin	One of the following: ciprofloxacin, 750 mg once a day for 1–3 days; azithromycin, 1,000 mg in a single dose; or rifaximin, 200 mg thrice daily for 3 days	
Shiga toxin–producing E. coli infection, including E. coli O157:H7 infection	None	None	
Cholera (due to Vibrio cholerae 01)	Doxycycline or tetracycline macrolide	Doxycycline, 300 mg in a single dose; or tetracycline, 500 mg four times a day for 3 days; or macrolide (erythromycin, 250 mg thrice daily; or azithromycin, 500 mg once a day) for 3 days	
Nontyphoid salmonellosis	None or FQ or macrolide	Levofloxacin, 500 mg (or other fluoroquinolone) once a day for 7–10 days; or azithromycin, 500 mg once a day for 7 days	Immunocompromised patients for 14 days
Enteric fever including typhoid fever	FQ or azithromycin	Levofloxacin, 500 mg (or other fluoroquinolone) once a day for 7 days; or azithromycin, 500 mg once a day for 7 days	
C. jejuni diarrhea	Macrolide	Azithromycin 500 mg once a day for 3 days, or erythromycin, 500 mg four times a day for 3 days	
Yersinia species	Antibiotics are often not required.	Doxycycline, aminoglycosides, TMP-SMZ, or fluoroquinolones	*Avoid FQ in children*

Table 49-7   Antimicrobial Therapy of Diarrhea: Nonbacterial Infections

Pathogen	First Choice	Second Choice	Comments
Entamoeba histolytica	Metronidazole 750 mg PO thrice daily for 10 days	Dehydroemetine 1 to 1.5 mg/kg/day IM for 5 days	A luminal amebicide for invasive intestinal infection and hepatic abscesses (iodoquinol 650 mg PO t.i.d. for 20 days or paromomycin 500 mg PO t.i.d. for 7 days); cyst passers without symptoms require luminicidal agent only.
Giardiasis	Metronidazole 250 mg PO thrice daily for 10 days	Tinidazole, quinacrine hydrochloride, furazolidone	Relapses may occur.
Cryptosporidium	No therapy proven effective	Nitazoxanide, paromomycin, TMP/SMX, azithromycin, or metronidazole	Benefit and duration of any therapy unclear, spontaneous resolution without specific therapy in immunocompetent hosts, and in HIV-infected individuals with CD4 counts above 150 cells/μL
Microsporidia	Albendazole 200–400 mg PO b.i.d. for 3 months		No treatment is determined in immunocompetent host. In immunocompromised host, albendazole is more effective for *Encephalitozoon intestinalis* than for *Enterocytozoon bieneusi*.
Isospora and *Cyclospora*	TMP/SMX 1 DS PO twice daily for 7–10 days		Maintenance therapy is required in immunocompromised patients.

- Boiled starches and cereals (e.g., potatoes, noodles, rice, wheat, and oats) with salt are indicated in patients with watery diarrhea; crackers, bananas, soup, and boiled vegetables may also be consumed. Foods with high fat content should also be avoided until the gut function returns to normal after a severe bout of diarrhea.
- Also note that *a secondary lactose malabsorption* is common following infectious diarrhea.
  - This might last for several weeks to months and should not be confused with a parasitic or other chronic diarrhea.
  - Consider temporary avoidance of lactose-containing foods until this resolves.
  - Attempting to repopulate the bowel flora with yogurt-containing live cultures or other probiotics has not been proven in adults.

SUGGESTED READINGS

Atmar RL, Bernstein DI, et al. Norovirus vaccine against experimental human Norwalk Virus illness. *N Engl J Med* 2011;365(23):2178–2187.
  This norovirus VLP vaccine provides protection against illness and infection after challenge with a homologous virus.
Beatty ME, Adcock PM, et al. Epidemic diarrhea due to enterotoxigenic *Escherichia coli. Clin Infect Dis* 2006;42(3):329–334.
  In the United States, where enterotoxigenic Escherichia coli is an emerging cause of foodborne disease, enterotoxigenic E. coli should be suspected in outbreaks of gastroenteritis when common bacterial or viral enteric pathogens are not identified.
Bresee JS, Widdowson MA, et al. Foodborne viral gastroenteritis: challenges and opportunities. *Clin Infect Dis* 2002;35(6):748–753.
Cohen ML. The epidemiology of diarrheal disease in the United States. *Infect Dis Clin North Am* 1988;2(3):557–570.
  Diarrheal disease remains an important health problem in the United States. The magnitude of this problem and the relative importance of bacterial, viral, and parasitic pathogens are examined. The often unique epidemiologic associations with specific organisms can be helpful not only in suggesting diagnoses in individual patients but also in the direction of public health action.
Dennehy PH. Acute diarrheal disease in children: epidemiology, prevention, and treatment. *Infect Dis Clin North Am* 2005;19(3):585–602.
DuPont HL. Guidelines on acute infectious diarrhea in adults. The Practice Parameters Committee of the American College of Gastroenterology. *Am J Gastroenterol* 1997;92(11):1962–1975.
DuPont HL, Flores Sanchez J, et al. Comparative efficacy of loperamide hydrochloride and bismuth subsalicylate in the management of acute diarrhea. *Am J Med* 1990;88(6A):15S–19S.
  An open-label, parallel comparison of loperamide hydrochloride (Imodium A-D) and bismuth subsalicylate (Pepto-Bismol) was conducted using nonprescription dosages in adult students with acute diarrhea (three or more unformed stools in the preceding 24 hours plus at least one additional symptom of enteric infection). For the 2-day study period, the daily dosage was limited to 8 mg (40 mL) for loperamide-treated subjects and to 4.9 g for bismuth subsalicylate–treated subjects. At these dosages, loperamide significantly reduced the average number of unformed bowel movements relative to bismuth subsalicylate. Following the initial dose of treatment, control of diarrhea was maintained significantly longer with loperamide than with bismuth subsalicylate. Time to last unformed stool was significantly shorter with loperamide than with bismuth subsalicylate. In providing overall subjective relief, subjects rated loperamide significantly better than bismuth subsalicylate at the end of the 24 hours. Both treatments were well tolerated, and none of the minor adverse effects reported resulted in discontinuation of therapy. It was concluded that loperamide is effective at a daily dosage limit of 8 mg (40 mL) for the treatment of acute nonspecific diarrhea and provides faster, more effective relief than bismuth subsalicylate.
Glass RI, Parashar UD, et al. Norovirus gastroenteritis. *N Engl J Med* 2009;361(18):1776–1785.

Guerrant RL, Van Gilder T, et al. Practice guidelines for the management of infectious diarrhea. *Clin Infect Dis* 2001;32(3):331–351.

Holmberg SD, Blake PA. Staphylococcal food poisoning in the United States. New facts and old misconceptions. *JAMA* 1984;251(4):487–489.

Hughes JM, Potter ME. Scombroid-fish poisoning. From pathogenesis to prevention. *N Engl J Med* 1991;324(11):766–768.

Imhoff B, Morse D, et al. Burden of self-reported acute diarrheal illness in FoodNet surveillance areas, 1998-1999. *Clin Infect Dis* 2004;38(suppl 3):S219–S226.

Johnson PC, Ericsson CD, et al. Comparison of loperamide with bismuth subsalicylate for the treatment of acute travelers' diarrhea. *JAMA* 1986;255(6):757–760.

Loperamide hydrochloride was compared with bismuth subsalicylate for the treatment of acute nondysenteric traveler's diarrhea in 219 students visiting seven countries in Latin America. Subjects whose condition was not improved with therapy could elect to take trimethoprim-sulfamethoxazole. Persons receiving loperamide passed fewer unformed stools when compared with the bismuth subsalicylate group during the first 4 hours of therapy, from 4 to 24 hours, and from 24 to 48 hours after therapy was initiated. Among subjects with disease due to enterotoxigenic E. coli, Shigella sp, other pathogens, and unknown agents, fewer unformed stools were passed by the loperamide-treated subjects than the bismuth subsalicylate–treated subjects for all time periods studied. No significant prolongation of disease was seen in subjects with shigellosis treated with loperamide. Eight of the loperamide-treated subjects experienced constipation compared with one in the bismuth subsalicylate–treated group; otherwise, there was no difference in minor side effects experienced between both treatment groups. We conclude that loperamide is a safe and effective alternative to bismuth subsalicylate for the treatment of nondysenteric traveler's diarrhea.

Le Loir Y, Baron F, et al. *Staphylococcus aureus* and food poisoning. *Genet Mol Res* 2003;2(1):63–76.

Lehane L, Olley J. Histamine fish poisoning revisited. *Int J Food Microbiol* 2000;58(1–2):1–37.

Lindsay JA. Chronic sequelae of foodborne disease. *Emerg Infect Dis* 1997;3(4):443–452.

Mead PS, Slutsker L, et al. Food-related illness and death in the United States. *Emerg Infect Dis* 1999;5(5):607–625.

Miller FH, Ma JJ, et al. Imaging features of enterohemorrhagic *Escherichia coli* colitis. *AJR Am J Roentgenol* 2001;177(3):619–623.

Morris JG Jr, Lewin P, et al. Clinical features of ciguatera fish poisoning: a study of the disease in the US Virgin Islands. *Arch Intern Med* 1982;142(6):1090–1092.

Cardiovascular signs and symptoms, including both hypotension and bradycardia, were noted in some acute cases. Therapy included antidiarrheal and antiemetic agents, intravenous fluids, atropine, and pralidoxime chloride. Efficacy of pralidoxime therapy could not be established on the basis of our data.

Musher DM, Musher BL. Contagious acute gastrointestinal infections. *N Engl J Med* 2004;351(23):2417–2427.

Outbreak of *Listeria monocytogenes* infections associated with pasteurized milk from a local dairy—Massachusetts, 2007. *MMWR Morb Mortal Wkly Rep* 2008;57(40):1097–1100.

Sandler RS, Everhart JE, et al. The burden of selected digestive diseases in the United States. *Gastroenterology* 2002;122(5):1500–1511.

Shandera WX, Tacket CO, et al. Food poisoning due to *Clostridium perfringens* in the United States. *J Infect Dis* 1983;147(1):167–170.

Siegler RL. The hemolytic uremic syndrome. *Pediatr Clin North Am* 1995;42(6):1505–1529.

Slutsker L, Ries AA, et al. *Escherichia coli* O157:H7 diarrhea in the United States: clinical and epidemiologic features. *Ann Intern Med* 1997;126(7):505–513.

Steffen R. Worldwide efficacy of bismuth subsalicylate in the treatment of travelers' diarrhea. *Rev Infect Dis* 1990;12(suppl 1):S80–S86.

Tarr PI, Gordon CA, et al. Shiga-toxin-producing *Escherichia coli* and haemolytic uraemic syndrome. *Lancet* 2005;365(9464):1073–1086.

The best way to prevent HUS is to prevent primary infection with Shiga toxin–producing bacteria.

Terranova W, Blake PA. *Bacillus cereus* food poisoning. *N Engl J Med* 1978;298(3):143–144.

Thornton AC, Jennings-Conklin KS, et al. Noroviruses: agents in outbreaks of acute gastroenteritis. *z* 2004;**2**(1):4–9.

This article provides an overview of noroviruses particularly as it relates to health care workers.

Wong CS, Jelacic S, et al. The risk of the hemolytic-uremic syndrome after antibiotic treatment of *Escherichia coli* O157:H7 infections. *N Engl J Med* 2000;342(26):1930–1936.

Antibiotic treatment of children with E. coli O157:H7 infection increases the risk of the HUS.

Zheng DP, Ando T, et al. Norovirus classification and proposed strain nomenclature. *Virology* 2006;346(2):312–323.

XII Intra-Abdominal Infections

50 Intra-Abdominal Infections

Jayalakshmi Kuseladass, Ashley Tyler, and Christopher Trabue

INTRODUCTION

Intra-abdominal infections represent a common and diverse group of infectious diseases. Appendicitis alone accounts for more than 300,000 hospital discharges annually. They are the second most common cause of sepsis and sepsis-related mortality behind pulmonary infections. **Identifying and controlling the source of such infections remains the cornerstone of management.**

EPIDEMIOLOGY AND CLASSIFICATION

I. UNCOMPLICATED—CONFINED TO HOLLOW VISCUS OF ORIGIN, 80% OF CASES

II. COMPLICATED—EXTENDS BEYOND HOLLOW VISCUS OF ORIGIN WITH ABSCESS FORMATION OR PERITONITIS

III. "HEALTH CARE ASSOCIATED" IS DEFINED AS EITHER

    a. Hospital onset (culture results >48 hours after hospital admission)

    b. Community onset in a patient with one of the following risk factors:

        i. Invasive device at the time of admission

        ii. History of methicillin-resistant *Staphylococcus aureus* (MRSA) infection or colonization

        iii. History of surgery, hospitalization, dialysis, or residence in a long-term care facility in past 12 months

IV. ETIOLOGY

    a. Appendicitis

    b. Pyogenic liver abscess

    c. Biliary infection

        i. Cholecystitis

        ii. Cholangitis

    d. Necrotizing pancreatitis

    e. Diverticulitis

    f. Health care–associated intra-abdominal infection (postoperative)

MICROBIOLOGY

I. COMMUNITY-ACQUIRED PATHOGENS

a. Enterobacteriaceae
  i. Microbiologic characteristics
    1. Gram-negative bacilli
    2. Facultative anaerobes (i.e., can survive in both aerobic and anaerobic conditions)
    3. Lactose fermenting
  ii. Examples: *Escherichia coli, Proteus mirabilis, Enterobacter* species, *Klebsiella* species
b. Obligate anaerobic bacteria
  i. Microbiologic characteristics: diverse
  ii. Examples: *Bacteroides fragilis, Clostridium* species, *Fusobacterium* species, *Peptostreptococcus* species
c. Gram-positive aerobic cocci
  i. Microaerophilic streptococci, including *Streptococcus anginosus* group bacteria
  ii. *Enterococcus* species
d. *Candida albicans*

II. HEALTH CARE–ASSOCIATED PATHOGENS—INCLUDES THE FOLLOWING, IN ADDITION TO COMMUNITY-ACQUIRED PATHOGENS:

a. Lactose-nonfermentative gram-negative bacilli
  i. *Pseudomonas aeruginosa*
  ii. *Serratia marcescens*
b. *S. aureus*, including MRSA
c. Extended-spectrum β-lactamase (ESBL)-producing Enterobacteriaceae
d. Vancomycin-resistant enterococcus (VRE)
e. Non-albicans *Candida* species

CLINICAL MANIFESTATIONS

I. ABDOMINAL PAIN

a. Localization to site of infection
b. A less sensitive predictor in elderly patients who may have nonspecific symptomatology (i.e., fever, malaise, weight loss)

II. SYSTEMIC INFLAMMATORY RESPONSE SYNDROME (SIRS) →TWO OR MORE OF THE FOLLOWING:

a. Temperature >38.5°C or <35.0°C
b. Heart rate of >90 beats/min
c. Respiratory rate of >20 breaths/min or $PaCO_2$ of <32 mm Hg
d. WBC count of >12,000 cells/mL, <4,000 cells/mL, or >10% immature (band) forms
e. Sepsis → SIRS plus infection

III. MISCELLANEOUS SYMPTOMS

    a. Abdominal distension

    b. Nausea/vomiting

    c. Malaise/fatigue

    d. Weight loss

    e. Constipation or obstipation

IV. SPECIFIC SYNDROMES

    a. Appendicitis

        i. Dull or vague periumbilical pain, followed by focal RLQ pain, followed by anorexia, nausea, and vomiting

        ii. Shorter duration of symptoms (<24 hours)

    b. Diverticulitis

        i. LLQ pain in >70% of patients

        ii. Longer duration of symptoms (>24 hours)

    c. Cholecystitis

        i. Epigastric pain and RUQ pain radiating to the right shoulder (tip of the scapula)

        ii. Biliary colic—transient RUQ pain following gallbladder contraction (i.e., after a fatty meal)

DIAGNOSTIC EVALUATION

I. HISTORY AND PHYSICAL EXAMINATION

    a. A thorough history and physical examination is usually sufficient to identify and in some cases localize an intra-abdominal infection.

    b. In addition to the clinical manifestations noted above, it is essential to discern any history of recent or remote surgery.

    c. Physical examination

        i. Vital signs and general appearance

        ii. SIRS manifestations

        iii. Must include rectal and genitourinary/pelvic examination

        iv. Abdominal examination

            1. General appearance

                a. Abdominal distension

                b. Skin findings

                    i. Wound appearance, if applicable

                        1. Erythema

                        2. Dehiscence

                        3. Drainage and characteristics of drainage

                            a. Purulence

                            b. Blood

                            c. Presence of a surgical drain (i.e., Jackson-Pratt, Hemovac)

Table 50-1	Physical Examination Findings in Patients with Peritonitis	
Sign	**Finding**	**Association**
Rebound tenderness	Worsening abdominal pain with release of palpation	Peritonitis
Psoas sign	Abdominal pain with extension of the right hip	Appendicitis with retrocecal appendix, psoas abscess
Obturator sign	Abdominal pain with internal rotation of the right thigh in flexion	Appendicitis with pelvic appendix
Rovsing sign	RLQ pain with palpation of the LLQ	Appendicitis
Murphy sign	Cessation or halting of breath with RUQ palpation, due to pain	Cholecystitis

        ii. Ecchymosis
           1. Periumbilical—Cullen sign
           2. Flank—Grey Turner sign
           3. Both are associated with intra-abdominal hemorrhage, classically in the context of hemorrhagic pancreatitis
    2. Auscultation for presence of bowel sounds
      a. May indicate ileus, which is common in the setting of intra-abdominal infection
    3. Percussion for presence of ascites
      a. Ascites may indicate the presence of peritonitis and could potentially be sampled to aid in the diagnosis.
    4. Palpation
      a. Tenderness
        i. Location
        ii. Quality
        iii. Severity
      b. Peritoneal signs (Table 50-1)
      c. Organomegaly

II. LABORATORY

    a. In general, laboratory tests alone cannot be used to diagnose intra-abdominal infection but may support such a diagnosis.
    b. Specific tests that support intra-abdominal infection
      i. Complete blood count and differential white blood cell count
        1. Leukocytosis
        2. Presence of immature neutrophils (i.e., band forms, "left shift")
        3. Thrombocytosis (or thrombocytopenia in the setting of sepsis or disseminated intravascular coagulation)
        4. Anemia of inflammation

    ii. Chemistries
        1. Decreased CO_2 and increased lactate level indicating a metabolic/lactic acidosis due to bowel ischemia
        2. Elevated creatinine indicating acute renal failure due to sepsis

III. MEDICAL IMAGING

    a. Diagnostic imaging is unnecessary for patients with peritonitis who merit immediate surgical intervention.
    b. Computerized tomography (CT) of the abdomen and pelvis
      i. Most useful diagnostic tool for localizing intra-abdominal infection
      ii. Superior sensitivity when compared to ultrasonography
      iii. Disadvantages include exposure to radiation and risk of contrast nephropathy.
    c. Abdominal ultrasonography
      i. Alternative diagnostic tool for localizing intra-abdominal infection
      ii. Noninvasive, low-risk modality
      iii. Limited by poor sensitivity, especially in the context of obesity

MANAGEMENT

I. SOURCE CONTROL

    a. Following identification of the source of infection, it is imperative that any focus of infection, including abscess or disruption of alimentary tract, be addressed.
    b. Methods of source control
      i. Percutaneous drainage utilizing interventional radiology
        1. Preferable to surgical drainage for localized fluid collections
        2. Minimizes surgical exposure and physiologic alterations associated with surgery
      ii. Surgery
        1. Laparotomy with drainage of abscesses and resection of bowel and fecal diversion through an ostomy
        2. For critically ill patients at risk for failed source control, laparotomy (i.e., open abdomen) and planned relaparotomy with reclosure may be utilized.
    c. Risk factors for failed source control
      i. Delay in intervention
      ii. APACHE II score >15
      iii. Advanced age
      iv. Significant comorbidities
      v. Hypoalbuminemia
      vi. Poor nutritional status
      vii. Severe peritonitis
      viii. Insufficient surgical debridement or drainage
      ix. Malignancy

II. FLUID RESUSCITATION

  a. Regardless of volume status, patients with intra-abdominal infection should be treated with intravenous fluids.
  b. Either crystalloid or colloid fluids may be used with the goal of maintaining a mean arterial pressure of ≥ 65 mm Hg.

III. ANTIMICROBIAL THERAPY (SEE TABLES 50-2 AND 50-3)

  a. Antibiotics are an adjunctive component of care to source control.
  b. Avoid any antimicrobial agent with a $\geq 10\%$ to 20% resistance rate for any common intra-abdominal pathogen. It is therefore imperative to be aware of local microbiology data and statistics (usually via institutional antibiogram).
  c. Antimicrobial agents should be tailored based on culture and susceptibility results.
  d. For uncomplicated appendicitis, 24 hours of antimicrobial therapy is sufficient.
  e. For complicated infections, the duration of treatment is 4 to 7 days, if source control is achieved.

Table 50-2	Empirical Antimicrobial Therapy for Community-Acquired Intra-Abdominal Infection

Mild-Moderate Illness	Comments
Moxifloxacin Ticarcillin-clavulanate Cefoxitin Ertapenem Tigecycline Cefazolin, cefuroxime, ceftriaxone, cefotaxime, levofloxacin, or ciprofloxacin plus metronidazole **Severe Illness** Piperacillin-tazobactam Antipseudomonal carbapenem[a] Cefepime, ceftazidime, ciprofloxacin, or levofloxacin, plus metronidazole	Avoid fluoroquinolones in areas where *E. coli* susceptibility is <90%. Tigecycline has no activity against *Pseudomonas* species or *Proteus* species and achieves poor serum levels (i.e., not suitable for bacteremic illness). Ertapenem has no activity against *Pseudomonas* species or *Enterococcus* species. Ampicillin-sulbactam is no longer recommended due to increased incidence of resistant *E. coli*. Cefotetan and clindamycin are no longer recommended for empiric treatment due to increased resistance to this agent in *B. fragilis*.

[a]Antipseudomonal carbapenems include imipenem-cilastatin, meropenem, and doripenem.

Table 50-3	Empirical Antimicrobial Therapy for Health Care–Associated Intra-Abdominal Infection

Antimicrobial Treatment	Comments
Piperacillin-tazobactam Antipseudomonal carbapenem[a] Ceftazidime or cefepime **plus** metronidazole	Aminoglycosides are not recommended as initial therapy unless clinical microbiology dictates otherwise.

Consider adding coverage of the following pathogens if at increased risk[b] or if grown from cultures:

Methicillin-resistant *Staphylococcus aureus* (MRSA)	Comments
Vancomycin Daptomycin Linezolid Tigecycline	Vancomycin is the preferred therapy for MRSA.

Vancomycin-resistant *Enterococcus faecium* (VRE)	
Linezolid Daptomycin Tigecycline	

Extended-spectrum β-lactamase (ESBL)-producing Enterobacteriaceae	
Antipseudomonal carbapenem	

Candida species	
An echinocandin[c] Fluconazole	Antifungal therapy is indicated only if *Candida* species are grown, or if the patient is critically ill, at risk for invasive candidiasis, and not responding to appropriate antibiotic therapy. Fluconazole is the recommended agent for infections due to *C. albicans*.

[a]Antipseudomonal carbapenems include imipenem-cilastatin, meropenem, and doripenem.
[b]Risk factors for MRSA infection include colonization with MRSA, recent antibiotic exposure, and recent hospitalization or residence in an intermediate care facility. Risk factors for VRE infection include receipt of vancomycin and cephalosporins, certain patient characteristics (ESRD, transplant recipient), and residence in a long-term care facility. Risk factors for invasive candidiasis include recent gastrointestinal surgery, total parenteral nutrition, presence of central venous catheter, colonization with *Candida* species, critical illness, broad-spectrum antibiotic use, and chronic or recent hemodialysis.
[c]Echinocandin antifungal agents include caspofungin, micafungin, and anidulafungin.

SUGGESTED READINGS

DeFrances CJ, Cullen KA, Kozak LJ. National Hospital Discharge Survey: 2005 annual summary with detailed diagnosis and procedure data. *Vital Health Stat* 2007;(165):1–209.

John H, Neff U, Kelemen M. Appendicitis diagnosis today: clinical and ultrasonic deductions. *World J Surg* 1993;17(2):243–249.

Mandell GL, et al. *Mandell, Douglas, and Bennett's principles and practice of infectious diseases.* 7th ed. New York: Elsevier/Churchill Livingstone; 2010:3111–3118.

Moss M. Epidemiology of sepsis: race, sex, and chronic alcohol abuse. *Clin Infect Dis* 2005;41(suppl 7):S490–S497.

Pappas PG, et al. Clinical practice guidelines for the management of candidiasis: 2009 update by the Infectious Diseases Society of America. *Clin Infect Dis* 2009;48(5):503–535.

Evidence-based guidelines for managing patients with intra-abdominal infection were prepared by an Expert Panel of the Surgical Infection Society and the Infectious Diseases Society of America. These updated guidelines replace those previously published in 2002 and 2003. The guidelines are intended for treating patients who either have these infections or may be at risk for them. New information, based on publications from the period 2003 to 2008, is incorporated into this guideline document. The panel has also added recommendations for managing intra-abdominal infection in children, particularly where such management differs from that of adults; for appendicitis in patients of all ages; and for necrotizing enterocolitis in neonates.

Podnos YD, Jimenez JC, Wilson SE. Intra-abdominal sepsis in elderly persons. *Clin Infect Dis* 2002;35(1):62–68.

Solomkin JS, Mazuski J. Intra-abdominal sepsis: newer interventional and antimicrobial therapies. *Infect Dis Clin North Am* 2009;23(3):593–608.

Solomkin JS, et al. Diagnosis and management of complicated intra-abdominal infection in adults and children: guidelines by the Surgical Infection Society and the Infectious Diseases Society of America. *Clin Infect Dis* 2010;50(2):133–164.

Complicated intra-abdominal infections are the second most common cause of septic death in the intensive care unit. Although there have been improvements in the outcome of sepsis regardless of etiology, this is even more striking for intra-abdominal infections. From observation, recent advances in interventional techniques, including more aggressive use of percutaneous drainage of abscesses and use of "open abdomen" techniques for peritonitis, have significantly affected the morbidity and mortality of physiologically severe complicated intra-abdominal infection.

Toorenvliet BR, et al. Colonic diverticulitis: a prospective analysis of diagnostic accuracy and clinical decision-making. *Colorectal Dis* 2010;12(3):179–186.

XIII Endemic Fungal Infections

Endemic Fungi

Paras Patel and James W. Myers

INTRODUCTION

- Blastomycosis, histoplasmosis, and coccidioidomycosis are the three common systemic and endemic mycoses in the United States.
- Even though most symptomatic cases of blastomycosis, coccidioidomycosis, and histoplasmosis *occur in patients without significant preexisting and predisposing disease,* individuals with defective cell-mediated immunity are at increased risk for these mycoses if they are exposed by living or traveling in the endemic areas.

EPIDEMIOLOGY AND PATHOGENICITY

- Blastomycosis, coccidioidomycosis, and histoplasmosis are caused, respectively, by the following dimorphic fungi: *Blastomyces dermatitidis, Coccidioides immitis* or *Coccidioides posadasii,* and *Histoplasmosis capsulatum.*
- Each species grows as a **mold in nature** or in the laboratory at temperatures below 98.6°F (37°C). On routine fungal culture media at 77°F to 86°F (25°C to 30°C), they produce mycelial colonies that vary in texture, pigment, and growth rate.
- Under the appropriate growth conditions in vitro, **they convert to a distinctive form of growth that is found in tissue.**
- Systemic fungal infections are acquired by inhalation of the airborne conidia of dimorphic, exogenous fungi. These fungi **convert to tissue forms** in the lungs, which subsequently disseminate to other organs as well as skin.
- The fungi that cause coccidioidomycosis and histoplasmosis are associated with dry soil, or soil mixed with guano.
- The agent of blastomycosis undoubtedly exists in nature, but its habitat has not been clearly defined.
- Inhalation of conidia of any of these fungi can lead to pulmonary infection, which may or may not become symptomatic.
- The organism may become dormant only to reactivate later.
- Some patients develop a progressive pulmonary disease, which can occasionally lead to systemic dissemination.
- These infections are **not contagious,** and they are not transmitted among humans or animals. No "Isolation Precautions" are needed in the hospital.

Table 51-1 compares some of the epidemiologic features of these systemic mycoses.

Table 51-1   Epidemiologic Features

Features	Blastomycosis	Histoplasmosis	Coccidioidomycosis
Geographic areas of high endemicity	Highly endemic in the **Mississippi and Ohio river basins,** areas surrounding the Great Lakes, and the St. Lawrence River valley	Highly endemic in the **Ohio and Mississippi river valleys.** Approximately 50% of adults in endemic areas have been infected.	Highly endemic in the southern **San Joaquin Valley of California and southern Arizona, New Mexico, Nevada, Texas, northern Mexico,** and parts of Central and South America
Saprophytic form (<95°F)	Hyaline, septate hyphae	Hyaline, septate hyphae	Hyaline, septate hyphae
Existence in environment	The moist soil enriched with decaying vegetation encourages the growth of the organism.	Possible exposure events include destroying chicken coops, cutting down trees, or spelunking in caves.	Exposure to the soil of the arid lower Sonoran Desert
Predominant tissue forms	Yeast	Yeast	Spherules
Mode of transmission	Inhalation of conidia from the environmental mold	Inhalation	Inhalation
Self-limited infection	Unknown	Yes	Yes
Approximate percentage of immunocompetent patients	More than 90	More than 90	More than 90
Approximate percentage of males among patients with disease	50–90	80–90	75–90
Relative frequency of disease among AIDS patients in the endemic areas	Rare	Common	Common
Approximate percentage of infections that are asymptomatic	>50	>65	>95

CLINICAL FEATURES

Blastomycosis

The most common manifestations are pulmonary, cutaneous, and bone infections.

- Infection is *asymptomatic* in more than 50% of infected individuals.
- The most common symptoms include cough, night sweats, weight loss, chest pain, skin lesions, fever, hemoptysis, myalgia, and dyspnea.
- Chest radiographs may reveal a patchy pneumonitis, a mass-like infiltrate, or nodules. **Often, it is confused with lung cancer.**
- Chronic cutaneous blastomycosis presents as one or more subcutaneous nodules that eventually ulcerate. **Skin lesions are often confused with skin cancers.**
  - Lesions are more common on exposed skin surfaces of body such as the face or extremities and may evolve over weeks or months into granulomatous lesions.
  - Aspiration or biopsy of leading edge of the skin lesion shows the active microabscesses and the typical yeast cells.
- When dissemination occurs, it may involve the genitourinary tract, central nervous system (CNS), spleen, **skin, bone,** and less commonly, the liver, lymph nodes, heart, and other viscera. Tables 51-2, 51-3 and 51-5 compare the features of the major endemic fungi.

Histoplasmosis Capsulatum

- Most infections are **asymptomatic.**
- Patients with **symptomatic pulmonary infection** usually have a *self-limited* illness that begins several weeks after exposure (2 weeks) to the fungus in a confined place such as a storm cellar, a chicken house, or a bat cave.
  - Patients with symptomatic disease usually present with fever, chills, fatigue, nonproductive cough, and myalgias.
  - Chest radiographs usually show a patchy lobar or multilobar nodular infiltrate.
  - Acute pulmonary infection can be associated with joint symptoms, especially in women.
    - Erythema nodosum
    - Erythema multiforme
    - Frank arthritis is rare.
    - Immunologic phenomena
- **Immunocompromised patients** with heavy exposure to *H. capsulatum* usually present with **life-threatening** acute pulmonary histoplasmosis.
  - Cases usually present with high spiking fevers, chills, prostration, dyspnea, and cough.
  - Chest radiograph reveals diffuse, reticulonodular pulmonary infiltrates.
- **Chronic cavitary pulmonary histoplasmosis** is a form of histoplasmosis, which mainly occurs in **elderly patients who have chronic obstructive pulmonary** disease.
  - Patients with chronic cavitary pulmonary histoplasmosis present with fever, fatigue, anorexia, weight loss, cough productive of purulent sputum, and hemoptysis.
  - Radiographs reveal unilateral or bilateral **upper lobe infiltrates** with multiple **cavities** and extensive **fibrosis** in the **lower** lobes.
- Pulmonary involvement with histoplasmosis has been associated with multiple complications such as mediastinal and hilar lymph nodes calcifications, granulomatous mediastinitis and fibrosing mediastinitis, and pericarditis.
  - **Enlarged mediastinal and hilar lymph nodes can cause pressure on adjacent structures, including the esophagus, airways, and blood vessels.**

- Pericarditis
  - 5%
  - Friction rub 75 %
  - 6 weeks after a respiratory illness
  - Yeast organisms uncommonly found
- **Acute disseminated histoplasmosis** occurs mainly in **immunocompromised patients such as HIV infected patients with CD4 counts lower than 150,** patients with an organ transplant, or patients taking corticosteroids or **tumor necrosis factor antagonists**.
  - Fever, chills, anorexia, weight loss, hypotension, dyspnea, **hepatosplenomegaly**, and skin and mucous membrane lesions. Ulcers are less common than in other forms.
  - **Pancytopenia, elevated alkaline phosphatase, diffuse pulmonary infiltrates on chest radiography** and computed Tomography (CT), findings of disseminated intravascular coagulation, and acute respiratory failure are common.
- **Subacute progressive disseminated** forms occur as well.
- Fever in approximately 50%
- Focal lesions in various organ systems
  - Gastrointestinal tract
    - Especially terminal ileum and cecum
  - Endovascular structures including the aortic valve and abdominal aorta. Difficult to grow in blood cultures
  - Adrenal glands. Addison disease in 10%
  - Hepatosplenomegaly, deep mucosal ulcers
  - CNS
    - Chronic meningitis. Lymphocytic, basilar location
    - Mass lesions
    - Cerebritis
- **Chronic progressive disseminated histoplasmosis** occurs mainly in middle-aged men who have no known immunosuppressive illness.
  - Fever (~30%), night sweats, weight loss, anorexia, and fatigue
  - The most common physical finding (~50%) is an **oropharyngeal ulcer** that is indurated and usually deep and painless.
  - Hepatosplenomegaly
  - Adrenal insufficiency may occur.
  - An increased erythrocyte sedimentation rate, elevated alkaline phosphatase, and pancytopenia are often noted.
  - Diffuse reticulonodular infiltrates on chest radiography and CT may be seen.
  - Granulomas, few yeasts on pathology specimens

  Histoplasma capsulatum var. *duboisii* causes **African histoplasmosis,** which differs in clinical presentation from the typical form.

- Larger yeast cells (10 microns vs. 2 microns)
- More skin and bone lesions and less pulmonary
- Giant cells (Tables 51-2 and 51-3)

Coccidioidomycosis

- Approximately 40% of people infected with *C. immitis* present with a flu-like symptom of cough, fever, night sweats, pleuritic chest pain, and shortness of breath **one to three weeks after inhalation** of spores.
- 60% of people remain asymptomatic.

Table 51-2	Comparison of Common Symptoms of the Endemic Fungi		
Clinical Features	**Blastomycosis**	**Histoplasmosis**	**Coccidioidomycosis**
Fever	Yes	Yes	Yes
Night sweats	Yes	Yes	Yes
Weight loss	Yes	Yes	Yes
Anorexia	Yes	Yes	Yes
Fatigue	Yes	Yes	Yes
Myalgia	Yes	Yes	Yes

- 5% of infected patients develop pulmonary lesions such as nodules or **thin-walled cavities** near the pleura.
- Less than 1% of patients develop disseminated disease.
- **Cutaneous coccidioidomycosis** presents with verrucous plaques, nodules, or papules.
- Commonly involve nasolabial folds or the sternoclavicular area
- Bones, joints, brain, spinal cord, thyroid, eye, larynx, or genitourinary tract may be involved as well.

Clinically significant illness may present as "valley fever" lasting weeks to months. Primary infections usually manifest as community-acquired pneumonia occurring **7 to 21** days after exposure.

- Chest pain, cough, and fever
- Cutaneous manifestations such as erythema nodosum and erythema multiforme
- Most pulmonary coccidioidal infections *resolve without complications* within several weeks to many months.
  - A few patients with infections develop pulmonary sequelae, and even less patients develop disseminated infection.
  - Pulmonary cavities usually are peripherally located and solitary. Over time, most develop a distinctive **thin-walled** cavity.

Table 51-3	Organ Involvement in Endemic Fungal Infections		
	Blastomycosis	**Histoplasmosis**	**Coccidioidomycosis**
Lungs	Yes	Yes	Yes
Skin	**Yes**	Yes	**Yes**
Skeleton and joints	**Yes**	Yes	**Yes**
Genitourinary system (the prostate, male genitalia, kidney, and adrenals)	Yes	Yes	Yes
Reticuloendothelial system (liver, spleen, lymph nodes)	Yes	**Yes**	Yes
CNS/meninges	Yes	Yes	**Yes**
Subcutaneous tissue	Yes	Yes	Yes
Mucous membrane	Yes	**Yes**	Yes

Immunodeficiency conditions such as the AIDS, Hodgkin lymphoma, organ transplantation, corticosteroid therapy, and tumor necrosis factor inhibitors increase the risk for dissemination of coccidioidal infection. In addition, risk of dissemination or progressive pulmonary disease is higher in certain racial groups (e.g., Filipinos, blacks) and pregnancy.

- **Disseminated coccidioidal infection involves joints, bones, skin, lymph nodes, and meninges.**
- Disseminated infections involving skin may present with superficial maculopapular lesions, subcutaneous fluctuant abscesses, or verrucous ulcers.
- Involvement of supraclavicular and cervical lymph nodes is common.
- Joint infections are associated with a prominent synovitis and effusion. **Knee joint is involved more frequently than any other joints**, followed by the joints of the hands and wrists, the feet and ankles, and the pelvis.
- Infection of the spine often involves multiple vertebra and produces anterior or posterior paraspinous soft tissue abscesses, or epidural abscesses.
- Coccidioidal meningitis **is the most serious form of disseminated infection**.
  - Approximately 50% of patients acquire CNS disease.
  - Common presenting symptoms are headache, vomiting, and altered mental status. Usually presents insidiously
  - Other presentations include focal neurologic deficits, coma, intention tremor, cranial nerve palsies, papilledema, gait abnormalities, hydrocephalus, and brain and spinal lesions.
  - In addition to cerebrospinal fluid (CSF) findings of an elevated white blood cell count, elevated protein levels, and a depressed glucose level, CSF **eosinophils are occasionally prominent** (up to 70%).
  - Complement fixation (CF) IgG is present in 90% of patients with coccidioidal meningitis. Occasionally, patients with meningitis have positive CSF CF titers with negative serum CF titers.

DIAGNOSIS

- Definitive diagnosis of fungal infections requires cultures or identification of the organism in the tissue or exudate (Table 51-4).
- Urinary antigen and serologic tests are also available for diagnosis of fungal infections but they are less sensitive. Chest x-ray reveals pulmonary infiltrates with ipsilateral adenopathy, pulmonary nodules, or cavities.
- Because skin tests for coccidioidomycosis remain positive for life, a result may not be related to the current illness.
- **Coccidioidal skin testing reagents are not available commercially.**
- Negative serial coccidioidin skin tests and a peak CF antibody titer of > or = 1:256 are independently associated with increased risk of relapse.
- IgM antibody against *Coccidioides* **is the most sensitive serologic indication** of early infection. It is detected in approximately 50% of infections by the first week and in 90% by 3 weeks but disappears by several weeks to 6 months. CF IgG antibodies are positive in approximately 90% of patients by 3 months after onset, persist for approximately 6 months, but disappear as the infection improves. Coccidioidal CF titers in the serum and CSF can be used to monitor disease and predict relapses.
- A CF titer >1:32 suggests active histoplasmosis infection.
  - Remain positive in 80% of chronic cases. 10% of cases of acute infection are positive within 3 weeks and up to 80% are positive by 6 weeks.
  - CF titers usually normalize after treatment of infection.

- Immunoprecipitating antibodies to histoplasmosis
  - 2 glycoproteins, H and M
  - Anti-M antibody remains positive for years in 60%. Anti-H antibody is **more specific** than anti-M, but it is less often positive (10% to 20%). Negative by 6 months.
- Antigenuria for histoplasmosis
  - 90% of cases with disseminated histoplasmosis
  - 80% with acute histoplasmosis
  - 30% with subacute histoplasmosis
  - Up to 88% with chronic pulmonary histoplasmosis

TREATMENT

Treatment recommendations for endemic fungal infections are summarized in Table 51-5. Table 51-6 highlights the therapy of histoplasmosis specifically.

- The preferred treatment for life-threatening endemic fungal infections is the **lipid formulation** of amphotericin B. The deoxycholate formulation of amphotericin B is an alternative in patients who are at a low risk for nephrotoxicity.
  - An **amphoteric** species is a molecule or ion that can react as acid as well as a base. Polyene antifungals associate with ergosterol, the main component of fungal cell membranes, forming a transmembrane channel that leads to monovalent ion leakage, which is the primary effect leading to fungal cell death but other mechanisms are postulated as well.
  - Because *mammalian and fungal membranes are similar in structure,* amphotericin B causes cellular toxicity in humans.
- Itraconazole inhibits the CYP-450–dependent synthesis of **ergosterol,** which is a vital component of fungal cell membranes.
  - The oral bioavailability of itraconazole is maximal when the capsules are given immediately after a **full meal**. Peak plasma levels are reached 3 to 4 hours following an oral dose. During chronic administration, steady state is reached after 1 to 2 weeks. Steady-state plasma concentrations of itraconazole 3 to 4 hours after drug intake are 0,4 mcg/mL (100 mg daily), 1,1 mcg/mL (200 mg daily), and 2,0 mcg/mL (200 mg twice daily). Elimination from plasma is biphasic with an elimination half-life of 1 to 1.5 days.
  - Itraconazole is extensively metabolized by the liver into a large number of metabolites. One of the metabolites is hydroxy-itraconazole, which has a comparable antifungal activity in vitro to itraconazole.
- Blood levels of itraconazole should be monitored to ensure adequate drug dose, and drug interactions should be assessed carefully. Generally, the initial plasma concentrations should be determined once the patient reaches steady-state levels (typically 1 to **2 weeks** after starting itraconazole therapy).
  - Note that the "bioassay" measurement overestimates itraconazole concentrations by perhaps five times because of the presence of the hydroxy-itraconazole metabolite. For clinical purposes, the bioassay may be sufficient to determine if the patient is adequately absorbing the drug. Itraconazole bioassay measures *total antifungal* effect/inhibition in the biologic test medium. The testing range for this itraconazole assay is from 0.5 to 20.0 mcg/mL.
  - High performance liquid chromatography (HPCL), an analytical method, is used to assay itraconazole levels for patients on **combination therapy (5-FC)** as well as for pharmacokinetic studies. The sensitivity range for HPLC is 0.01 to 5.0 mcg/mL. The HPLC result is reported in terms of the *parent* drug, itraconazole, and also itraconazole's *largest metabolite,* hydroxy-itraconazole.
  - It has been well documented that the two methods, bioassay and HPLC, do not correlate; hence, bioassay values are approximately **three times higher** due to the active metabolite (please see Tables 51-5 to 51-8 for more additional information).

Table 51-4	Diagnostic Testing		
Tests	Blastomycosis	Histoplasmosis	Coccidioidomycosis
Specimens for cultures	Sputum, pus exudates, urine, and biopsies from lesions	Sputum, urine, scrapings from superficial lesions, **bone marrow aspirates,** and buffy coat blood cells	Sputum, exudate from cutaneous lesions, **spinal fluid,** blood, urine, and tissue biopsies
Microscopic examination	Wet mount of specimens may show **broad-based budding cell on thick-walled yeast cells.**	The **small ovoid cells** may be observed within macrophages in histologic sections stained with fungal stains.	Materials should be examined fresh for typical spherules. KOH or calcofluor white stain will be useful in seeing the **spherules and endospores.**
Culture	**Colonies usually develop within 2 weeks** on Sabouraud or enriched blood agar at 30°C. The identification is confirmed by detection of B. dermatitidis specific antigen or by a specific DNA probe.	Specimens are cultured in the rich media such as glucose cysteine blood agar at 37°C and on Sabouraud agar or inhibitory mold agar at 25–30°C after **incubation for at 4–8 weeks:** 1.15% positive in acute disease 2.60 % positive in chronic pulmonary Histoplasmosis is a slow grower.	Cultures on inhibitory mold agar, Sabouraud agar, or blood agar slants can be incubated at room temperature or at 37°C. Suspicious cultures are examined only in a biosafety cabinet. **Grows in 3–7 days** Arthroconidia **PCR amplification** has been used to identify the highly specific *Ag2/PRA* antigen gene of *C. posadasii* in appropriate samples of sputum.
Serology	Antibodies can be measured by complement fixation of ID tests. **Overall serologic tests are not as useful** for the diagnosis of blastomycosis.	Complement fixation tests for histoplasma antibodies become positive within **2–5 weeks** after infection. CF titers rise during progressive disease and then decline to very low levels when the disease is inactive. A radioassay or enzyme immunoassay for serum or **urinary antigen of** *H. capsulatum* is most sensitive.	A latex agglutination, complement fixation or immunodiffusion test detect antibodies to **coccidioidin.** Titer will decline with the resolution of primary infection. In contrast, titer will continue to rise in case of progressive disease. **Titer more than 1:32 is indication of progressive disease.** AIDS patients may have negative serologic tests.

Table 51-5 Treatment of Endemic Fungi

Clinical Manifestation	Blastomycosis	Histoplasmosis[a]	Coccidioidomycosis	Duration of Treatment
Asymptomatic	Close monitoring is needed and treated if patient will develop progressive disease.	No treatment	No treatment is required but close monitoring should be done every 1–3 months up to 1 year or longer is advised with physical and radiographic examination as well as serologic testing.	
Acute pulmonary infection— life threatening	Amphotericin B followed by itraconazole	Amphotericin B followed by itraconazole	Treat with amphotericin B followed by oral azole	Duration of treatment is 12 months.
Acute pulmonary infection—mild to moderate	Treat with itraconazole or ketoconazole or fluconazole	Itraconazole	Itraconazole	Duration of treatment is 6–12 months.
Chronic pulmonary infection	Amphotericin B followed by itraconazole once patient is stabilized. Those patients with less severe infection can be treated with ketoconazole, itraconazole, or fluconazole.	Most cases do not require treatment; however, it should be considered in immunosuppressed patients or those with underlying lung disease.	If asymptomatic, only close monitoring is needed, with consideration of resection if there are complications, enlargement, or persistence of the lesion after 2 years. If there is symptomatic disease, treat with fluconazole or itraconazole for at least 1 year. Voriconazole and posaconazole are other options for therapy. Surgical resection may need to be considered for refractory lesions.	• Treatment duration is at least 6 months for blastomycosis. • Treatment duration for at least 1 year for coccidioidomycosis.
Disseminated infection	Same as chronic pulmonary infection	Liposomal amphotericin B, changing to itraconazole	Treat with fluconazole or itraconazole or amphotericin B	Therapy should be continued for at least 6–12 months.
CNS involvement	Treat with amphotericin B, with the total dosage at least 2 g	Liposomal amphotericin B followed by itraconazole or posaconazole for at least 1 year of therapy	Treat with fluconazole or itraconazole. Consider intrathecal amphotericin for those who do not respond to azoles. Other measures include ventriculoperitoneal (VP) shunting in cases with obstructive hydrocephalus.	Azole therapy is continued for life in case of coccidioidomycosis.

[a]Discontinuation of maintenance therapy in HIV patients may be safe if patients on stable ART >6 months with CD4 >150, serum Ag <2 units, and have completed induction and minimum of 12 months of maintenance antifungal therapy. Resume if CD4 <150.

407

Table 51-6　Treatment of Histoplasmosis

Histoplasmosis	Treatment Indicated or Not	Treatment Regimen
Mild to moderate, acute pulmonary—self-limited	No treatment for most cases	Itraconazole (200 mg three times daily for 3 days and then 200 mg once or twice daily for 6–12 weeks) is recommended for patients who continue to have symptoms for 1 month.
Severe—acute pulmonary histoplasmosis	Indicated	Amphotericin B +/– corticosteroids, followed by itraconazole for a total of 6–12 weeks of therapy Lipid formulation of amphotericin B (3.0–5.0 mg/kg daily intravenously for 1–2 weeks) followed by itraconazole (200 mg three times daily for 3 days and then 200 mg twice daily, for a total of 12 weeks) is recommended. Methylprednisolone (0.5–1.0 mg/kg daily intravenously) during the first 1–2 weeks of antifungal therapy is recommended for patients who develop respiratory complications.
Mediastinal lymphadenopathy	Although no therapy is usually necessary, treatment should be initiated if symptoms will persist.	Itraconazole, 200 mg three times daily for 3 days, followed by 200 mg once or twice daily for 6–12 weeks for those who have symptoms greater that 1 month Prednisone (0.5–1.0 mg/kg daily [maximum, 80 mg daily] in tapering doses over 1–2 weeks) is recommended in severe cases with obstruction or compression of contiguous structures.
Mediastinal fibrosis	No consensus on optimal treatment	Surgery, corticosteroids, and antifungal agents have been used in the treatment of this condition, with minimal success. The placement of intravascular stents is recommended for selected patients with pulmonary vessel obstruction. Itraconazole (200 mg once or twice daily for 12 weeks) is recommended if clinical findings cannot differentiate **mediastinal fibrosis from mediastinal granuloma,** which is treated with itraconazole (200 mg three times daily for 3 days and then once or twice daily for 6–12 weeks) that is recommended for symptomatic cases. Azoles after surgery have been proposed, but the usefulness of this approach is debatable.
Chronic cavitary histoplasmosis	Those who have thick-walled cavities, progressive pulmonary infiltrate, or persistent cavities associated with declining respiratory function should be treated.	Oral itraconazole, 200 mg three times daily for 3 days, followed by once or twice daily, should be given for 12–24 months. Relapse is common. Monitor levels of itraconazole.

Condition		
Acute pericarditis following acute histoplasmosis	No treatment is indicated in most cases.	Nonsteroidal anti-inflammatory agents for 2–12 weeks Use corticosteroids if patients fail to respond to NSAIDs • Itraconazole, 200 mg three times daily for 3 days, followed by 200 mg once or twice daily for 6–12 weeks, **should be included if corticosteroids are necessary.**
Endocarditis	Treatment initiated	If the valve is involved alone, treatment with a lipid formulation or the deoxycholate preparation for 2 weeks following surgical extraction may be sufficient.
Meningitis	Treatment indicated	Liposomal amphotericin B, 3–5 mg/kg/day for 4–6 weeks, followed by itraconazole, 200 mg two or three times daily for at least 1 year
Acute progressive disseminated histoplasmosis—not HIV infected	Treatment indicated	Amphotericin B followed by itraconazole for a total of 12 months for severe cases Liposomal amphotericin B (3.0 mg/kg daily) is recommended for 1–2 weeks, followed by oral itraconazole (200 mg three times daily for 3 days and then 200 mg twice daily for a total of at least 12 months). Itraconazole alone 200 mg b.i.d. may be given for 12 months for mild or moderate cases.
Acute progressive disseminated histoplasmosis—non-AIDS	Treatment indicated	Amphotericin B followed by itraconazole for lifelong Although there are no reliable data to make this decision, it may be reasonable to discontinue itraconazole in patients who have been on HAART, a CD4 count more than 150/L for 6 months, and undetectable viral load and if patient had received at least 12 months of antifungal therapy with a negative test for *Histoplasma* antigen in urine.
Broncholithiasis	No antimicrobials	Bronchoscopic or surgical removal
Pulmonary nodules	No treatment	
Rheumatologic syndromes	Treatment sometimes indicated	Nonsteroidal anti-inflammatory therapy is recommended in mild cases.
Presumed ocular histoplasmosis syndrome	No treatment	

Table 51-7	IDSA Guidelines

Fungus	IDSA Guidelines PMID Number
Cryptococcus	20047480
Histoplasmosis	17806045
Blastomycosis	18462107
Candida	19191635
Sporotrichosis	17968818
Coccidioidomycosis	16206093
Aspergillus	18177225

Table 51-8	Fungal Resources

| Dr Fungus | http://www.doctorfungus.org/ |
| Miravista Diagnostics | http://www.miravistalabs.com/ |

SUGGESTED READINGS

Bariola JR, Hage CA, et al. Detection of Blastomyces dermatitidis antigen in patients with newly diagnosed blastomycosis. *Diagn Microbiol Infect Dis* 2011;69(2):187–191.
B. dermatitidis antigen was detected in most of the patients with blastomycosis and can be a useful tool for timely diagnosis.
Bercovitch RS, Catanzaro A, et al. Coccidioidomycosis during pregnancy: a review and recommendations for management. *Clin Infect Dis* 2011;53(4):363–368.
This article summarizes the data on these issues and offers guidance on the management of coccidioidomycosis during pregnancy.
Body BA. Cutaneous manifestations of systemic mycoses. *Dermatol Clin* 1996;14(1):125–135.
Bonifaz AVazquez-Gonzalez D, et al. Endemic systemic mycoses: coccidioidomycosis, histoplasmosis, paracoccidioidomycosis and blastomycosis. *J Dtsch Dermatol Ges* 2011;9(9): 705–714; quiz 715.
In this article, the authors provided up-to-date epidemiologic, clinical, diagnostic, and therapeutic data on the four most important imported systemic mycoses in Europe.
Bradsher RW Jr. Pulmonary blastomycosis. *Semin Respir Crit Care Med* 2008;29(2):174–181.
Itraconazole is now considered to be the agent of choice with fluconazole, voriconazole, and posaconazole having a role in selected patients. In a patient with life-threatening or central nervous system blastomycosis, amphotericin B should be given, at least initially.
Chapman SW, Dismukes, WE et al. Clinical practice guidelines for the management of blastomycosis: 2008 update by the Infectious Diseases Society of America. *Clin Infect Dis* 2008;46(12):1801–1812.
Evidence-based guidelines for the management of patients with blastomycosis were prepared by an expert panel of the Infectious Diseases Society of America.
Conces DJ Jr. Endemic fungal pneumonia in immunocompromised patients. *J Thorac Imaging* 1999;14(1):1–8.
Crampton TL, Light RB, et al. Epidemiology and clinical spectrum of blastomycosis diagnosed at Manitoba hospitals. *Clin Infect Dis* 2002;34(10): 1310–1316.
This study provides a summary of the current status of blastomycosis in this area of endemicity in Canada.

Hage CA, Connolly P, et al. Investigation of the efficacy of micafungin in the treatment of histoplasmosis using two North American strains of Histoplasma capsulatum. *Antimicrob Agents Chemother* 2011;55(9):4447–4450.

Micafungin appears to be ineffective in treatment of histoplasmosis.

Hage CA, Kirsch EJ, et al. Histoplasma antigen clearance during treatment of histoplasmosis in patients with AIDS determined by a quantitative antigen enzyme immunoassay. *Clin Vaccine Immunol* 2011;18(4):661–666.

Histoplasma antigenemia decreases more rapidly than antigenuria, providing a more sensitive early laboratory marker for response to treatment. Antigenuria declines earlier with amphotericin B than with itraconazole.

Hage CA, KnoxKS, et al. Antigen detection in bronchoalveolar lavage fluid for diagnosis of fungal pneumonia. *Curr Opin Pulm Med* 2011;17(3):167–171.

Fungal antigen testing of BAL specimens is recommended if bronchoscopy is performed for diagnosis of pulmonary infiltrates in patient groups at risk for aspergillosis or the endemic mycoses if the diagnosis cannot be established by evaluation of sputum specimens or detection of antigen in the urine or serum.

Hage CA, Ribes, JA. et al. A multicenter evaluation of tests for diagnosis of histoplasmosis. *Clin Infect Dis* 2011;53(5):448–454.

The sensitivity of antigen detection in disseminated histoplasmosis is higher in immunocompromised patients than in immunocompetent patients and in patients with more severe illness. The sensitivity for detection of antigenemia is similar to that for antigenuria in disseminated infection.

Howard DH. The epidemiology and ecology of blastomycosis, coccidioidomycosis and histoplasmosis. *Zentralbl Bakteriol Mikrobiol Hyg A* 1984;257(2):219–227.

Kim MM, VikramHR. et al. Treatment of refractory coccidioidomycosis with voriconazole or posaconazole. *Clin Infect Dis* 2011;53(11):1060–1066.

Voriconazole and posaconazole are reasonable but not infallible options for salvage treatment of refractory coccidioidomycosis. Prospective comparative trials are required to provide further insights into their efficacy and utility.

Krupp PJ, St Romain, MJ. Vaginal fungi during pregnancy. *J La State Med Soc* 1960;112:176–177.

Limper AH, Knox, KS, et al. An official american thoracic society statement: treatment of fungal infections in adult pulmonary and critical care patients. *Am J Respir Crit Care Med* 2011;183(1):96–128.

Martynowicz MA, Prakash UB. Pulmonary blastomycosis: an appraisal of diagnostic techniques. *Chest* 2002;121(3):768–773.

Commonly used serologic assays are insensitive and are not useful for diagnostic screening.

Mathisen G, Shelub A, et al. Coccidioidal meningitis: clinical presentation and management in the fluconazole era. *Medicine (Baltimore)* 2010;89(5):251–284.

Despite the clear advantages of azole treatment in CM, new therapeutic approaches are needed to provide definitive cure and to reduce the need for long-term suppressive therapy.

Saccente M, Woods GL. Clinical and laboratory update on blastomycosis. *Clin Microbiol Rev* 2010;23(2):367–381.

Although a long course of amphotericin B is usually curative, itraconazole is also highly effective and is the mainstay of therapy for most patients with blastomycosis.

Schein R, Homans, J, et al. Posaconazole for chronic refractory coccidioidal meningitis. *Clin Infect Dis* 2011;53(12):1252–1254.

Coccidioidal meningitis is a potentially lethal infection. Disease progression while taking fluconazole is a common complication and safe, effective, alternative treatments are limited. Posaconazole therapy resulted in symptomatic and laboratory improvement in 2 patients and clinical improvement in a third patient with chronic, previously unresponsive coccidioidal meningitis.

Ta M, Flowers, SA, et al. The role of voriconazole in the treatment of central nervous system blastomycosis. *Ann Pharmacother* 2009;43(10):1696–1700.

Further studies are needed to fully elucidate the role of voriconazole in the treatment of CNS blastomycosis. It nonetheless may be considered as an azole option for either follow-up therapy after liposomal amphotericin B therapy or as salvage therapy in patients intolerant of amphotericin B or other azoles.

Vergidis P, WalkerRC, et al. False-positive Aspergillus galactomannan assay in solid organ transplant recipients with histoplasmosis. *Transpl Infect Dis* (2011).

False-positive tests for Aspergillus GM can occur in immunosuppressed patients who have histoplasmosis, and may obscure the correct diagnosis.

Wheat LJ. Laboratory diagnosis of histoplasmosis: update 2000. *Semin Respir Infect* 2001;16(2):131–140.

Wheat, LJ. Approach to the diagnosis of the endemic mycoses. *Clin Chest Med* 2009;30(2):379–389, viii.

Wheat LJ, Garringer, T, et al. Diagnosis of histoplasmosis by antigen detection based upon experience at the histoplasmosis reference laboratory. *Diagn Microbiol Infect Dis* 2002;43(1):29–37.

XIV Antimicrobial Therapy

52

Interpreting Sensitivity Reports

Paul Lewis and James W. Myers

INTRODUCTION

Since the discovery of sulfonamides and penicillin, clinicians have attempted to predict the success or failure of treatment with antimicrobial resistance testing (AST). One of the first tools utilized was the minimum inhibitory concentration (MIC).

MIC is defined as the lowest concentration of antibiotic that inhibits visible growth of bacteria. We now know that MIC alone is insufficient to guide antimicrobial selection. For example, a clinician who selects one agent because of a reported MIC of 2 over another agent with an MIC of 8 may not have selected the best agent. The agent with an MIC of 2 may only achieve plasma concentrations of 1, while the agent with MIC of 8 may maintain plasma concentration 5 times that MIC. For this reason, breakpoints are established. A breakpoint, simply put, is the drug concentration that separates organisms into resistant or susceptible categories. This takes into account the microbiologic data as well as pharmacodynamic and pharmacokinetic data to predict the likelihood of success. As our knowledge of the relationship between pharmacokinetics and pharmacodynamics continues to grow, so does the effect of antimicrobial susceptibility testing. Animal models and statistical or mathematical models such as the Monte Carlo simulation further assist in the prediction of success.

ANTIMICROBIAL SUSCEPTIBILITY TESTING

There are two categories of susceptibility testing: qualitative and quantitative.

1. Qualitative resistance testing such as disk diffusion will allow for a susceptible (S), intermediate (I), or resistant (R) interpretation. Qualitative testing is usually performed by Kirby-Bauer disk diffusion. While sufficient for less complicated conditions such as urinary tract infections, the lack of MIC data is often a limitation to qualitative testing.

2. Quantitative methods include broth macrodilution, broth microdilution, agar dilutions, E-test, and several automated systems, which yield the MIC of the antimicrobial to the organism tested. The dilutions are time consuming, cumbersome, and not practical for use in clinical practice. Oftentimes, they are used to validate other methods including automated methods.

Kirby-Bauer Disk Diffusion

- A standard concentration of bacteria in a broth or saline solution is spread confluently and uniformly over a blood or Mueller-Hinton agar.
- Antibiotic-impregnated disks are placed on the plate and then incubated.
- The antibiotic diffuses out, establishing a concentration gradient.

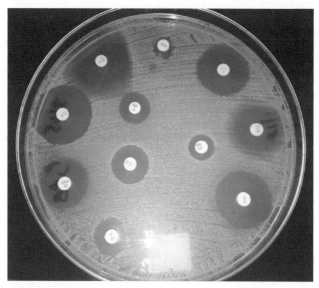

Figure 52-1. Kirby-Bauer disk diffusion allows antibiotic-impregnated disks to create a zone of inhibition. The zones are measured in millimeters and are compared to standard references to determine susceptible (S), intermediate (I), or resistant (R).

- At a certain point, the antibiotic concentration is insufficient to inhibit the growth of the bacteria forming a ring or zone of inhibition.
  - See Figure 52-1
- The zone of inhibition is measured and recorded.
- Based on predefined set points, the antimicrobial is classified as S, I, or R.
- Advantages include simplicity, inexpensiveness, and customizability of antimicrobials tested.
- Disadvantages include the lack of an MIC, being time consuming to the microbiologist, and a possibility of interpretation error by the microbiologist manually measuring the zone.

Dilution Testing
- Macrobroth uses test tubes with serial dilutions of antibiotic concentrations.
- Microbroth uses serial concentration in a well plate.
- Agar dilution uses plates of serial concentrations.
- All are inoculated with a standard concentration and incubated.
- The MIC is determined by the highest concentration that contains no visible growth.
- The advantage is reliability as it is the gold standard for MIC testing.
- The disadvantage is that these methods are time consuming and too labor-intensive for clinical practice.

Epsilometer Test (E-test)

- Uses an antibiotic-containing strip with a numeric concentration gradient.
- Bacteria are plated in a uniform manner with strips placed in a radial manner and allowed to incubate.
- Bacteria will grow in an elliptical pattern based on the concentration gradient.
- The MIC is determined by the point at which the ellipse crosses the strip.
  - See Figure 52-2
- Since the strips can be placed on a wide range of media, fastidious organisms and other organisms requiring special growth media can be tested.
- Strips may be supplemented with additional agents to detect certain resistance mechanisms.
- Other advantages include simplicity and flexibility, useful with rarely tested antibiotics.
- The disadvantage is that it is relatively expensive.

Spiral Gradient Endpoint Method

- Uses an agar with increasing antibiotic concentrations spiraling out from the center of the plate.
- An organism is streaked from the center of the plate outward.
- The distance of growth determines susceptibility.
- Although the method is expensive, inefficient, and rarely used, it may be valuable in detecting heteroresistance to vancomycin.

ESTABLISHING BREAKPOINTS

- Breakpoints are established by a number of different organizations.
  - Food and Drug Administration (FDA)
    - Establishes the baseline breakpoints at the time of drug approval

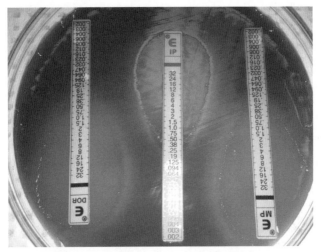

Figure 52-2. The E-strip contains a gradient of concentrations. The MIC is determined by visualizing where the ellipse crosses the strip.

- ◦ Pharmaceutical companies play a major role in the contribution of data.
- ◦ Rarely reevaluates
- • The Clinical and Laboratory Standards Institute (CLSI)
  - ◦ Formerly the National Committee for Clinical Laboratory Standards (NCCLS)
  - ◦ Nonprofit organization that develops consensus standards for the healthcare community.
  - ◦ Information regarding resistance mechanisms is also taken into consideration, often not available at the time of FDA approval.
- • The European Committee on Antimicrobial Susceptibility Testing (EUCAST)
  - ◦ Component of the European Society of Clinical Microbiology and Infectious Diseases
  - ◦ Publishes clinical breakpoints and available for download at www.eucast.org.
- • Both CLSI and EUCAST continuously update breakpoints on a yearly basis and as needed throughout the year.
  - ◦ The tables provide the MIC susceptibility breakpoint for Enterobacteriaceae (Table 52-1), *Pseudomonas aeruginosa* (Table 52-2), *Acinetobacter* spp. (Table 52-3), *Staphylococcus aureus* (Table 52-4), and *Streptococcus pneumoniae* (Table 52-5).
- • The establishment of clinical breakpoints is traditionally based on three key components: the distribution of the MIC's, the pharmacokinetic/pharmacodynamic data, and the clinical outcomes
  - • The distribution of MICs
    - ◦ Wild-type population without acquired resistance
    - ◦ Non–wild-type that may be harboring resistance patterns
  - • Pharmacokinetic data of the antimicrobial agent
    - ◦ In vitro drug characteristics
      - – Such as stability, MIC, and zone diameters
      - – Site of action—ribosome, cell wall, cell membrane, DNA
      - – Model for killing—time > MIC, AUC:MIC ratio, or concentration dependent
      - – Post-antibiotic effect—present if the drug continues to kill despite undetectable levels
      - – Bacteriostatic versus bacteriocidal
    - ◦ In vivo data such as pharmacokinetic properties and blood and tissue penetration bioavailability (if oral)
      - – Serum peak concentration (Cmax)
      - – Serum trough concentrations (Cmin)
      - – Volume of distribution (Vd)
        - • Tissue penetration
        - • Cerebrospinal fluid penetration
        - • Alveolar fluid penetration for pneumonia
        - • Body fluids pertaining to the type of infection
      - – Protein binding
      - – Metabolism
      - – Clearance
      - – Elimination half-life
      - – Special populations: renal and hepatic failure, obesity
  - • The clinical outcomes
    - ◦ Must have at least 500 isolates
    - ◦ Clinical and microbiologic cure rates
    - ◦ Clinical correlation is useful; however, extremely difficult to evaluate due to the multitude of confounders.

Table 52-1	Breakpoints for Enterobacteriaceae		
Antibiotic	**EUCAST**	**CLSI**	**Comments**
Ampicillin	8	8	Used for amoxicillin
Ampicillin-sulbactam	8/4	8/4	
Piperacillin-tazobactam	8/4	16/4	
Ticarcillin-clavulanate	8	16/2	
Cefazolin	R	2	Based on 2 g q8
Ceftriaxone	1	1	Based on 1 g q24
Ceftazidime	1	4	Based on 1 g q8
Cefepime	1	8	Based on 1 g q8 or 2 q12
Doripenem	1	1	Based on 500 mg q8
Ertapenem	0.5	2	Based on 1 q24
Imipenem-cilastatin	2	4	Low-level resistance common in *Morganella*, *Proteus*, and *Providencia*
Meropenem	2	4	
Aztreonam	1	4	Based on 1 g q8
Levofloxacin	1	2	
Gentamicin	2	4	Based on high-dose extended interval dosing
Tobramycin	2	4	Based on high-dose extended interval dosing
Amikacin	8	16	Based on high-dose extended interval dosing
Tigecycline	1	ND	Limited activity against *Proteus*, *Providencia*, and *Morganella*
Colistin	2	ND	
Trimethoprim-sulfamethoxazole	2/38	2/38	
Fosfomycin	32	64	*E. coli* urinary tract isolates only
Nitrofurantoin	64	32	Urinary isolates only

R, should be reported as resistant without testing; ND, not defined.

- Deterministic approach versus probabilistic approach to establishing breakpoints.
  - **Deterministic approach**
    - Breakpoints established by adjusting the mean population pharmacokinetic parameters to the susceptibility of different pathogens
    - Many of the pharmacokinetic/pharmacodynamic properties are not taken into consideration.
    - Tends to yield potentially higher breakpoints than what is feasible in clinical practice
  - Probabilistic
    - A newer approach to breakpoint establishment that takes into account pharmacokinetic modeling
    - Attempts to what is likely to happen, not simply what could possibly happen
    - Tends to result in lower than previously established breakpoints

Table 52-2	Breakpoints for *Pseudomonas aeruginosa*		
Antibiotic	**EUCAST**	**CLSI**	**Comments**
Piperacillin-tazobactam	16	16/4	Based on 4.5 g q6
Ticarcillin-clavulanate	16	16/2	Based on 3.1 g q6h
Cefepime	8	8	Based on 2 g q12 (CLSI) and q8 (EUCAST)
Ceftazidime	8	8	Based on 2 g q8
Doripenem	1	2	500 mg q8
Imipenem	4	2	Based on 1g q6 (EUCAST) and q8 (CLSI)
Meropenem	2	2	1 g q8
Aztreonam	1	8	
Levofloxacin	1	2	
Gentamicin	4	4	Based on high doses (5–7 mg/kg)
Tobramycin	4	4	Based on high doses (5–7 mg/kg)
Amikacin	8	16	Based on high doses (15–21 mg/kg)
Colistin	4	2	

Table 52-3	Breakpoints for *Acinetobacter* spp.		
Antibiotic	**EUCAST**	**CLSI**	**Comments**
Piperacillin-tazobactam	IE	16/4	
Ticarcillin-clavulanate	IE	16/2	
Ceftriaxone	R	8	
Cefepime	R	8	
Ceftazidime	R	8	
Doripenem	1	NR	
Imipenem	2	4	Based on 1 g q6
Meropenem	2	4	
Levofloxacin	1	2	
Gentamicin	4	4	Based on high doses (5–7 mg/kg)
Tobramycin	4	4	Based on high doses (5–7 mg/kg)
Amikacin	8	16	Based on high doses (15–21 mg/kg)
Colistin	2	2	
Trimethoprim-sulfamethoxazole	2	2/38	
Tigecycline	IE	NR	

IE, insufficient evidence to define a breakpoint; R, should be reported as resistant without testing; NR, not reported.

Table 52-4	Breakpoints for *Staphylococcus aureus*		
Antibiotic	**EUCAST**	**CLSI**	**Comments**
Penicillin	0.12	0.12	MIC <0.12 should be confirmed with disk diffusion.
Oxacillin	2	2	
Ceftaroline	NR	NR	Resistant isolates not discovered
Vancomycin	2	2	MIC of 2 may have reduced response
Daptomycin	1	1	
Tetracycline	1	4	If isolate susceptible, assume susceptible to doxycycline and minocycline
Minocycline	0.5	4	May be still be active even if resistant to tetracycline
Doxycycline	1	4	May be still be active even if resistant to tetracycline
Levofloxacin	1	1	
Clindamycin	0.25	0.5	If D-test negative
Trimethoprim-sulfamethoxazole	2	2/38	
Linezolid	4	4	
Nitrofurantoin	NR	32	
Telavancin	1	NR	
Tigecycline	0.5	NR	

NR, not reported.

- o The Monte Carlo simulation, for example, uses computer-generated model to create multiple scenarios.
  - o The probability from low to high of achieving the desired outcome is reported.
  - o Continuously updated as knowledge of pharmacokinetics and pharmacodynamics continues to increase and as new resistance mechanisms are introduced into the environment
- Normalized MIC distributions
  - MIC reported in terms of standard deviations away from the wild-type mode of distributions
  - Takes into consideration that breakpoints are drug-species dependent and would allow for direct comparison between agents
  - Would allow direct comparison between agents
  - This may one day play an important role in objectifying antimicrobial susceptibility results.

Other factors that contribute to the success of an antimicrobial therapy

- Host immune response
  - Single most important factor
  - Many disease states and medications contribute to suppression of the immune system.
  - May also be inhibited by virulence factors of certain microorganisms

Table 52-5	Breakpoints for *Streptococcus pneumoniae*		
Antibiotic	**EUCAST**	**CLSI**	**Comments**
Penicillin (meningitis)	0.06	0.06	
Penicillin (other)	2	2	With high doses (12 million units/day)
Ceftriaxone	0.5	0.5	CLSI: 1 for nonmeningitis
Cefepime	1	0.5	CLSI: 1 for nonmeningitis
Meropenem (meningitis)	0.25	0.25	
Meropenem (other)	2	See comment	CLSI—predicted by penicillin susceptibility
Levofloxacin	2	2	High dose (750 mg)
Vancomycin	2	1	
Linezolid	2	2	
Azithromycin	0.25	0.5	CLSI—susceptibility predicted by erythromycin ≤0.25
Clindamycin	0.5	0.25	
Doxycycline	1	See comment	CLSI: susceptibility predicted by tetracycline MIC ≤2
Trimethoprim-sulfamethoxazole	1	0.5/9.5	

- Site of infection
  - Drug-tissue penetration must be considered.
  - Immune system response may be insufficient in certain sites (central nervous system).
- Source control of infection
  - Antibiotics may not penetrate avascular fluid collections.
  - Abscesses and fluid collections must be drained in conjunction with antibiotics.
- Bacterial burden
  - Overwhelming sepsis by organisms may not respond appropriately to antibiotics.
- Appropriate dosing
  - Concentration-dependent drugs need to achieve sufficient concentrations at the site of infection.
  - Time above MIC-dependent drugs needs to sustain effective concentration for a sufficient period of time at the site of infection.

COMMON BACTERIA

Appropriate empiric antibiotic selection should target the most likely organisms to cause a certain infection. When considering an organism, an antimicrobial regimen should be selected based on the knowledge of common resistance patterns in conjunction with local susceptibilities such as a hospital antibiogram.

An **antibiogram** is a summary organism specific susceptibilities submitted to the hospital's microbiology and published periodically. Upon attainment of a culture and sensitivity report, the clinician can further target appropriate dosing or if needed, select a different agent with a higher likelihood of success. While the culture and sensitivity report is the most useful tool to guide treatment selection, there are certain pearls and pitfalls in susceptibility testing that must be considered. Many of these are organism specific. Also noted, certain Infectious Diseases Society of America (IDSA) guidelines have drug-organism specific treatment recommendations, which have been included.

- *Staphylococcus aureus*
  - Leading cause of nosocomial infections
  - Penicillin resistance is due to the production of a penicillinase.
    - Defined as MIC >0.12
    - Preferred beta-lactams include nafcillin, oxacillin, beta-lactam/beta-lactamase inhibitor combinations, first-generation cephalosporins, and carbapenems.
  - Methicillin resistance is due to alteration of the penicillin binding protein 2a (PBP2a) encoded on the mecA gene
    - Defined as MIC >2
    - The mecA gene frequently codes for resistance to aminoglycosides, macrolides, and fluoroquinolones.
    - Tetracyclines, trimethoprim-sulfamethoxazole, and clindamycin may still remain active against many strains of MRSA.
  - Macrolides, clindamycin, and streptogramin resistance is generally coded for by ermA and ermC, responsible for a ribosomal modification.
    - Resistance may be always constitutive or inducible.
    - For erythromycin-resistant, clindamycin-susceptible strains, a D-test should be performed to detect inducible clindamycin resistance.
    - This involves placing a clindamycin disk (CC) between 15 and 26 mm away from an erythromycin disk.
      - Circular growth indicates no inducible resistance.
      - D-shaped growth indicates inducible clindamycin resistance and clinical failure is likely.
      - See Figure 52-3
  - Vancomycin still maintains reliable activity against *Staphylococcus* although concern for MIC "creep" has emerged.
    - Still the preferred treatment for serious or life-threatening infections
    - MIC creep is a slow trend toward higher MIC's and has been associated with treatment failure, though the debate is controversial.
    - IDSA recommends selecting an alternative agent for vancomycin MIC >1 mcg/dL.
    - Vancomycin-intermediate *S. aureus* is related to a thickening of the cell wall resulting in reduced penetration of vancomycin to the site of action.
    - Vancomycin-resistant *S. aureus* is extremely rare.
      - There have been eight reported cases at the time of this writing in the United States.
      - Has been shown in vitro and in vivo that *Enterococcus faecalis* can transfer the vanA gene to *S. aureus* resulting in an alteration to the D-alanine-D-alanine binding site.
    - Alternative agents include linezolid, daptomycin, tigecycline, ceftaroline, telavancin, and quinupristin/dalfopristin.
- **Coagulase-negative staphylococci**
  - Common colonizers of the skin; true infection is often difficult to determine
  - Resistance patterns are similar to *S. aureus*.

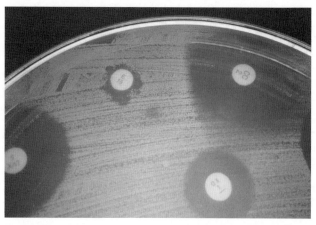

Figure 52-3. In a D-test positive isolate, the CC is placed within proximity of the erythromycin disk (E). The resistant erythromycin diffuses into the zone of clindamycin inducing resistance and giving the appearance of a D. Clindamycin should not be selected for treatment.

- Since resistance mechanisms are expressed at lower levels, lower breakpoints to oxacillin have been established.
  ○ MIC breakpoint for oxacillin set at 0.5 mcg/L, except for *Staphylococcus lugdunensis*
  ○ To assume oxacillin susceptible, multiple cultures are needed to confirm.
  ○ Cefoxitin is often used as a surrogate as it is more accurately detects the mecA-mediated resistance to beta-lactam.
- *S. lugdunensis* in the blood warrants attention and cardiac workup.
  ○ Often beta-lactamase–negative and oxacillin susceptible
  ○ MIC breakpoint set at 2
  ○ Can be confused with MSSA as it can be coagulase-positive if the slide test is used without the tube test confirmation
  ○ Not a contaminant!
- *Staphylococcus saprophyticus* is a pathogen in the urine and should be treated accordingly.
  ○ Second leading cause of urinary tract infections in young, sexually active females
  ○ Novobiocin resistance distinguishes from other nonpathogenic CNS.
  ○ Resistant strains are treated similar to *S. aureus.*
- **Enterococci**
  - Common colonizers of the gastrointestinal tract
  - Intrinsically resistant to cephalosporins, clindamycin, trimethoprim-sulfamethoxazole, and ticarcillin
  - Altered penicillin binding protein affinity responsible for penicillin, ampicillin, piperacillin, and imipenem resistance
  - *E. faecalis* capable of producing a beta-lactamase although not routinely tested
    ○ If detected, a beta-lactamase/beta-lactamase inhibitor combination may be used.
  - vanA and vanB confer high-level vancomycin resistance, seen predominantly in *E. faecalis* and *E. faecium*.

- vanC is a low-level resistance and is mostly seen in *Enterococcus gallinarum, Enterococcus flavescens*, and *Enterococcus casseliflavus.*
  - May still be susceptible to ampicillin!
- vanD, vanE, and vanG confer low-level resistance and not as commonly encountered.
- While not active as monotherapy, aminoglycosides are useful in serious infections when used synergistically with a cell-wall active agent.
  - Gentamicin is preferred due to simplicity of serum concentration testing.
    - Gentamicin resistance is most often the result of plasmid-mediated aminoglycoside-modifying enzymes (AMEs) that result in adenylation, acetylation, or phosphorylation.
  - Streptomycin may be used in certain gentamicin-resistant strains.
    - Not susceptible to AMEs
    - Resistance due to ribosomal modification
  - Other aminoglycosides are often intrinsically resistant and should not be used.
- Linezolid, daptomycin, and tigecycline seem to have activity against vancomycin-resistant enterococci, although breakpoints are not established.
- Quinupristin/dalfopristin is active against **E. faecium** but not **E. faecalis.**
- *Streptococcus pneumoniae*
  - Gram-positive diplococci found in the respiratory tract and leading cause of community-acquired pneumonia and bacterial meningitis
  - Increase in serotypes displaying a higher level of antibiotic resistance, such as 19A
  - Penicillin resistance due to alterations of the penicillin binding protein emerging worldwide
  - May also acquire resistance to macrolides due to ermB, tetracyclines due to TetM, and aminoglycosides due to aphA3, all contained on the transposon Tn1546
  - MefA also codes for efflux pump conferring resistance to macrolides.
  - Multidrug-resistant strains may still be susceptible to fluoroquinolones (not ciprofloxacin), vancomycin, and linezolid.
  - Different MIC values exist for meningitis and nonmeningitis isolates.
  - In the setting of meningitis, only penicillin, ceftriaxone, cefotaxime, meropenem, and vancomycin are reported.
  - **For meningitis, IDSA recommends the following based on the penicillin MIC.**
    - MIC <0.1:
      - Penicillin 4 million units every 4 hours
      - Ampicillin 2 g every 4 hours
    - MIC 0.1 to 1.0:
      - Third-generation cephalosporin (ceftriaxone 2 g every 12 hours)
    - MIC of 2 or greater or ceftriaxone MIC 1 or greater
      - Vancomycin plus a third-generation cephalosporin
      - May also consider adding rifampin if the ceftriaxone MIC is >2
  - **For community-acquired pneumonia, IDSA recommends the following based on the penicillin MIC.**
    - MIC <2:
      - Penicillin G or amoxicillin
    - MIC of 4 or greater
      - Third-generation cephalosporin (not ceftazidime)
      - Respiratory fluoroquinolone (not ciprofloxacin)

- MIC of 4 or less, may consider
  - Amoxicillin 1 g every 8 hours
  - Penicillin at doses of 18 to 24 million units/day
- *Streptococcus* **groups A, B, C, and G**
  - Beta-lactam susceptibility is inferred from penicillin susceptibility.
  - Resistance to penicillin (MIC >0.25) is rare and not yet reported.
  - Beta-lactamase inhibitors is unnecessary as groups A, B, C, and G do not produce beta-lactamases.
  - Susceptibility to erythromycin screens for susceptibility to azithromycin and clarithromycin
    - Macrolide resistance emerging
  - Inducible clindamycin resistance can be detected using a D-test.
  - While levofloxacin and moxifloxacin susceptibility may be inferred from a norfloxacin screen, ciprofloxacin has little activity against streptococci.
  - While tetracycline susceptibility implies susceptibility to doxycycline and minocycline, resistance does not always translate to doxycycline or minocycline resistance.
    - An MIC method (E-test) should be performed on tetracycline-resistant isolates.
  - Other reliable options include vancomycin, tigecycline, daptomycin, and linezolid.
  - Common organisms
    - *Streptococcus pyogenes* **(group A streptococci)**
      - Common cause of bacterial pharyngitis, cellulitis, and other skin and soft tissue infections
      - Also the cause of acute rheumatic fever and acute glomerulonephritis
      - Virulence is dependent upon the presence of several proteins.
      - Tetracyclines and trimethoprim-sulfamethoxazole are not reliable treatment options.
    - *Streptococcus agalactiae* **(group B streptococci)**
      - Common pathogen in neonatal sepsis/meningitis, septic arthritis, and skin and soft tissue infections
      - More common in elderly and those with comorbidities (diabetes)
      - Often resistant to clindamycin
- **Viridans group streptococci**
  - Normal flora of the mucosa, gastrointestinal tract, upper respiratory tract, and skin in healthy humans
  - Often contaminants and should only be considered pathogens in sterile sites
  - Species known to cause infections in humans.
    - Anginosus group
      - *Streptococcus anginosus, Streptococcus constellatus*, and *Streptococcus intermedius*
      - Formerly known as *Streptococcus milleri*
      - May cause certain purulent infections
    - Bovis group
      - *S. gallolyticus, S. pasteurianus, S. infantarius*, and *S. lutetiensis*
      - May be a cause of endocarditis
      - Linked to colonic malignancy, related to the portal of entry
    - Mutans group
      - *Streptococcus mutans* and *Streptococcus sobrinus*
      - Associated with endocarditis and dental caries
    - Salivarius group
      - *Streptococcus salivarius* and *Streptococcus vestibularis*
      - Mostly seen in immunocompromised hosts

○ Mitis group
  - *Streptococcus mitis, Streptococcus oralis, Streptococcus sanguis*, and *Streptococcus gordonii*
  - May be seen in endocarditis and neutropenic infections
- Beta-lactam susceptibility can be inferred from penicillin susceptibility.
  ○ Isolates reported as resistant to penicillin should be tested for individual agents
  ○ Disk diffusion is unreliable for beta-lactams; E-test should be performed.
- As with *S. aureus*, inducible clindamycin resistance can be detected using a D-test.
- May develop increased MIC's to penicillin
- **For endocarditis, IDSA recommends the following treatments based on MIC.**
  ○ MIC ≤0.12 (highly sensitive)
    - Penicillin 12 to 18 million units per day for 4 weeks
  ○ MIC 0.25 to 0.5 (relatively resistant)
    - Penicillin 24 million units per day for 4 weeks
      · Add gentamicin for serious infections for 2 weeks
    - Ceftriaxone 2 g/day for 4 weeks
      · Add gentamicin for serious infections for 2 weeks
    - Vancomycin 15 mg/kg every 12 hours for 4 weeks
  ○ MIC >0.5 (resistant)
    - Penicillin 18 to 30 million units plus gentamicin for 6 weeks
    - Ampicillin plus gentamicin for endocarditis for 6 weeks
    - Vancomycin 15 mg/kg every 12 hours for 6 weeks
- **Nutritionally variant streptococci**
  - Includes *Abiotrophia defectiva* and *Granulicatella* species
  - Difficult to grow, may be considered in "culture-negative" endocarditis
  - Require supplementation with pyridoxine or cysteine
  - Determination of susceptibilities is difficult and not reliable.
  - Should be treated like enterococci
    ○ Non-endocarditis: ampicillin or vancomycin
    ○ Endocarditis: add gentamicin
- **Enterobacteriaceae**
  - Family containing many species of aerobic and facultatively anaerobic gram-negative bacilli.
  - Common colonizers of the gastrointestinal tract
  - Leading cause of urinary tract infections and a major source of nosocomial infections
  - Common pathogenic Enterobacteriaceae include *Escherichia, Enterobacter, Klebsiella, Proteus, Providencia,* and *Salmonella.*
  - Less pathogenic Enterobacteriaceae include *Citrobacter, Edwardsiella, Erwinia, Hafnia, Serratia, Shigella,* and *Yersinia.*
  - Resistance can be innate or acquired.
    ○ Innate (or intrinsic resistance) is shown in Table 52-6.
    ○ Acquired resistance becoming increasingly common; therapy should be guided by susceptibility testing for clinically significant organisms.
    ○ Resistance to aminoglycosides, tetracyclines, chloramphenicol, fluoroquinolones, and trimethoprim-sulfamethoxazole also common; however, standard testing is generally accurate in detecting resistance.
  - Beta-lactamase production is a constantly increasing and evolving issue.
    ○ TEM-1 and TEM-2: resistance to ampicillin in *Escherichia coli*
    ○ SHV-1: resistance to ampicillin in *Klebsiella* spp.

Table 52-6	Innate Resistance of Enterobacteriaceae							
Organism	Ampicillin	Ampicillin-sulbactam	Piperacillin	Cefazolin	Cefuroxime	Tetracyclines	Colistin
Citrobacter freundii	R	R		R	R		
Citrobacter koseri	R	R	R				
Enterobacter spp.	R	R		R	R		
Klebsiella pneumoniae	R						
Morganella morganii	R			R	R	R	R
Proteus mirabilis						R	R
Proteus vulgaris	R			R	R	R	R
Providencia stuartii	R	R		R	R	R	R
Serratia marcescens	R	R		R	R		R

R, denotes intrinsic resistance by the organism. If reported as susceptible, caution is advised in interpretation.

○ Class A (Bush 2b): resistance to penicillin and aminopenicillins
○ **Extended spectrum beta-lactamase (ESBL):**
  - Derivatives of the TEM and SHV genes
  - Confer resistance to all penicillins, cephalosporins, and aztreonam
  - May show in vitro susceptibility to cefoxitin
  - Automated systems have variable sensitivity and specificity for the detection of ESBL.
  - Manual tests include the addition of clavulanic acid to cefotaxime or ceftazidime.
    • A decrease of three MIC dilutions or more or a zone diameter decrease of >5 mm confirms ESBL.
    • Enhanced activity of amoxicillin-clavulanate placed at 30 mm from third-generation cephalosporin may also be a screening too.
  - Broth dilution confirmation is concluded by a threefold or greater MIC reduction by the addition of clavulanate to a third-generation cephalosporin.
  - Additional automated systems (VITEK) or DNA probes are also available.
  - While beta-lactam inhibitors are active against ESBLs, the hyperproduction may overwhelm the inhibitor and therapeutic failure may occur.
  - Carbapenems or tigecycline may be used.
○ AmpC:
  - Class I inducible beta-lactamase
  - Present in almost all *Enterobacter, Serratia, Providencia, Morganella morganii, Citrobacter freundii, Hafnia alvei,* and *Aeromonas*
  - Not susceptible to beta-lactamase inhibitors (cefoxitin will show as resistant)
  - May not express until 3 to 4 days of therapy with a third-generation cephalosporin
  - AmpC presence may result in false-negative ESBL detection.
  - AmpC is much less active on cefepime, which may be used as a screening tool for detection.
  - Carbapenems or tigecycline may be used.
○ Carbapenemases
  - May be chromosomal or plasmid mediated
  - Confer resistance to all beta-lactams including penicillins, cephalosporins, and carbapenems
  - Class A carbapenemases
    • Require *serine* at the active position to account for beta-lactam hydrolysis
    • Notable enzymes include
      • Serratia marcescens enzyme (SME) seen in *Serratia marcescens*
      • Imipenem hydrolyzing enzyme (IMI) seen in *Enterobacter*
      • Not metalloenzyme carbapenemase (NMC) seen in *Enterobacter*
    • Klebsiella pneumoniae carbapenemases (KPCs) detected on a number of Enterobacteriaceae as well as *P. aeruginosa*
    • Detected by increasing MICs to carbapenems with ertapenem and perhaps meropenem being the most sensitive
    • Confirmation tests include the modified Hodge test and broth microdilution.
      • See Figure 52-4
  - Class B carbapenemases
    • Also known as metallo-beta-lactamases (MBL)
    • Require zinc (instead of serine) for hydrolysis of beta-lactams
    • May naturally occur in organisms such as *Aeromonas hydrophila* and *Stenotrophomonas maltophilia*

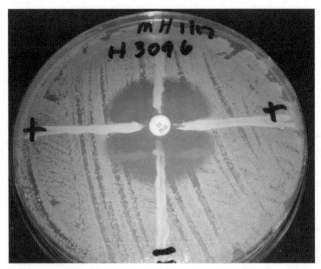

Figure 52-4. In a modified Hodge test, a carbapenem susceptible strain of *E. coli* is confluently and uniformly spread on a Mueller-Hinton plate. A carbapenem disk is placed in the center of the plate. Above, two positive controls (+), a negative control (–), and the tested isolate (3096) are streaked from the edge of the disk to the outside of the plate. After incubation, the positive controls and the tested isolate show growth of the *E. coli* along the streak line giving the appearance of a cloverleaf. The negative control shows no growth along the streak line.

- Notable enzymes include:
  - New Delhi MBL (NDM-1)
    ○ First isolated in India
    ○ Has a high propensity to spread
  - Verona integron-encoded MBL (VIM)
  - Others include IMP, VIM, GIM, SPM, and SIM
  - May appear susceptible in vitro and are difficult to detect
  - EDTA, a chelating agent, may play a role in detection due to the dependence on zinc for activity.
  - Class D carbapenemases
  - Includes the OXA-type enzymes
  - Mostly seen in *Acinetobacter*
  - There are no screening methods.
  - Colistin or tigecycline may be considered for therapy.
- *Pseudomonas aeruginosa*
  - Strict aerobe commonly colonizing hospital equipment and a common cause of nosocomial infections
  - Intrinsically resistant to narrow-spectrum penicillins, first- and second-generation cephalosporins, and trimethoprim-sulfamethoxazole
  - May possess inducible resistance to many antibiotics and repeat cultures should be retested for susceptibilities

- Capable of producing a exopolysaccharide biofilm further complicating treatment
- Therapeutic options include piperacillin, ticarcillin, ceftazidime, cefepime, carbapenems except ertapenem, aminoglycosides, levofloxacin, and ciprofloxacin.
- Aztreonam may be an alternative treatment option in a patient with severe beta-lactam allergy although resistance rates are rising.
- Of the aminoglycosides, amikacin has the highest activity, followed by tobramycin, and lastly, gentamicin.
- Colistin and polymyxin B are considered last-line agents for multidrug-resistant strains; however, MIC interpretive criteria are not established.
- *Stenotrophomonas maltophilia*
  - Increasing cause of nosocomial infections in immunocompromised or debilitated patients with limited treatment options
  - Commonly a colonizer in immunocompetent hosts
  - Intrinsically resistant to many beta-lactams including carbapenems and aminoglycosides
  - Mechanisms of resistance include beta-lactamases, decreased outer membrane permeability, and efflux pumps.
  - Treatment of choice is trimethoprim-sulfamethoxazole.
  - Other therapeutic options include newer fluoroquinolones (levofloxacin and moxifloxacin), minocycline, ticarcillin-clavulanate, aztreonam, and tigecycline.
- *Acinetobacter* **spp.**
  - Strict aerobic gram-negative rod and common cause of nosocomial infections
  - May be difficult to gram stain resulting in a falsely reported gram-positive cocci
  - Known to acquire a multitude of resistance mechanisms including beta-lactamases, efflux pumps, and altered membrane proteins
  - Disk diffusion methods may be inconsistent for certain beta-lactams such as ticarcillin-clavulanate and piperacillin-tazobactam.
  - Carbapenems are generally considered to be the preferred therapy.
  - Tigecycline is often used for multidrug-resistant strains; however, no breakpoints exist.
  - Colistin and polymyxin B have established breakpoints and should be considered as last-line therapy.
  - While ampicillin has little activity, sulbactam does possess direct antimicrobial activity against *Acinetobacter* and may be considered for last-line therapy.
  - The addition of rifampin to a therapeutic regimen may be considered for persistent infections.
- *Burkholderia cepacia*
  - Mostly seen in cystic fibrosis, however, emerging as a nosocomial pathogen
  - Highly resistant and difficult to test
  - Therapeutic options include trimethoprim-sulfamethoxazole, fluoroquinolones, and minocycline.
  - Though controversial, synergy testing may be considered.
- **Miscellaneous**
  - *Listeria monocytogenes*
    - Opportunistic organism associated with child birth and age >50
    - Treatment of choice is ampicillin with or without gentamicin.
    - Alternatives include meropenem and sulfamethoxazole-trimethoprim.
    - Possibly consider the use of zyvox.

- *Haemophilus influenzae*
  - Growth requires two factors…both present on a chocolate agar
  - Up to 40% produce a beta-lactamase (TEM-1) resistant to ampicillin
  - Beta-lactamase–positive organisms still remain susceptible to third-generation cephalosporins (ceftriaxone), macrolides, and fluoroquinolones.
  - Trimethoprim-sulfamethoxazole resistance emerging
  - Of the macrolides, azithromycin is more active in vitro than clarithromycin.
- *Moraxella catarrhalis*
  - Beta-lactamase producer, similar to *H. influenzae*
  - Sulfamethoxazole-trimethoprim and tetracycline resistance may also be an issue.
  - Second- or third-generation cephalosporins are the treatment of choice.
- *Neisseria*
  - *Neisseria gonorrhoeae*
    - Resistance testing is not practical and rarely performed.
    - May produce a beta-lactamase or have altered penicillin binding protein, however, still susceptible to third-generation cephalosporins
    - **Fluoroquinolones are no longer recommended due to resistance.**
  - *Neisseria meningitidis*
    - E-test has demonstrated variable results.
    - Fluoroquinolone resistance becoming an issue
    - Penicillin MIC should be considered when treating.
    - **For meningitis, IDSA recommends the following based on the penicillin MIC.**
      - <0.1
        - Penicillin 4 million units every 4 hours
        - Ampicillin 2 g every 4 hours
      - MIC 0.1 to 1.0
        - Third-generation cephalosporin (ceftriaxone 2 g every 12 hours)
- Coryneform bacteria
  - Frequent contaminants
  - Club-shaped gram-positive rods on gram stain often said to mimic Chinese letters
  - Includes *Corynebacterium, Arcanobacterium, Brevibacterium, Dermabacter, Microbacterium, Rothia, Turicella, Arthrobacter,* and *Oerskovia*
  - May cause infection in immunocompromised hosts and in hospitalized patients
  - Notable pathogens
    - *Corynebacterium jeikeium* and *Corynebacterium amycolatum*
      - Often multidrug resistant
      - May be treated with vancomycin
    - *Corynebacterium urealyticum*
      - Usually resistant to beta-lactams, aminoglycosides, and trimethoprim-sulfamethoxazole
      - Variable susceptibility to fluoroquinolones, macrolides, and tetracyclines
      - Remains susceptible to vancomycin
    - *Corynebacterium striatum* may be resistant to penicillin but is often susceptible to other beta-lactams and vancomycin.

- *Bacillus*
  - Environmental contaminants
  - *Bacillus cereus* produces a broad-spectrum beta-lactamase and may be treated with clindamycin, gentamicin, vancomycin, or a carbapenem.
- *Chryseobacterium* spp.
  - Soil and water inhabitants and can survive treatment with chlorine
  - Usually low virulence
  - *Chryseobacterium meningosepticum* may cause hospital-acquired infections or infection in immunocompromised hosts.
  - Resistant to most antibiotics and no established breakpoints by CLSI
  - Therapeutic options may include levofloxacin, trimethoprim-sulfamethoxazole, vancomycin, and minocycline.
  - Rifampin appears to be active and may be added for combination therapy.
- Anaerobes
  - Common source of normal flora
  - May be associated with intra-abdominal infections, infections of the oral cavity, empyema, aspiration pneumonia, pelvic inflammatory disease, diabetic foot infections, gas gangrene, and abscess formation
  - Gram-positive anaerobes include *Clostridium, Peptostreptococcus,* Peptococcus, *Actinomyces,* and *Propionibacterium.*
  - Gram-negative anaerobes include *Bacteroides, Prevotella, Fusobacterium, Porphyromonas,* and *Veillonella.*
  - Resistance primarily due to beta-lactamases, although other mechanisms reported
  - **Routine susceptibility testing rarely performed**
    - Global surveillance susceptibilities should guide therapy.
    - Tables 52-7 and 52-8 provide susceptibilities based on surveillance cultures.
  - When clinically necessary, E-test should be performed as disk diffusion is not reliable.
  - For *Bacteroides fragilis*, clindamycin and moxifloxacin may not be reliable.
  - For *Propionibacterium acnes*, metronidazole is not reliable.

Antimicrobial susceptibility testing is an important part of antibiotic selection but must be used in conjunction with several other factors such as tissue penetration and host immunity. Breakpoints have been established to assist clinicians in assessing culture and sensitivity reporting. There are many limitations to antimicrobial susceptibility testing, and clinical knowledge of the organisms is crucial to avoid therapeutic failure. As our knowledge of pharmacokinetics and pharmacodynamics and the impact of antimicrobial therapy continues to grow, breakpoints are adapted to provide the highest quality of care.

Table 52-7	Percent Resistance of Bacteroides Group Organisms Against Selected Organisms from 2008 to 2009							
Species	Ampicillin-sulbactam	Piperacillin-tazobactam	Cefoxitin	Meropenem	Tigecycline	Clindamycin	Moxifloxacin	Metronidazole
B. fragilis	3.2	1.3	7.4	2.5	5.4	29.9	39.9	0
B. ovatus	1.4	0	14.1	0	4.7	36	71.9	0
B. thetaiotaomicron	2.7	0.5	20.9	1.8	2.3	43.2	56.9	0
B. vulgatus	4.4	0	5.8	1.4	4.3	43.9	71	0
B. distasonis	11.1	0	16.6	0	0	37	38.9	0
B. uniformis	3.6	0	7.1	0	3.6	35.8	57.2	0

Table 52-8	Percent Resistance of Non-Bacteroides Group Organisms Against Selected Organisms from 2007 to 2009							
Species	Ampicillin-sulbactam	Piperacillin-tazobactam	Cefoxitin	Meropenem	Penicillin	Clindamycin	Moxifloxacin	Metronidazole
Prevotella	1	1	1	1	49	39	24	0
Clostridium perfringens	0	0	0	0	0	0	1	0
Other Clostridium spp.	0	0	26	0	9	21	12	0
Fusobacterium nucleatum-necrophorum	0	0	0	0	0	0	5	0
Veillonella spp.	0	7	0	0	28	7	11	11
Proprionibacterium acnes	0	0	0	0	0	3	0	97
Gram-positive anaerobes[a]	1	0	0	0	3	20	11	1

[a]Includes *Peptococcus, Peptostreptococcus, Finegoldia, Peptoniphilus*, and *Anaerococcus*. (Clinical and Laboratory Standards Institute. *Performance Standards for Antimicrobial Susceptibility Testing; Twenty-Second Informational Supplement. CLSI document M100-S22.* Clinical and Laboratory Standards Institute, Wayne, Pennsylvania, USA; 2012.

SUGGESTED READINGS

Ambrose PG. Antimicrobial susceptibility breakpoints: PK-PD and susceptibility breakpoints. *Treat Respir Med* 2005;4(suppl 1):5–11.

Baddour LM, Wilson WR, et al. Infective endocarditis: diagnosis, antimicrobial therapy, and management of complications: a statement for healthcare professionals from the Committee on Rheumatic Fever, Endocarditis, and Kawasaki Disease, Council on Cardiovascular Disease in the Young, and the Councils on Clinical Cardiology, Stroke, and Cardiovascular Surgery and Anesthesia, American Heart Association: endorsed by the Infectious Diseases Society of America. *Circulation* 2005;111(23):e394–e434.

Carattoli A. Resistance plasmid families in Enterobacteriaceae. *Antimicrob Agents Chemother* 2009;53(6):2227–2238.

Clinical and Laboratory Standards Institute. *Performance Standards for Antimicrobial Susceptibility Testing; Twenty-Second Informational Supplement. CLSI document M100-S22.* Clinical and Laboratory Standards Institute. Wayne, Pennsylvania, USA; 2012.

Dalhoff A, Ambrose PG, et al. A long journey from minimum inhibitory concentration testing to clinically predictive breakpoints: deterministic and probabilistic approaches in deriving breakpoints. *Infection* 2009;37(4):296–305.

EUCAST. Breakpoint tables for interpretation of MICs and zone diametersVersion 2.0, valid from 2012-01-01. Available at http://www.eucast.org/clinical_breakpoints. Accessed January 17, 2012.

Holland TL, Woods CW, et al. Antibacterial susceptibility testing in the clinical laboratory. *Infect Dis Clin North Am* 2009;23(4):757–790, vii.

Jacoby GA. AmpC beta-lactamases. *Clin Microbiol Rev* 2009;22(1):161–182, Table of Contents.

Kanj SS, Kanafani ZA. Current concepts in antimicrobial therapy against resistant gram-negative organisms: extended-spectrum beta-lactamase-producing Enterobacteriaceae, carbapenem-resistant Enterobacteriaceae, and multidrug-resistant *Pseudomonas aeruginosa. Mayo Clin Proc* 2011;86(3):250–259.

Kronvall G. Normalized resistance interpretation as a tool for establishing epidemiological MIC susceptibility breakpoints. *J Clin Microbiol* 2010;48(12):4445–4452.

Normalized resistance interpretation (NRI) utilizes the fact that the wild-type population on the sensitive side is not affected by resistance development, and therefore, a normalized reconstruction of the peak can be performed. This method offers a new tool in comparative susceptibility studies such as global surveillance of resistance as well as in quality control in individual laboratories.

Kronvall G, Giske CG, et al. Setting interpretive breakpoints for antimicrobial susceptibility testing using disk diffusion. *Int J Antimicrob Agents* 2011;38(4):281–290.

Leclercq R, Canton R, et al. EUCAST expert rules in antimicrobial susceptibility testing. *Clin Microbiol Infect* 2011 Oct21.doi:10.1111/j.1469–0691.2011.03703.x. [Epub ahead of print].

MacGowan A. Breakpoints for extended-spectrum beta-lactamase-producing Enterobacteriacae: pharmacokinetic/pharmacodynamic considerations. *Clin Microbiol Infect* 2008;14(suppl 1):166–168.

With ESBL-producing strains of Enterobacteriacae, it is known that MIC, and hence T>MIC, for beta-lactams predicts outcome.

Schreckenberger PC, Binnicker MJ. Optimizing antimicrobial susceptibility test reporting. *J Clin Microbiol* 2011;49:S15–S19.

Stass H, Dalhoff A. The integrated use of pharmacokinetic and pharmacodynamic models for the definition of breakpoints. *Infection* 2005;33(suppl 2):29–35.

Stratton CW. In vitro susceptibility testing versus in vivo effectiveness. *Med Clin North Am* 2006;90(6):1077–1088.

Tunkel AR, Hartman BJ, et al. Practice guidelines for the management of bacterial meningitis. *Clin Infect Dis* 2004;39(9):1267–1284.

Yang K, Guglielmo BJ. Diagnosis and treatment of extended-spectrum and AmpC beta-lactamase-producing organisms. *Ann Pharmacother* 2007;41(9):1427–1435.

53 Case Examples in MIC Interpretation

Paul Lewis and James W. Myers

Bacterial cultures are tested for minimum inhibitory concentrations (MICs) and given an interpretation of susceptible (S), intermediate (I), or resistant (R) based on the breakpoints established in the previous chapter. Antibiotic reports are often a better source of determining which agents should not be used rather than predicting which agents will be successful.

For mild to moderate infections, the S, I, or R interpretation may be all that is needed in selecting an antimicrobial agent. In general, a serum level of >10 times the MIC usually means the organism is S. Around four times the MIC means the organism is intermediate and less than four often means the organism is resistant.

However, for serious infections, other more stringent criteria must be considered when selecting a drug and a dose. It is important to note that the lowest MIC is not always the drug of choice. The MICs cannot be directly compared without knowing the pharmacokinetics and pharmacodynamics of the drug. Table 53-1 provides many of the important parameters useful in evaluating MIC criteria. Table 53-2 provides recommendations to assist in selecting an antimicrobial regimen. There is often more than one correct choice, and clinical experience should always be considered. The following cases discuss the results susceptibility reports and the rationale in selecting an antimicrobial regimen.

CASE 1

Patient X is a 72-year-old female admitted for sepsis with gram-negative rod bacteremia. Patient had nausea and vomiting for a day almost 4 days back, which improved, but after that she stayed lethargic with decreased oral intake. She also complained of dysuria and left flank pain so her daughter took her to the primary care doctor where she was found to have leukocytosis and acute renal failure and was sent into the hospital for admission. Blood cultures are positive for gram-negative rods; however, culture and susceptibilities are pending. The urine culture returned the following results:

Specimen number: #####
Specimen source: Urine—Clean Catch
Culture:
Escherichia coli
>100,000 cfu/mL

Antibiotic	*E. coli*
Ampicillin	≥32 R
Ceftriaxone	≤1 S
Gentamicin	4 S
Imipenem	≤1 S
Levofloxacin	4 I
Nitrofurantoin	≤16 S
Trimethoprim-sulfa	≥320 R

Table 53-1	Pharmacokinetic Parameters Affecting Plasma Concentrations		
Antibiotic	**Peak (mcg/mL)**	**Half-Life in Nonrenal Impairment (Hours)**	**Pharmacokinetic Model**
Piperacillin 3 g	240	1	T > MIC
Piperacillin 4 g	300	1	T > MIC
Cefazolin 1 g	180	2	T > MIC
Ceftriaxone 1 g	150	8	T > MIC
Cefepime 1 g	80	2	T > MIC
Cefepime 2 g	160	2	T > MIC
Imipenem 500 mg	40	1	T > MIC
Doripenem 500 mg	23	1	T > MIC
Levofloxacin 500 mg	7	7	AUC:MIC
Levofloxacin 750 mg	12	7	AUC:MIC
Gentamicin 2 mg/kg	8	2	Peak:MIC
Gentamicin 7 mg/kg	28	2	Peak:MIC
Amikacin 8 mg/kg	32	2	Peak:MIC
Amikacin 15 mg/kg	60	2	Peak:MIC
Tigecycline 50 mg	0.6	42	AUC:MIC
Vancomycin 20 mg/kg	40	6	AUC:MIC
Linezolid 600 mg	15	5	AUC:MIC
Daptomycin 6 mg/kg	60	9	Peak:MIC

T > MIC: time above MIC dependant killing; AUC:MIC: area under the curve (total drug exposure) dependant killing; Peak:MIC: concentration dependant killing

Ampicillin and trimethoprim-sulfamethoxazole are reported as R and should not be used. Levofloxacin is reported as I. If the patient did not show signs of sepsis, then levofloxacin may be considered since the concentration in the urine is extremely high. However, a 750-mg dose of levofloxacin IV achieves a plasma level of approximately 12 mcg/mL. This would not be sufficient to achieve adequate killing in the plasma and should not be used. Nitrofurantoin is reported as S with an MIC ≤16. While this number may seem high, even at 32, nitrofurantoin achieves a high enough concentration in the urine to be considered for cystitis but does not treat infections such as pyelonephritis or urosepsis. Therefore, nitrofurantoin should not be used. *E. coli* does not possess any intrinsic resistance, and further workup is not needed unless allergies warrant alternative agents. The remaining antibiotics include two beta-lactams (ceftriaxone and imipenem) and an aminoglycoside, gentamicin. If the infection were only in the urine, either of the three would be fine. However, gentamicin with an MIC of four would be a poor choice for a bloodstream infection. When dosed as 2 mg/kg, the peak plasma level is approximately 8 mcg/mL. When dosed using 7 mg/kg, the peak plasma concentration would be approximately 28 mcg/mL. Both imipenem and ceftriaxone achieve very high plasma levels and would be good options even with the bloodstream infection; however, ceftriaxone has a narrower spectrum and would be preferred. Susceptibilities to tobramycin and amikacin may be requested if an aminoglycoside were needed. Turnaround time is generally 24 hours but should be considered if the patient's condition worsens.

Table 53-2	Tips for Selecting an Antimicrobial Agent Based on an MIC Report

1. Avoid any drugs reported as R or I.
2. Avoid any drugs that are not likely to get to the source of infection (moxifloxacin or tigecycline in the urine, clindamycin or tigecycline in the blood, daptomycin in the lungs, levofloxacin or piperacillin-tazobactam in the brain).
3. Avoid drugs for which the organism is known to have intrinsic resistance (see table in previous chapter).
4. Consider whether further testing is needed to detect inducible resistance (clindamycin D-test, ESBL detection probe, modified Hodge test for carbapenemase).
5. If there are multiple organisms, consider whether single agent can cover multiple organisms.
6. Of the remaining agents, consider pharmacokinetic/pharmacodynamic data (from table in previous chapter: drug peak, half-life, and killing model). Compare the MIC with the most appropriate killing model:
   a. Will the drug level be maintained above the MIC for a sufficient amount of time (at least 40%–70%) for beta-lactams and other time above MIC dependant killers?
   b. Can a sufficient peak to MIC ratio (5–10×) be achieved for aminoglycosides and other concentration dependant killers?
   c. Will the total 24-hour drug exposure compared to the MIC be sufficient for fluoroquinolones and other AUC:MIC dependant killers?
7. Of the remaining agents, beta-lactams are generally preferred. If no beta-lactam is available, consider what agents are appropriate for the site of infection (aminoglycosides for urine).
8. Select the narrowest spectrum agent if possible.

CASE 2

Patient Y is a 62-year-old male with a past medical history significant for obesity, diabetes mellitus type 2, hypertension, and peripheral neuropathy. He is admitted to a general medicine floor for a complicated diabetic foot ulcer involving the right foot with fever of 39.4°C, chills, gangrenous little toe with purulent discharge, and redness involving the little toe. A culture is taken from the discharge, and the patient is empirically started on ceftriaxone and metronidazole. The following report appears 2 days later.

Specimen number:######
Specimen Source: Wound—Leg, Left
Gram stain: moderate (3+) gram-positive cocci and moderate (3+) gram-negative rods
Culture:
Aerobic plate: *Staphylococcus aureus, Pseudomonas aeruginosa*
Susceptibility to follow
Anaerobic plate: *Bacteroides fragilis*

Antibiotic	S. aureus	P. aeruginosa
Amikacin		4 S
Amoxicillin-clav		

(Continued)

Cefazolin		
Cefepime		8 S
Ceftriaxone		
Clindamycin	≤0.25 R	
Erythromycin	≥8 R	
Gentamicin	≤0.5 S	8 I
Imipenem		≤1 S
Levofloxacin		1 S
Oxacillin	≥4 R	
Penicillin	≥0.5 R	
Piperacillin-tazo		4 S
Tetracycline	≤1 S	
Tobramycin		4 S
Trimethoprim-sulfa	≤10 S	
Vancomycin	1 S	
Clindamycin D-test	Positive	

This culture contains three different organisms. Anaerobic cultures are rarely tested for susceptibilities. Treatment should be guided by national surveillance reports and general knowledge of antimicrobial cover. Metronidazole is the gold standard for *Bacteroides* group organisms. Alternatives include beta-lactam/beta-lactamase inhibitor combinations, carbapenems, and tigecycline. Double coverage is not needed. Clindamycin, moxifloxacin, and cefoxitin are also active against many anaerobes but resistance is possible.

The *S. aureus* is penicillin and oxacillin or methicillin resistant (MRSA). Oxacillin resistance implies resistance to all beta-lactams so no other beta-lactams are reported. Ceftaroline is the exception to this as it is active against MRSA; however, *in vitro* testing is not routinely performed. In the setting of clindamycin susceptible (MIC ≤ 0.25) and erythromycin resistance, a D-test is automatically performed. A positive result corrected the clindamycin from S to R due to the presence of inducible clindamycin resistance. Since the organism is D-test–positive, clindamycin is not an option, despite the presence of a low MIC. Susceptibility to gentamicin suggests that it may be used for synergy dosing but not as the primary agent. Tetracycline susceptibility also predicts doxycycline and minocycline susceptibility. The MIC to vancomycin is 1 suggesting that vancomycin may be used assuming that sufficient dosing (15 to 20 mg/kg) is given to target vancomycin troughs of 15 to 20 mcg/mL. If MIC were 2, it would still appear as susceptible; however, alternative agents should be considered based on the 2009 Infectious Diseases Society of America vancomycin guidelines. Alternative agent such as linezolid, daptomycin, telavancin, or tigecycline should be considered. These agents may also be considered if the wound fails to respond to current therapy. MIC reports may be off by 1 dilution in either direction; therefore, a reported MIC of 1 may truly be 0.5 or 2.

For *P. aeruginosa* the MICs reported from *in vitro* testing is reliable. Comparison of MIC data with simple pharmacokinetics should be taken into consideration to ensure that the appropriate drug concentrations reach the site of infection. Three beta-lactams were tested: cefepime, piperacillin-tazobactam, and imipenem. Since beta-lactams are time above MIC dependant killers, therapy is designed to maintain consistent levels of drug at the site of infection for the most amount of time.

Piperacillin 4-g dose achieves a peak concentration of 300 mcg/mL and has a half-life of 1 hour in normal renal function. By the end of a 6-hour dosing interval, the plasma concentration will still remain above the MIC. If an 8-hour interval were incorrectly chosen, the level would drop below the MIC, unless an extended dosing interval was used. Cefepime 2-g dose achieves a peak concentration of 160 mcg/mL and has a half-life of 2 hours. The after 8 hours would still be sufficient to provide effective killing however would be insufficient after 12 hours. If 1 g every 12 hours were incorrectly chosen, the plasma level would not be sufficient to drop to roughly 1 mcg/mL, with most of the dosing time below the MIC. The imipenem MIC is reported as ≤1, meaning that the test sensitivity does not go below 1 for that drug-organism combination. Essentially, this is not needed since a carbapenem with an MIC of 1 or less will be effective. Since most diabetic foot infections require multiple courses of antibiotics in conjunction with wound care and surgical intervention, the carbapenem should be reserved for treatment failure.

Gentamicin (I) and tobramycin (S) would not be good options. Amikacin would be the preferred aminoglycoside. When comparing MICs of the aminoglycosides, it is important to consider that amikacin is dosed at a higher dose (15 to 21 mg/kg) and achieves higher peak concentrations (60 mcg/mL) than gentamicin and tobramycin (5 to 7 mg/kg) with serum peak concentrations of 28 mcg/mL. This is reflected in the breakpoints established by CLSI being 4 for gentamicin and tobramycin and 16 for amikacin. Therefore, an MIC of 4 for amikacin would be preferred over a tobramycin MIC of 4. It is also important to note that the MIC breakpoints are based on high-dose extended interval dosing. The traditional dosing method of 1 to 2 mg/kg only achieves serum peak concentration of 4 to 8 mcg/mL and would be ineffective for organisms with MICs greater than 1. Amikacin (in addition to a carbapenem) may be needed if the patient's condition worsens.

Since the fluoroquinolones are a completely different class with different pharmacokinetics, directly comparing the MIC of levofloxacin to gentamicin or cefepime cannot be performed. As discussed above, levofloxacin 750 mg IV only achieves a serum peak concentration of 12 mcg/mL. The CLSI breakpoint for levofloxacin is 2 for *Pseudomonas*. This may not be the best option initially but may be considered for step down therapy.

After review of the culture and sensitivity report, ceftriaxone and metronidazole are discontinued and piperacillin-tazobactam and vancomycin are started. While metronidazole is the preferred treatment for Bacteroides group organisms, beta-lactamase inhibitor combinations also have excellent coverage. Vancomycin is still the gold standard for serious MRSA infections. Upon clinical improvement of the infection, the patient may be switched to doxycycline, minocycline, or trimethoprim-sulfamethoxazole.

CASE 3

Patient Z is a 77-year-old male admitted to the hospital 5 days ago complaining of generalized weakness, fever, and some cough for the past 1 week. According to him, he had chemotherapy for the above-mentioned condition about a week ago, and after that, he started feeling weak and generalized malaise. He now complains of increased cough with white to yellowish color phlegm, shortness of breath, and chest pain. Chest x-ray is consistent with a new infiltrate. Sputum culture returns the following results.

Specimen ######
Specimen Source: Sputum—Expectorated
Gram stain: many (4+) gram-negative rods
Culture:
Aerobic plate: *Enterobacter cloacae*
Susceptibility to follow

Antibiotic	*E. cloacae*
Amikacin	
Amoxicillin-clav	≥32 R
Cefazolin	≥64 R
Cefepime	8 S
Ceftriaxone	8 I
Gentamicin	4 S
Imipenem	≤1 S
Levofloxacin	2 S
Piperacillin-tazo	≥32 R
Tetracycline	≥16 R
Tobramycin	≥1 S
Trimethoprim-sulfa	≤20 S

After reviewing the sensitivities, amoxicillin-clavulanate, cefazolin, ceftriaxone, piper-acillin-tazobactam, and tetracycline can be eliminated from therapeutic consideration. Furthermore, *E. cloacae* is inherently resistant to cefazolin and amoxicillin-clavulanate and reporting is unnecessary. This organism is also known to produce an inducible AmpC beta-lactamase, which may not be observed on the initial culture. Resistance to a beta-lactam/beta-lactamase inhibitor is suggestive of an inducible AmpC since tazobactam has no effect on AmpC. Elevated MICs to ceftriaxone and cefepime also contribute to the suspicion. Antibiotic selection should take this into consideration. In mild to moderate infections, cefepime may still be considered although a chance of treatment failure still exists. In the setting of pneumonia or bloodstream infection, a carbapenem would be preferred.

Oftentimes, the microbiology lab will suppress the results of amikacin due to the susceptibility to gentamicin and tobramycin. This is often part of an antimicrobial stewardship effort to steer prescribers away from using amikacin so that it may be reserved for more resistant organisms. While gentamicin and tobramycin are both S, tobramycin would be preferred since their pharmacokinetics are almost identical and tobramycin has an MIC of ≤1. This is one of the few exceptions when the MIC between agents can be directly compared. Since amikacin is not reported on the *Enterobacter*, the physician may ask the microbiology lab to test this if multiple organisms are present. For instance, if the sputum culture also grew the *Pseudomonas* present in case 2 above, gentamicin and tobramycin would not be good options. If the test has not been performed, the result is usually available in 24 hours.

The levofloxacin MIC is 2. According to CLSI, this organism is still suscep-tible; however, the organism would be considered intermediate by the EUCAST breakpoint. This may not be the best choice of antibiotics despite it being reported as S. Trimethoprim-sulfamethoxazole has no activity against *Pseudomonas* but may be active against many of the *Enterobacteriaceae*. The MIC is reported as ≤20, empha-sizing again that MIC alone is insufficient in making a clinical decision. While an

MIC of 20 may seem high (especially in reference to the MIC of 2 to levofloxacin), trimethoprim-sulfamethoxazole would be fully active and could certainly be considered, particularly in the urine. In the setting of pneumonia, however, a beta-lactam would still be preferred.

CONCLUSION

When selecting an antimicrobial regimen, there is often more than one correct choice. Interpretations of S, I, or R are provided based on breakpoints established as discussed in the previous chapter. For mild to moderate infections, agents that are reported as S will likely be effective assuming the drug penetrates the infected tissue. For severe infections, knowledge of pharmacokinetic parameters can greatly assist in the interpretation of MICs. Agents with the lowest MIC are not always the best choice, and simply selecting the lowest MIC will likely result in a suboptimal regimen. Following the steps in Table 53.2 will also assist in narrowing the therapeutic options. Beta-lactams are usually preferred if more than one class is available. If more than one beta-lactam is available, the narrowest spectrum that still treats the infection should be considered. This is to reserve the broader agents in the event of a treatment failure or recurrent infection. If a beta-lactam is not available, expert consultation is advised.

54

Therapeutic Drug Monitoring

Paul Lewis and James W. Myers

INTRODUCTION

As antimicrobial resistance issues continue to rise and with very few novel antimicrobials in the pipeline, the emphasis on using the current agents more effectively becomes increasingly important. Understanding the *pharmacokinetics,* what the body does to the drug, and the *pharmacodynamics,* what the drug does to the body or organism, will assist in dose optimization. In conjunction with a solid understanding of the pharmacokinetic/pharmacodynamic (PK/PD) relationship is the use of therapeutic drug monitoring (TDM) (Table 54-1).

TDM has been around since the early 1970s and continues to play a role in antimicrobial management today. Several conditions support TDM. Serum drug concentration correlates with therapeutic efficacy or toxicity or both. The drug has a *narrow therapeutic index,* defined as less than a twofold difference between the minimum toxic concentration and the minimum effective concentration in blood. Interpatient variability in pharmacokinetics is larger than the therapeutic range. Little variation exists at steady state within an individual patient. The drug effect is difficult to assess clinically. Finally, drug assays are available to assist in dosage alteration. The most notable antibiotics utilizing TDM are the aminoglycosides and vancomycin. However, many additional antimicrobials have data to support TDM including antifungals, antiretrovirals, and antimycobacterials. This chapter evaluates current dosing strategies involving the use of TDM.

REASONS TO MONITOR DRUG LEVELS

The goal of TDM is to maximize efficacy of the antibiotic while minimizing the toxicity. Differences in patient pharmacokinetic characteristics necessitate individualized dosing. Plasma concentrations are used as a surrogate marker of therapeutic effect. This must be in conjunction with knowledge of tissue penetration. For instance, in meningitis, an antibiotic with limited penetration into the central nervous system will likely not be successful despite therapeutic plasma concentrations. Many reasons exist for monitoring of drug levels.

- Plasma concentration is often a better predictor of success than dose alone.
- Variation in population pharmacokinetics exists.
- Many drug level assays are readily available with quick turnaround time.
- Drug levels can determine if a medication is being taken correctly (compliance with antiretrovirals and antimycobacterials).
- Drug-drug interactions may alter pharmacokinetics requiring dosage changes (rifampin may induce the metabolism of voriconazole).
- Drug-food interactions may alter pharmacokinetics (food significantly enhances the absorption of posaconazole).

| Table 54-1 | **Common Terms and Abbreviations** |

Therapeutic Drug Monitoring (TDM): The measurement and interpretation of drug concentration in the plasma to tailor dosing regimens for the safety and efficacy of drug therapy

Minimum Inhibitory Concentration (MIC): The minimum concentration of an antibiotic that will inhibit visible growth of an organism

Peak Concentration (Cmax): The maximum concentration of a drug; it is the time immediately following the end of infusion for an IV medication.

Trough Concentration (Cmin): The minimum concentration of a drug; it is the time immediately prior to the administration of an IV medication.

Area Under the Curve (AUC): The area under the plasma drug concentration vs. time (per 24 hours) curve; this is related to total drug exposure.

Elimination Rate Constant (K): For first-order kinetics, the fraction of drug removed from the body over a period of time (usually 1 hour); can be used to calculate a **random concentration (C_t)** at the **elapsed time (t)** so long as the **initial concentration (C_0)** is known ($C_t = C_0 * e^{-Kt}$)

Half-Life ($t_{1/2}$): The amount of time needed for a drug concentration to decrease by half; $t_{1/2} = 0.693/K$

Volume of Distribution (Vd): A theoretical term, the apparent volume in which a drug distributes; highly lipophilic medications or medications highly distributed into tissue can have Vds greater than the total volume of the body; Vd = total dose/initial drug concentration

Timing of Levels

- Peak
  - Peaks are usually performed at least 1 hour after the end of an infusion.
  - Should not be drawn immediately postdose due to the alpha distribution phase or tissue distribution
  - Extrapolated peak can be calculated using the observed peak and the elimination rate constant (K).
    - True peak = observed Peak * e^{Kt}
    - t being the time in hours after the end of infusion
  - Most useful for measuring concentration-dependant antibiotics (aminoglycosides)
  - Primarily influenced by the dose
- Trough
  - Drawn just prior to the start of a dose
  - If not drawn immediately prior to dose, an extrapolated trough can be drawn using the observed trough and the elimination rate constant.
    - True trough = observed trough * e^{-Kt}
    - t being time in hours prior to when the next dose is due
  - Useful when measuring time above minimum inhibitory concentration (MIC)-dependant antibiotics or area under the curve (AUC)-dependant antibiotics when volume of distribution is stable (vancomycin) (Table 54-2)
  - Primarily influenced by the dosing frequency
- Random level
  - Drawn without regard to dosing interval
  - May be useful with pulse dosing (vancomycin in severe renal failure) or in antibiotics with extremely long half-lives (itraconazole)

Table 54-2	Pharmacodynamic Model Predicting Efficacy	
T > MIC	**Cmax/MIC**	**AUC/MIC**
(Time Dependant)	**(Concentration Dependant)**	**(Total Drug Exposure)**
Penicillins	Aminoglycosides	Azithromycin
Cephalosporins	Fluoroquinolones	Clindamycin
Carbapenems	Daptomycin	Tetracyclines
Aztreonam	Metronidazole	Tigecycline
Erythromycin	Telithromycin	Linezolid
Clarithromycin	Echinocandins	Vancomycin
Flucytosine	Amphotericin	Triazole antifungals

- Used in various nomograms to predict dosing frequency (Hartford nomogram with aminoglycosides)
- Used with a second level (peak or trough) to calculate a patient-specific elimination rate constant (K)
  - $K = (Ln (C_2/C_1))/\Delta T$
  - C_2 and C_1 are two serum concentrations not separated by a dose.
  - ΔT is the time difference between C_2 and C_1.

VANCOMYCIN

Vancomycin is the workhorse for many gram-positive infections, including those resistant to beta-lactams. A glycopeptide, vancomycin was first isolated in 1953 from *Amycolatopsis orientalis* and finally reached market in 1958. Due to the inability of organisms to develop resistance of the original compound, this new drug was said to vanquish infection and was coined vancomycin. Originally, vancomycin contained many impurities which earned it the term "Mississippi Med." Concern for nephrotoxicity and ototoxicity limited the use in its early use. As methicillin-resistant *Staphylococcus aureus* continues to rise, vancomycin has become the mainstay for empiric coverage of hospital-acquired and health care–associated infections. Concern for nephrotoxicity and ototoxicity still exist, though some would argue the toxicities were due to the impurities seen with the earlier preparations. The Infectious Diseases Society of America (IDSA) published guidelines for the therapeutic monitoring of vancomycin in 2009 and serve as the basis for the following recommendations (Table 54-3).

- For systemic infections, vancomycin should be given IV.
  - To avoid red-man syndrome (a histamine-related adverse reaction), vancomycin should not be administered faster than 1 g/hr.
- Vancomycin displays a two-compartment model:
  - A central compartment (serum) with high perfusion
  - A peripheral compartment (muscle and fat) with less perfusion
- Drug is only eliminated from the serum compartment.
  - Drug must leave the tissue and enter back into the serum to be eliminated.

Table 54-3	Recommended Vancomycin Trough Concentration
<10 mg/L	No therapeutically accepted indication
10–15 mg/L	Complicated urinary tract infections (including pyelonephritis) cellulitis
	Complicated skin and soft tissue infections
15–20 mg/L	Bacteremia/endocarditis
	Line infections
	Pneumonia
	Meningitis/CNS infections
	Osteomyelitis
	Sepsis
	Bone and joint infections
	Intra-abdominal infections
	Febrile neutropenia
	A known pathogen with an MIC = 1 mg/L

- Due to the two-compartment model, vancomycin also distributes in two phases.
  - The alpha phase lasts 30 minutes to an hour and mostly involves rapid distribution into the tissue.
  - During the beta phase, the drug reenters the plasma and is eliminated by the kidneys at a logarithmic rate.
- Volume of distribution is roughly 0.65 L/kg (range 0.4 to 1 L/kg).
- Based on Matzke equation, the elimination rate constant (K) can be calculated.
  - $K = 0.00083*CrCl + 0.0044$
- Vancomycin displays AUC:MIC-dependant killing.
- For systemic infections, vancomycin is given as intermitted intravenous infusion.
  - Continuous infusion is not likely to significantly impact efficacy.
- Dosing should target an AUC:MIC of 400 or greater for greatest chance at clinical success.
- Serum trough concentrations are the most accurate and practical measures for efficacy.
- Troughs should be considered when therapy is likely to exceed 72 hours.
- Troughs should be drawn prior to the fourth dose to ensure steady state has been reached.
  - Troughs drawn prior to steady state are not recommended.
- Regardless of indication, serum troughs should never drop below 10 mg/L to avoid the development of resistant organisms.
- Complicated infections such as bacteremia, endocarditis, osteomyelitis, meningitis, and hospital-acquired pneumonia should target serum troughs of 15 to 20 mg/L.
- Any organism with an MIC known to be 1 mg/L, a serum trough level of 15 to 20 mg/L, is needed to attain the target AUC:MIC, regardless of indication.
- For patients with normal renal function, doses 15 to 20 mg/kg of actual body weight given every 8 to 12 hours are necessary to achieve the target serum trough.
- Loading doses of 25 to 30 mg/kg may be considered for complicated infections.
- As renal function declines, dosage adjustments should be made (see Table 54-4 below).
- Peak concentrations are rarely needed.
  - A peak may be needed to determine volume of distribution, if needed.
  - A peak may be drawn to calculate an elimination coefficient for difficult to dose patients (obesity, amputees, significantly underweight).

| Table 54-4 | Vancomycin Dosing Nomogram | | | |

Dose Recommendation   **Interval Recommendations**

Weight[a] (kg)	Load[b] (mg)	Maintenance (mg)	Creatinine Clearance[c] (mL/min)	Dosing Interval[d] (h)
<40 kg	25–30 mg/kg	500		
40–59	1,250	750	>80	12
60–74	1,500	1,000	40–79	24
75–89	1,750	1,250	20–39	48
90–110	2,000	1,500	<20	Pulse dosing or consult pharmacokinetics service if available
111–125	2,000	1,750		
>126	2,000	2,000		

[a]Based on actual body weight.
[b]Consider loading dose in seriously ill patients.
[c]Based on Cockcroft-Gault equation.
[d]May consider a more aggressive interval (every 8 h) for seriously ill patients.
Modified from McCluggage L, Lee K, Potter T, et al. Implementation and evaluation of vancomycin nomogram guidelines in a computerized prescriber-order-entry system. *Am J Health Syst Phar* 2010;67(1):70–75.

- *S. aureus* with an MIC equal to 2 should be treated with an alternative agent as the goal AUC:MIC of 400 or greater is not attainable with conventional dosing.
- Oral and rectal administration should not affect the serum levels of vancomycin since very little of the drug is absorbed.

AMINOGLYCOSIDES

The aminoglycosides were first introduced into practice in 1943 with the isolation of streptomycin from a species of *Streptomyces*. In the 1960s, gentamicin, isolated from *Micromonospora*, entered the market with enhanced coverage of many gram-negative bacilli including *Pseudomonas aeruginosa*. Tobramycin and amikacin were subsequently introduced with increasing coverage of gram-negative bacilli. Concern for nephrotoxicity and ototoxicity has limited their use. With little previous exposure and rapidly cidal effect, aminoglycosides may be the only option in certain multidrug-resistant organisms. They also may be considered as a therapeutic option for synergy when combined with a beta-lactam for difficult-to-treat gram-positive organisms such as *S. aureus* and *Enterococcus* spp.

- Only available IV over 30 minutes to an hour for systemic infections
- Only gentamicin and streptomycin are used for synergy in gram-positive organisms.
- Amikacin has the highest gram-negative activity followed by tobramycin, then gentamicin.
- Aminoglycosides follow a three-compartment model.
  - The alpha phase involves tissue distribution.

- The beta phase involves elimination from the serum.
- The gamma phase, typically beginning 16 hours postdose, involves the tissue release of the drug.
  - Due to the complexity of a three-compartment model, a one-compartment model is typically used for predicting serum levels.
- Volume of distribution is roughly 0.26 L/kg (range 0.2 to 0.4).
- Based on population parameters, the elimination rate constant (K) can be calculated.
- K= 0.00293*CrCl + 0.014
- Ideal body weight (or adjusted body weight for obesity) should be used in dose calculation.
- Aminoglycosides display concentration-dependant killing and are noted to have postantibiotic effect.
- Nephrotoxicity and ototoxicity appear to be saturable at low levels.
  - Higher peaks do not result in greater toxicity.
  - Drug-free periods may allow for recovery of toxicity.
- Two common dosing strategies exist, traditional and high-dose extended interval.
- Traditional dosing method
  - Involves 1 to 2 mg/kg per (7 to 8 mg/kg for amikacin) dose and given multiple times daily, or less frequently for renal impairment
  - For target peak and troughs, see Table 54-5.
  - Most commonly used for synergy and in patients who do not meet criteria for high-dose extended interval
  - Upon attainment of a peak and trough
    o To adjust peak, change the dose.
    o To adjust trough, change the frequency.
- The high-dose extended interval method
  - Involves 5 to 7 mg/kg for gentamicin and tobramycin (15 to 21 mg/kg for amikacin) and is given every 24, 36 or 48 hours based on renal function
  - Shown to be at least as efficacious as the traditional method with less nephrotoxicity
  - Recommended for all patients who do not meet any of the exclusion criteria (see Table 54-6)
  - Interval is determined by plotting a randomly drawn concentration between 6 and 14 hours after the initial dose on the Hartford nomogram.
    o Based on 7 mg/kg for gentamicin and tobramycin; all other doses should be corrected using a ratio before plotting.

Table 54-5	Exclusion Criteria for High-Dose Extended-Interval Aminoglycosides
Pregnancy	
Age >70 years	
Extensive burns (>20% of the body surface area)	
Severe liver disease involving ascites	
Severe renal disease (CrCl <30 mL/min)	
Dialysis	
Cystic fibrosis	
Synergistic use gram-positive organisms	
History of hearing loss or vestibular toxicity	

Table 54-6 Recommended Therapeutic Goals, Dosing, and Monitoring for Aminoglycosides

		Traditional		Extended Interval	
	Indication	Gent/Tobra	Amikacin	Gent/Tobra	Amikacin
Therapeutic Goals	Goal Peak (mg/L) Synergy[a]	3–4	NA	NA	NA
	Mild	4–6	20–25	16–20	40–50
	Severe	8	25–30	24–28	60–70
	Goal Trough (mg/L) Synergy	<1	NA	<1	NA
	Mild	<1.5	<4	<1	<4
	Severe	<2	<8	<1	<4
Initial Dosing Interval	CrCl				
	>60 mL/min	Q8h		Q24h	
	41–60 mL/min	Q12h		Q36h	
	31–40 mL/min	Q18h		Q48h	
	20–30 mL/min	Q24h		Use traditional method	
	<20 mL/min	Use pulse dosing and follow random levels			
	Hemodialysis	See renal dosing chapter			
Initial Dose	Loading dose (mg/kg) Synergy	1	NA	NA	NA
	Mild	2	8	5	15
	Severe	3	10	7	20
	Maintenance dose (mg/kg) Synergy	1	NA	NA	NA
	Mild	1.5	7	5	15
	Severe	2	8	7	20
	Round to the nearest 10 mg for gentamicin and tobramycin and 25 mg for amikacin				
Monitoring	Initial	Peak following third dose Trough prior to fourth dose		Random level 6–14 hours after first dose	
	Following a dose change	Peak and trough with fourth dose		Trough prior to fourth dose	
	Stable regimen	Weekly trough		Weekly trough	

[a] When treating enterococcal infections.

- The plotted serum concentration on the x-axis should correlate with the dosing interval on the y-axis.
- The Hartford nomogram can be found on many Web sites; a few are listed below.
  - http://ugapharmd.com/calculators/gentldei.htm (includes amikacin)
  - http://www.nicpld.org/online/antimicro/images/hartford.gif
  - http://www.rxkinetics.com/amino.html
- Subsequent monitoring includes only a weekly trough.
- Target trough is <1 mg/L (less than four for amikacin).
  - If needed, the interval should be changed to achieve the target trough.
- Therapeutic monitoring has shown a reduction in side effects, lower costs, shorter stays, and reduced mortality.

BETA-LACTAMS

Typically, beta-lactams do not require TDM. Pharmacodynamic modeling supports that the time above MIC-dependant antibiotics should be maintained above the MIC between 40% and 70% of the time for optimal performance. Retrospective reviews in critically ill patients suggest that longer times may be needed. Roberts et al. conducted a single-arm study in the intensive care unit targeting a steady-state trough of 4 to 10 times the MIC. Dosage adjustments were made in 74.2% of patients based on twice weekly levels. Though no comparator group exists, a positive outcome defined as completion of treatment course without the need of a regimen change or addition was observed in 87.3% of patients suggesting that further research is needed.

ANTIFUNGALS

The incidence of invasive fungal disease continues to rise in immunocompromised patients. The need for long-term antifungal agents has increased. The narrow range of therapeutic efficacy and toxicity has necessitated the investigation into TDM.

- Amphotericin
  - Benefit from TDM has not been demonstrated.
- Fluconazole
  - Highly predictable pharmacokinetics and specific dosing recommendations based off clearance
  - Well absorbed orally and not affected by food
  - TDM not necessary
- Itraconazole
  - Poorly absorbed
  - Influenced by food and stomach pH
  - Drug interactions may affect also concentration.
  - Two formulations
    - Oral capsules
      - Needs acidic environment for absorption, caution with acid-suppressing agents
      - Recommended to be taken with food or cola
    - Oral solution
      - Contains cyclodextrin to increase absorption
      - Recommended to be taken on an empty stomach

- Not influenced by acid-suppressing agents
- Serum concentrations approximately 30% higher than with capsules
  - Dose conversion is 100 mg capsule = 50 mg solution.
- Monitoring is useful, especially in long-term therapy such as histoplasmosis and blastomycosis (Table 54-7).
- Blood concentrations >0.5 mg/L have been associated with therapeutic efficacy.
- Levels should be drawn at steady state, which takes approximately 2 weeks.
- Due to the long half-life, there is little difference between peak and trough; the level can be drawn at any time throughout the day.
- When measured by high performance liquid chromatography (HPCL), the therapeutic level is the sum of itraconazole and its active metabolite, hydroxy-itraconazole.
- Voriconazole
  - Variable absorption, 60% to 100%
  - Absorption decreased with food, as much as 22%
  - Drug interactions may affect drug metabolism.
  - Metabolized by CYP2C19, a liver isoenzyme known to display genetic polymorphism
    - Ultra-rapid metabolizers will have lower than predicted levels.
    - Poor or slow metabolizers will have higher than predicted levels.
  - The elimination half-life is 6 to 9 hours and may increase as the dose increases.
  - Steady state is often achieved in 5 to 7 days.
  - Retrospective studies have suggested that low voriconazole levels are associated with therapeutic failure and high levels are associated with neurologic and ocular adverse events.

Table 54-7	Therapeutic Monitoring for Antifungal Agents		
Drug	**What to Draw**	**Therapeutic Range**	**Toxicity**
Itraconazole plus hydroxy-itraconazole	Random level 2 weeks after therapy	Therapeutic: >1 mg/L Prophylaxis: >0.5 mg/L Toxic: >10 mg/L	Hepatic, electrolytes, neurologic
Voriconazole	Trough after 5 days	Therapeutic: >0.5 mg/L Prophylaxis: ND[a] Toxicity: >5 mg/L	Ocular, hepatic, and neurologic
Posaconazole	Random after 5 days	Treatment: >1.5 mg/L Prophylaxis: ND[a]	Hepatic, electrolytes, neurologic
Flucytosine	Peak after 3–5 days, drawn 2 hours postdose	Treatment: 30–80 mg/L Toxicity: >100 mg/L	Bone marrow suppression, renal, hepatic, electrolytes

[a]The goals for prophylaxis are not defined but may be lower than the treatment dose similar to itraconazole.
ND, not defined.

- Monitoring should be considered in patients on long-term therapy such as aspergillosis.
- Recommended monitoring is a trough approximately 5 days into therapy.
- Posaconazole
  - Absorption highly dependent upon food, increased fat intake is recommended.
  - Absorption is saturable, requiring it to be administered multiple times daily.
  - Lower absorption observed in patients receiving proton pump inhibitors
  - Absorption may also be decreased by the presence of mucositis.
  - High lipophilicity and large distribution suggestive of tissue concentrations higher than plasma concentrations
  - Metabolism different from that of itraconazole and voriconazole, uses glucuronidation
  - Half-life extremely long, >24 hours
  - Therapeutic efficacy has been observed with increasing levels.
  - While TDM has yet to be fully established and further research is needed, reasonable recommendations can be made based on limited data.
  - A random level should be drawn after 5 days of therapy.
- Flucytosine
  - Narrow therapeutic index as it gets deaminated to 5-fluorouracil, used for chemotherapy
  - Weight-based dosing 100 to 150 mg/kg/day in four divided doses
  - Absorption ranges from 78% to 90%.
  - Relatively short half-life, 3 to 6 hours
  - Greater than 90% cleared unchanged in urine
  - Studies have shown a strong relationship between TDM and toxicity and efficacy.
  - Maximal killing should target serum concentrations greater than the MIC for only 50% of the dosing interval based on pharmacokinetic studies.
  - In a recent retrospective review of more than 1,000 patients, only 20% had a therapeutic peak.
  - A peak is recommended after at least 3 days of therapy.
- Echinocandins
  - Not absorbable, only available intravenously
  - Limited drug-drug interactions
  - Limited pharmacokinetic variability, predictable dose-exposure relationships
  - TDM not likely to be necessary

ANTIMYCOBACTERIALS

- Leading cause of death from a curable disease worldwide
- Low serum concentrations can be the result of poor absorption, inaccurate dosing, altered metabolism, or drug interactions.
- Majority of research done worldwide, with little access to TDM
- Centers for Disease control (CDC) tuberculosis guidelines mention TDM as optional consideration.
- Appropriately responding patients not likely to benefit from TDM
- Slow response to therapy may be an indication for TDM.
- Recommended monitoring includes a 2-hour postdose (C_{2hr}) (Table 54-8).

Table 54-8	Reference Ranges for Antimycobacterials

Drug	Therapeutic Range
Isoniazid[a]	Daily: 3–6 mg/L
	Twice weekly: 9–18 mg/L
Rifampin[a]	8–24 mg/L
Rifabutin[a]	0.3–0.9 mg/L
Ethambutol[a]	2–6 mg/L
Pyrazinamide[a]	20–50 mg/L
Streptomycin[b]	Peak: 25–50 mg/L
	Trough: <5 mg/L

[a]Drawn 2 hours postdose.
[b]Peak drawn 1 hour postdose and trough drawn 30 min prior to dose.

ANTIRETROVIRALS

Multiple difficulties exist concerning treatment with antiretrovirals. Lack of adherence, drug resistance, toxicity, drug-drug interactions, and drug-food interactions all influence the possibility of success with therapy. Large prospective randomized trials are needed to fully determine the role of TDM in antiretrovirals. Protease inhibitors and non-nucleoside reverse transcriptase inhibitors have shown a dose-response relationship and are gaining support for TDM. Darunavir, etravirine, and raltegravir continue to be evaluated; however, no formal recommendation can be made (Table 54-9). The CCR5 antagonist, maraviroc, has shown a concentration-response relationship; however, a formal recommendation is lacking. The nucleoside reverse transcriptase inhibitors do not have an established concentration-response relationship, and monitoring should be considered for research purposes only. While the World Health

Table 54-9	Suggested Minimum Trough Concentrations for Antiretrovirals		
Susceptible Virus		**Resistant Virus**	
Drug	**Concentration (ng/mL)**	**Drug**	**Concentration (ng/mL)**
Amprenavir[a]	400	Maraviroc	>50
Atazanavir	150	Tipranavir	20,500
Indinavir	100	Darunavir[c,d]	3,300 (1,255–7,368)
Lopinavir	1,000	Etravirine[d]	275 (81–2,980)
Nelfinavir[b]	800	Raltegravir[d]	72 (29–118)
Saquinavir	100–250		
Efavirenz	1,000		
Nevirapine	3,000		

[a]Also fosamprenavir.
[b]Measurable active metabolite.
[c]Evaluated as 600 mg twice daily.
[d]Reported from clinical trials as the median (range).

Organization does not support the use of TDM, the 2011 United States HIV-1 Adult and Adolescent guidelines support TDM for the following selected populations.

- Multidrug regimens with high likelihood for drug-drug interactions
- Patients with gastrointestinal alterations affecting absorption
- Hepatic or renal dysfunction
- Pregnancy
- Heavily pretreated populations with previous virologic failure
- Regimens not observed in clinical trials
- Known concentration-dependant drug toxicities observed
- Lack of expected virologic response
- The 2011 Pediatric HIV-1 guidelines also support the role of TDM in selected circumstances.

CONCLUSION

For drugs meeting criteria, TDM can be a powerful tool to assist clinicians in optimizing treatment regimens. While much of the data involve vancomycin and aminoglycosides, other agents have special circumstances that may benefit. The body of medical literature supporting TDM continues to grow as the need for dose optimization becomes increasingly important due to issues of resistance. Prospective trials are needed to assess the impact of TDM on clinical outcomes.

SUGGESTED READINGS

American Thoracic Society; CDC; Infectious Diseases Society of America. Treatment of tuberculosis. *MMWR Recomm Rep* 2003;52(RR-11):1–77.

Andes D. In vivo pharmacodynamics of antifungal drugs in treatment of candidiasis. *Antimicrob Agents Chemother* 2003;47(4):1179–1186.

Andes D, Pascual A, et al. Antifungal therapeutic drug monitoring: established and emerging indications. *Antimicrob Agents Chemother* 2009;53(1):24–34.

Dodds Ashley ES, Lewis R, Lewis JS, et al. Pharmacology of systemic antifungal agents. *Clin Infect Dis* 2006;43:S28–S39.

Heysell SK, Moore JL, et al. Therapeutic drug monitoring for slow response to tuberculosis treatment in a state control program, Virginia, USA. *Emerg Infect Dis* 2010;16(10):1546–1553.

Diabetes was associated with slow response (p<0.001), and persons with diabetes were more likely than persons without diabetes to have low rifampin levels (p = 0.03). Dosage adjustment of rifampin was more likely to elevate serum concentration to the target range than adjustment of isoniazid given in daily doses (p = 0.01).

Holland DP, Hamilton CD, et al. Therapeutic drug monitoring of antimycobacterial drugs in patients with both tuberculosis and advanced human immunodeficiency virus infection. *Pharmacotherapy* 2009;29(5):503–510.

Low serum concentrations of antituberculous drugs, which suggest malabsorption, are common among patients with advanced HIV who also have tuberculosis but can be overcome with higher doses. TDM may be an effective tool to optimize therapy but needs further study.

Hussaini T, Ruping MJ, et al. Therapeutic drug monitoring of voriconazole and posaconazole. *Pharmacotherapy* 2011;31(2):214–225.

Reviewed the pharmacokinetic and pharmacodynamic characteristics of voriconazole and posaconazole in the context of clinical indications for TDM. In addition, the most recent evidence examining the relationship between serum concentrations of voriconazole and posaconazole and their efficacy or toxicities was evaluated. This information was then integrated to formulate recommendations for use of TDM in clinical settings.

Nicolau DP, Freeman CD, et al. Experience with a once-daily aminoglycoside program administered to 2,184 adult patients. *Antimicrob Agents Chemother* 1995;39(3):650–655.
Classic article.

Owens RC, Jr, Shorr AF. Rational dosing of antimicrobial agents: pharmacokinetic and pharmacodynamic strategies. *Am J Health Syst Pharm* 2009;66(12 suppl 4):S23–S30.
Optimizing the dose and duration of antimicrobial therapy via PK/PD principles is one strategy to reduce antimicrobial resistance. PK/PD-based dosing provides patient- and pathogen-specific therapy and has the potential to make antimicrobial therapy safer and more effective by accounting for factors such as renal function, underlying pathogen, and local patterns of resistance.

Panel on Antiretroviral Therapy and Medical Management of HIV-Infected Children. Guidelines for the Use of Antiretroviral Agents in Pediatric HIV Infection. August 11, 2011; 1–268. Available at http://aidsinfo.nih.gov/ContentFiles/PediatricGuidelines.pdf.

Panel on Antiretroviral Guidelines for Adults and Adolescents. Guidelines for the use of antiretroviral agents in HIV-1-infected adults and adolescents. Department of Health and Human Services. October 14, 2011;1–167. Available at http://www.aidsinfo.nih.gov/ContentFiles/AdultandAdolescentGL.pdf.

Pagkalis S, Mantadakis E, et al. Pharmacological considerations for the proper clinical use of aminoglycosides. *Drugs* 2011;71(17):2277–2294.

Pretorius E, Klinker H, et al. The role of therapeutic drug monitoring in the management of patients with human immunodeficiency virus infection. *Ther Drug Monit* 2011;33(3): 265–274.
The best pharmacokinetic measures of drug exposure such as trough and peak concentrations or concentration ratios have not been unambiguously established.

Roberts JA, Ulldemolins M, et al. Therapeutic drug monitoring of beta-lactams in critically ill patients: proof of concept. *Int J Antimicrob Agents* 2010;36(4):332–339.

Rybak M, Lomaestro B, et al. Therapeutic monitoring of vancomycin in adult patients: a consensus review of the American Society of Health-System Pharmacists, the Infectious Diseases Society of America, and the Society of Infectious Diseases Pharmacists. *Am J Health Syst Pharm* 2009;66(1):82–98.

Smith J, Andes D. Therapeutic drug monitoring of antifungals: pharmacokinetic and pharmacodynamic considerations. *Ther Drug Monit* 2008;30(2):167–172.
This review summarizes the current literature on TDM for these antifungal agents.

Tod MM, Padoin C, et al. Individualising aminoglycoside dosage regimens after therapeutic drug monitoring: simple or complex pharmacokinetic methods? *Clin Pharmacokinet* 2001;40(11):803–814.

Touw DJ, Neef C, et al. Cost-effectiveness of therapeutic drug monitoring: a systematic review. *Ther Drug Monit* 2005;27(1):10–17.

Wheat LJ, Freifeld AG, et al. Clinical practice guidelines for the management of patients with histoplasmosis: 2007 update by the Infectious Diseases Society of America. *Clin Infect Dis* 2007;45(7):807–825.

Antibiotic Dosing in Obesity

Paul Lewis and James W. Myers

INTRODUCTION

The WHO recognizes obesity as a global health problem. As of 2005, 400 million people worldwide were obese with 1.6 billion overweight. Epidemiologic studies have linked obesity to a number of comorbidities including hypertension, coronary artery disease, stroke, type 2 diabetes mellitus, osteoarthritis, depression, and several forms of cancer. Although obese patients are encountered frequently in practice, very little data exist concerning drug dosing and obesity. In fact, many researchers exclude obese patients during clinical trials. Most of the data describing the pharmacokinetics and pharmacodynamics of the majority of drugs come from case reports and small case series.

DEFINING BODY COMPOSITION

There are several different means to measure and classify body composition.

- **Direct quantification**
  - Underwater weighing, skinfold measurement, and bioelectric impedance
  - Most accurate
  - *Difficult and impractical*
- **Indirect measures**
  - **Body mass index (BMI)**
    - Calculated as weight in kilograms divided by square of the height in meters
    - The WHO classification
      - underweight as BMI <18.5 kg/m^2
      - normal weight 18.5 to 24.99 kg/m^2
      - **overweight as 25 to 29.99 kg/m^2**
      - obese class I as 30 to 34.99 kg/m^2
      - obese class II as 35 to 39.99 kg/m^2
      - obese class III or morbid obesity as >40 kg/m^2.
  - Percentage of ideal body weight (IBW) as a function of height
    - For a man, IBW equals 50 kg plus 2.3 kg for every inch above 5 feet
    - For a woman, IBW equals 45.5 kg plus 2.3 kg for every inch above 5 feet
    - Classification
      - Underweight <80% of IBW
      - Normal weight is 80% to 124% of IBW
      - **Obesity is 125% to 190% of IBW**
      - Morbid obesity is >190% of IBW

EFFECTS OF OBESITY ON PHARMACOKINETICS

When compared to the bacterial minimum inhibitory concentration (MIC), three pharmacodynamic principals predict therapeutic response: peak concentration (C_{max}), area under the concentration-time curve/24 hours (AUC), and time above MIC (T>MIC). However, these parameters fail to capture the complete picture due to many unknowns such as bound versus free drug, blood versus tissue levels, and interstitial versus intracellular concentrations (please see Table 55-1). **In the absence of a more substantial model, most of pharmacokinetics is simplified to two parameters: volume of distribution (Vd) and drug clearance (Cl).** Volume of distribution plays an important role in loading and maintenance doses, while drug clearance more affects the frequency of administration.

- **Volume of distribution**
  - Affected by many factors including body composition, regional blood flow, drug lipophilicity, and plasma protein binding
  - Maximum blood flow into adipose tissue is <5% of cardiac output.
  - **Hydrophilic drugs should not be significantly affected by increased body weight.**
  - For a list of hydrophilic versus lipophilic drugs, see Table 55-2.
  - **Drugs bound to albumin are also not likely to be significantly affected by obesity.**
  - However, antibiotics bound to α_1-acid glycoprotein may have changes in volume of distribution.
  - For hydrophilic drugs, IBW tends to be a better measure.
  - **For lipophilic drugs, measurements that include added mass (total bodyweight [TBW] or adjusted body weight [ABW]) for obesity may be a better descriptor.**
  - For lipophilic drugs given at a flat dose such as fluoroquinolones, macrolides, linezolid, sulfonamides, and fluconazole, it is not unreasonable to consider higher doses to attain more appropriate levels (please see Table 55-3).
- **Drug clearance**
  - Accomplished primarily by the liver and kidney
  - Metabolism of drugs primarily performed by the liver
    - Phase I consists of oxidation, reduction, and hydrolysis.
    - Phase II consists of glucuronidation and sulfation.
    - **Both of which can increase in obesity**
  - Elimination occurs primarily by the kidneys.
    - Most antibiotics are renally eliminated.
    - Clearance involving the kidney occurs through a variety of mechanisms: glomerular filtration, tubular secretion, and tubular reabsorption.
    - **One report states that obesity may result in a state of glomerular hyperfiltration, similar to the early stages of diabetic nephropathy.**
    - Another study using [^{125}I]Na iothalamate CL showed a higher GFR in obese females than normal-weight controls, although the results were not significant.

Table 55-1 **Dosing Adjustments for Obesity**

Drug Class	Effect on Obesity	Recommendation
Aminoglycosides	9%–58% increase in Vd 15%–91% increase in clearance	Use ABW **ABW = IBW + 0.4** **(TBW – IBW)**
Vancomycin	49% increase in Vd 131%–156% increase in clearance	Use *total* body weight
Cephalosporins		
Cefotaxime	42%–68% increases in Vd	Dose increases may be warranted but data are lacking
Cefazolin	14%–63% increase in clearance Increases in Vd observed	**2 g doses may be needed for prophylaxis**
Carbapenems		
Ertapenem	Vd increase 17%–39%	No formal recommendation
Meropenem	38% increase in Vd 28% increase in clearance	No change recommended
Penicillins		
Nafcillin	Increased Vd, decreased clearance	**May consider 3 g q6h**
Piperacillin	167 kg patient had C_{max} of 67.4 mg/L compared to population of 242 mg/L	Higher doses needed organism MIC >16 mg/L to maintain T>MIC for >50% of interval
Fluoroquinolones		
Ciprofloxacin	–5%–23% change in Vd –9%–21% change in clearance	Higher doses may be needed
Levofloxacin	Variable AUC and clearance	Use **750** mg dose
Moxifloxacin	Distributes to adipose tissue	Dosage adjustment not likely
Daptomycin	26% increase C_{max} 35% increase in AUC24	Dose on **total** body weight
Linezolid	**Conflicting data**	No change in dose Consider 600 mg q8 for pathogens with MIC >2 mcg/mL
Quinupristin-dalfopristin	25% increase in C_{max}	Use **total** body weight although, an ABW may be needed
Fluconazole	Limited data	Higher doses may be needed
Amphotericin		
Lipid-associated	Limited data	Dose on **lean body** weight
Acyclovir		Manufacturer recommends **IBW, but may consider ABW** in severe cases
Ganciclovir	Limited data	Use **adjusted** body weight
Clindamycin		Consider 900 mg q8

Vd, volume of distribution; ABW, adjusted body weight; TBW, total body weight; IBW, ideal body weight; MIC, minimum inhibitory concentration; C_{max}, maximum concentration; T>MIC, time above MIC

Table 55-2	Water Versus Fat Soluble Characteristics of Antibiotics by Class
Hydrophilic	**Lipophilic**
Penicillins	Fluoroquinolones
Cephalosporins	Macrolides
Monobactams	Clindamycin
Carbapenems	Linezolid
Glycopeptides	Tetracyclines
Aminoglycosides	Glycylcyclines
Polymyxins	Trimethoprim-sulfamethoxazole
Fosfomycin	Rifamycins
Daptomycin	Chloramphenicol

The degree of hydrophilicity may vary between agents in each drug class.

In summary, obesity affects many of the parameters used in dosing medications. Due to limitations in testing, little data exist regarding the dosing of antibiotics. Volume of distribution is highly dependent on the physiochemical properties of the drug, such as hydrophilicity and protein binding. In contrast, clearance is more dependent on physiologic processes of the body such as measured renal and hepatic function. The approach to dosing in obesity must take into consideration all available factors before making a final decision.

Table 55-3	Weight-Based Drugs	
Ideal Body Weight	**Actual Body Weight**	**Adjusted Body weight**
Acyclovir	Amphotericin (conventional)	Acyclovir (severe CNS)
Amphotericin (lipid-associated)	Daptomycin	Amikacin
Ethambutol	Quinupristin-dalfopristin	Ganciclovir
Flucytosine	Telavancin	Gentamicin
Isoniazid	Vancomycin	Streptomycin
Pyrazinamide	Voriconazole	Tobramycin
Rifampin		Trimethoprim-sulfamethoxazole

SUGGESTED READINGS

Alffenaar JW, van der Werf T. Dosing ethambutol in obese patients. *Antimicrob Agents Chemother* 2010;54(9):4044;author reply 4044–4045.

Bearden DT, Rodvold KA. Dosage adjustments for antibacterials in obese patients: applying clinical pharmacokinetics. *Clin Pharmacokinet* 2000;38(5):415–426.

The apparent volume of distribution (Vd) and total body clearance of vancomycin are increased in obese patients and have a better correlation with TBW than with IBW.

Boullata JI. Drug disposition in obesity and protein-energy malnutrition. *Proc Nutr Soc* 2010;69(4):543–550.

Until more data are available, routine monitoring by the clinician of the protein-energy malnourished or obese patient receiving weight-based drug regimens is necessary.

Chen M, Nafziger AN, et al. Comparative pharmacokinetics and pharmacodynamic target attainment of ertapenem in normal-weight, obese, and extremely obese adults. *Antimicrob Agents Chemother* 2006;50(4):1222–1227.

The results suggest that the standard 1-g ertapenem dose may not provide adequate drug exposure for any BMI classification for MICs in excess of 0.25 to 0.5 mcg/mL.

Davis RL, Quenzer RW, Weller S, et al. Acyclovir pharmacokinetics in morbid obesity. In: *31st Interscience Conference on Antimicrobial Agents and Chemotherapy*, Sept 29–Oct 2. Chicago, IL: American Society for Microbiology; 1991.

Erstad BL. Dosing of medications in morbidly obese patients in the intensive care unit setting. *Intensive Care Med* 2004;30(1):18–32.

There is clearly a need for more investigations involving dosing regimens of medications in the morbidly obese population. Until such studies are available, the clinician must try to derive the best dosing regimens for medications based on the limited pharmacokinetic data available for some agents and clinical judgment.

Falagas ME, Karageorgopoulos DE. Adjustment of dosing of antimicrobial agents for body-weight in adults. *Lancet* 2010;375(9710):248–251.

Gillum JG, Johnson M, et al. Flucytosine dosing in an obese patient with extrameningeal cryptococcal infection. *Pharmacotherapy* 1995;15(2):251–253.

Hall RG, Swancutt MA, et al. Fractal geometry and the pharmacometrics of micafungin in overweight, obese, and extremely obese people. *Antimicrob Agents Chemother* 2011;55(11):5107–5112.

The authors previously demonstrated that overweight patients exhibit higher micafungin systemic clearance (SCL) than leaner patients. Furthermore, micafungin SCL continues to increase as weight increases, with no obvious plateau. This leads to a requirement for strategies to determine individualized dosing levels for obese and extremely obese patients.

Hanley MJ, Abernethy DR, et al. Effect of obesity on the pharmacokinetics of drugs in humans. *Clin Pharmacokinet* 2010;49(2):71–87.

Excellent review article.

Hollenstein UM, Brunner M, et al. Soft tissue concentrations of ciprofloxacin in obese and lean subjects following weight-adjusted dosing. *Int J Obes Relat Metab Disord* 2001;25(3):354–358.

Kees MG, Weber S, et al. Pharmacokinetics of moxifloxacin in plasma and tissue of morbidly obese patients. *J Antimicrob Chemother* 2011;66(10):2330–2335.

The pharmacokinetics of moxifloxacin is not significantly affected by morbid obesity. No dose adjustment seems to be necessary in this particular population.

Newman D, Scheetz MH, et al. Serum piperacillin/tazobactam pharmacokinetics in a morbidly obese individual. *Ann Pharmacother* 2007;41(10):1734–1739.

Pai MP, Bearden DT. Antimicrobial dosing considerations in obese adult patients. *Pharmacotherapy* 2007;27(8):1081–1091.

As obesity continues to increase in prevalence throughout the world, it becomes important to explore the effects that obesity has on antimicrobial disposition. Excellent review.

Pai MP, Norenberg JP, et al. Influence of morbid obesity on the single-dose pharmacokinetics of daptomycin. *Antimicrob Agents Chemother* 2007;51(8):2741–2747.

Stein GE, Schooley SL, et al. Pharmacokinetics and pharmacodynamics of linezolid in obese patients with cellulitis. *Ann Pharmacother* 2005;39(3):427–432.

One treatment concern would be an obese patient receiving oral linezolid who was infected with a less susceptible (MIC > or = 4.0 mcg/mL) strain of Staphylococcus aureus.

Yuk J, Nightingale CH, et al. Pharmacokinetics of nafcillin in obesity. *J Infect Dis* 1988;157(5):1088–1089.

56 Dosing Patients in Renal Failure

Paul Lewis and James W. Myers

INTRODUCTION

The majority of antibiotics are cleared via renal elimination and will require adjustment for those patients who have renal impairment. Nevertheless, there are several important antibiotics that do not require a dosage adjustment during renal impairment (see Table 56-1).

Renal impairment or failure affects many different pharmacokinetic parameters including absorption, distribution, metabolism, and elimination. Renally eliminated medications do not need to be avoided in patients with impaired renal function; however, a dosing reduction to prevent toxicity may be needed in order to appropriately treat the patient (see Table 56-2). Dosage reduction is usually accomplished by either a decrease in dose or frequency of administration or both.

Hemodialysis also plays a critical role in drug removal. There are multiple methods for administering hemodialysis including intermittent, continuous, and peritoneal dialysis. It is important to determine the type of dialysis as it plays a significant role in drug removal and the need for replacement dosing. It is also important to determine the type of filter being used. For instance, high-flux filters allow for the clearance of larger molecules such as vancomycin warranting a replacement dose after a standard 4-hour session. Peritoneal dialysis uses the body's own peritoneum as the filter, which does not allow for the passage of larger molecules. Physicians also have the option of dosing antibiotics intravenously or via the intraperitoneal route. This chapter provides a reference for the various dosing strategies for the various degrees of renal dysfunction and for the types of dialysis, including intraperitoneal dosing in peritoneal dialysis.

IMPACT OF RENAL IMPAIRMENT ON PHARMACOKINETICS

Absorption
- Multiple factors contribute to lower absorption such as nausea, vomiting, gastroparesis, intestinal edema, and delayed gastric emptying.
- Increases in stomach pH may decrease absorption.
- Presence of antacids phosphate binders may decrease absorption.

Distribution
- Protein binding may be limited, increasing the amount of "free drug" at the binding site and at the points of elimination (dialysis or hepatic metabolism).
- Presence of edema or ascites will **increase** the volume of distribution of highly protein bound and water soluble medications.
- Muscle mass loss and dehydration can **reduce** volume of distribution.

Table 56-1	Antibiotics Without Renal Adjustments	
Amphotericin	Linezolid	Oxacillin
Azithromycin	Metronidazole	Rifampin
Ceftriaxone	Micafungin	Rifabutin
Clindamycin	Minocycline	Rifaximin
Doxycycline	Moxifloxacin	Tigecycline
Itraconazole	Nafcillin	**Voriconazole (PO)**

Metabolism

- Uremia can reduce the amount of first-pass metabolism increasing drug levels.
- Cytochrome P450 isoenzymes 2C6, 2C11, 3C11, 3A1, and 3A2 may be down-regulated due to the accumulation of endogenous inhibitors.
- Glucuronidation, sulfated conjugation, and oxidation **not likely to be affected** by uremia

Elimination

- Drug removal is accomplished by glomerular filtration and tubular secretion.
- Drugs may also be reabsorbed into circulation.
- When glomerular filtration decreases, tubular secretion may be enhanced.
- Renal impairment reduces both glomerular filtration and tubular secretion.

Estimating Renal Function

- 24-hour urine collection
  - Most accurate, however often impractical to do in the clinical setting
- Serum creatinine
  - Endogenous amino acid derivative freely filtered by the glomerulus and secreted by the proximal tubules
  - **Body composition** plays a large role as creatinine is a function of muscle mass.
  - Dietary intake may account for variations seen in different age, race, ethnic, and geographic groups.
  - **Age** also plays a role as advanced age results in decreased muscle mass and lower creatinine levels.
  - **Trimethoprim** and cimetidine may **inhibit tubular secretion of creatinine** causing a falsely elevated serum creatinine.
  - Not useful as a single marker
- **Cockcroft-Gault formula**
  - Preferred method for measuring creatinine clearance (CrCl) due to ease of use and historical experience
  - Basis for **manufacturer** recommendations regarding renal adjustments
  - **Of note, Cockcroft-Gault is only valid in "stable" serum creatinine levels!**
  - **In patients with oliguria or rapidly rising serum creatinine, consider the CrCl to be <10 mL/min.**

Table 56-2	Antibiotic Dosage Adjustments in Renal Impairment not on Dialysis[a]	
Creatinine Clearance	**Moderate to Severe**	**Severe to Life Threatening**
Ampicillin		
CrCl >50 mL/min	2 g q6h	2 g q4h
CrCl 10–50 mL/min	2 g q8h	2 g q6h
CrCl <10 mL/min	2 g q12h	2 g q8h
Ampicillin-sulbactam		
CrCl >30 mL/min	1.5 g q6h	3 g q6h
CrCl 15–29 mL/min	1.5 g q12h	3 g q12h
CrCl <15 mL/min	1.5 g q24h	3 g q24h
Aztreonam		
CrCl >50mL/min	1 g q8h	2 g q6–8h
CrCl 10–50 mL/min	1 g q12h	2 g q12h
CrCl <10 mL/min	1 q q24h	2 g q24h
Cefazolin		
CrCl >35 mL/min	1 g q8h	2 g q8h
CrCl 11–34 mL/min	500 mg q12h	1 g q12h
CrCl <10 mL/min	500 mg q24h	1 g q24h
Cefepime		
CrCl >60 mL/min	2 g q12h	2 g q8h
CrCl 30–60 mL/min	2 g q24h	2 g q12h
CrCl <30 mL/min	1 g q24h	2 g q24h
Cefoxitin		
CrCl >50 mL/min	1 g q6h	2 g q6h
CrCl 30–50 mL/min	1 g q8h	2 g q8h
CrCl 10–30 mL/min	1 g q12h	2 g q12h
CrCl <10 mL/min	500 mg q24h	1 g q24h
Ceftazidime		
CrCl >50 mL/min	1 g q8h	2 g q8h
CrCl 30–50 mL/min	1 g q12h	2 g q12h
CrCl 10–30 mL/min	1 g q24h	2 g q24h
Ciprofloxacin		
CrCl >30 mL/min	400 mg q12h	400 mg q8h
CrCl <30 mL/min	400 mg q24h	400 mg q12h
Colistin		
CrCl >50 mL/min	2.5 mg/kg q12h	2.5 mg/kg q12h
CrCl 30–50 mL/min	1.5 mg/kg q12h	1.5 mg/kg q12h
CrCl 10–30 mL/min	2.5 mg/kg q24h	2.5 mg/kg q24h
CrCl <10 mL/min	1.5 mg/kg q24h	1.5 mg/kg q24h
Daptomycin		
CrCl >30 ml/min	4 mg/kg q24h	6–10 mg/kg q24h
CrCl <30 mL/min	4 mg/kg q48h	6–10 mg/kg q48h

(Continued)

Table 56-2	Antibiotic Dosage Adjustments in Renal Impairment not on Dialysis[a] *(Continued)*	
Creatinine Clearance	**Moderate to Severe**	**Severe to Life Threatening**
Doripenem		
CrCl >50 mL/min	500 mg q8h	500 mg q8h
CrCl 30–50 mL/min	250 mg q8h	250 mg q8h
CrCl <30 mL/min	250 mg q12h	250 mg q12h
Ertapenem		
CrCl >30 mL/min	1 g q24h	1 g q24h
CrCl <30 mL/min	500 mg q24h	500 mg q24h
Imipenem-cilastatin		
CrCl >70 mL/min	500 mg q6–8h	1 g q6–8h
CrCl 41–70 mL/min	500 mg q8h	500 mg q6h
CrCl 20–40 mL/min	250 mg q6h	500 mg q8h
CrCl <20 mL/min	250 mg q12h	500 mg q12h
Levofloxacin		
CrCl >50 mL/min	500 mg q24h	750 mg q24h
CrCl 20–50 mL/min	250 mg q24h	750 mg q48h
CrCl <20 mL/min	250 mg q48h	500 mg q48h
Meropenem		
CrCl >50 mL/min	1 g q8h	2 g q8h
CrCl 25–50 mL/min	1 g q12h	1 g q8h
CrCl 10–25 mL/min	500 mg q12h	1 g q12h
CrCl <10 mL/min	500 mg q24h	1 g q24h
Penicillin		
CrCl >50 mL/min	2 million units q4h	4 million units q4h
CrCl 10–50 mL/min	1–1.5 million units q4h	2–3 million units q4h
CrCl <10 mL/min	1 million units q6h	2 million units q6h
Piperacillin-tazobactam		
CrCl >40 mL/min	3.375 g q6h	4.5 g q6h
CrCl 20–40 mL/min	2.25 g q6h	3.375 g q6h
CrCl <20 mL/min	2.25 g q8h	2.25 g q6h
Telavancin		
CrCl >50 mL/min	10 mg/kg q24h	10 mg/kg q24h
CrCl 30–50 mL/min	7.5 mg/kg q24h	7.5 mg/kg q24h
CrCl <30 mL/min	10 mg/kg q48h	10 mg/kg q48h
Ticarcillin-clavulanic acid		
CrCl >60 mL/min	3.1 g q6h	3.1 g q4h
CrCl 30–60 mL/min	2 g q4–6h	2 g q4h
CrCl 10–30 mL/min	2 g q8–12h	2 g q8h
CrCl <10 mL/min	2 g q12h	2 g q12h
Trimethoprim-sulfamethoxazole		
CrCl >30	5 mg/kg q12h	5 mg/kg q8h
CrCl 10–30	2.5 mg/kg q12h	5 mg/kg q12h
CrCl <10	Avoid	2.5 mg/kg q12h

[a]Vancomycin and aminoglycosides are discussed in the therapeutic drug monitoring chapter.

- Formula for calculating CrCl (mL/min)
  ○ For males,

$$CrCl = \frac{(140 - age) \times Body \ Weight \ in \ Kg}{(72 \times SCr \ (in \ mg/dL))}$$

  ○ **For females, multiply this value by 85%.**
  ○ Ideal body weight (IBW) using the **Devine method** has been proposed over total body weight.
    - Male IBW = 50 Kg + 2.3 Kg for each inch over 5 feet in height
    - Female IBW = 45 Kg + 2.3 Kg for each inch over 5 feet in height
  ○ Adjusted body weight (IBW + **40% of the difference** between ideal and total weight) has been proposed for obesity.
  ○ Consider rounding the serum creatinine to 0.8 to 1 mg/dL in age >65
- Modification of Diet in Renal Disease (**MDRD**) formula
  - Developed in 1999 and reexpressed in 2005 using a standardized creatinine
  - **Normalized for body surface area (BSA)**
  - Currently only useful in the staging of renal impairment
  - FDA now recommending that future pharmacokinetic studies evaluate MDRD in addition to Cockcroft-Gault
  - GFR (mL/min/1.73 m^2) = 175 × (standardized creatinine)$^{-1.154}$ × (age)$^{-0.203}$ × 0.742 (if female) and × 1.212 (if black)
  - To convert from the BSA normalized MDRD to mL/min:
    ○ GFR (mL/min/1.73 m^2 × estimated BSA ÷ 1.73 m^2)
    ○ BSA = (weight in kg)$^{0.425}$ × (height in cm)$^{0.725}$ × 0.007184

DOSING IN RENAL IMPAIRMENT

A multitude of antibiotics are cleared primarily by the kidney and are affected by the reduced renal function.

- **Initial doses may require a load** or larger load due to increased volume of distribution, especially when therapeutic levels are needed quickly.
- Maintenance dosing may be adjusted by **decreasing the dose or extending the interval.**
- Time>MIC-dependent antibiotics are often given as a reduced dose.
- Concentration-dependant antibiotics are usually adjusted by increasing the interval of administration.

Drugs that display a time above MIC-dependant killing model such as the beta-lactams typically involve a *decrease in dose* (doripenem reduced from 500 mg every 8 hours to 250 mg every 8 hours). Drugs that display a concentration-dependant killing model typically involve a *reduction in frequency* (daptomycin changed to every 48 hours from every 24 hours).

DOSING IN DIALYSIS

Intermittent hemodialysis (IHD) is still the most common method for renal replacement therapy in patients with end-stage kidney disease (ESRD). For patients with unstable hemodynamics and unable to tolerate IHD, **continuous renal replacement therapies** typically consist of continuous venovenous hemofiltration (CVVH), continuous venovenous hemodialysis (CVVHD), or continuous venovenous diafiltration (CVVHDF).

Drug removal is accomplished by two main principles, convection and diffusion. **Convection** involves the removal of solvent *independent* of concentration gradient. Plasma water is pushed across a membrane filter as a result of a pressure gradient. As fluid is removed, drug is dragged with the fluid.

Diffusion involves the passive movement across a membrane from an area of high concentration (blood) to low concentration (extracorporeal dialysate fluid). For recommended doses, see Table 56-3.

Factors affecting drug removal during dialysis

- Residual renal function
  - Noted by the presence of urine output
  - Nonrenal clearance may increase during acute renal failure.
- Drug properties
  - Molecular size—**smaller molecules have higher diffusion.**
  - Ionic charge—negatively charged molecules more likely to pass through membrane
  - Lipophilicity—**hydrophilic molecules more readily dialyzable**
  - Protein binding—only unbound drug is removed.
  - Volume of distribution—drugs with **high volumes of distribution** have a higher concentration in tissues and less likely to be dialyzed.
- Dialyzer properties
  - Blood flow rate—small variations have limited affect on drug removal.
  - Membrane surface area—larger membrane should increase elimination, however likely insignificant.
  - Membrane permeability—"high flux" membranes allow larger molecules to pass, such as **vancomycin.**

Intermittent Hemodialysis

- Typical duration is 3 to 4 hours.
- Usually performed thrice weekly
- Goal blood flow rates are typically around 400 mL/hr.
- **Drug removal accomplished by diffusion**
- Due to the risk of dialysis disequilibrium syndrome, blood flow rates and duration of therapy are considerably lower, resulting in much **less drug** removal.

Continuous Venovenous Hemofiltration

- Continuous ultrafiltration with the least amount of drug removal
- Characterized by large volumes of IV replacement fluids
- Fluid replacement rates around 3 to 4 L/hr
- **Drug removed by convection**

Continuous Venovenous Hemodialysis

- Continuous ultrafiltration with second most amount of drug removal
- Characterized by extracorporeal dialysate
- **Drug removed by diffusion into the dialysate**

Table 56-3 Antibiotic Dosing in IHD and Continuous Renal Replacement Therapy

Agent	IHD	LD for CRRT	Maintenance for CRRT CVVH	CVVHD	CVVHDF
Acyclovir	2.5–5 mg/kg q24	None	5–10 mg/kg q24h	5–10 mg/kg q12–24h	5–10 mg/kg q12–24h
Amikacin	7.5 mg/kg q72h	10 mg/kg	7.5 mg/kg when level drops below 10 mg/L		
Ampicillin	1–2 g q12–24h	2 g	2 g q12h	2 g q8h	2 g q6h
Ampicillin–sulbactam	1.5–3 g q12–24h	3 g	3 g q12h	3 g q8h	3 g q6h
Aztreonam	500 mg q12h	2 g	1–2 g q8h	1 g q8h	1 g q8h
Cefazolin	0.5–1 g q24h	2 g	1–2 g q12h	2 g q12h	2 g q12h
Cefepime	0.5–1 g q24h	2 g	1–2 g q12h	2 g q12h	2 g q12h
Cefotaxime	1–2 g q24h	None	1–2 g q8–12h	1–2 g q8h	1–2 g q6h
Ceftazidime	1 g q24h	2 g	1–2 g q12h	2 g q12h	2 g q12h
Ciprofloxacin	200–400 mg q24	None	400 mg q24h	400 mg q12h	400 mg q12h
Colistin	1.5 mg/kg q24–48h	None	2.5 mg/kg q48h	2.5 mg/kg q48h	2.5 mg/kg q48h
Daptomycin	4–6 mg/kg q48h	4–8 mg/kg q48h			
Fluconazole	200–400 mg q48 100–200 mg q24	400–800 mg	200–400 mg q24h	400–800 mg q24h	800 mg q24h
Gentamicin	2.5 mg/kg X1, then	2–3 mg/kg, then			
UTI/synergy	1 mg/kg q48–72	1 mg/kg q24–36h, redose when level <1 mg/L			
Severe	2 mg/kg q48–72	2 mg/kg q24–48h, redose when level <3 mg/L			
Imipenem–cilastatin	500 mg q12h	None	500 mg q6h	500 mg q8h	500 mg q8h
Levofloxacin 500 mg	250 mg q48h	500 mg	250 mg q24h	250 mg q24h	500 mg q24h
Levofloxacin 750 mg	500 mg q48h	750 mg	500 mg q48h	500 mg q24h	750 mg q24h
Meropenem	500 mg q24h	1 g	1 g q12h	1 g q8h	1 g q8h
Piperacillin–tazobactam	2.25 g q12h	None	2.25 g q6h	2.25 g q6h	3.375 g q6h

(Continued)

Table 56-3   Antibiotic Dosing in IHD and Continuous Renal Replacement Therapy *(Continued)*

Agent	IHD	LD for CRRT	CVH	Maintenance for CRRT CVHD	CVHDF
Piperacillin-tazobactam (HAP)	2.25 g q8	None	3.375 g q6h	3.375 g q6h	3.375 g q6h
Ticarcillin-clavulanate	2 g q8h	3.1 g	2 g q6h	3.1 g q6h	3.1 g q6h
Tobramycin	Same as gentamicin	Same as gentamicin			
Trimethoprim-sulfa-methoxazole (PCP)	10 mg/kg q24h	None	7.5 mg/kg (TMP) q12h		
Vancomycin	15–25 mg/kg X1, then 5–10 mg/kg after each dialysis	25 mg/kg 10 mg/kg q24–48h Redose when level drops below 20 mg/L		, 15 mg/kg q24h/7.5 mg/kg q12h	10 mg/kg q12h

IHD, intermittent hemodialysis; CRRT, continuous renal replacement therapy; CVH, continuous venovenous hemofiltration; CVHD, continuous venovenous hemodialysis; CVHDF, continuous venovenous diafiltration; UTI, urinary tract infection; HAP, hospital acquired pneumonia; PCP, pneumocystis carinii (jiroveci) pneumonia; TMP, trimethoprim.

Continuous Venovenous Diafiltration

- Continuous ultrafiltration with the *most* amount of drug removal
- Characterized by the use of large volume of IV replacement fluid and extracorporeal dialysate
- Drug removed by **diffusion and by convection**
- Has the most amount of drug removal

Peritoneal Hemodialysis

- Form of dialysis in which the peritoneal membrane selectively filters solute and waste from the blood
- Dialysate is instilled into the peritoneal cavity, allowed to "dwell," and then drained periodically.
- Forms include
  - Continuous ambulatory peritoneal dialysis (CAPD)
    - Most common form of PD
    - **Dialysate is manually exchanged three to four times per day.**
    - Usually involves exchanging 2 L of dialysate per exchange
    - **In most cases, it involves a long dwell overnight.**
  - Continuous cycling peritoneal dialysis (CCPD) or automated peritoneal dialysis (APD)
    - Uses special machinery called a **cycler** to exchange dialysate throughout the night
    - **Does not require exchanges during the day**
    - Only a few drugs have been studied (see Table 56-4).
- Routes of administration for antibiotics
  - Intravenous
    - **Use dosing recommendation for CrCl <10 mL/min.**
    - Use therapeutic drug level monitoring whenever possible.
  - Intraperitoneal (see Table 56-5).
    - May be given intermittently
      - Given *once daily* with the longest dwell
      - Requires at least *6 hours* of dwell time
      - Dosing is usually in mg/kg of body weight.

Table 56-4	Dosing of Antibiotics Using an Automated Cycler
Antibiotic	**Dosing Recommendation**
Cefazolin	20 mg/kg IP daily, given during the longest dwell
Cefepime	1 g IP daily, given as a single dose
Fluconazole	200 mg IP every 24–48 hours, given as a single dose
Tobramycin	LD 1.5 mg/kg IP, MD 0.5 mg/kg IP daily, given as a single dose in longest dwell
Vancomycin	LD 30 mg/kg IP, MD 15 mg/kg IP every 3–5 days, use therapeutic drug level monitoring to maintain serum trough greater 15 mcg/mL

Table 56-5	Intraperitoneal Dosing of Antibiotics During Peritoneal Dialysis	
Antibiotic	**Intermittent**	**Continuous**
	Added to Longest Dwell (Overnight)	**All Exchanges (Dose per Liter)**
Amikacin	2 mg/kg	LD 25 mg, MD 12 mg
Amphotericin	ND	MD 1.5 mg
Ampicillin	ND	MD 125 mg
Ampicillin-sulbactam	2 g every 12 hours	LD 1,000 mg, MD 100 mg
Aztreonam	ND	LD 1,000 mg
Cefazolin	15 mg/kg	LD 500 mg, MD 125 mg
Cefepime	1,000 mg	LD 500 mg, MD 125 mg
Ceftazidime	1,000 mg	LD 500 mg, MD 125 mg
Ciprofloxacin	ND	LD 50 mg, MD 25 mg
Daptomycin	ND	LD 100 mg, MD 20 mg
Fluconazole	200 mg every 24–48 hours	ND
Gentamicin	0.6 mg/kg	LD 8 mg, MD 4 mg
Imipenem-cilastatin	1 g every 12 hours	LD 250 mg, MD 50 mg
Nafcillin	ND	MD 125 mg
Tobramycin	0.6 mg/kg	LD 8 mg, MD 4 mg
Vancomycin	15–30 mg/kg every 5–7 days	LD 1,000 mg, MD 25 mg

For residual renal function >100 mL/day, increase empiric dose by 25%.

- May be given continuously
  - With **all** exchanges (maintenance or MD)
  - Oftentimes, a loading dose (LD) is required.
  - Dosing is usually in mg/L of dialysate.
  - Some drugs have no data (ND) available for intermittent dosing.

OTHER CONSIDERATIONS WHEN DOSING IN RENAL IMPAIRMENT:

- While there are several methods for estimating renal function, Cockcroft-Gault CrCl is preferred since the renal adjustments provided by the manufacturers are based on this formula.
- A risk:benefit ratio should be considered when deciding between two dosing recommendations (wide therapeutic window drugs such as beta-lactams should be dosed more aggressively, while narrower drugs like aminoglycosides should be dosed more conservatively).
- For narrow therapeutic window drugs, the use of therapeutic drug monitoring should be utilized whenever possible.
- The functional CrCl of a patient with no urine output is 0 mL/min, regardless of the reported serum creatinine.
- Patients initiated on cimetidine or trimethoprim may have falsely elevated serum creatinine levels and dosage adjustments are not needed.

- Due to the complications associated with hemodialysis, very few infections are considered uncomplicated or mild. Antimicrobial dosing should target the *higher end* of a reference range.
- **Considerably more drug is removed during continuous renal replacement therapy than IHD.** *When a patient switches modalities, the dosing should be reevaluated for changes.*
- While many manufacturers recommend a "supplemental" dose following dialysis (0.75 g of piperacillin-tazobactam), scheduling the full dose (piperacillin-tazobactam 2.25 g) immediately following dialysis eliminates the need for the supplemental dose!
- When treating methicillin-sensitive *Staphylococcus aureus*, consider using cefazolin 2 g after dialysis Monday and Wednesday (or Tuesday and Thursday) and **3 g after dialysis on Friday** (or Saturday) if possible.
- Upon resolution of symptoms when treating *Pseudomonas aeruginosa* and other gram-negative enterics, consider using cefepime 2 g or ceftazidime 2 g after dialysis for the remainder of the duration.
- For vancomycin, a substantial LD (15–25 mg/kg) **is still required** to get the patient up to a therapeutic level. The maintenance dose should be based on the type of dialysis and dialysis filter being used. **For high flux filters, about one-third of the dose is cleared**. A 75-kg patient would need a 1500 mg (20 mg/kg) LD and 500 mg after each hemodialysis.
- While voriconazole is not renally eliminated, the **vehicle used in the IV formulation** is cleared by the kidneys. The LD may be given IV, but the maintenance doses should be oral.
- Lipid-associated preparations of amphotericin B are preferred over conventional amphotericin B deoxycholate, especially in renal impairment due to less nephrotoxicity.

EXAMPLE CASE

Patient X is a 56-year-old female admitted to intensive care unit with fever of 39.4°C, heart rate of 125 beats per minute, blood pressure of 110/70 mm Hg, and breathing at a rate of 30 breaths per minute. Urinalysis is positive for many bacteria. Serum creatinine is 3.6 mg/dL, yielding an estimated CrCl <20 mL/min. Piperacillin-tazobactam is started at 2.25 g IV every 8 hours, renally adjusted down from 3.375 g IV every 6 hours. Renal function continues to decline and hemodialysis is initiated. Blood cultures turn positive and gram-positive cocci in clusters is seen on gram stain. Piperacillin-tazobactam is discontinued and vancomycin is initiated. Based on a patient weight of 83 kg, the patient is given vancomycin 1.75 g X1 dose, approximately 20 mg/kg rounded to the nearest 250 mg. The first dialysis session lasts approximately 2 hours with a blood flow rate of 200 mL/hr. Due to the reduced duration and limited extraction, a supplemental vancomycin dose is not needed. On the second hemodialysis, the blood flow rate is increased to 400 mL/hr and the session lasts 3 hours. Vancomycin 500 mg supplemental dose is given, approximately one-third of the LD to replace what was removed during dialysis. Overnight, the patient's blood pressure drops to 74/40 mm Hg nonresponsive to fluid boluses and vasopressors are initiated. Nephrology elects to change to CVVHD. Vancomycin is changed to 1,250 mg IV every 24 hours and piperacillin-tazobactam is added back at 3.375 g IV every 6 hours.

SUGGESTED READINGS

Chaijamorn W, Jitsurong A, Wiwattanawongsa K, et al. Vancomycin clearance during continuous venovenous haemofiltration in critically ill patients. *Int J Antimicrob Agents* 2011;38(2):152–156.

The maintenance dose of vancomycin, calculated from parameters from patients in this study, would be 500–750 mg every 12 hours to provide a steady-state trough concentration of 15–20 mg/L. Owing to alterations in clinical conditions, serum vancomycin concentrations must be closely monitored in critically ill patients.

Choi G, Gomersall CD, Tian Q, et al. Principles of antibacterial dosing in continuous renal replacement therapy. *Crit Care Med* 2009;37(7):2268–2282.

Details dose optimization strategies for continuous renal replacement therapy. There is an excellent description of drug removal including illustrations.

Churchwell MD, Mueller BA. Drug dosing during continuous renal replacement therapy. *Semin Dial* 2009;22(2):185–188.

This drug dosing review highlights factors that clinicians should consider when determining a pharmacotherapy regimen for a patient receiving continuous renal replacement therapy (CRRT).

Gilbert B, Robbins P, Livornese LL. Use of antibacterial agents in renal failure. *Infect Dis Clin N Am* 2009;23:899–924.

A great review of the impact of renal failure on the changes in pharmacokinetics, including multiple dosing tables, and a closer look at vancomycin and aminoglycosides.

Heintz BH, Matzke GR, Dager WE. Antimicrobial dosing concepts and recommendations for critically ill adult patients receiving continuous renal replacement therapy or intermittent hemodialysis. *Pharmacotherapy* 2009;29(5):562–577.

Li PK, Szeto CC, Piraino B, et al. Peritoneal dialysis-related infections recommendations: 2010 update. *Perit Dial Int* 2010;30(4):393–423.

Nikitidou O, Liakopoulos V, Kiparissi T, et al. Peritoneal dialysis-related infections recommendations: 2010 update. What is new? *Int Urol Nephrol* 2012;44(2):593–600.

Nyman HA, Dowling TC, Hudson JQ, et al. Comparative evaluation of the cockcroft-gault equation and the modification of diet in renal Disease (MDRD) study equation for drug dosing: an opinion of the nephrology practice and research network of the american college of clinical Pharmacy. *Pharmacotherapy* 2011;31(11):1130–1144.

Patel N, Scheetz, MH, Drusano GL, et al. Determination of antibiotic dosage adjustments in patients with renal impairment: elements for success. *J Antimicrob Chemother* 2010;65(11):2285–2290.

This review describes a methodology for optimally identifying dosage adjustments in patients with impaired renal function using extended-infusion piperacillin-tazobactam as an illustrative example.

Trotman RL, Williamson, JC, Shoemaker DM, et al. Antibiotic dosing in critically ill adult patients receiving continuous renal replacement therapy. *Clin Infect Dis* 2005;41(8):1159–1166.

Ververs TF, van Dijk A, Vinks SA, et al. Pharmacokinetics and dosing regimen of meropenem in critically ill patients receiving continuous venovenous hemofiltration. *Crit Care Med* 2000;28(10):3412–3416.

Vilay AM, GrioM, Depestel DD, et al. Daptomycin pharmacokinetics in critically ill patients receiving continuous venovenous hemodialysis. *Crit Care Med* 2011;39(1):19–25.

Antimicrobial Use and Pregnancy

Paul Lewis and James W. Myers

INTRODUCTION

More than 10 million women are either pregnant or lactating at one time. These women make up a unique population with special considerations. In addition to traditional adverse effects that may be experienced by both the mother and the fetus, there is the added risk of teratogenesis to the fetus. There are limited data regarding the use of antimicrobials and pregnancy. Most of the data come from registry reports and postmarketing surveillance. Clinicians must utilize what little information is available with the clinical picture of the patient to optimize care while minimizing harm.

FETAL DEVELOPMENT

- Fetal development occurs in three stages: fertilization/implantation, embryonic period, and the fetal period.
  - Fertilization and implantation lasts from conception until about 17 days' gestation. During this time, exposure to toxins will *typically result in death followed by spontaneous abortion.*
  - The embryonic stage starts at the end of implantation and lasts through about 55 days' gestation. *Organogenesis occurs during this period* and represents a crucial time when teratogenesis is likely to occur.
  - During the fetal stage, the fetus has a higher barrier of resistance to the effects of teratogens. However, reductions in cell size or number can occur leading to intrauterine growth retardation.
- See Table 57-1 for a classification of drugs used in pregnancy.

ANTIMICROBIAL CONSIDERATIONS

Antibacterial Agents

- Beta-lactams (with the exception of imipenem-cilastatin) are pregnancy category B and should be considered first line whenever possible.
- Macrolides, clindamycin, daptomycin, and fosfomycin are also pregnancy category B.
- Nitrofurantoin, while pregnancy category B, should be *avoided near term* due to possible hemolytic anemia.
- While trimethoprim-sulfamethoxazole has been teratogenic to rats and its use should be cautioned, a number of observational studies support its safety and should be used if necessary.
- Chloramphenicol should be avoided near term due to the potential for "gray baby syndrome."

Table 57-1   Drug Classifications

	Category B	Category C	Category D/X
Antibacterial	Azithromycin Beta-lactams Clindamycin Daptomycin Erythromycin Fosfomycin Metronidazole[a] Nitrofurantoin Polymyxin Quinupristin- Dalfopristin[b]	Bacitracin Chloramphenicol[c] Clarithromycin Colistin Fluoroquinolones Linezolid Sulfamethoxazole Sulfadiazine[d] Telavancin[e] Telithromycin Trimethoprim Vancomycin Methenamine	Aminoglycosides Neomycin Tetracyclines Tigecycline
Antiviral	Famciclovir Telbivudine Tenofovir Valacyclovir	Acyclovir Cidofovir Entecavir Foscarnet Ganciclovir Lamivudine Oseltamivir Rimantadine Valganciclovir Zanamivir	Ribavirin—X
Antifungal	Amphotericin Nystatin Terbinafine	Echinocandins Fluconazole Flucytosine Itraconazole Posaconazole	Voriconazole
Antiparasitic	Nitazoxanide Permethrin	Albendazole Atovaquone Chloroquine Dapsone Ivermectin Mebendazole Mefloquine Primaquine[f] Pyrimethamine[g] Quinidine Quinine Tinidazole	
Antituberculosis	Ethambutol Rifabutin	Isoniazid Rifampin Rifapentine Pyrazinamide[h]	Streptomycin

[a]Contraindicated during first trimester.
[b]Manufacturer does not recommend.
[c]Should not be used near delivery due to gray baby syndrome.
[d]Contraindicated near delivery due to risk of kernicterus.
[e]May cause fetal harm; avoid during pregnancy.
[f]Risk of hemolytic anemia if fetus is G6PD deficient, defer treatment until after delivery.
[g]Supplement with folinic acid 5 mg daily if used.
[h]CDC does not recommend during pregnancy.

Table 57-2	Pregnancy Category Definitions
Pregnancy Category	**Description**
A	Well-controlled studies showing no adverse events in humans
B	Well-controlled studies showing no adverse events in humans; however animal data showing adverse events OR no well-controlled studies in humans; however no adverse events seen in animal studies
C	Human data lacking with adverse events seen in animals OR no data in animals or humans
D	Adverse events demonstrated in humans; benefit may outweigh risk
X	Adverse events demonstrated in humans, risk clearly outweighs benefit

- Fluoroquinolones are associated with arthropathies and should be used with caution.
- **Vancomycin is associated with fetal ototoxicity and should be avoided unless benefit outweighs the risk.**
- Aminoglycosides are linked to eighth cranial nerve toxicity, especially in the first trimester, and should be used only when the benefit outweighs the risk.
- Tetracyclines are generally contraindicated due to liver toxicity to the mother and tooth and bone toxicities in the fetus (please see Table 57-2).

Antifungals

- Topical agents such as nystatin and terbinafine should be considered first line for **superficial** infections.
- Serious fungal infections warrant treatment with amphotericin. If amphotericin is required, appropriate monitoring of serum electrolytes, vital signs, and infusion-related symptoms is particularly important.
- While many uncertainties and inconsistencies exist, the azole antifungals have several proposed mechanisms of teratogenicity, including disruption of the *embryonic retinoic acid* pathway.
- Little is known regarding the use of the echinocandins in pregnancy.

Antivirals

- There is an increased risk of death and complications with influenza in pregnancy. The CDC recommends that the antiviral medications, oseltamivir and zanamivir, be used.
- It is estimated that 30% to 65% of pregnant women are infected with herpes simplex virus (HSV). Because of the symptoms associated with infection, it is recommended that recently acquired genital HSV be treated with oral acyclovir or valacyclovir and intravenous acyclovir for severe HSV.
- Congenital cytomegalovirus (CMV) can lead to hearing loss and mental retardation. While the effectiveness of prenatal antiviral therapy has not been conclusive, CMV-specific hyperimmune globulin may have some benefit. If therapy with ganciclovir is warranted, limited data in humans have shown no adverse events. Foscarnet should only be used in life-threatening conditions.
- Ribavirin and interferon should be avoided if at all possible in pregnant women.

Antiparasitics

- Malaria can have great impact on the well-being of a pregnant woman and the unborn baby, yet treatment may be hindered by the fears of adverse reactions to antimalarial medications.
- The less severe, *Plasmodium vivax*, is associated with maternal anemia and low birth weight.
  - For pregnant women requiring malaria prophylaxis, chloroquine or hydroxychloroquine is recommended. If traveling to a chloroquine-resistant region, mefloquine is recommended. One review suggests that atovaquone-proguanil may be an alternative; however, the CDC does not recommend it.
  - The CDC recommends chloroquine or hydroxychloroquine for the treatment of uncomplicated malaria caused by *P. vivax, Plasmodium ovale, Plasmodium malariae*, or chloroquine-sensitive *Plasmodium falciparum*.
- *P. falciparum* can cause maternal anemia, low birth weight, preterm delivery, and substantially increased mortality.
  - For chloroquine-resistant *P. falciparum*, the CDC recommends quinine plus clindamycin.
- Chloroquine-resistant *P. vivax* should be treated with quinine alone.
- Severe malaria should be treated with intravenous quinidine.
- Eradication of liver hypnozoites caused by *P. vivax* and *P. ovale* with primaquine should be *deferred until after* pregnancy.
- Tetracyclines should be avoided if at all possible.

VACCINES

- Inactivated vaccines are generally safe during pregnancy.
  - The trivalent inactivated influenza vaccine should be offered to **all pregnant women.**
  - No firm data exist regarding Tdap.
    - ○ Defer until after pregnancy for now.
    - ○ If needed, Td may be given to appropriate patients if the previous booster was given >10 years ago.
- **The pneumococcal, meningococcal, hepatitis A, and hepatitis B vaccines may be given during pregnancy if another indication warrants their use.**
- Rabies vaccine should be given if the risk for exposure is substantial.
- No recommendation exists regarding the use of human papillomavirus vaccines in pregnancy; **defer until after** pregnancy.
- No data are available regarding Japanese encephalitis; pregnant women required to travel to an endemic region should be vaccinated.
- Inactivated polio should be given if traveling to an endemic region.
- Typhoid polysaccharide *is preferred over the live bacterial* typhoid as a theoretical transmission risk is possible.
- Live vaccines are generally contraindicated during pregnancy due to the risk of transmission to the fetus.
  - *Varicella, zoster, and MMR are contraindicated during pregnancy.*
- Live attenuated influenza should **not** be given during pregnancy; use the inactivated.
- Yellow fever vaccine is a live attenuated vaccine.
  - ○ If travel to an endemic region is required and risk for yellow fever **outweighs vaccination risk, vaccination may be given.**

- The infant should be monitored after birth for evidence of adverse events or congenital infection.
    - Serologic testing to confirm immune response should be considered due the potential for the vaccine to interfere with the immune system.
- Tuberculosis (BCG) is contraindicated.
- Immune globulins pose no known threat to the fetus and should be given **if indicated.**

LACTATION

- The majority of medications transfer into breast milk via passive diffusion down a concentration gradient.
- The amount of diffusion is proportional to the concentration gradient.
- **Small, nonionized, non–protein-bound, lipophilic molecules are the most likely to cross into breast milk.**
- Drugs with large volume of distributions and short half-lives tend to have lower serum concentrations leading to lower concentrations in breast milk.
- If plasma concentration drops below the concentration in the breast milk, the drug may passively diffuse back to the serum.
- There are several tips that assist in drug selection to minimize potential risk:
  - Use topical whenever possible.
  - **Medications that are safe for infants are usually safe for breast-feeding.**
  - Choose medications with short half-lives and high protein binding.
  - Choose medications that have poor oral absorption and low lipid solubility.
  - If possible, select a once daily medication and schedule the medication just before the longest sleep interval (after bedtime feeding).
  - For multiple daily dosing, breast-feeding should take place just before the medication is due.
- Penicillins, aminopenicillins, clavulanic acids, and cephalosporins **are generally safe** although there is a small risk of allergic reaction.
- Macrolides are excreted into breast milk. Erythromycin is considered safe. Limited data exist regarding azithromycin and clarithromycin, although no adverse events are likely to occur.
- Vancomycin is poorly absorbed in the GI tract and is likely to be safe.
- Daptomycin use in breast-feeding has not been reported but is likely to be safe.
- Tigecycline **is not recommended** during breast-feeding due to gut flora interference.
- **Linezolid is not recommended during breast-feeding due to myelosuppression**.
- Metronidazole has been associated with mutagenicity in older studies. However, no adverse events have been reported though breast milk. While single high-dose metronidazole should be avoided, low dose is considered safe. A topical preparation does exist for certain clinical situations.
- Sulfamethoxazole should not be used within the first 2 months due to hyperbilirubinemia leading to kernicterus according to the FDA. However, no strong evidence exists, and the American Academy of Pediatrics (AAP) does not place limitation on lactating women.
- **Fluoroquinolones have been linked to arthropathies and phototoxicity and should not be used first line.**
- Tetracycline is excreted in very small amounts due to the calcium limiting the absorption. Minocycline and doxycycline have higher absorption than tetracycline **and should be avoided**.

- Fluconazole, often used for nipple yeast infections, is likely to be safe.
- Acyclovir and valacyclovir, often used to treat herpes in neonates, are likely to be safe.
- Chloroquine, hydroxychloroquine, and quinine are safe in breast-feeding. **Mefloquine is found in breast milk. Given the long half-life, it is possible for doses sufficient to cause side effects may accumulate**. Little is known about other antimalarial medications.
- Antihelminthics have no data during pregnancy. Breast-feeding should be held following administration.

SUGGESTED READINGS

CDC. Antiviral Agents for the Treatment and Chemoprophylaxis of Influenza. *MMWR Recomm Rep* 2011;60:1–24.

CDC. Treatment of Malaria (http://www.cdc.gov/MALARIA/)

CDC. Travelers' Health (Pregnant Travelers). (http://wwwnc.cdc.gov/travel/yellowbook/2012/chapter-8-advising-travelers-with-specific-needs/pregnant-travelers.htm)

Corey L, Wald D. Maternal and neonatal herpes simplex virus infections. *N Engl J Med* 2009;361:1376–1385.

Davis TM, Mueller I, Rogerson SJ. Prevention and treatment of malaria in pregnancy. *Future Microbiol* 2010;5:1599–1613.

Edwards MS. Antibacterial therapy in pregnancy and neonates. *Clin Perinatol* 1997:24;251–266.

Money DM. Antiviral and antiretroviral use in pregnancy. *Obstet Gynecol Clin North Am* 2003;30:731–749.

Moudgal VV, Sobel JD. Antifungals in pregnancy: a review. *Expert Opin Drug Saf* 2003;5:147–183.

Nahum GG, Uhl K, Kennedy DL. Antibiotic use in pregnancy and lactation. *Obstet Gynecol* 2007;107:1120–1138.

Spencer JP, Gonzalez LS, Barnhart DJ. Medications in the breast-feeding mother. *Am Fam Physician* 2001;64:119–126.

Yinon T, Farine D, Yudin MH. Screening, diagnosis, and management of cytomegalovirus infection in pregnancy. *Obstet Gynecol Surv* 2011;65:736–743.

58 Choosing an Antifungal

Paul Lewis and James W. Myers

Fungal infections are becoming increasingly common, mostly as a result of medical progression. Broad-spectrum antibiotics, aggressive surgeries, central lines, and immunosuppression are among the risk factors predisposing patients to fungal invasion. Risk factors are listed in Table 58-1. Susceptibility testing is available, usually as a send-out lab. *Candida* testing can be performed on some automated systems. This is usually not necessary, and treatment is generally guided by the knowledge of resistance patterns. For example, the majority of *Candida* species are susceptible to fluconazole; however, *Candida krusei* is inherently resistant and an alternative agent should be selected. This chapter focuses on selecting the most appropriate antifungal agent empirically and organism directed.

MORPHOLOGIES

Fungi come in a variety of shapes and sizes. Many fungi are noninvasive to humans and include organisms such as mushrooms, rusts, smuts, puffballs, truffles, and morels. Some fungi can cause infection in a normal host; however, most are opportunistic organisms taking advantage of a weakened immune system. Fungi that are invasive to humans usually come in three forms: yeasts, molds, and dimorphic fungi.

- Yeasts
  - Unicellular spherical organisms
  - Reproduce via binary fission or budding
  - Common organisms
    ○ *Candida*
      - Most common cause of invasive fungal disease.
      - Candidemia is the fourth leading cause of nosocomial bloodstream infections.
      - Noted species
        · *Candida albicans*
        · *Candida tropicalis*
        · *Candida parapsilosis*
        · *Candida glabrata*
        · *C. krusei*
        · *Candida lusitaniae*
        · *Candida guilliermondii*
    ○ Cryptococcus
      - Encapsulated organism
      - Notable species
        · *Cryptococcus neoformans*
        · *Cryptococcus gattii*

Table 58-1	Risk Factors for Fungal Infections

Broad-spectrum antibiotics
Central venous catheters
Total parenteral nutrition
Immunosuppression
   Transplants
   Antineoplastics and neutropenia
   HIV/AIDS
   Chronic steroid use
Prosthetic valves and devices
Aggressive surgeries
Renal replacement therapy
Diabetes mellitus

- Molds
  - Complex in nature and exist as higher order structures
  - Filamentous fungi ubiquitously found in soil and decaying material
  - Contain filamentous branching structures known as hyphae
  - Notable species
    - *Aspergillus*
      - *Aspergillus fumigatus*
      - *Aspergillus niger*
      - *Aspergillus terreus*
    - *Zygomycetes*
      - Order of *Mucorales*
        - *Rhizopus*
          - *Rhizopus arrhizus*
          - *Rhizopus microsporus*
        - *Absidia corymbifera*
        - *Rhizomucor pusillus*
        - *Mucor racemosus*
        - *Cunninghamella bertholletiae*
    - *Scedosporium*
      - *Scedosporium apiospermum*
        - *Pseudallescheria boydii* (sexual form or teleomorph)
      - *Scedosporium prolificans*
    - *Fusarium*
      - *Fusarium solani*
      - *Fusarium moniliforme*
      - *Fusarium oxysporum*
    - *Cladosporium*
    - *Penicillium marneffei*
    - *Paecilomyces lilacinus*
- Dimorphic fungi
  - Exist in both the yeast and mold form depending on the temperature
  - In the human body, these organisms present as yeasts.

- These organisms also tend to be endemic to certain regions.
- Common organisms
  - *Histoplasma*
    - Endemic to central and eastern United States covering the Ohio and Mississippi River valleys as well as Central and South America, the Caribbean islands, and temperate regions of Asia
    - Notable species
      - *Histoplasma capsulatum*
  - *Blastomyces*
    - Endemic to the southeastern and south central states adjacent to the Mississippi and Ohio Rivers, the midwestern states that border the Great Lakes, and parts of New York adjacent to the St. Lawrence Seaway, as well as parts of Canada adjacent to large waterways
    - Notable species
      - *Blastomyces dermatitidis*
  - *Coccidioides*
    - Endemic to southern Arizona, central or other areas of California, southern New Mexico, and West Texas
    - Most common clinical presentation is a self-limited subacute community-acquired pneumonia presenting 1 to 3 weeks after contact
    - May progress to an acute infection in select populations
    - Notable species
      - *Coccidioides immitis*
      - *Coccidioides posadasii*
  - *Sporothrix*
    - Found throughout the world in decaying vegetation, sphagnum moss, soil, and digging animals, such as armadillos
    - Notable species
      - *Sporothrix schenckii*

DIAGNOSIS

While diagnosis of superficial fungal infections can be accomplished easily by direct examination (thrush), invasive fungal infections can be difficult with limited available tests. Fungal cultures are available although sensitivity can be lacking. Blood cultures are only positive in about 50% of cases. Biopsies still play an important role if feasible, though many critical conditions prevent the attainment of reliable biopsies. In the absence of biopsy or culture-guided therapy, serologic markers, antigen testing, and nucleic acid testing have become increasingly common. Imaging and radiographic evidence also assist in diagnosis.

- Fungal cultures
  - Single best method for detecting fungal pathogens
  - Generally require aeration and agitation
  - Can be taken from blood, skin, mucosa, tissues, CSF, and secretions
  - Yeasts grow easily on a variety of media.
    - Sometimes contain antibacterials to enhance fungal growth
    - Candida may be differentiated on plates such as the CHROMagar.

- Molds can be determined by macroscopic and microscopic growth.
- Advantages
  - Identifies species
  - Can be used to perform susceptibility testing
- Disadvantages include
  - Cannot differentiate pathogen versus colonization
    - *Candida* in sputum or urine
    - *Aspergillus* in respiratory secretions
  - Long-time incubation period
- Microscopic examination of tissue samples and fluids
  - Common stains on exudates and fluids
    - Gram stain
    - Potassium hydroxide (KOH)
    - Giemsa stain
    - Wright stain
  - Wet mounts with or without KOH
    - Budding yeast cells with hyphae indicate *C. albicans.*
    - Yeast with a "figure eight" or broad budding pattern is characteristic of *B. dermatitidis.*
    - Encapsulated cells indicate *C. neoformans.*
    - Large cells with endospores indicate *C. immitis.*
    - Septate hyphae with acute-angle branching indicate molds such as *Aspergillus, Mucor, Fusarium, Penicillium, Pseudallescheria, and Scopulariopsis.*
  - Special stains
    - India ink stain—used for *C. neoformans*
    - Mucicarmine stain—also used for *C. neoformans*
    - Gomori methenamine silver (GMS)—useful for *H. capsulatum*
    - Hematoxylin-eosin (H&E)—shows dematiaceous fungi
    - Periodic acid-Schiff—used to stain internal structures
  - Advantages
    - Practicality and sensitivity
    - Rapid detection
  - Disadvantages
    - Cannot differentiate pathogen from colonization
- Biochemical markers
  - Serologies
    - Relies on immune system to form antibodies to pathogens
    - Not useful in clinical practice
      - Immunocompromised may not produce antibodies.
      - Positive results may only indicate exposure.
  - Antigen testing
    - Detects fungal component in blood, urine, or CSF
    - Advantages
      - Quick turnaround time
      - Specificity
    - Disadvantages
      - Potential for crossover between species
      - Not available for many organisms
  - Molecular testing
    - Uses nucleic acid amplification technology such as polymerase chain reaction (PCR) to detect individual genetic material

- ○ Advantages
  - − Highly sensitive and specific
- ○ Disadvantages
  - − Not universally available
  - − Expensive
  - − Cannot distinguish from contamination
- See Table 58-2 for a list of biochemical markers
- Imaging
  - Plays an important role, especially when more invasive diagnostic testing is not available
  - Some of the more common findings are listed below, though this list is far from all-inclusive
- Pulmonary aspergillosis
  - ○ Plain radiographs are relatively insensitive
  - ○ CT scan much more reliable
    - − "Tree-in-bud" pattern or branching linear opacities
    - − "Halo sign" macronodules surrounded by ground glass opacity
    - − "Air-crescent" sign and cavitary nodules
      - • Resulting from necrotic tissue separating from surrounding lung tissue
      - • May develop into a thin wall cavity and become secondarily infected
- Pulmonary mucormycosis
  - ○ Chest radiograph shows rapidly progressive lobar or segmental consolidation.
  - ○ Upper lung lobes most commonly affected.
  - ○ Other findings include multilobar consolidation, nodules or masses, lymphadenopathy, and pleural effusions.
  - ○ CT findings similar to aspergillosis.
- Pulmonary cryptococcosis
  - ○ Radiography may show diffuse interstitial opacities, especially in HIV+.
  - ○ Immunocompromised may also show cavitation, miliary disease, pleural effusions, and lymphadenopathy.
- Pulmonary coccidioidomycosis
  - ○ Acute disease may present as airspace opacities and consolidation.
  - ○ May also show as multifocal, ill-defined pulmonary nodules
- Acute pulmonary histoplasmosis
  - ○ Radiographs may be normal or minimal parenchymal opacities.
  - ○ In severe cases, may show bilateral diffuse reticulonodular opacities.

ANTIFUNGAL AGENTS

Unlike bacteria, fungi are eukaryotic organisms. Many of the cellular structures are similar to mammalian cells. Due to the overlap, many of the fungal targets create significant toxicities limiting their use. Ergosterol, the fungal cell membrane equivalent of cholesterol, is the target of the polyene antifungals and azole antifungals. The first in class agent, ketoconazole, also inhibited several enzymes in mammalian steroid metabolism leading to many of the adverse events. Newer azoles have greater specificity for fungal targets and have less toxicity than older agents. Flucytosine gets deaminated to 5-fluorouracil inside the fungal cell resulting in similar toxicity. Fungi also contain a cell wall, unlike mammalian cells. This is the target of the newest class of antifungals known as the echinocandins with minimal adverse effects. For a comparison of toxicity, see Table 58-3.

Table 58-2	Non–Culture-Based Laboratory Tests for Invasive Fungal Diseases				
Assay	**Organisms**	**Source**	**Accuracy (%)**	**Advantages**	**Disadvantages**
1,3-β-D-glucan (Fungitec)	Multiple	Serum, BAL	Sen 85–90 Spec 95–100	Rapid turnaround	Does not detect *Cryptococcus* or *Zygomycetes*
PCR	Multiple	Many	Sen 64–100 Spec 64–95	Able to detect species	False positives (contamination)
Mannan Ag/Ab α/β-Ag	*Candida*, except *C. krusei* and *C. parapsilosis*	Serum	Sen 80–85 Spec 93–95	Good for surveillance	Does not differentiate species
D-arabinitol assay	*Candida* except *C. krusei*	Serum, urine	Sen 58–100 Spec 86–91	Good for surveillance	Poor sensitivity for *C. glabrata*
FISH	*C. albicans C. glabrata*	Gram stain	Sen 95–100 Spec 100	Differentiates organisms	Limited detection threshold
Antibodies	Multiple	Serum	Poor	None	Poor performance
Galactomannan	*Aspergillus*	Serum	Sen 22–90 Spec 84–93	Surveillance in high-risk groups	False positives with piperacillin-tazobactam or ampicillin/sulbactam
D-mannitol	*Aspergillus*	BAL, serum	No data		Animal studies only
Cryptococcal Ag	*Cryptococcus*	Many	Sen 71–100 Spec 97–100	Very good for CSF, serum, BAL	Does not differentiate species, false positives
Coccidioido-mycosis IgM	*C. immitis C. posadasii*	Many	Sen 56–83 Spec 75–10	IgG can track treatment	Delayed antibody response
Histoplasma Ag	*H. capsulatum*	Many	Sen 70–95 Spec 99	Antigen levels follow treatment response	Poor sensitivity for subacute disease
Blastomyces Ag	*B. dermatitidis*	Many	Sen 80–93 Spec 79	Good performance	Cross reactivity with other fungi

BAL, bronchoalveolar lavage; Sen, sensitivity; Spec, specificity; PCR, polymerase chain reaction; FISH, fluorescent in situ hybridization; Ag, antigen; CSF, cerebrospinal fluid; Ab, antibody

Table 58-3	Adverse Reactions of Antifungal Agents		
Amphotericin	**Azoles**	**Echinocandins**	**Flucytosine**
Infusion-related reactions: fever, chills, rigors, myalgias, arthralgias, nausea, vomiting, headaches, sweating and bronchospasm	Hepatotoxicity Skin rash Hypokalemia QTc prolongation	Histamine-mediated symptoms: rash, pruritus, facial swelling	(Similar to 5-fluorouracil) Gastrointestinal intolerance (diarrhea)
Nephrotoxicity: potassium- and magnesium-wasting azotemia, renal tubular acidosis, and impaired urinary concentration	*Voriconazole*: transient visual disturbance (photopsia), CNS disturbances	Increased LFTs, bilirubin Phlebitis Anaphylaxis (rare)	Bone marrow suppression Pruritus Peripheral neuropathy
Hepatotoxicity Bone marrow suppression Hypocalcemia Anemia Phlebitis Rash Hypotension Hypertension Tachycardia Metallic taste	*Itraconazole*: CHF exacerbation		

- Polyenes
  - Binds directly to ergosterol resulting in increased permeability across the cellular membrane leading to leakage of intracellular components
  - Also binds to the mammalian equivalent to ergosterol, cholesterol, resulting in toxicity
- Nystatin
  - Available as a topical cream and powder, oral suspension, and vaginal tablet
  - Uses include oropharyngeal, vulvovaginal, and cutaneous candidiasis
  - Dosing
    - Thrush: one to two tablets or 5 to 10 mL swish and swallow 4× day.
    - Vaginitis: one vaginal tablet (100,000 units) daily
    - Topical candidiasis: Apply cream, ointment, or powder to affected areas twice daily.
- Amphotericin
  - Broadest coverage of any antifungal
  - Mainstay of fungal treatment since the 1950s

- ○ Generally reserved for severe or life-threatening fungal infections
- ○ Conventional formulation
- ○ Use is limited by infusion-related reactions and nephrotoxicity.
- ○ Still used for symptomatic urinary tract infections
- ○ Dosing ranges from 0.3 to 0.7 mg/kg actual body weight daily.
- ○ In renal dysfunction, consider switching to lipid agent.
- ○ No hepatic adjustment
- ○ Three lipid-associated formulations (Lipid AmB) now available
  - – Less nephrotoxicity
  - – Still associated with infusion-related toxicities
  - – Dosing
    - • Amphotericin B cholesteryl sulfate complex (ABCD) 3 to 7 mg/kg/day
    - • Amphotericin B lipid complex (ABLC) 5 mg/kg/day
    - • Amphotericin B liposomal (Liposomal AmB) 3 to 5 mg/kg/day
      - • Doses as high as 15 mg/kg used for zygomycosis
  - – ABCD has the highest rate of infusion reactions of the three lipid products.
  - – Liposomal AmB has shown less nephrotoxicity and fewer infusion-related toxicity than ABLC.
- ○ Saline loading 250 to 500 mL before and after amphotericin is nephroprotective.
- ○ Hydrocortisone 10 to 50 mg and acetaminophen 650 mg can be given prior to dose to reduce fever and chills.
- ○ Meperidine 25 mg IV every 15 minutes, up to 100 mg total can be given for rigors.
- Azoles
  - • Inhibit 14-α-demethylase, a crucial step in the formation of ergosterol, leading to altered cell membrane function and cell death
  - • Significant drug interactions may limit use.
    - ○ See Table 58-4 for specific enzymes.
    - ○ Immunosuppressants (cyclosporine, tacrolimus, and sirolimus) are associated with increased risk of fungal infections and have significant drug interactions.
      - – Fluconazole and itraconazole do not require an initial dosage adjustment; however, careful monitoring of the immunosuppressant is recommended.
      - – Upon initiation of voriconazole, cyclosporine should be reduced by 50% and tacrolimus by 67%.

Table 58-4	CYP Interactions with Triazole Antifungals			
	Fluconazole	**Itraconazole**	**Voriconazole**	**Posaconazole**
Inhibitor				
CYP2C19	Minimal	None	Substantial	None
CYP2C9	Moderate	Minimal	Moderate	None
CYP3A4	Moderate	Substantial	Moderate	Substantial
Substrate				
CYP2C19	None	None	Substantial	None
CYP2C9	None	None	Minimal	None
CYP3A4	Minimal	Substantial	Minimal	None

- Upon initiation of posaconazole, cyclosporine should be reduced by 25% and tacrolimus by 67%.
    - Posaconazole and voriconazole should not be used with sirolimus.
  - Other common medication and medication classes that may interact
    - Antiretrovirals
    - Rifampin and rifabutin
    - Benzodiazepines (midazolam and diazepam)
    - Methadone and fentanyl
    - Anticonvulsants
    - Warfarin
    - Statins (simvastatin and lovastatin)
- Fluconazole
  - Available IV and oral
  - Bioavailability approximately 90% and not affected by food or gastric pH
  - Greatest penetration into CNS, vitreous body, and urine
  - Dosing ranges from 100 to 2000 mg/day depending on indication.
    - Primarily cleared by kidneys and requires renal adjustment
      - CrCl <50 mL/min: reduce daily dose by 50%
      - Intermittent hemodialysis: usual dose given post dialysis
      - CVVDH: 400 mg daily
      - Peritoneal dialysis: reduce daily dose by 50%
  - Standard of therapy for oropharyngeal, esophageal, and vaginal candidiasis.
- Itraconazole
  - Available as an oral liquid and oral capsules
  - Dosing
    - Mild infections: 200 mg q12 to 24h.
    - Severe infections: 200 mg PO 3× day for 3 days, then 200 mg b.i.d.
    - Does not require renal or hepatic adjustment.
    - Therapeutic drug monitoring is recommended for long-term therapy; see Therapeutic Drug Monitoring chapter for recommendations.
  - Variable absorption
    - Capsules enhanced by acidic environment
    - Suspension better absorbed on an empty stomach
    - Conversion: 100 mg suspension = 200 mg capsules
  - Drug of choice for mild to moderate or step-down therapy for dimorphic fungi and esophagitis in patients failing fluconazole
- Voriconazole
  - Available IV and oral
  - Good penetration into CNS and vitreous body
  - Bioavailability is approximately 90% and is not affected by gastric pH.
  - Should be given on empty stomach since food decreases absorption
  - Dosing
    - Severe infections: 6 mg/kg IV q12h × 2 doses, then 4 mg/kg q12h, then transition to 200 mg PO q12h
    - Patients <40 kg: consider 100 mg PO q12h.
    - Inadequate response: consider increasing dose to 300 mg PO q12h.
    - Requires hepatic adjustment

- Decrease dose to 2 mg/kg IV 12h or 100 mg PO q12h.
  - Coadministration with efavirenz
    - Increase dose to 400 mg PO q12h.
    - Decrease efavirenz to 300 mg daily.
  - Coadministration with phenytoin
    - Increase oral dose to 400 mg PO q12h or IV to 5 mg/kg q12h.
  - While renal dosing is not needed, the IV formulation should not be used in CrCl < 50 mL/min due to accumulation of sulfobutylether-cyclodextrin vehicle.
  - Due to genetic polymorphism, may consider therapeutic drug monitoring; see Therapeutic Drug Monitoring chapter for recommendations.
  ○ Drug of choice for aspergillosis
- Posaconazole
  ○ Available as oral suspension only
  ○ Must be given with food (preferably high-fat) to enhance absorption
  ○ Dosing:
    - Prophylaxis of invasive fungal infections: 200 mg q8h
    - Treatment of invasive fungal infections: 200 mg q6h or 400 mg q12h
    - Does not require dosage adjustments
  ○ May have potential for zygomycosis
- Echinocandins
  - Inhibit 1,3-beta-glucan synthase, responsible for the formation of the fungal cell wall
  - Newest class of antifungal agents
  - Similar pharmacokinetics between agents and interchangeable depending on availability
  - Only available IV
  - Caspofungin
    ○ Dosing
      - Invasive fungal disease: 70 mg × 1, then 50 mg daily
      - Coadministration with rifampin, nevirapine, efavirenz, carbamazepine, dexamethasone, or phenytoin
        - Increase dose to 70 mg daily.
      - Only echinocandin that must be dose adjusted for hepatic dysfunction
        - Child-Pugh 7 to 9: Decrease daily dose to 35 mg daily.
        - Severe impairment: no data
    ○ Also must be dose adjusted if given with rifampin
  - Micafungin
    ○ Only echinocandin that does not require a loading dose
    ○ Dosing
      - Prophylaxis: 50 mg daily
      - Invasive fungal disease: 100 to 150 mg daily
  - Anidulafungin
    ○ Similar to caspofungin and micafungin
    ○ Dosing
      - Serious infections: 200 mg × 1, then 100 mg daily
      - Oropharyngeal or esophageal candidiasis: 100 mg × 1 then 50 mg daily
- Antimetabolites
  - Flucytosine
  - Pyrimidine analogue that works by inhibiting thymidylate synthase
  - Only available orally

- Dosing
  - In addition to AmB: 25 mg/kg q6h
  - Dosage adjustment required for renal impairment
    - CrCL 10 to 50 mL/min decrease interval to q12 to 24h
    - CrCl <10 mL/min decrease interval to q24 to 48h
    - Hemodialysis: dose after dialysis
    - Peritoneal dialysis: 500 mg q24h
- Should not be used as a single agent except possibly in the urine

TREATMENT

While susceptibility testing is available in certain cases, antifungal therapy is generally guided by species identification and knowledge of preferred treatment. Due to the low occurrence rate of some fungal infections, most recommendations are based on guidelines of best practice. The Infectious Diseases Society of America (IDSA) publishes guidelines periodically that are available for download. The recommendations are summarized here.

- Empiric therapy
  - Immunocompromising conditions predispose patients to opportunistic infections.
  - Diagnostic testing can have limited yields and still lack sensitivity.
  - Fluconazole and the echinocandins are the predominant agents used for empiric therapy when targeting yeast infections.
  - Voriconazole and amphotericin are the predominant agents used for empiric therapy when targeting mold infections.

Table 58-5	Empiric Antifungal Therapy Based on Location		
Infection	**First Line**	**Second Line**	**Other Alternatives**
Systemic, life-threatening	Amphotericin		
Throat/mouth	Nystatin	Fluconazole	Itraconazole Echinocandin
Esophagus	Fluconazole	Itraconazole	Echinocandin
Urine	Fluconazole	Amphotericin	Amphotericin bladder washes
Lungs, life-threatening	Amphotericin	Voriconazole	Organism specific
Lungs, mild to moderate	Voriconazole	Echinocandin	Amphotericin
Lungs, endemic travel	Amphotericin	Itraconazole	
Brain/CNS	Amphotericin ± flucytosine	Fluconazole	
Bloodstream (sepsis)	Echinocandin	Amphotericin	Fluconazole
Heart (endocarditis)	Amphotericin	Echinocandin	
Peritoneum	Amphotericin + flucytosine	Echinocandin	Azole (if susceptible)

Table 58-6	Empiric Antifungal Therapy Based on Organism		

C. albicans
    C. tropicalis
	Fluconazole	Echinocandin	Voriconazole,
			    itraconazole,
			    posaconazole,
			    amphotericin

C. glabrata	Echinocandin	Amphotericin	

C. kruseii	Echinocandin	Voriconazole	Amphotericin,
			    itraconazole,
			    posaconazole

C. lusitaniae
    (amphotericin-resistant)
	Fluconazole	Echinocandin	Voriconazole,
			    itraconazole

A. fumigatus
Aspergillus flavus
A. niger
	Voriconazole	Amphotericin	Echinocandin,
			    posaconazole,
			    itraconazole

A. terreus
    (amphotericin-resistant)
	Voriconazole	Echinocandin	Posaconazole,
			    itraconazole

Mucormycosis	Amphotericin	Posaconazole	
Blastomycosis	Amphotericin	Itraconazole	Fluconazole
Histoplasmosis	Amphotericin	Itraconazole	Fluconazole
Coccidioidomycosis	Fluconazole	Amphotericin	Itraconazole
Sporotrichosis	Amphotericin	Itraconazole	Fluconazole
Fusariosis	Amphotericin	Voriconazole	Posaconazole
Scedosporiosis	Voriconazole	Posaconazole	

- Tables 58-5 and 58-6 provide recommendations for empiric therapy based on infection location or suspected species.
- Organism guided
  - Upon attainment of culture, histology, or biologic marker, therapy can be directed based on organism and indication.
  - Yeasts
    ○ Candidiasis
      – Fluconazole
        • Preferred for mild to moderate infections
        • Should not be used if resistant organism is identified (*C. glabrata or C. krusei*)
      – Echinocandins
        • Preferred for
          • Severe infections
          • Neutropenia
          • Recent azole exposure
        • Step down to fluconazole if organism is known to be susceptible.
        • See Table 58-7 for resistance patterns
      – Voriconazole
        • May be considered for *C. krusei* as an oral step-down to the echinocandins
        • *C. glabrata* can be resistant to voriconazole; susceptibility testing is needed prior to initiating therapy.
      – Amphotericin

Table 58-7	Susceptibility of Antifungal Agents to *Candida* Species					
	Fluconazole	**Itraconazole**	**Voriconazole**	**Posaconazole**	**Amphotericin**	**Candins**
C. albicans	S	S	S	S	S	S
C. tropicalis	S	S	S	S	S	S
C. parapsilosis	S	S	S	S	S	S or R
C. glabrata	DD to R	DD to R	DD to R	DD to R	S to I	S to R
C. krusei	R	DD to R	S	S	S to I	S
C. lusitaniae	S	S	S	S	S to R	S

S, susceptible; I, intermediate; R, resistant; DD, dose-dependant susceptible; resistance may be overcome by increasing doses.

- May also be considered if other agents are not available
- *C. lusitaniae* can be resistant to amphotericin; consider susceptibility testing.
- – Superficial infections can be treated with nystatin or topical azoles.
  - Systemic therapy can be considered for severe cases.
- – For treatment based on indication, see Table 58-8.
- – Additional measures
  - Patients with candidemia should undergo an ophthalmologic examination to evaluate for Candida endophthalmitis.
  - Remove all intravascular catheters, if possible.
  - Treat 14 days after first negative blood culture result and resolution of signs and symptoms associated with candidemia.
  - If treatment failure occurs, consider susceptibility testing, especially *C. glabrata*.
- ○ Cryptococcosis
  - – Severe infections including CNS are treated with lipid-associated amphotericin plus flucytosine.
  - – CNS disease may need frequent lumbar puncture for pressure relief.
  - – Mild to moderate infections can be treated with fluconazole.
  - – Alternative agents include conventional amphotericin.
  - – HIV-infected patients
    - Initiate HAART 2 to 10 weeks after completion of induction
    - Concern for immune reconstitution syndrome
    - Prophylactic antifungal therapy should continue after completion of therapy until immune reconstitution
      - Fluconazole preferred
      - Alternatives include itraconazole and weekly amphotericin, although less effective.
      - Duration is at least 12 months and CD4 count >100 cells/mcL with undetectable viral load for at least 3 months.
  - – *C. gattii* should be treated the same as *C. neoformans*.
  - – For specific recommendations, see Table 58-9.
- • Molds
  - ○ Aspergillosis
    - – Drug of choice for most infection is voriconazole.
    - – Alternative agents include amphotericin, echinocandins, itraconazole, and posaconazole.
    - – For specific recommendations, see Table 58-10.
  - ○ Zygomycosis
    - – Drug of choice has traditionally been high-dose amphotericin.
    - – Posaconazole has developed a role in the treatment of certain species.
  - ○ Fusariosis
    - – Treatment should be based on species identification.
    - – *F. solani* is the more resistant species and should be treated with amphotericin.
    - – *Fusarium verticillioides* is susceptible to posaconazole.
    - – *F. moniliforme* and *F. oxysporum* may be treated with voriconazole.
    - – Echinocandins do not have activity.
  - ○ Scedosporiosis
    - – Resistant to amphotericin and echinocandins
    - – *S. apiospermum* should be treated with voriconazole.
      - Posaconazole may be considered as a second line.

Table 58-8	Preferred Antifungal Therapy for Candidiasis Based on Indication		

Indication	Preferred	Alternative	Duration
Candidemia			
Severe or neutropenic	Echinocandin	Amphotericin	Treat 14 days after first negative blood culture
Mild to moderate	Fluconazole 800 mg × 1, then 400 mg daily	Echinocandin	
Symptomatic cystitis			
Fluconazole susceptible	Fluconazole 200 mg daily	Amphotericin (nonlipid)	7–14 days
Fluconazole resistant	Amphotericin bladder wash		1–5 days
Pyelonephritis	Fluconazole 400 mg daily	Amphotericin	2 weeks
Vulvovaginal candidiasis	Fluconazole 150 mg × 1	Topical agents	Variable
Osteomyelitis	Fluconazole 400 mg daily	Echinocandin	6–12 months
Septic arthritis	Fluconazole 400 mg daily	Echinocandin	6 weeks or longer
CNS candidiasis	Liposomal AmB 3–5 mg daily plus flucytosine 25 mg/kg q6h with step-down to fluconazole	Fluconazole	Until symptom and CSF resolution
Endophthalmitis	Liposomal Amb 3–5 mg/kg daily plus flucytosine 25 mg/kg q6h	Fluconazole	4–6 weeks or longer depending on treatment response
Vitreitis	Surgery		
Endocarditis	Liposomal Amb 3–5 mg/kg daily plus flucytosine 25 mg/kg q6h	Echinocandin	6–12 months, consider chronic suppression if valve not replaced
Oropharyngeal			
Moderate to severe	Fluconazole 200 mg daily	Itraconazole Fluconazole	7–14 days
Mild	Clotrimazole troches 10 mg 5× day or nystatin suspension 5 mL 4× day		
Esophageal	Fluconazole 200–400 mg daily	Echinocandin	14–21 days
Peritonitis, dialysis related	Fluconazole 200 mg IP q24–48 h	Amphotericin Echinocandin	4–6 weeks
Candida in sputum	No treatment		

Table 58-9	Preferred Antifungal Therapy for Cryptococcosis Based on Indication	

Indication	Regimen	Duration
Meningoencephalitis in HIV+		
Induction	Liposomal AmB (3–4 mg/kg), daily plus flucytosine 25 mg/kg q6h	2 weeks 2 weeks
Consolidation	Fluconazole 400 mg daily	8 weeks
Maintenance	Fluconazole 200 mg daily	At least 1 year, longer if no HAART
Meningoencephalitis in transplant recipient		
Induction	Liposomal AmB (3–4 mg/kg), daily plus flucytosine 25 mg/kg q6h	2 weeks 2 weeks
Consolidation	Fluconazole 400–800 mg daily	4–6 weeks
Maintenance	Fluconazole 200–400 mg daily	6–12 months
Meningoencephalitis in non-HIV, nontransplant		
Induction	Liposomal AmB (3–4 mg/kg), daily plus flucytosine 25 mg/kg q6h	2–4 weeks, longer if yeast grows in CSF after 2 weeks
Consolidation	Fluconazole 400–800 mg daily	8 weeks
Maintenance	Fluconazole 200–400 mg daily	6–12 months
Cryptococcemia	Same as meningoencephalitis	12 months
Pulmonary cryptococcosis		
Mild to moderate	Fluconazole 400 mg daily	6–12 months
Severe	Same as meningoencephalitis	12 months
Other infections	Fluconazole 400 mg daily	6–12 months

- *Scedosporium prolificans* has shown resistance to almost all antifungals.
  - May consider voriconazole
- Addition of terbinafine to voriconazole has shown some benefit in vitro.
- Dimorphics
  - Blastomycosis
    - Mild to moderate infections can usually be treated with itraconazole.
    - Moderately severe to severe infections should be initiated with amphotericin and stepped down to itraconazole.

Table 58-10	Preferred Antifungal Therapy for Aspergillus Infections Based on Indication		
Indication	**Preferred**	**Alternative**	**Duration**
Aspergillosis, invasive pulmonary, invasive sinus, tracheobronchial, CNS, endocarditis, myocarditis, pericarditis, osteomyelitis, septic arthritis, cutaneous infection, peritonitis	Voriconazole 6 mg/kg IV q12h × 2 doses, then 4 mg/kg IV q12h; transition to 200 mg PO q12h when appropriate	Amphotericin Echinocandin Posaconazole Itraconazole	Not defined, based on site of infection, treatment response, surgical intervention, level of immunosuppression, and reversal of immunosuppression
Aspergillosis, infections of the eye	Intraocular AmB plus surgical intervention	Voriconazole Echinocandin	
Aspergilloma, single lesion	Surgical resection	Itraconazole	
Aspergilloma, chronic cavitary	Itraconazole 200 mg t.i.d. × 3 days then, 200 mg b.i.d. Voriconazole	Amphotericin Echinocandin	
Aspergillosis, allergic bronchopulmonary (ABPA)	Itraconazole	Voriconazole Posaconazole	

- Fluconazole may be used at higher doses (400 to 800 mg/day) in CNS infections.
- Voriconazole and posaconazole have activity in vitro; however, their role is uncertain.
○ Histoplasmosis
- Mild pulmonary infections may spontaneously resolve, especially in immunocompetent host.
- Mild infections should be treated with itraconazole.
- Severe infections should be treated with amphotericin with step-down to itraconazole.
○ Coccidioidomycosis
- Mild infections are usually self-limiting.
- Other infections are treated with an azole.
- Severe infections should be initially treated with amphotericin.
○ Sporotrichosis
- Treatment options include local hyperthermia, super saturated potassium iodide (SSKI), azoles (itraconazole preferred), amphotericin, and terbinafine.
- Mild infections are preferentially treated with itraconazole.
- Severe infections should be initially treated with amphotericin.
○ See Table 58-11 for specific recommendations.

Table 58-11	Preferred Antifungal Therapy for Dimorphic Fungi Based on Indication	

Indication	Regimen	Duration
Blastomycosis, mild	Itraconazole 200 mg t.i.d. × 3 days then 200 mg b.i.d.	6–12 months
Blastomycosis, moderate to severe (pulmonary or disseminated)		
Induction	Lipid AmB 3–5 mg/kg/day	1–2 weeks
Consolidation	Itraconazole 200 mg t.i.d. × 3 days then 200 mg b.i.d.	6–12 months
Blastomycosis, CNS		
Induction	Lipid AmB 5 mg/kg/day	1–2 weeks
Consolidation	Itraconazole 200 mg t.i.d. OR fluconazole 800 mg daily	6–12 months 6–12 months
Histoplasmosis, mild to moderate pulmonary	None	
Symptoms <4 weeks		
Symptoms >4 weeks	Itraconazole 200 mg q12–24h	6–12 weeks
Histoplasmosis, severe pulmonary		
Induction	Lipid AmB 3–5 mg/kg/day	1–2 weeks
Consolidation	Itraconazole 200 mg b.i.d.	12 weeks total
Histoplasmosis, chronic cavitary pulmonary	Itraconazole 200 mg q12–12h	>12 months
Histoplasmosis, pericarditis		
Moderate to severe	Itraconazole 200 mg q12–24h plus prednisone	6–12 weeks
Mild	NSAIDS	
Coccidioidomycosis, mild pulmonary	Treatment not necessary	
Coccidioidomycosis, severe pulmonary, chronic pulmonary, or disseminated	Lipid AmB 2–5 mg/kg/day OR fluconazole 400–800 mg daily OR Itraconazole 200 mg q8–12h	3–6 months
Sporotrichosis, cutaneous or lymphocutaneous	Itraconazole 200 mg daily	2–4 weeks after symptom resolution
Sporotrichosis, osteoarticular	Itraconazole 200 mg q12h OR Lipid AmB 3–5 mg/kg daily	>12 months
Sporotrichosis, pulmonary or disseminated		
Severe	Lipid AmB 3–5 mg/kg daily	Until response
Mild to moderate or step-down	Itraconazole 200 mg q12h	>12 months
Sporotrichosis, meningeal		
Initial	Lipid AmB 5 mg/kg daily	4–6 weeks
Step-down	Itraconazole 200 mg q12h	>12 months

CONCLUSION

Choosing an antifungal agent can be an empirical decision based on patient risk factors or pathogen directed upon attainment of a specific diagnosis. Regardless of how the decision was made, knowledge of drug-bug matchups often guides therapy as susceptibility testing is rarely performed. Drug interactions and dose-limiting toxicities should be carefully monitored during therapy and adjustments made when necessary.

SUGGESTED READINGS

Badiee P, Alborzi A. Invasive fungal infections in renal transplant recipients. *Exp Clin Transplant* 2011;9:355–362.

Barberán J, Mensa J, Llamas JC, et al. Recommendations for the treatment of invasive fungal infection caused by filamentous fungi in the hematological patient. *Rev Esp Quimioter* 2011;24:263–270.

Caira M, Trecarichi EM, Mancinelli M, et al. Uncommon mold infections in hematological patients: epidemiology, diagnosis and treatment. *Expert Rev Anti Infect Ther* 2011;9:881–892.

Chapman SW, Dismukes WE, Proia LA, et al. Clinical practice guidelines for the management of blastomycosis: 2008 update by the Infectious Diseases Society of America. *Clin Infect Dis* 2008;46:1801–1812.

Enoch DA, Aliyu SH, Sule O, et al. Posaconazole for the treatment of mucormycosis. *Int J Antimicrob Agents* 2011;38:465–473.

Galgiani JN, Ampel NM, Blair JE, et al. Coccidioidomycosis. *Clin Infect Dis* 2005;41:1217–1223.

Hsu JL, Ruoss SJ, Bower ND, et al. Diagnosing invasive fungal disease in critically ill patients. *Crit Rev Microbiol* 2011;37:277–312.

Islam A, Mody CH. Management of fungal lung disease in the immunocompromised. *Ther Adv Respir Dis* 2011;5:305–324.

Kauffman CA, Bustamante B, Chapman SW, et al. Clinical practice guidelines for the management of sporotrichosis: 2007 update by the Infectious Diseases Society of America. *Clin Infect Dis* 2007;45:1255–1265.

Lewis, RE. Current concepts in antifungal pharmacology. *Mayo Clin Proc* 2011;86:805–817.

Moen MD, Lyseng-Williamson KA, Scott LJ. Liposomal amphotericin B: a review of its use as empirical therapy in febrile neutropenia and in the treatment of invasive fungal infections. *Drugs* 2009;69:361–392.

Mohr J, Johnson M, Cooper T, et al. Current options in antifungal pharmacotherapy. *Pharmacotherapy* 2008;28:614–645.

Muhammed M, Coleman JJ, Carneiro HA, et al. The challenge of managing fusariosis. *Virulence* 2011;2:91–96.

Nivoix Y, Ubeaud-Sequier G, Engel P, et al. Drug-drug interactions of triazole antifungal agents in multimorbid patients and implications for patient care. *Curr Drug Metab* 2009;10:395–409.

Pappas PG, Kauffman CA, Andes D, et al. Clinical practice guidelines for the management of candidiasis: 2009 update by the Infectious Diseases Society of America. *Clin Infect Dis* 2009;48:503–535.

Perfect, JR, Dismukes WE, Dromer F, et al. Clinical practice guidelines for the management of cryptococcal disease: 2010 update by the Infectious Diseases Society of America. *Clin Infect Dis* 2010;50:291–322.

Walsh TJ, Asaissie EJ, Denning DW, et al. Treatment of aspergillosis: clinical practice guidelines of the Infectious Diseases Society of America. *Clin Infect Dis* 2008;46:327–360.

Wheat JL, Freifeld AG, Kleiman MB, et al. Clinical practice guidelines for the management of patients with histoplasmosis: 2007 update by the Infectious Diseases Society of America. *Clin Infect Dis* 2007;45:807–825.

XV Vaccination

59 Vaccination of Healthy Adults

Waseem Ahmad and Paras Patel

INTRODUCTION

An effective means of preventing infectious diseases is immunization, the act of artificially inducing immunity or providing protection from disease; it can be active or passive. The goal of active immunization of a vaccine or toxoid is to stimulate the host to produce a primary immune response. Passive immunization involves administration of antibodies.

Vaccines may be live attenuated organisms, dead/inactivated organisms, or purified products derived from them. Commonly employed killed vaccines include influenza vaccine, cholera vaccine, bubonic plague vaccine, inactivated polio vaccine, hepatitis A vaccine, and rabies vaccine. Major live attenuated vaccines include influenza vaccine (FluMist), yellow fever, measles, rubella, mumps, varicella, typhoid and BCG.

CDC recommends routine vaccination to prevent 17 vaccine-preventable diseases that occur in infants, children, adolescents, or adults. Optimal response to a vaccine depends on multiple factors, including the type of vaccine, age of the recipient, and immune status of the recipient. Certain products, including inactivated vaccines, toxoids, recombinant subunit vaccines, polysaccharide conjugate vaccines, and live vaccines, require ≥2 doses to elicit an adequate antibody response. Tetanus and diphtheria toxoids require booster doses to maintain protective antibody concentrations. See Table 59-1 for a summary of recommendations.

SPECIFIC KEY VACCINES

Influenza Vaccination

- Annual vaccination against influenza is recommended for all persons aged 6 months and older, including all adults.
- Healthy, nonpregnant adults aged <50 years without high-risk medical conditions can receive either intranasally administered live, attenuated influenza vaccine (FluMist) or inactivated vaccine.
- Other persons should receive the inactivated vaccine. Adults aged 65 years and older can receive the standard influenza vaccine or the high-dose (Fluzone) influenza vaccine.

Tetanus, Diphtheria, and Acellular Pertussis Vaccination

- Administer a one-time dose of tetanus, diphtheria, and acellular pertussis (Td/Tdap) to adults aged <65 years who have not received Tdap previously or for whom vaccine status is unknown to replace one of the 10-year Td boosters and as soon as feasible to all (i) postpartum women, (ii) close contacts of infants younger than age 12 months (e.g., grandparents and child-care providers), and (iii) healthcare personnel with direct patient contact.

Table 59-1	Vaccines for Adults		
Vaccine	**Doses**	**Recommendation**	**Comment**
Measles-mumps-rubella (MMR)	One or two doses	High-risk groups such as college students, healthcare workers, and international travelers should receive two doses; others should receive one dose.	Adults born before 1956 have innate immunity and do not require vaccine.
Tetanus-diphtheria and tetanus-reduced diphtheria-acellular pertussis (Tdap)	Td every 10 years	All adults should receive a Td every 10 years after completion of primary series.	Adults ages 19 to 64 should receive a single dose of Tdap in place of a Td booster if their last dose of Td was 10 years previously or earlier.
Influenza	One dose every year	All adults every year	Allergic hypersensitivity to egg proteins is a contraindication for vaccine.
Pneumococcal vaccine, poly-saccharide[a]	One or two doses	• All adults age ≥65 years of age • Adults 19 through 64 years of age who are smokers or have asthma or any long-term health conditions • Residents of nursing homes or long-term care facilities	A second dose is recommended for people 65 years and older who got their first dose when they were younger than 65 and it has been 5 or more years since the first dose.
Varicella	Two doses 28 days apart	High-risk adults who never had chickenpox or not received chickenpox vaccine	Healthcare professionals, teachers, child-care workers, residents and staff in the long-term care facilities, nonpregnant women of childbearing age, college students
Zoster vaccine	Single dose	Adults 60 years old or older, whether or not the patient reported a prior episode of shingles. Persons with chronic medical conditions may be vaccinated unless a contraindication or precaution exists for their condition.	Not if allergic to neomycin and gelatin, immunocompromised pts, pregnant women, active untreated tuberculosis (until resolved), children, or adolescents

Hepatitis A	Two-dose series	Adults in high-risk groups	High-risk group that includes international travelers, residents of communities with high rates of infection (Native Americans, Alaskan natives, and Pacific Islanders), homosexual and bisexual men, injection-drug users, persons with chronic liver disease, and food handlers
Hepatitis B	Three-dose series at 0, 1, and 6 months	Universal infant vaccination and catch-up vaccination of nonimmune older children, adolescents, and high-risk individuals	High-risk groups include healthcare workers, residents and staff of long-term care facilities or prisons, homosexual or bisexual men or heterosexuals with multiple partners, injection-drug users, recipients of clotting factor concentrates, household or sexual contacts of HBV carriers.
HPV vaccine	Three doses series at 0, 1, and 6 months	For girls ages 11–12 years, with catch-up vaccination for girls and women ages 13–26 years	Advisory Committee on Immunization Practices (ACIP) provided guidance that HPV4 may be given to males aged 9 through 26 years to reduce their likelihood of acquiring genital warts; ACIP does not recommend HPV4 for routine use among males.
Meningococcal vaccine	Two doses. The first dose at 11 or 12 years of age, with a booster dose at age 16	Adolescents 11 through 18 years of age, college freshmen living in dormitories, microbiologists who are routinely exposed to isolates of *Neisseria meningitidis*, military recruits, people who have terminal complement component deficiencies and have anatomic or functional asplenia	Covers serogroups A, C, Y, and W-135, but not B

[a]The FDA approved a 13-valent, conjugate pneumococcal vaccine for adults >50 in December 2011 but this has not been added to the vaccine schedule to date.

- Adults aged 65 years and older who have not previously received Tdap and who have close contact with an infant aged <12 months also should be vaccinated.
- Other adults aged 65 years and older may receive Tdap. Tdap can be administered regardless of interval since the most recent tetanus or diphtheria-containing vaccine.
- Adults with uncertain or incomplete history of completing a three-dose primary vaccination series with Td-containing vaccines should begin or complete a primary vaccination series.
- For unvaccinated adults, administer the first two doses at least 4 weeks apart and the third dose 6 to 12 months after the second. If incompletely vaccinated (i.e., <3 doses), administer remaining doses. Substitute a one-time dose of Tdap for one of the doses of Td, either in the primary series or for the routine booster, whichever comes first.
- If a woman is pregnant and received the most recent Td vaccination 10 or more years previously, administer Td during the second or third trimester. If the woman received the most recent Td vaccination <10 years previously, administer Tdap during the immediate postpartum period. At the clinician's discretion, Td may be deferred during pregnancy and Tdap substituted in the immediate postpartum period, or Tdap may be administered instead of Td to a pregnant woman after an informed discussion with the woman.

Varicella Vaccination

- All adults without evidence of immunity to varicella should receive two doses of single-antigen varicella vaccine if not previously vaccinated or a second dose if they have received only one dose, unless they have a medical contraindication.
- Special consideration should be given to those who (i) have close contact with persons at high risk for severe disease (e.g., healthcare personnel and family contacts of persons with immunocompromising conditions) or (ii) are at high risk for exposure or transmission (e.g., teachers; child-care employees; residents and staff members of institutional settings, including correctional institutions; college students; military personnel; adolescents and adults living in households with children; nonpregnant women of childbearing age; and international travelers).
- Evidence of immunity to varicella in adults includes any of the following:
  1. Documentation of two doses of varicella vaccine at least 4 weeks apart
  2. US-born before 1980 (although for healthcare personnel and pregnant women, birth before 1980 should not be considered evidence of immunity)
  3. History of varicella based on diagnosis or verification of varicella by a health-care provider (for a patient reporting a history of or having an atypical case, a mild case, or both, healthcare providers should seek either an epidemiologic link with a typical varicella case or to a laboratory-confirmed case or evidence of laboratory confirmation, if it was performed at the time of acute disease)
  4. History of herpes zoster based on diagnosis or verification of herpes zoster by a healthcare provider
  5. Laboratory evidence of immunity or laboratory confirmation of disease
- Pregnant women should be assessed for evidence of varicella immunity. Women who do not have evidence of immunity should receive the first dose of varicella vaccine upon completion or termination of pregnancy and before discharge from the healthcare facility. The second dose should be administered 4 to 8 weeks after the first dose.

Human Papilloma Virus Vaccination

- Human papillomavirus (HPV) vaccination with either quadrivalent (HPV4) vaccine or bivalent vaccine (HPV2) is recommended for females at age 11 or 12 years and catch-up vaccination for females aged 13 through 26 years.
- Ideally, vaccine should be administered before potential exposure to HPV through sexual activity; however, females who are sexually active should still be vaccinated consistent with age-based recommendations. Sexually active females who have not been infected with any of the four HPV vaccine types (types 6, 11, 16, and 18, all of which HPV4 prevents) or any of the two HPV vaccine types (types 16 and 18, both of which HPV2 prevents) receive the full benefit of the vaccination. Vaccination is less beneficial for females who have already been infected with one or more of the HPV vaccine types.
- HPV4 or HPV2 can be administered to persons with a history of genital warts, abnormal Papanicolaou test, or positive HPV DNA test, because these conditions are not evidence of previous infection with all vaccine HPV types.
- HPV4 may be administered to males aged 9 through 26 years to reduce their likelihood of genital warts. HPV4 would be most effective when administered before exposure to HPV through sexual contact. A complete series for either HPV4 or HPV2 consists of three doses. The second dose should be administered 1 to 2 months after the first dose; the third dose should be administered 6 months after the first dose.

Hepatitis A Vaccination (See Accompanying Chapter 8 on Hepatitis Prevention)

- Vaccinate persons with any of the following indications and any person seeking protection from hepatitis A virus (HAV) infection:
  - Men who have sex with men and persons who use injection drugs
  - Persons working with HAV-infected primates or with HAV in a research laboratory setting
  - Persons with chronic liver disease and persons who receive clotting factor concentrates
  - Persons traveling to or working in countries that have high or intermediate endemicity of hepatitis A
  - Unvaccinated persons who anticipate close personal contact (e.g., household or regular babysitting) with an international adoptee during the first 60 days after arrival in the United States from a country with high or intermediate endemicity
- The first dose of the two-dose hepatitis A vaccine series should be administered as soon as adoption is planned, ideally 2 or more weeks before the arrival of the adoptee.
- Single-antigen vaccine formulations should be administered in a two-dose schedule at either 0 and 6 to 12 months (Havrix), or 0 and 6 to 18 months (Vaqta). If the combined hepatitis A and hepatitis B vaccine (Twinrix) is used, administer three doses at 0, 1, and 6 months; alternatively, a four-dose schedule may be used, administered on days 0, 7, and 21 to 30, followed by a booster dose at month 12.

Hepatitis B Vaccination (See Accompanying Chapter 8 on Hepatitis Prevention)

- Vaccinate persons with any of the following indications and any person seeking protection from hepatitis B virus (HBV) infection:

- Sexually active persons who are not in a long-term, mutually monogamous relationship (e.g., persons with more than one sex partner during the previous 6 months)
- Persons seeking evaluation or treatment for a sexually transmitted disease (STD)
- Current or recent injection-drug users
- Men who have sex with men
- Healthcare personnel and public-safety workers who are exposed to blood or their potentially infectious body fluids
- Persons with end-stage renal disease, including patients receiving hemodialysis
- Persons with HIV infection
- Persons with chronic liver disease
- Household contacts and sex partners of persons with chronic HBV infection
- Clients and staff members of institutions for persons with developmental disabilities
- International travelers to countries with high or intermediate prevalence of chronic HBV infection
- Administer missing doses to complete a three-dose series of hepatitis B vaccine to those persons not vaccinated or not completely vaccinated. The second dose should be administered 1 month after the first dose; the third dose should be given at least 2 months after the second dose (and at least 4 months after the first dose).
- If the combined hepatitis A and hepatitis B vaccine (Twinrix) is used, administer three doses at 0, 1, and 6 months; alternatively, a four-dose Twinrix schedule, administered on days 0, 7, and 21 to 30, followed by a booster dose at month 12 may be used.
- Adult patients receiving hemodialysis or with other immunocompromising conditions should receive 1 dose of 40 mcg/mL (Recombivax HB) administered on a three-dose schedule or two doses of 20 mcg/mL (Engerix-B) administered simultaneously on a four-dose schedule at 0, 1, 2, and 6 months.

Haemophilus Influenzae Type B (Hib) Vaccine

- One dose of Haemophilus influenzae type b (Hib) vaccine should be considered for persons who have sickle cell disease, leukemia, or HIV infection or who have had a splenectomy, if they have not previously received Hib vaccine.

IMMUNOCOMPROMISING CONDITIONS

Inactivated vaccines generally are acceptable (e.g., pneumococcal, meningococcal, influenza [inactivated influenza vaccine]) and live vaccines generally are avoided in persons with immune deficiencies or immunocompromising conditions. HIV-infected individuals with CD4+ T cell counts >200 cells/mm^3 may receive live, attenuated vaccines.

CONTRAINDICATIONS AND PRECAUTIONS

The only contraindication applicable to all vaccines is a history of a severe allergic reaction (i.e., anaphylaxis) after a previous dose of vaccine or to a vaccine component (unless the recipient has been desensitized; see Special Situations section). In addition, severely immunocompromised persons generally should not receive live vaccines. Children who experienced encephalopathy within 7 days after administration of a previous dose of diphtheria and tetanus toxoids and whole-cell pertussis vaccine (DTP), DTaP, or Tdap not attributable to another identifiable cause should not receive additional doses of a vaccine that contain pertussis. Because of the theoretical risk to the fetus, women known to be pregnant generally should not receive live, attenuated virus vaccines.

SUGGESTED READINGS

American Academy of Pediatrics. Committee on Infectious Diseases. Policy statement: recommended childhood and adolescent immunization schedules—United States, 2010. *Pediatrics* 2010;125:195–196.

CDC. Prevention of herpes zoster: recommendations of the Advisory Committee on Immunization Practices. *MMWR Recomm Rep* 2008;57(RR-5):1–30.

CDC. Recommendations from the Advisory Committee on Immunization Practices (ACIP) regarding administration of combination MMRV vaccine. *MMWR Recomm Rep* 2010;59(RR-3):1–12.

CDC. Prevention and control of seasonal influenza with vaccines: recommendations of the Advisory Committee on Immunization Practices (ACIP), 2010. *MMWR Recomm Rep* 2010;59(RR-8):1–62.

This document provided clear recommendations for control of seasonal influenza, including issues such as initial therapy and infection control.

CDC. Recommended immunization schedules for persons aged 0 through 18 years—United States, 2011. *MMWR Morb Mortal Wkly Rep* 2011;60(5):1–4.

CDC. Recommended adult immunization schedule—United States, 2011. *MMWR Morb Mortal Wkly Rep* 2011;60(4):1–4.

This CDC publication outlines the currently recommended immunizations based on a review of the safety and efficacy data. These recommendations frequently change, and the CDC website should be accessed regularly for the most up-to-date recommendations.

CDC vaccine schedule 2012: http://www.cdc.gov/vaccines/recs/schedules/downloads/adult/mmwr-adult-schedule.pdf

Vaccination of Healthcare Personnel

Waseem Ahmad and Paras Patel

- Healthcare personnel (HCP) are defined as all paid and unpaid persons working in healthcare settings who have the potential for exposure to patients and/or to infectious materials, including body substances, contaminated medical supplies and equipment, contaminated environmental surfaces, or contaminated air.
- HCP might include (but are not limited to) physicians, nurses, nursing assistants, therapists, technicians, emergency medical service personnel, dental personnel, pharmacists, laboratory personnel, autopsy personnel, students and trainees, contractual staff not employed by the healthcare facility, and persons (e.g., clerical, dietary, housekeeping, laundry, security, maintenance, administrative, billing, and volunteers) not directly involved in patient care but potentially exposed to infectious agents that can be transmitted to and from HCP and patients.
- Maintenance of immunity is therefore an essential part of prevention and infection control programs for HCP.
- On the basis of documented nosocomial transmission, HCP are considered to be at substantial risk for acquiring or transmitting immunization-preventable diseases, including hepatitis B, influenza, measles, mumps, rubella, pertussis, and varicella.
- See Table 60-1 for current recommendations for vaccination for HCP.

HEPATITIS B

- HCP who perform tasks that may involve exposure to blood or body fluids should receive a three-dose series of hepatitis B vaccine at 0-, 1-, and 6-month intervals.
- Test for hepatitis B surface antibody (anti-HBs) to document immunity 1 to 2 months after dose #3.
- If anti-HBs is at least 10 mIU/mL (positive), the patient is immune. No further serologic testing or vaccination is recommended.
- If anti-HBs is <10 mIU/mL (negative), the patient is unprotected from hepatitis B virus (HBV) infection; revaccinate with a three-dose series. Retest anti-HBs 1 to 2 months after dose #3.
- If anti-HBs is positive, the patient is immune. No further testing or vaccination is recommended.
- If anti-HBs is negative after six doses of vaccine, the HCP is a nonresponder.
- HCP who are nonresponders should be considered susceptible to HBV and should be counseled regarding precautions to prevent HBV infection and the need to obtain HBIG prophylaxis for any known or probable parenteral exposure to hepatitis B surface antigen (HBsAg)-positive blood.
- See Table 60-2 for postexposure prophylaxis for HBV.

Table 60-1	Recommendations for Vaccination of HCP		
Vaccine	**Available Form(s) of Vaccine**	**Dose**	**Recommendation/Comments**
Hepatitis B	Single-antigen vaccine available as Recombivax HB or Engerix-B	Three-dose series at 0, 1, and 6 months	All healthcare workers should receive a three-dose series and obtain anti-HBs titer 1–2 months after third dose.
Influenza	Inactivated trivalent injectable vaccine; live attenuated	One dose annually	All healthcare workers should receive influenza vaccine annually.
MMR	Monovalent vaccine of measles, rubella, and mumps as well as combinations of measles-mumps-rubella (MMR), measles-rubella (MR), and rubella-mumps are available.	Two doses given 4 weeks apart, SC	Two doses of MMR vaccine to unvaccinated healthcare workers born before 1957 who do not have serologic evidence of immunity as well as all adults born after 1956 with no evidence of immunity
Varicella	Available as a single-antigen varicella vaccine and a combination MMR and varicella vaccine	Two doses given 4 weeks apart, SC	Healthcare professionals, teachers, child-care workers, residents and staff in long-term care facilities, nonpregnant women of childbearing age, college students
Td/Tdap	Tdap is available as Boostrix, Adacel	Td every 10 years intramuscularly (IM)	All adults should receive a one-time dose of Tdap and a Td booster every 10 years.
Meningococcal vaccine	MCV4	One dose IM or SC	Microbiologists who are routinely exposed to isolates of *N. meningitidis*

Table 60-2	Postexposure Prophylaxis for HBV		
	Status of Source		**Status of Source Unknown**
Status of Exposed Person	**HbsAg Positive**	**HbsAg Negative**	**High Risk**
No vaccine	HBIG + vaccine	Initiate vaccine series	Initiate vaccine series
Vaccine responder	No treatment	No treatment	No treatment
Vaccine nonresponder	HBIG + vaccine	Vaccine	HBIG + vaccine, no need for revaccination for low-risk exposure
Nonresponder status post revaccination	HBIG × 2	No treatment	HBIG × 2 for high-risk exposure, no treatment for low-risk exposure
Response unknown	If anti-HbsAb negative, give HBIG + vaccine	No treatment	If anti-HBsAb negative, initiate vaccine series and follow up anti-HbsAb

HBIG, hepatitis B immunoglobulin; HbsAg, hepatitis B surface antigen; HbsAb, hepatitis B surface antibody.

INFLUENZA

- All HCP should receive annual vaccination against influenza.
- Live, attenuated influenza vaccine (LAIV) may only be given to nonpregnant, healthy HCP aged 49 years and younger.
- Inactivated, injectable influenza vaccine (TIV) is preferred over LAIV for HCP who are in close contact with severely immunosuppressed persons (e.g., stem cell transplant patients) when patients require protective isolation.

MEASLES, MUMPS, RUBELLA

- HCP who work in medical facilities should be immune to measles, mumps, and rubella (MMR).
- HCP born in 1957 or later can be considered immune to measles, mumps, or rubella only if they have documentation of
  - laboratory confirmation of disease or immunity (HCP who have an "indeterminate" or "equivocal" level of immunity upon testing should be considered nonimmune) or
  - appropriate vaccination against MMR (i.e., two doses of live measles and mumps vaccines given on or after the first birthday, separated by 28 days or more, and at least one dose of live rubella vaccine)

- Although birth before 1957 generally is considered acceptable evidence of MMR immunity, healthcare facilities should consider recommending two doses of MMR vaccine routinely to unvaccinated HCP born before 1957 who do not have laboratory evidence of disease or immunity to measles and/or mumps, and should consider one dose of MMR for HCP with no laboratory evidence of disease or immunity to rubella. For these same HCP who do not have evidence of immunity, healthcare facilities should recommend two doses of MMR vaccine during an outbreak of measles or mumps and one dose during an outbreak of rubella.

VARICELLA

- It is recommended that all HCP be immune to varicella. Evidence of immunity in HCP includes documentation of two doses of varicella vaccine given at least 28 days apart, history of varicella or herpes zoster based on physician diagnosis, laboratory evidence of immunity, or laboratory confirmation of disease.

TETANUS/DIPHTHERIA/PERTUSSIS (TD/TDAP)

- All HCP who have not or are unsure if they have previously received a dose of Tdap should receive a one-time dose of Tdap as soon as feasible, without regard to the interval since the previous dose of Td. Then, they should receive Td boosters every 10 years thereafter.

DISEASES FOR WHICH VACCINATION MIGHT BE INDICATED

MENINGOCOCCUS

- Nosocomial transmission of *Neisseria meningitidis* is rare, but HCP have become infected after direct contact with respiratory secretions of infected persons (e.g., managing of an airway during resuscitation) and in a laboratory setting.
- Vaccination is recommended for microbiologists who are routinely exposed to isolates of *N. meningitidis*.
- Use of MCV4 is preferred for persons aged 55 years or younger; give intramuscularly (IM). Use MPSV4 only if there is a permanent contraindication or precaution to MCV4. Use of MPSV4 (not MCV4) is recommended for HCP older than age 55; give SC.
- Postexposure management of exposed HCP
  - Postexposure prophylaxis is advised for all persons who have had intensive, unprotected contact (i.e., without wearing a mask) with infected patients (e.g., via mouth-to-mouth resuscitation, endotracheal intubation, or endotracheal tube management), including HCP who have been vaccinated with either the conjugate or polysaccharide vaccine.
  - Antimicrobial prophylaxis can eradicate carriage of *N. meningitidis* and prevent infections in persons who have unprotected exposure to patients with meningococcal infections.
  - Rifampin, ciprofloxacin, and ceftriaxone are effective in eradicating nasopharyngeal carriage of *N. meningitidis*.

- In areas of the United States where ciprofloxacin-resistant strains of *N. meningitidis* have been detected (as of August 30, 2011, only parts of Minnesota and North Dakota), ciprofloxacin should not be used for chemoprophylaxis. Azithromycin can be used as an alternative. Ceftriaxone can be used during pregnancy.

TYPHOID FEVER

- Microbiologists and others who work frequently with *S. typhi* should be vaccinated with either of the two licensed and available vaccines. Booster vaccinations should be administered on schedule according to the manufacturers' recommendations.

POLIOMYELITIS

- Vaccination is recommended for HCP who are at greater risk for exposure to polio-viruses than the general population, including laboratory workers who handle specimens that might contain polioviruses and HCP who have close contact with patients who might be excreting wild polioviruses, including HCP who travel to work in areas where polioviruses are circulating.
- Unvaccinated HCP should receive a three-dose series of inactivated polio vaccine (IPV), with dose 2 administered 4 to 8 weeks after dose 1 and dose 3 administered 6 to 12 months after dose 2. HCP who have previously completed a routine series of poliovirus vaccine and who are at increased risk can receive a lifetime booster dose of IPV if they remain at increased risk for exposure. Available data do not indicate the need for more than a single lifetime booster dose with IPV for adults.

TRAVEL VACCINATION

Please refer to the chapter on prophylaxis for infections in travelers.

- Hospital personnel and other HCP who perform research or healthcare work in foreign countries might be at increased risk for acquiring certain diseases that can be prevented by vaccines recommended in the United States (e.g., hepatitis B, influenza, MMR, Tdap, poliovirus, varicella, and meningococcal vaccines) and travel-related vaccines (e.g., hepatitis A, Japanese encephalitis, rabies, typhoid, or yellow fever vaccines).

WORK RESTRICTIONS FOR SUSCEPTIBLE HEALTHCARE PERSONNEL AFTER EXPOSURE TO VACCINE-PREVENTABLE DISEASE

- Postexposure work restrictions ranging from restriction of contact with high-risk patients to complete exclusion from duty appropriate for HCWs who are not immune to certain vaccine-preventable diseases are listed in Table 60-3.

Table 60-3 Work Restrictions for HCP Exposed to or Infected with Certain Vaccine-Preventable Diseases and Conditions

Disease	Status of Health Care Worker	Work Restriction	Duration of Work Furlough
Hepatitis B	Acute or chronic antigenemia	Recommend expert panel consultation for HCP who perform invasive procedures	Per expert panel recommendation
Hepatitis A	Active disease	Avoid patient contact and food handling	7 days after jaundice appears
Influenza/upper respiratory infection	Active disease	Exclude from work	Until symptoms resolve
Measles	Active disease	Exclude from work	7 days after rash appears
	Postexposure	Exclude from work	5th day post first exposure to 21st day post last exposure or 7 days after rash appears
Mumps	Active disease	Exclude from work	9 days after onset of symptoms
	Postexposure	Exclude from work	12th day post first exposure to 26th day post last exposure or 9 days after onset of symptoms
Pertussis	Active disease	Exclude from work	Beginning of catarrhal stage through 3rd week after onset of paroxysms or until 5 days after start of effective antimicrobial therapy
	Postexposure: symptomatic	Exclude from work	5 days after start of effective antimicrobial therapy
	Postexposure:asymptomatic	No restriction	No antimicrobial therapy

(Continued)

Table 60-3 Work Restrictions for HCP Exposed to or Infected with Certain Vaccine-Preventable Diseases and Conditions *(Continued)*

Disease	Status of Health Care Worker	Work Restriction	Duration of Work Furlough
Rubella	Active disease	Exclude from work	5 days after rash appears
	Postexposure susceptible person	Exclude from work	7th day post first exposure to 21st day post last exposure/5 days after rash appears
Varicella	Active disease	Exclude from work	Until all skin lesions are dry and crusted
	Postexposure susceptible person	Exclude from work	10th day post first exposure to 21st day (28th day if VZIG administered) post last exposure
Herpes zoster	Active disease	Cover lesions and avoid care of immunocompromised patients and neonates.	Until all skin lesions are dry and crusted
	Postexposure susceptible person	Avoid contact with patient	10th day post first exposure to 21st day post last exposure

SUGGESTED READINGS

Bolyard EA, Tablan OC, Williams WW, et al. Guideline for infection control in health care personnel, 1998. Hospital Infection Control Practices Advisory Committee. *Infect Control Hosp Epidemiol* 1998;19(6):407–463.

Centers for Disease Control and Prevention (CDC). General recommendations on immunization: recommendations of the Advisory Committee on Immunization Practices (ACIP). *MMWR Morb Recomm Rep* 2011;60(2):1–64.

Centers for Disease Control and Prevention (CDC). Hospital-associated measles outbreak-Pennsylvania, March-April 2009. *MMWR Morb Mortal Wkly Rep* 2012;61(2):30–32.

Henderson DK, Dembry L, Fishman NO, et al. SHEA guideline for management of healthcare workers who are infected with hepatitis B virus, hepatitis C virus, and/or human immuno-deficiency virus. *Infect Control Hosp Epidemiol* 2010;31(3):203–232.
This article discusses the often difficult situations involving HCP who are infected with chronic viruses that are transmissible in the healthcare setting.

Immunization of Health-Care Personnel: recommendations of the Advisory Committee on Immunization Practices (ACIP). *MMWR Recomm Rep* 2011;60(RR-07):1–45.
These guidelines represent the most recent update on preventing infection in HCP.

Immunization of health-care workers: recommendations of the Advisory Committee on Immunization Practices (ACIP) and the Hospital Infection Control Practices Advisory Committee (HICPAC). *MMWR Recomm Rep* 1997;46(RR-18):1–42.

Kretsinger K, Broder KR, Cortese MM, et al.; Centers for Disease Control and Prevention; Advisory Committee on Immunization Practices; Healthcare Infection Control Practices Advisory Committee. Preventing tetanus, diphtheria, and pertussis among adults: use of tetanus toxoid, reduced diphtheria toxoid and acellular pertussis vaccine recommendations of the Advisory Committee on Immunization Practices (ACIP) and recommendation of ACIP, supported by the Healthcare Infection Control Practices Advisory Committee (HICPAC), for use of Tdap among health-care personnel. *MMWR Recomm Rep* 2006;55(RR-17):1–37.

Marin M, Güris D, Chaves SS, et al. Prevention of varicella: recommendations of the Advisory Committee on Immunization Practices (ACIP). *MMWR Recomm Rep* 2007;56 (RR-4):1–40.
This guideline provides specific recommendations on handling the issue of varicella immunity in HCP.

Watson JC, Hadler SC, Dykewicz CA, et al. Measles, mumps, and rubella—vaccine use and strategies for elimination of measles, rubella, and congenital rubella syndrome and control of mumps: recommendations of the Advisory Committee on Immunization Practices (ACIP). *MMWR Recomm Rep* 1998;47(RR-8):1–57.

XVI Bioterrorism

61 Bioterrorism

Anil Mathew and Jonathan P. Moorman

The United States public health system and primary health care providers must be prepared to address various biologic agents, including pathogens that are rarely seen in the United States. High-priority agents (**Category A agents, Table 61-1**) include organisms that pose a risk to national security because they

- Can be easily disseminated or transmitted from person to person
- Result in high mortality rates and have the potential for major public health impact
- Might cause public panic and social disruption
- Require special action for public health preparedness

BOTULISM TOXIN

- Botulinum toxin is the most poisonous substance known. A single gram of crystalline toxin adequately dispersed has the potential to kill more than 1 million people.
- As a bioterrorist attack, botulinum toxin would be dispersed as an aerosol or by contamination of food supply.

Microbiology

- Botulinum toxin is produced by *Clostridium botulinum*, a gram-positive, spore-forming anaerobe.
- The toxin exists in seven distinct antigenic types, designated letters A to G.
- Antitoxin directed against one type will have little activity against the other types (absence of cross neutralization).
- The toxin types can also serve as epidemiologic markers.

Clinical Features

- All forms of botulism result from absorption of botulinum toxin into the circulation from either a mucosal surface (gut, lung) or a wound.
- Once the toxin is absorbed into the bloodstream, it binds irreversibly to neuromuscular junctions at peripheral cholinergic synapses. The toxin enters the cell and enzymatically blocks acetylcholine release.
- Botulism causes an **acute, afebrile, descending flaccid paralysis** that begins in bulbar musculature, initially developing multiple cranial nerve palsies.
- Prominent bulbar palsies result in diplopia, dysarthria, dysphonia, and dysphagia.
- Findings of dry mouth, ptosis, dilated pupils, fatigue, and weakness in extremities, with clear sensorium
- Severe cases may result in generalized weakness and hypotonia requiring intubation and mechanical ventilation.
- Recovery may take weeks to months, requiring regeneration of new motor neuron synapses with the muscle cell.
- Diagnosis is based on clinical suspicion and confirmed by mouse bioassay or toxin immunoassay.

Table 61-1	Category A Agents of Bioterrorism	
Agent	**Signs and Symptoms**	**Treatment**
Anthrax	Fever, headache, muscle aches, which progress to shortness of breath, chest discomfort, shock, and death Chest imaging reveals characteristic findings of mediastinal widening and pleural effusions.	Ciprofloxacin 400 mg IV q12h Or Doxycycline 100 mg IV q12h Plus Clindamycin 900 mg IV q8h and/or Rifampin 300 mg IV q12h Switch to PO when stable and continue treatment for 60 days total.
Botulism	Acute, afebrile, descending flaccid paralysis that begins in bulbar musculature, initially developing multiple cranial nerve palsies Findings of dry mouth, ptosis, dilated pupils, fatigue, weakness in extremities, with clear sensorium Severe cases may result in generalized weakness and hypotonia requiring intubation and mechanical ventilation.	Supportive care, may require intubation, mechanical ventilation, and parenteral nutrition. Equine antitoxin, optimally used as soon as possible after diagnosis, may minimize subsequent nerve injury and severity of disease, but will not reverse existent paralysis.
Plague	Fever, cough, and dyspnea, with rapid progression to severe pneumonia with chest pain and hemoptysis. Gastrointestinal symptoms, including nausea, vomiting, abdominal pain, and diarrhea, may also occur. Chest x-ray findings of pulmonary infiltrates and consolidations, commonly bilateral, would be expected.	Gentamicin 2.0 mg/kg IV loading then 1.7 mg/kg q8h IV Or Streptomycin 1 g q12h IM or IV Alternatives: Doxycycline 100 mg IV or PO b.i.d. Or Chloramphenicol 500 mg IV or PO q.i.d.

Tularemia	Febrile illness with development of pleuritis, pneumonitis, and hilar lymphadenitis. Chest imaging may demonstrate bronchopneumonia, pleural effusions, and hilar lymphadenopathy.	Streptomycin 1 g IM q12h × 10 days Or Gentamicin 5 mg/kg/day IV × 10 days Alternatives: Doxycycline 100 mg IV q12h Or Chloramphenicol 1 g IV q6h Or Ciprofloxacin 400 mg IV q12h May switch to PO when stable. Treat for 14–21 days.
Smallpox	Symptoms most often begin 12–14 days after infection, with high fever, malaise, headache, and backache. A maculopapular rash begins on the face and extremities and spreads to the trunk (centripetal). Lesions are all in the same stage of development. Initially maculopapular, then vesicular, pustules, and scab over on day 8 or 9.	Supportive measures Consider cidofovir, antivaccinia immunoglobulin. Prophylaxis: vaccinia immunization
Viral Hemorrhagic Fevers	Fever, rash, body aches, headaches; later signs of progressive hemorrhagic diathesis develop with petechiae, mucous membrane and conjunctival hemorrhage, hematuria, hematemesis, and melena. Disseminated intravascular coagulation and circulatory shock may follow.	Supportive measures Consider ribavirin and interferon. Yellow fever vaccination

Treatment

- Person-to-person spread of botulism does not occur; no isolation is necessary.
- Supportive care: may require intubation, mechanical ventilation, parenteral nutrition
- Equine antitoxin, optimally used as soon as possible after diagnosis, may minimize subsequent nerve injury and severity of disease, but will not reverse existent paralysis.

ANTHRAX

Microbiology

- *Bacillus anthracis* is a gram-positive, aerobic, nonmotile, spore-forming rod.
- Found in soil and predominantly causes disease in cattle, goats, and sheep.
- Anthrax spores can survive for decades in the environment.

Clinical Features

- Inhalational anthrax
  - Most likely form after bioterrorist aerosol attack with *B. anthracis*.
  - Inhalation of spores into alveolar spaces which are phagocytosed by macrophages. Surviving spores are transported to the mediastinal and peribronchial lymph nodes via lymphatics, where they germinate after a variable duration of time.
  - Replicating bacilli elaborate edema toxin and lethal toxin, which result in edema, hemorrhage, and necrosis.
  - Initial symptoms include fever, headache, and muscle aches, which progress to shortness of breath, chest discomfort, shock, and death. Chest imaging reveals characteristic findings of mediastinal widening and pleural effusions.
- Cutaneous anthrax
  - Initial lesion begins as a papule resulting from introduction of spores through skin, especially through a cut or abrasion. The papule evolves into a painless blister/vesicle, followed by a black eschar often with surrounding edema.
- Gastrointestinal anthrax
  - Rarely seen and unlikely to result from a bioterrorist attack.
  - Typically occurs due to ingestion of contaminated meat. The oropharyngeal form results in an oral or esophageal ulcer with development of regional lymphadenopathy and edema. The intestinal form results in lesions in the terminal ileum or cecum, with symptoms of nausea and vomiting, which may progress to bloody diarrhea, acute abdomen, and shock.
- **Diagnosis** can be confirmed by culture, gram stain, PCR, and/or Wright stain of peripheral smear.

Treatment

- Active disease:
  - No need for special isolation procedures for inhalational anthrax. Patients are not contagious.
  - Ciprofloxacin 400 mg IV q12h
    Or
  - Doxycycline 100 mg IV q12h
    Plus

- Clindamycin 900 mg IV q8h and/or rifampin 300 mg IV q12h
- Switch to PO when stable and continue treatment for 60 days total.
- Postexposure prophylaxis:
  - Ciprofloxacin 500 mg PO b.i.d. × 60 days
    Or
  - Doxycycline 100 mg PO b.i.d. × 60 days
    Or
  - Amoxicillin 500 mg PO q8h (if strain is proved to be susceptible)

PLAGUE

Microbiology

- *Yersinia pestis* is an aerobic, nonmotile, gram-negative bacillus that exhibits bipolar "safety pin" appearance on staining with Wright, Giemsa, and Wayson stains.

Clinical Features

- Primary pneumonic plague is the form likely to occur from a bioterrorist, aerosol attack.
- Following inhalation, symptoms would begin to occur in 1 to 6 days.
- First signs are fever, cough, and dyspnea, with rapid progression to severe pneumonia with chest pain and hemoptysis.
- Gastrointestinal symptoms, including nausea, vomiting, abdominal pain, and diarrhea, may also occur.
- Chest x-ray findings of pulmonary infiltrates and consolidations, commonly bilateral, would be expected.
- Bubonic plague, the form mostly seen currently, is the result of a flea bite. After inoculation into the skin, the bacteria travel through cutaneous lymphatics to regional lymph nodes, where they are phagocytosed but not destroyed. They multiply rapidly, leading to inflammation and painful lymphadenopathy with necrosis, resulting in "buboes," fever, septicemia, and death.
- **Diagnosis** can be confirmed by culture, gram stain, direct fluorescent antibody, and PCR.

Treatment

- Active disease:
  - Preferred:
    - Pneumonic plague patients should be placed on droplet and contact precautions.
    - Gentamicin 2.0 mg/kg IV loading then 1.7 mg/kg q8h IV
      Or
    - Streptomycin 1 g q12h IM or IV
  - Alternatives:
    - Doxycycline 100 mg IV or PO b.i.d.
      Or
    - Chloramphenicol 500 mg IV or PO q.i.d.
- Postexposure prophylaxis:
  - Doxycycline 100 mg PO b.i.d.
    Or
  - Ciprofloxacin 500 mg PO b.i.d.

TULAREMIA

- As a bioterrorist attack, *Francisella tularensis* would be dispersed as an aerosol.

Microbiology

- *F. tularensis* is a nonmotile, aerobic, gram-negative coccobacillus.
- Hardy non–spore-forming organism that can survive for weeks at low temperatures in water, soil, hay, straw, and decaying animal carcasses.
- Considered a lab hazard. Notify lab when submitting suspected specimens.

Clinical Features

- A nonspecific febrile illness beginning 3 to 5 days after inhalation
- Subsequent development of pleuritis, pneumonitis, and hilar lymphadenitis
- Chest imaging may demonstrate bronchopneumonia, pleural effusions, and hilar lymphadenopathy.

Treatment

- Not spread by person to person transmission. No isolation necessary.
  - Preferred:
    - Streptomycin 1 g IM q12h × 10 days
    Or
    - Gentamicin 5 mg/kg/day IV × 10 days
  - Alternatives:
    - Doxycycline 100 mg IV q12h
    Or
    - Chloramphenicol 1 g IV q6h
    Or
    - Ciprofloxacin 400 mg IV q12h
- May switch to PO when stable. Treat for 14 to 21 days.

SMALLPOX

- Smallpox is a highly contagious and deadly disease caused by variola virus.
- As a bioterrorist attack, variola virus would be dispersed as an aerosol.
- Variola virus can spread from person to person.
- No widely available licensed treatment
- High fatality rate (10% to 30% mortality in unimmunized individuals)
- Global population is extremely vulnerable to the disease, since routine smallpox immunization ceased in the United States in 1972 and throughout the world in 1980.

Microbiology

- Smallpox is a double strand DNA virus and a member of the Poxviridae family.

Clinical Features

- Symptoms most often begin 12 to 14 days after infection, with high fever, malaise, headache, and backache.
- A maculopapular rash begins on the face and extremities and spreads to the trunk (centripetal).

- **Lesions are all in the same stage of development**: initially maculopapular, then vesicles, pustules, and scabbing over on day 8 or 9.
- Two highly virulent atypical forms: hemorrhagic and malignant
  - Hemorrhagic form is uniformly fatal, presenting with a severely prostrating illness with high fevers, headache, back pain, and abdominal pain. A dusky erythema develops with petechiae and hemorrhages into the skin and mucous membranes.
  - Malignant form is frequently fatal, with a similar onset to the hemorrhagic form, but with confluent skin lesions (flat), never progressing to the pustular stage.
- Infected persons are considered contagious from the time the rash appears to the time it heals.
- **Diagnosis** is by clinical suspicion of characteristic rash and confirmed by culture, PCR, and electron microscopy.

Treatment

- Suspected smallpox patients should be placed on airborne and contact isolation.
- Supportive measures. Consider cidofovir, antivaccinia immunoglobulin.
- Prophylaxis: vaccinia immunization

VIRAL HEMORRHAGIC FEVERS

- The hemorrhagic fever viruses are organisms capable of causing clinical disease with febrile illness, rash, bleeding diathesis, and shock.
- As a bioterrorist attack, viral hemorrhagic fever (VHF) viruses would be dispersed as an aerosol.

Microbiology

RNA viruses belonging to the following families:

1. Filoviridae: Ebola and Marburg viruses
2. Arenaviridae: Lassa fever and New World Arenaviruses (e.g., Junin, Machupo, Guanarito, and Sabia viruses)
3. Bunyaviridae: Crimean-Congo hemorrhagic fever virus, Rift Valley fever virus, and agents of hemorrhagic fever with renal syndrome
4. Flaviviridae: dengue, yellow fever, Omsk hemorrhagic fever, Kyasanur forest disease

Clinical Features

- Symptoms would likely occur 2 to 21 days after infection, depending on the virus involved.
- Patients may present with fever, rash, body aches, headaches; later signs of progressive hemorrhagic diathesis develop with petechiae, mucous membrane and conjunctival hemorrhage, hematuria, hematemesis, and melena.
- Disseminated intravascular coagulation and circulatory shock may follow.
- Diagnosis may be confirmed by PCR, serologic testing, and virus isolation by CDC.

Treatment

- Suspected VHF patients should be placed on droplet and contact precautions.
- Supportive measures. Consider ribavirin, interferon, and yellow fever vaccination.

Second highest priority agents, or **Category B agents**, include those that

- Are moderately easy to disseminate
- Result in moderate morbidity rates and low mortality rates
- Require specific enhancements of CDC's diagnostic capacity and enhanced disease surveillance

CATEGORY B AGENTS/DISEASES

- Brucellosis (*Brucella* species)
- Epsilon toxin of *Clostridium perfringens*
- Food safety threats (e.g., *Salmonella* species, *Escherichia coli* O157:H7, *Shigella*)
- Glanders (*Burkholderia mallei*)
- Melioidosis (*Burkholderia pseudomallei*)
- Psittacosis (*Chlamydia psittaci*)
- Q fever (*Coxiella burnetii*)
- Ricin toxin from *Ricinus communis* (castor beans)
- Staphylococcal enterotoxin B
- Typhus fever (*Rickettsia prowazekii*)
- Viral encephalitis (alphaviruses [e.g., Venezuelan equine encephalitis, eastern equine encephalitis, western equine encephalitis])
- Water safety threats (e.g., *Vibrio cholerae*, *Cryptosporidium parvum*)

Third highest priority agents, or **Category C agents**, include emerging pathogens that could be engineered for mass dissemination in the future because of

- Availability
- Ease of production and dissemination
- Potential for high morbidity and mortality rates and major health impact

Category C Agents/Diseases
- Emerging infectious diseases such as Nipah virus and Hantavirus

SUGGESTED READINGS

Arnon SS, Schechter R, Inglesby TV, et al.; Working Group on Civilian Biodefense. Botulinum toxin as a biological weapon: medical and public health management. *JAMA* 2001;285(8):1059–1070.
   This article is one of a series of excellent, comprehensive review articles published in JAMA and addressing the issues of the agents of bioterrorism. See the below references for other specific agents.
Borio L, Inglesby T, Peters CJ, et al.; Working Group on Civilian Biodefense. Hemorrhagic fever viruses as biological weapons: medical and public health management. *JAMA* 2002;287(18):2391–2405.
CDC Web site: cdc.gov
Dennis DT, Inglesby TV, Henderson DA, et al.; Working Group on Civilian Biodefense. Tularemia as a biological weapon: medical and public health management. *JAMA* 2001;285(21):2763–2773.
Henderson DA, Inglesby TV, Bartlett JG, et al.; Smallpox as a biological weapon: medical and public health management. Working Group on Civilian Biodefense. *JAMA* 1999;281(22):2127–2137.
Inglesby TV, O'Toole T, Henderson DA, et al.; Working Group on Civilian Biodefense. Anthrax as a biological weapon, 2002: updated recommendations for management. *JAMA* 2002;287(17):2236–2252.
Inglesby TV, Dennis DT, Henderson DA, et al.; Plague as a biological weapon: medical and public health management. Working Group on Civilian Biodefense. *JAMA* 2000;283(17):2281–2290.

XVII Infections in Pregnancy

62 Infections in Pregnancy and the Perinatal Period

Amanda Guedes de Morais and Jonathan P. Moorman

INTRODUCTION

Pregnancy is by no means considered a pathologic state, and throughout history, the ability to conceive has been considered synonymous with good health. However, there are well-described physiologic and hormonal changes that make the gestational and the perinatal periods very unique from the medical standpoint. The goal of this chapter is to concisely review the most important infections that are associated with this period.

VIRAL DISEASES

Genital Herpes Simplex (HSV 1 and HSV2)

- 20% to 30% of women may be infected with herpes simplex virus type 2 (HSV2), the serotype responsible for approximately 85% of cases of genital herpes infections.
- It is estimated that 30 million people are currently infected in the United States.
- Transmission is usually through sexual contact with mucosal membranes or eroded skin.
  - Viral shedding can occur even during the prodromal stage, when the patient has neuralgia/tingling/itching, but the skin lesions are not yet visible.
  - In discordant couples, the only way to prevent disease transmission is wearing condoms consistently.
- Clinical diagnosis is often inaccurate, as the lesions may present atypically. The Tzanck smear showing intranuclear inclusions and multinucleated giant cells has a sensitivity of only 65%. The commercially available serologic assays are not reliable to differentiate the serotypes 1 and 2. Western blot and PCR are more specific techniques, but are not widely distributed.
- Primary genital HSV infection is the development of genital herpes lesions in a patient with no preexisting antibodies to either HSV1 or HSV2. If a patient develops compatible lesions for the first time, but is known to have positive herpes serology (latent disease), the appropriate term to be used is first-episode, nonprimary infection. Recurrent episodes can be painless and therefore go unnoticed.
- Pregnant women are at increased risk of acquiring HSV due to hormonal changes. They can present with a more severe course of a primary HSV infection than nonpregnant females, including development of disseminated disease, with meningitis or hepatitis. If the infection is acquired in the first trimester, there is an increased risk of spontaneous abortion, but no embryopathy has been described. When acquired in the second/third trimesters, infection has been associated with preterm labor, intrauterine growth restriction (IUGR) and neonatal infection.

- This risk of transmission to the infant during vaginal delivery is variable.
  - If the mother has a symptomatic first episode lesion (primary or nonprimary), it is approximately 50%.
  - If the first episode is asymptomatic, the risk drops to 33%.
  - If there is fetal exposure to a recurrent lesion, the risk falls to 4%.
  - If there are no identifiable lesions or symptoms, the risk is as low as 0.04%.
  - **Currently, abdominal delivery is recommended by the American College of Obstetrics and Gynecology (ACOG) in the setting of any active genital lesion or reported prodromal symptoms**.
- Neonatal herpes presents as disseminated disease in 20% of the newborns, which carries a 50% mortality rate. The disease is limited to the central nervous system (CNS) in 35% of the cases and is limited to skin and mucous membranes in 45%. The latter carries the best prognosis, with 100% survival and 5% sequelae.
- Antiviral management is indicated for females with more than six recurrences per year and for females whose initial herpes diagnosis happened during pregnancy. The drug of choice is still acyclovir 400 mg orally three times daily. There are currently no vaccines approved for prevention of HSV infections.

Varicella (Varicella-Zoster Virus)

- **Varicella-zoster virus** (VZV) is a DNA virus from the herpes family; primary infection presents as a diffuse exanthema termed varicella or chickenpox. After rash resolution, VZV remains latent in the sensory ganglia and can secondarily reactivate, usually following a dermatomal pattern and termed herpes zoster or shingles.
- This virus is highly contagious through contact with skin lesions and respiratory droplets.
  - The incubation period is 10 to 21 days.
    The prodomes are fever, headache, and malaise followed by a widespread typical rash (macules→ papules → vesicles → crusts). The rash occurs in waves, with skin lesions in different stages at a given time, or "lesion polymorphism."
    The disease lasts 6 to 10 days, but the contagious period starts 2 days before the first skin lesion appears till complete crusting of all lesions.
  - The diagnosis is clinical, based on the characteristic skin lesions. All primary infections are thought to confer immunity.
- Varicella in pregnancy is relatively rare in the United States, (~5 cases/10,000 gestations), but the complications can be devastating, including maternal pneumonia, disseminated disease, fetal malformations, and neonatal infection.
    In case of exposure, pregnant females without a positive history of chickenpox should be tested for antibody detection. Most patients will have a positive antibody, but if the result is negative or no antibody test is available, it is recommended to administer varicella-zoster immunoglobulin (VZIG) within 96 hours of exposure. The dose is 125 U (1 vial) per 10 kg, with a maximum of 625 U administered.
- If a pregnant woman is diagnosed with varicella, she should be isolated from other potentially nonimmune persons. The live attenuated varicella vaccine is not recommended in pregnancy.
- If there is development of pneumonia symptoms and signs (tachydyspnea, cough, hemoptysis, cyanosis, chest pain, chest x-ray with classical bilateral nodular infiltrates) or the skin lesions are not appropriately crusting, hospitalization is recommended to start antiviral therapy with acyclovir 7.5 mg/kg intravenously every 8 hours.

- Even in the setting of appropriated therapy, up to 40% of the patients with varicella pneumonia may progress to respiratory failure requiring ventilator support.
- Congenital varicella presents with CNS lesions, limb hypoplasia, joint contractures, skin scarring, hypopigmented lesions, and other miscellaneous changes. The contamination is transplacental. If the mother develops the rash within 5 days before delivery up to 2 days after, there is increased likelihood of transmission due to a lack of maternal IgG production. All neonates delivered within this period should receive VZIG 125 U as an attempt to prevent the disease.
- There are no reports of congenital varicella in the setting of maternal herpes zoster. If the eruption does not involve the breast, breast-feeding is considered safe.

Cytomegalovirus

- Cytomegalovirus (CMV) is a DNA virus in the herpes family. It has the ability to remain latent after the primary infection, which allows it to be endemic.
- 50% of the pregnant females are seropositive for CMV antibodies and maternal immunity does not protect against recurrences or transmission to the fetus.
- CMV is the most common cause of congenital viral infection in the United States, affecting 40,000 infants per year.
- Transmission among adults happens in the setting of close contact. Fetal transmission is thought to be transplacental, but it can also be acquired during breast-feeding.
- The risk of transmission to the fetus is higher if the mother acquires the primary infection during pregnancy (~30% to 40%)
  - If the mother experiences a reactivation, the risk of transmission drops to 0.2% to 1.8%.
  - Due to high prevalence, most neonatal infections are acquired during reactivation; however, the ones secondary to primary infection are more severe.
- Only 10% of the infected neonates are symptomatic at birth.
  - Present with microcephaly, ventriculomegaly, periventricular calcifications, pneumonia, hepatosplenomegaly, high bilirubin, retinitis, and IUGR
  - Mortality rate is high among symptomatic newborns, reaching 20% to 30%, and the ones who survive usually have CNS sequelae.
- Diagnosis in an immunocompetent adult is difficult, as most patients are asymptomatic.
  - May present as a mononucleosis-like syndrome (fever, myalgias, arthralgias, and enlarged lymph nodes) or rarely as a more disseminated disease
  - Diagnosis is confirmed by serology, usually ELISA, with specimens collected 4 weeks apart to detect an IgG rise.
  - IgM titer can also be checked, but it can persist for up to 18 months, and it is not as specific, with 20% of the primary infections negative for IgM to CMV.
  - The use of PCR to detect the viral DNA has become more available and is a very reliable diagnostic tool.
  - Viral cultures have been used in the past but demand too much time and trained personnel.
- Currently, there is no well-studied, effective treatment for CMV during pregnancy. Also, there is no way to predict the clinical severity of the neonatal disease. Elective abortions are not recommended, even in the case of proven maternal primary infection. It is not recommended to routinely screen the pregnant population to CMV immunity. Women of childbearing age should be educated about CMV infection and contact hygiene precautions, particularly if there is exposure to immunocompromised hosts or young children.

Parvovirus B19

Parvoviruses are the smallest DNA virus that can affect mammals.

- It is a causative organism for aplastic crisis in sickle cell patients, and it is linked to erythema infectiosum or fifth disease in children.
- Parvovirus infection in the pregnant population has been associated with nonimmune hydrops fetalis and fetal death.
- It is a common childhood infection, which confers immunity. As opposed to the herpes family viruses, there are no reports of recurrence.
- It is very contagious, spreads by respiratory and mouth secretions contact. Infected blood products can also be a source. It is more prevalent in spring months (March to May), and epidemics occur cyclically every 4 to 5 years.
- The symptoms of erythema infectiosum are usually mild, including fever, headache, coryza, nausea, and diarrhea, followed by the classic "slapped cheek rash" in 2 to 5 days. A maculopapular body rash may then appear.
- Adult females may present with severe polyarthropathy that can last for months.
  - Acute anemia is not uncommon, although rarely symptomatic, unless there is an underlying hemoglobinopathy. In those cases, a transient aplastic crisis may occur.
  - If infection occurs during pregnancy, asymptomatic transmission to the fetus happens in 1/4 to 1/3 of the cases. On follow-up, most of these infants did well, with no associated sequelae. Up to 5% of fetuses may develop a transient aplastic crisis, which can be severe given their shortened fetal red blood cell life span and accelerated red blood cell production. They become severely anemic, develop a high output heart failure, hydrops, and possibly death. Second trimester pregnancies are particularly vulnerable.
- If a gravida is exposed to a patient with parvovirus infection, she should have her IgM and IgG antibody titers checked.
  - If both are positive, this indicates that exposure was over the past 6 months.
  - If IgG is positive and IgM is negative, this female is previously immune.
  - If both antibody subclasses are negative, this patient is at risk, and a repeat IgM titer should be drawn in 3 to 4 weeks to detect acute infection.
  - PCR may be useful in immunocompromised patients who cannot mount an antibody response or in the fetal blood.
  - An elevation of the maternal serum alphafetoprotein may be a diagnostic clue to anticipate development of fetal hydrops.
- Once a gestational infection is confirmed, serial weekly obstetric ultrasounds should be done for 8 weeks to look for early signs of hydrops: If no signs of hydrops, the pregnancy should be uneventful. If it develops, intrauterine blood transfusion through cordocentesis and IVIG may be indicated.
- During epidemics, it may be appropriate to screen females of childbearing age who work with small children and possibly relocate the seronegative gravid women, but otherwise, there is no role for universal female screening.
- There are currently no vaccines to prevent parvovirus infections. Avoidance of contact with small children if at all possible remains the best prevention strategy.

German Measles (Rubella)

- Rubella virus is a unique virus from the Togavirus family. It is the only one transmitted via the respiratory route and causes rubella or German measles. It is highly contagious, but the incidence of rubella in North America has decreased markedly since the introduction of routine childhood rubella vaccination.

- In the absence of pregnancy, it is usually a mild, self-limited infection of childhood. However, during pregnancy, the virus can have devastating effects on the developing fetus, being directly responsible for congenital malformations.
- The incubation period for rubella is 12 to 23 days. The infectious period is from 7 days before to 5 to 7 days after rash onset.
  - Asymptomatic in 25% to 50% of cases, but some patients may have mild prodromal symptoms such as low-grade fever, conjunctivitis, sore throat, coryza, headaches, malaise, and tender lymphadenopathy.
  - The typical scarlatiniform rash is mildly pruritic and usually starts on the face and spreads to trunk and extremities, following 1 to 5 days after the prodrome.
  - Resolves within 3 days in the same order in which it appeared
  - Polyarthritis and polyarthralgia are potential sequelae, developing mostly in adolescent and adult women (60% to 70%) about 1 week after the rash, and may last for 4 weeks.
  - Other rare manifestations are tenosynovitis, carpal tunnel syndrome, thrombocytopenia, postinfectious encephalitis, myocarditis, hepatitis, hemolytic anemia, and hemolytic uremic syndrome.
- Congenital rubella syndrome (CRS) is fetal infection acquired hematogenously, and the rate of transmission varies with the gestational age at which maternal infection occurs.
  - If the exposure happens in the first trimester, fetal infection rates are near 80%, but only 25% in the late second trimester and varies from 35% at 27 to 30 weeks' gestation to nearly 100% beyond 36 weeks' gestation.
  - The risk of congenital defects is primarily limited to exposure in the first 16 weeks. After the first 20 weeks, the fetus can present with IUGR.
- After infecting the placenta, the rubella virus spreads through the vascular system of the developing fetus, causing cytopathic damage to blood vessels and ischemia in developing organs.
  - The most common congenital defects associated with rubella are audiologic anomalies including deafness, cardiac defects (pulmonary stenosis, patent ductus arteriosus, ventricular septal defect), ophthalmic defects (retinopathy, cataracts, microphthalmia, glaucoma), and CNS defects (mental retardation, microcephaly, meningoencephalitis).
  - Later, the child may develop diabetes mellitus, thyroiditis, growth hormone deficit, and behavioral problems.
- If a pregnant woman develops signs or symptoms of a rubella-like illness or has recently been exposed to rubella, gestational age should be determined as well as her state of immunity.
  1. Known immune >12 weeks of gestation: no further testing is necessary. CRS has not been reported after maternal reinfection beyond 12 weeks' gestation.
  2. Known immune <12 weeks of gestation: if these women demonstrate a significant rise in rubella IgG antibody titer without detection of IgM antibody, they should be informed that reinfection is likely to have occurred. Fetal risk for congenital infection after maternal reinfection during the first trimester has been estimated at 8%. Appropriate counseling should be provided.
  3. Nonimmune or immunity unknown:
     a. Gestational age ≤16 weeks: acute and convalescent IgG and IgM should be obtained. If IgM antibodies are positive or if there is significant increase in IgG titers 2 to 4 weeks apart, it indicates rubella infection and counseling should be provided.

b. Gestational age between 16 and 20 weeks: CRS between 16 and 20 weeks' gestation are rare (<1%) and may be manifested by sensorineural deafness (often severe) in the newborn. Appropriate counseling is indicated.

c. Gestational age ≥20 weeks: no studies have documented CRS after 20 weeks. Reassurance is recommended.

- Currently, there is no effective treatment for rubella. The Centers for Disease Control recommend limiting the use of rubella immunoglobulin to women with known rubella exposure who decline pregnancy termination.
- Prevention through vaccination remains the key to avoid CRS.

The recommendations of the Society of Obstetricians and Gynaecologists of Canada (SOGC) Clinical Guidelines on rubella and pregnancy from 2008 are summarized below:

1. Since the effects of CRS vary with the gestational age at the time of infection, accurate gestational dating should be established, as it is critical to counseling.
2. The diagnosis of primary maternal infection should be made by serologic testing.
3. In a pregnant woman who is exposed to rubella or who develops signs or symptoms of rubella, serologic testing should be performed to determine immune status and risk of congenital rubella syndrome.
4. Rubella immunization should not be administered in pregnancy but may be safely given postpartum.
5. Women who have been inadvertently vaccinated in early pregnancy or who become pregnant immediately following vaccination can be reassured that there have been no cases of CRS documented in these situations.
6. Women wishing to conceive should be counseled and encouraged to have their antibody status determined and undergo rubella vaccination if needed.

AIDS: Adult Immunodeficiency Syndrome (Human Immunodeficiency Virus: HIV)

- HIVs 1 and 2 are members of the lentivirus subfamily of Retroviridae group, which is characterized by the presence of a RNA-dependent DNA polymerase or reverse transcriptase enzyme to direct viral DNA synthesis after infecting a host cell. This ability allows the virus to cause disease by inserting genomes on the host cell that can induce malignant transformation and/or creating an immunodeficiency state that ultimately leads to opportunistic infections and neoplasms.
- According to CDC's data, at the end of 2008, an estimated 1,178,350 persons aged 13 and older were living with HIV infection in the United States. Of those, 20% had undiagnosed HIV infections.
- In 2009, there were an estimated 48,100 new HIV infections in the United States, and 11,200 of those infections were among women. That year, women comprised 51% of the US population and 23% of those newly infected with HIV. 57% occurred in blacks, 21% were in whites, and 16% were in Hispanics/Latinas. This raises our awareness to the increasing risk of pregnancy- and perinatal-related HIV.
- Females can transmit HIV to the fetus during pregnancy through the placenta, via direct blood contact during delivery or through breast milk. Nearly all AIDS cases in US children are secondary to maternal exposure, so it is **recommended to screen all pregnant females to HIV in the very first obstetric visit**. Retesting in the third trimester (preferably before 36 weeks' gestation) is recommended for women at high risk for acquiring HIV infection (e.g., women who use illicit drugs, have sexually transmitted diseases (STDs) during pregnancy, have multiple sex partners during pregnancy, live in areas with high HIV prevalence, or have HIV-infected partners).

- If not treated, about 25% of pregnant women with HIV will transmit the virus to their babies. This transmission rate can be reduced to <2% if the mother receives appropriated antiretroviral (ARV) treatment during pregnancy and delivery.
- Regardless of plasma HIV RNA copy number or CD4 cell count, all pregnant HIV-infected women should receive a combination antepartum ARV drug regimen to prevent perinatal transmission. A combination regimen is recommended both for women who require therapy for their own health and for prevention of perinatal transmission in those who would not yet require therapy.
- ARV drug-resistance studies should be performed before starting ARV drugs, with the exceptional cases when HIV is diagnosed late in pregnancy and ARV should be initiated pending results of resistance testing.
- The current NIH guidelines from September 2011 provide "Recommendations for Use of Antiretroviral Drugs in Pregnant HIV-1-Infected Women for Maternal Health and Interventions to Reduce Perinatal HIV Transmission in the United States."
  - There are several combination regimens available. Nucleoside reverse transcriptase inhibitors (NRTIs) are recommended for use as a backbone of combination regimens, usually including two NRTIs with either a non–nucleoside reverse transcriptase inhibitor (NNRTI) or one or more protease inhibitor (PI).
  - Lamivudine (3TC) has been used extensively in pregnancy in combination with zidovudine (ZDV), and this is the recommended dual-NRTI backbone for pregnant women.
  - Abacavir (ABC) is an alternative NRTI for dual-NRTI backbone of combination regimens or can be used with ZDV and 3TC as triple-NRTI regimen.
  - Emtricitabine (FTC) and tenofovir (TDF) are alternative NRTIs for dual-NRTI backbone of combination regimens. TDF would be a preferred NRTI in combination with 3TC or FTC in women with chronic HBV infection. Because of potential for renal toxicity with TDV, renal function should be monitored.
  - Stavudine (d4T) and didanosine (ddI) are also alternative NRTIs for dual-NRTI backbone of combination regimens. However, ddI should never be used with d4T as there is increased risk of lactic acidosis.
  - The preferred NNRTI is nevirapine (NVP). However, it should only be initiated in pregnant women with CD4 counts >250 cells/mm^3 if the benefits clearly outweigh risk because of the increased risk of potentially life-threatening hepatotoxicity in women with high CD4 cell counts. Women who enter pregnancy on NVP regimens and are tolerating them well may continue therapy, regardless of CD4 count.
  - **Efavirenz (EFV) is a FDA pregnancy category class D**, as it was associated with malformations (anencephaly, anophthalmia, cleft palate) in monkeys and humans. Use of EFV should be avoided in the first trimester. After the first trimester, it can be considered if this is the best/only choice for a specific woman. If EFV is to be continued postpartum, adequate contraception must be assured as it decreases oral contraceptive blood levels.
  - There is insufficient date to recommend use of rilpivirine (RPV) or etravirine (ETR).
  - Lopinavir + ritonavir (LPV/r) is the preferred PI combo to be used in combination regimens with two NRTI drugs. PK studies suggest that the dose should be increased to 600 mg/150 mg b.i.d. during the second and third trimester, especially in PI-experienced patients, to keep appropriated levels. Once-daily LPV/r dosing is not recommended during pregnancy.

- Atazanavir + ritonavir (ATV/r) and saquinavir + ritonavir (SQV/r) are alternative regimens to be used with in combination regimens with two NRTI drugs. There is no need for dose adjustment with ATV/r, but SQV/r requires a twice-daily dose, and unboosted SQV is not recommended.
- Indinavir (IDV) should only be used when preferred and alternative agents cannot be used. Also, during pregnancy, it has to be used in combination with low-dose ritonavir. Nelfinavir (NFV) has been extensively used in pregnancy. It can be considered in special circumstances for prophylaxis of transmission in women in whom therapy would not otherwise be indicated, when alternative agents are not tolerated due to proven lower viral response when compared to LPV/r- or EFV-based regimens.
- There are insufficient data to recommend use of darunavir (DRV), fosamprenavir (FPV), and tipranavir (TPV).
- There is also lack of data regarding the use of other ARV classes during pregnancy, as the integrase inhibitor raltegravir (RAL) and the entry inhibitors enfuvirtide (T20) or maraviroc (MVC).
- Counseling during pregnancy is extremely important and should emphasize the importance of adherence to the ARV drug regimen. A multidisciplinary approach with health services, social support, mental health services, and drug abuse treatment may be necessary. Good communication between HIV specialists and obstetrical providers is imperative. HIV-related questions during pregnancy can be addressed by the "National Perinatal HIV Hotline" (1-888-448-8765). This is a federally funded service providing free clinical consultation to providers caring for HIV-infected women and their infants.

Recommendations regarding mode of delivery:

- Abdominal delivery or C-section is recommended to prevent perinatal transmission for women with HIV RNA >1,000 copies/mL or unknown near the time of delivery, regardless of administration of antepartum ARV.
- In women receiving ARV and HIV RNA <1,000 copies, the decision about the mode of delivery should be individualized. There are insufficient studies to evaluate the benefits of scheduled C-section in this group. The risks of this surgical procedure and the possible benefits to the neonate need to be weighted.
- After rupture of the membranes, it is unclear if C-section is of any benefit in preventing HIV transmission.

Special Considerations for HIV-2 Infection During Pregnancy

- HIV-2 infection should be suspected in pregnant women who are from—or have partners from—countries in which the disease is endemic (Angola; Mozambique; Cape Verde, Ivory Coast, Gambia, Guinea-Bissau, Mali, Mauritania, Nigeria, Sierra Leone, Benin, Burkina Faso, Ghana, Guinea, Liberia, Niger, Nigeria, Sao Tome, Senegal, and Togo; and in parts of India) and in patients who are HIV antibody positive on an initial enzyme-linked immunoassay screening test, and who have repeatedly indeterminate results on HIV-1 Western blot and an HIV-1 RNA viral load at or below the limit of detection.
  - NNRTIs and enfurvitide are not active against HIV 2; therefore, they should not be used for treatment or prophylaxis for this infection.
  - If the pregnant woman requires HIV-2 treatment for their own health because they have significant clinical disease or CD4 counts <500 cells/mm^3, it is recommended to use a regimen with two NRTIs and a boosted PI.
  - If CD4 counts ≥500 cells/mm^3 and the patient has no significant clinical disease, experts recommended the following prophylactic regimens:

○ A boosted PI-based regimen (two NRTIs plus lopinavir/ritonavir) for prophylaxis, with the drugs stopped postpartum

○ ZDV Prophylaxis alone during pregnancy and intrapartum

- All infants born to HIV-2–infected mothers should receive the standard 6-week ZDV prophylactic regimen (BIII).

- In the United States, breast-feeding is not recommended for infants of HIV-2–infected mothers.

BACTERIAL DISEASES

- During pregnancy, the fetus is physically protected against bacterial infections by the chorioamniotic membranes and the placenta. The amniotic fluid itself has anti-bacterial properties. Some bacteria, however, have the ability to bypass these barriers and infect the fetus transplacentally, such as *Listeria monocytogenes* and *Treponema pallidum*. Others will affect the newborn shortly after delivery.

- Neonatal sepsis can be divided in early-onset (infection that happens within the first 7 days of life) and late-onset (infection that manifests in between the 7th day and the 28th day of life).

- The most common bacteria associated with neonatal sepsis are Group B *Streptococcus* (GBS), *Escherichia coli*, *L. monocytogenes*, *Enterococcus*, and group A *Streptococcus*. This chapter will focus on the first three ones.

Group B *Streptococcus* (*Streptococcus agalactiae*)

- GBS is a gram-positive bacteria that causes invasive disease primarily in infants, pregnant or postpartum women, and older adults, with the highest incidence among young infants.

- GBS can be classified based on specific polysaccharides, and the serotypes I to VI are known to cause human disease, being the serotype III found in 85% of the cases of neonatal infections.

- 20% to 25% of pregnant women are colonized with GBS on the lower vaginal/anorectal area.

- About 50% of infants of women colonized with GBS will become colonized themselves, before, during, or after birth. However, only 1% to 2% of infants born to colonized women will develop early disease.

- The well-known risk factors for GBS infections are gestational age <37 completed weeks, longer duration of membrane rupture (>18 hours), peripartum fever, intra-amniotic infection, young maternal age, black race, and low maternal levels of GBS-specific anticapsular antibody. Previous delivery of an infant with invasive GBS disease is a risk factor for early-onset disease in subsequent deliveries. GBS bacteriuria is a marker for heavy genital tract colonization and is associated with higher rates of infant colonization and infection as well.

- Early-onset GBS disease usually develops in the first 24 to 48 hours of life, more commonly during the first 8 hours. The classic clinical manifestations are pneumonia, septicemia without a focus, and meningitis. It can deteriorate rapidly and progress to respiratory failure and shock in hours.

- Identification of the pregnant females who are colonized with GBS is crucial to prevent neonatal colonization and early infection.

The MMWR "Prevention of Perinatal Group B Streptococcal Disease Revised Guidelines from CDC, 2010" recommends for all pregnant woman to be screened for group B strep with a vaginal/rectal swab culture at 35 to 37 weeks of pregnancy. Prevention of GBS disease can be done in two ways:

- Antibiotic prophylaxis: Penicillin is the drug of choice, ampicillin is a reasonable alternative. Women with history of nonanaphylactic penicillin allergy should receive cefazolin instead. Due to a recent increase in GBS resistance to clindamycin, this drug should be reserved for situations when the susceptibility panel is available.
- Pregnant women with GBS bacteriuria at any time on current pregnancy or history of previous infant with invasive GBS disease should receive antibiotic prophylaxis and do not need third trimester screening for GBS colonization.
- At the time of labor or rupture of membranes, intrapartum antibiotic prophylaxis should be given to all pregnant women who tested positive for GBS colonization, except in the instance of cesarean delivery performed before onset of labor on a woman with intact amniotic membranes.
- For circumstances in which screening results are not available at the time of labor and delivery, intrapartum antibiotic prophylaxis should be given to women who are <37 weeks and 0 days' gestation, have a duration of membrane rupture ≥18 hours, or have a temperature of ≥100.4°F (≥38.0°C).
- In the absence of GBS urinary tract infection, antimicrobial agents should not be used before the intrapartum period to eradicate GBS genitorectal colonization, because such treatment is not effective in eliminating carriage or preventing neonatal disease and can cause adverse consequences.
- The use of perioperative prophylactic antibiotics to prevent infectious complications of cesarean delivery should not be altered or affected by GBS status. Women expected to undergo cesarean deliveries should undergo routine vaginal and rectal screening for GBS at 35 to 37 weeks' gestation because onset of labor or rupture of membranes can occur before the planned cesarean delivery, and under those circumstances, GBS-colonized women should receive intrapartum antibiotic prophylaxis.
- Healthcare providers should inform women of their GBS screening test result and the recommended interventions.
- Immunoprophylaxis: One study showed that 57% of immunized pregnant females at 31 weeks' gestation with a type III polysaccharide group B streptococcus vaccine mounted an antibody response and passed that on to their infants. Nevertheless, polysaccharides alone are poorly immunogenic, and further studies are needed.

Escherichia coli

- *E. coli* is the most common type of gram-negative bacteria that cause sepsis in newborn infants. Sources for newborn colonization are either direct contact with the maternal genital tract or nosocomial spread through nurse personnel.
- The only specific risk factor for development of *E. coli* identified so far is prematurity.
- The capsular subtype K1 is present in 40% of the cases, which may be explained by the fact that it is poorly immunogenic, and so there is little, if any, maternal antibody production to be passively transmitted to the newborn.
- Antibiotic treatment can be guided by the antibiogram, but most *E. coli* are susceptible to penicillins and cephalosporins. Some prevention can be achieved by following standards of hand hygiene in the neonatal unit.

Listeria monocytogenes

- *L. monocytogenes* is a gram-positive rod usually found in sheep and cattle, but rarely pathogenic to humans, except for pregnant females, newborns, and immunocompromised hosts. This infection is foodborne, associated with intake of contaminated undercooked meat or unpasteurized cheese.
- Certain serotypes (1/2a, 1/2b, 1/2c, and 4b) are associated with most human diseases and have caused several outbreaks, which are usually manifested as a self-limiting gastroenteritis in immunocompetent host.
- In pregnant females, this infection manifests initially as flu-like symptoms, but within days it affects the fetoplacental unit and results in a high incidence of premature deliveries and stillbirths.
- In the newborn population, it can present as early-onset sepsis (first 7 days) with amniotic fluid stained with meconium, pneumonia, hepatosplenomegaly, thrombocytopenia, and skin rash or late-onset listeriosis (after the first 7 days), with more of a meningitis type of picture. The mortality rate in neonates can be up to 15%.
- The antibiotic of choice for treatment of listeriosis is ampicillin, usually associated with gentamicin for synergism, but sulfatrimethoprim is an alternative for penicillin allergic patients.
- This potentially fatal infection can be prevented with simple measures, as thoroughly cooking animal source food and washing raw vegetables before eating; avoiding unpasteurized milk and food from unpasteurized milk; washing hands, utensils, and cutting boards used with uncooked food; and keeping ready-to-eat food cold. Pregnant females are advised to avoid consuming soft, unpasteurized cheeses.

Treponema pallidum (Syphilis)

- Syphilis is a STD caused by the spirochete *T. pallidum*, but it can also be acquired through nonsexual personal contact; transplacentally, contaminated blood transfusion; and organ transplantation.
- The prevalence of this disease has declined significantly after the advent of penicillin, but since 1997, there have been an increased number of new reported cases in the United States, primarily among MSM.
- The disease is characterized by alternating periods of relapse and latency. Following an average incubation period of 21 days, a painless lesion appears at the inoculation site—the chancre—characterizing primary syphilis. It will spontaneously heal in 4 to 6 weeks. Secondary syphilis consists in the generalized parenchymal, constitutional, mucosal, and skin lesions that appear after 6 to 8 weeks after the chancre resolves. If this constellation of symptoms goes undiagnosed, the patient becomes asymptomatic in 2 to 6 weeks and enters the latent stage. The latter can last for many years and about a third of the infected patients will actually develop clinically significant tertiary lesions as gummas (granuloma formations), cardiovascular changes as aortic aneurysm, and neurosyphilis.
- Congenital syphilis is a major concern due to the possible devastating fetal outcomes. If maternal syphilis is not treated, there may be a rate of fetal loss of 40% (including stillbirths and abortions).
  - Few infants are born with fulminant congenital syphilis, which carries a poor prognosis, but most infected infants will appear healthy at birth and progressively develop symptoms.
  - The early manifestations appear during the first 2 years and resemble secondary syphilis systemic manifestations as rhinitis, mucocutaneous disease, bone changes,

hepatosplenomegaly, jaundice, lymphadenopathy, bone marrow changes, and CNS manifestations.

- Late symptoms appear after 2 years and are usually subclinical (cardiovascular, neurologic, deafness, arthropathies, periostitis). The classic stigmata as Hutchinson teeth, saddle nose, and saber shins are uncommon.
- Screening of all pregnant women for syphilis is recommended at the first prenatal visit. Women who are at higher risk, live in areas of high syphilis morbidity, or are previously untested should be screened again at 28 weeks' gestation and at delivery. Infants should not be discharged from the hospital unless the syphilis serologic status of the mother has been determined at least one time during pregnancy and preferably again at delivery. Any woman who delivers a stillborn infant should be tested for syphilis.
- All pregnant women who have syphilis should be also tested for HIV infection.
- According to CDC 2006 guidelines, **penicillin is the only approved treatment for syphilis in pregnancy**. If the patient has a penicillin allergy, desensitization is recommended. After treatment completion, a quantitative nontreponemal test should be repeated monthly, and if there is not a fourfold decrease over 3 months, the patient should be retreated. Appropriate maternal treatment before 16 weeks should prevent all fetal damage and completion of the treatment before the third trimester should adequately treat the infected fetus.
- The diagnosis of congenital syphilis is complicated by the transplacental transfer of maternal nontreponemal and treponemal IgG antibodies to the fetus. This transfer of antibodies makes the interpretation of reactive serologic tests for syphilis in infants difficult. The decision to treat an infant is based on the following aspects:
  1. Diagnosis of syphilis in the mother
  2. Adequacy of maternal treatment
  3. Presence of clinical, laboratory, or radiographic evidence of syphilis in the infant
  4. Comparison of maternal (at delivery) and infant nontreponemal serologic titers by using the same test and preferably the same laboratory
- All infants born to mothers who have reactive nontreponemal and treponemal test results should be evaluated with a quantitative nontreponemal serologic test (RPR or VDRL) performed on infant serum because umbilical cord blood can become contaminated with maternal blood and could yield a false-positive result. Conducting a treponemal test (i.e., TP-PA or FTA-ABS) on a newborn's serum is not necessary. No commercially available immunoglobulin (IgM) test can be recommended.
- All infants born to women who have reactive serologic tests for syphilis should be carefully examined for signs of congenital syphilis. Pathologic examination of the placenta or umbilical cord by using specific fluorescent antitreponemal antibody staining is suggested. Dark field microscopic examination or DFA staining of suspicious lesions or body fluids (e.g., nasal discharge) also should be performed.
- Penicillin is also the drug of choice to treat congenital syphilis and the recommendations to treat an infant at birth are the following:
  1. Unknown serologic status of the mother
  2. Mother has received inappropriate nonpenicillin treatment
  3. Mother has received penicillin treatment on the third trimester
  4. Infant may be difficult to follow

If there is a suspicion for congenital syphilis, the infant's CSF should be evaluated before treatment to obtain baseline values.

- The recommended regimens and dosing are variable according to the infant's risk factors, serologic tests, and changes on physical exam and may be obtained at the CDC's website: www.cdc.gov.

Protozoa

Toxoplasma gondii (T. gondii): Toxoplasmosis

- Toxoplasmosis is considered one of the neglected parasitic infections. According to the CDC, more than 60 million men, women, and children in the United States have been contaminated, but most commonly, the immunocompromised hosts are the only individuals who actually develop symptoms. Of particular concern is the possibility of maternal-fetal transmission, because of the potentially serious consequences to the fetus.
- *T. gondii* is a parasite that can infect most mammals, but its definite host is the feline. The life cycle starts with shedding of unsporulated oocysts from acutely infected cat's feces. Oocysts take 1 to 5 days to sporulate in the environment and become infective. Intermediate hosts in nature (including birds and rodents) become infected after ingesting soil, water, or plant material contaminated with oocysts. They transform into tachyzoites shortly after ingestion, which will localize in neural and muscle tissue and develop into tissue cyst bradyzoites. Animals bred for human consumption as lamb or pigs may become infected after ingestion of sporulated oocysts in the environment. Cats can become infected by ingestion of tissue cysts from other mammals or oocysts from the environment. Humans can become infected by any of several routes:
  - Eating undercooked meat of animals harboring tissue cysts
  - Consuming food or water contaminated with cat feces or by contaminated environmental samples (such as fecal-contaminated soil or changing the litter box of a pet cat)
  - Blood transfusion or organ transplantation
  - Transplacentally from mother to fetus
- Both the incidence of placental transmission and severity of congenital disease depend on gestational age at which maternal seroconversion occurs. Although transmission rates from mother to fetus tend to be low early in pregnancy, fetal disease severity is highest when the fetus is infected early in gestation. The greatest overall risk appears to occur with maternal seroconversion between 24 and 30 weeks' gestation. During this time, there is a 10% risk of having a congenitally infected child with early clinical disease detectable in utero or with early neonatal signs.
- Serologic tests to determine maternal seroconversion are available; however, to accurately diagnose an acute toxoplasmosis infection can be rather challenging.
- Maternal serologic screening is possible via IgG and IgM antibody testing. Successful secondary prevention programs based on universal maternal screening are available in countries with high disease incidence as France and Austria. Toxoplasmosis is much less prevalent in the United States, so our current practice suggests that maternal screening should be considered in the following cases:
  - If abnormal fetal findings are detected on ultrasound as hydrocephaly, anatomic abnormalities of the CNS, symmetric fetal growth restriction, and nonimmune hydrops
  - All HIV-infected pregnant women, emphasizing the ones with CD4 count <200
  - Immunocompetent women with lymphadenopathy who have negative mononucleosis tests

Testing for maternal IgM antibodies is the most common method used worldwide in the attempt to determine if and when a pregnant woman has experienced acute infection with toxoplasmosis. They appear at the time of infection, but may also persist for many years. A negative IgM test rules out the presence of acute infection, but a positive result requires thorough interpretation. False positives are a major concern because they generate anxiety during pregnancies, expose fetuses to unnecessary procedural risks of diagnosis and side effects of treatment, and may ultimately lead to termination of a noninfected pregnancy.

The table below summarizes the interpretation of the most common combinations for IgG/IgM results.

IgG	IgM	Interpretation
Negative	Negative	Woman has not been infected with toxoplasma and is at risk for primary infection during pregnancy.
Positive	Negative	Most likely represents infection acquired before the pregnancy, except when test done during third trimester.
Negative	Positive or equivocal	Can represent early acute infection and should be followed by confirmatory test at a reference laboratory
Positive	Positive or equivocal	Can represent early acute infection and should be followed by confirmatory test at a reference laboratory

- Recent studies showed that the IgG avidity test may help to differentiate patients with acute infection from those with chronic infection better than assays that measure IgM antibodies, but it is most useful when performed early in gestation. IgG produced early in infection is less avid and binds to *T. gondii* antigens weaker than antibodies produced later in the course of infection. High antibody avidity indicates an older infection. A long-term pattern occurring late in pregnancy does not exclude the possibility that the acute infection may have occurred during the first months of gestation.
- When there is uncertainty as to the diagnosis, the CDC recommends referral to "The Toxoplasma Serology Laboratory at Palo Alto Medical Foundation Research Institute was established by Dr. Jack S. Remington," as it is recognized as the reference laboratory in this country. This laboratory is now using a panel of tests, the Toxoplasma Serological Profile (TSP), to provide more comprehensive confirmatory testing.
- Confirmed positive maternal serologic screening should be accompanied by fetal diagnosis, which requires a combination of ultrasound, amniocentesis, and funipuncture. PCR from the amniocentesis is currently the gold standard test. The PCR provides earlier testing and more rapid results, allowing couples to initiate in utero treatment as soon as possible or to consider pregnancy termination prior to 24 weeks' gestation.
- Treatment is indicated for pregnant women with possible acute infection determined by the above-mentioned serology panel. The drug of choice is spiramycin, a macrolide that achieves higher concentration in the placenta. It is estimated that

it reduces maternal-fetal transmission in about 60%. It is not available for retail sale in the United States; therefore, the FDA has to be contacted and will provide this medication based on a case-to-case review. The recommended dose is 1 gm orally every 8 hours without food. It has few side effects, primarily gastrointestinal upset.

- Spiramycin does not cross the placenta well, so if the amniocentesis demonstrates fetal infection, the treatment of choice for the fetus is pyrimethamine 50 mg daily and sulfadiazine 3 gm daily. Alternating this combination with spiramycin every 3 weeks seems to be a reasonable option when side effects of marrow suppression become an issue.
- Therapeutic abortion can be considered when both the amniocentesis and the fetal ultrasound show compatible fetal abnormalities.
- If there is a suspicion for congenital infection, cord blood has to be sent for toxoplasma serology and PCR, and the infant should be started on treatment with folinic acid, sulfadiazine, and pyrimethamine. If the diagnosis of neonatal toxoplasmosis is confirmed, the infant should be treated for 1 year to prevent further neurologic and visual complications.

SUGGESTED READINGS

Genital Herpes Simplex (HSV 1 and HSV2)
American College of Obstetricians and Gynecologists (ACOG). Management of herpes in pregnancy. Washington (DC): American College of Obstetricians and Gynecologists (ACOG); 2007 Jun. 10 p. (ACOG practice bulletin; no. 82).

Prober CG, Corey L, Brown ZA, et al. The management of pregnancies complicated by genital infections with herpes simplex virus. *Clin Infect Dis* 1992;15:1031.

Mertz GJ, Benedette J, Ashley R, et al. Risk factors for the sexual transmission of genital herpes. *Ann Intern Med* 1992;116:197.

Nahmias AJ, Josey WE, Naib ZM, et al. Perinatal risk associated with maternal genital herpes simplex infection. *Am J Obstet Gynecol* 1971;110:825–837.

Varicella
http://www.cdc.gov/ncbddd/pregnancy_gateway/infections-chickenpox.html

Rouse DJ, Gardner M, Allen SJ, et al. Management of the presumed susceptible varicella (chickenpox) exposed gravida: a cost effectiveness-cost benefit analysis. *Obstet Gynecol* 1996;87:932–936.

Server JA, White LR. Intrauterine viral infections. *Annu Rev Med* 1969;19:471–486.

CMV
The 2010 SOGC Clinical Practice Guidelines in Cytomegalovirus Infection in Pregnancy: http://www.sogc.org/guidelines/documents/gui240CPG1004E.pdf
http://www.cdc.gov/cmv/risk/preg-women.html

Parvovirus B 19
Anderson LJ. Role of parvovirus B19 in human disease. *Pediatr Infect Dis J* 1987;6:711–718.

Anderson MJ, Higgins PG, Davis LR, et al. Experimental parvoviral infection in humans. *J Infect Dis* 1985;152:257–265.

Rubella
The 2008 SOGC Clinical Practice Guidelines in Rubella in Pregnancy. http://www.sogc.org/guidelines/documents/guiJOGC203CPG0802.pdf

HIV 1

http://www.cdc.gov/hiv/topics/women/index.htm
http://aidsinfo.nih.gov/guidelines/html/3/perinatal-guidelines

HIV 2

http://aidsinfo.nih.gov/guidelines/html/3/perinatal-guidelines/161/special-situations—
   hiv-2-infection-and-pregnancy

Group B strep

http://www.cdc.gov/groupbstrep/guidelines/guidelines.html
Baker C, Edwards M. Group B streptococcal infections: perinatal impact and prevention methods. *Ann NY Acad Sci* 1988;549:193–202

Escherichia coli

Robbins J, McCraken G Jr, Gotschuch E, et al. Escherichia coli K1 capsular polysaccharide
   associated with neonatal meningitis. *N Engl J Med* 1974;290:1216–1220.

Listeria monocytogenes

http://www.cdc.gov/ncbddd/pregnancy_gateway/infections-listeria.html
Baud D, Greub G. Intracellular bacteria and adverse pregnancy outcomes. *Clin Microbiol Infect*
   2011;17(9):1312–1322.
Mylonakis E, et al. Listeriosis during pregnancy: a case series and a review of 222 cases. *Medicine*
   (Baltimore) 2002;81:260–269.

Syphilis

http://www.cdc.gov/std/treatment/2006/congenital-syphilis.htm
http://www.cdc.gov/std/treatment/2010/specialpops.htm#pregwomen

Toxoplasmosis

http://www.cdc.gov/parasites/toxoplasmosis/
Iqbal J, Khalid N. Detection of acute Toxoplasma gondii infection in early pregnancy by IgG
   avidity and PCR analysis. *J Med Microbiol* 2007;56(Pt 11):1495–1499.
Montoya JG, Remington JS. Management of Toxoplasma gondii infection during pregnancy.
   Clin Infect Dis 2008;47(4):554–566.

XVIII Mycobacterial Infections

63 Mycobacterium Tuberculosis

Melanie Gerrior, Cassandra D. Salgado, and L.W. Preston Church

INTRODUCTION

- Almost one-third of the world's population is infected with tuberculosis (TB). In 2010, nearly nine million people developed TB associated illness and 1.4 million succumbed to TB-related death.
- TB continues to be a leading cause of mortality among patients with human immunodeficiency virus (HIV). Others at increased risk are inmates in correctional facilities, the elderly, the homeless, and foreign-born persons.
- In the United States, 10,521 cases of TB (3.4 cases per 100,000 persons) were reported in 2011, which was a 6.4% decline compared to 2010. Incident TB among foreign-born persons in the United States was 12 times greater than US-born persons, and Asians surpassed Hispanics as the largest racial/ethnic group represented. Most foreign-born persons with TB have latent TB infection (LTBI) acquired abroad.
- Despite continued decline in US TB cases, this still falls short of the 2010 goal of TB elimination set in 1989.

PATHOGENESIS

- TB spreads from person to person through the air by droplet nuclei (1 mm to 5 mm) containing *Mycobacterium tuberculosis*. Infectious droplets are produced when persons with pulmonary or laryngeal TB cough, sneeze, or speak. Additionally, procedures that generate aerosols such as sputum induction, bronchoscopy, and processing infectious specimens may spread TB.
- After inhalation, infectious droplet nuclei may reach respiratory bronchioles or alveoli. Depending on bacterial virulence and the inherent host defense mechanisms of the alveolar macrophages, infection may be established and replication may ensue.
- The tubercle bacillus grows slowly, dividing every 25 to 32 hours within the macrophage. Initially, there is no host response until a sufficient number of organisms are produced (2 to 12 weeks). Then there is a cellular immune response that can be detected by reaction to the tuberculin skin test (TST).
- Before cellular immunity develops, bacilli spread via lymphatics to hilar lymph nodes and through the bloodstream to distant sites. Sites with favorable microenvironments for replication of the organism include the upper lungs, kidneys, bones, and brain.
- For most individuals with normal cell-mediated immune function, proliferation of *M. tuberculosis* is halted through collections of activated T cells and macrophages that form granulomas. Small numbers of viable organisms exist in the center of the granulomas, which may become necrotic.
- Sometimes a primary complex is seen on chest imaging; however, the majority of pulmonary TB infections are clinically and radiographically inapparent. Most often, a positive TST is the only sign that infection with *M. tuberculosis* has occurred.

- Individuals who successfully halt replication of TB and thus do not have active disease are classified as having LTBI. These individuals cannot transmit the organism to other persons; however, it is estimated that approximately 10% of individuals with LTBI will develop active disease. Thus, for adequate control and possible elimination of TB, preventive treatment for this group is needed.

LATENT TUBERCULOSIS INFECTION

- Persons with increased risk for developing TB include those who have had recent infection with *M. tuberculosis* and those who have clinical conditions that are associated with an increased risk for progression of LTBI to active TB such as HIV, intravenous drug use, diabetes, chronic renal failure, or immunosuppression.
- Persons with LTBI who are considered to be at high risk for developing active TB should be offered treatment irrespective of age and irrespective of bacille Calmette-Guérin (BCG) immunization.

Diagnosis of Latent Tuberculosis

- For more than a century, the diagnosis of LTBI has depended on the intradermal injection of purified protein derivative, the TST. Guidelines for interpretation are regularly updated by the Centers for Disease Control (CDC) (Table 63-1).

Table 63-1	Criteria for a Positive Tuberculin Skin Test	
Induration ≥5 mm	**Induration ≥10 mm**	**Induration ≥15 mm**
HIV-positive persons	Residents and employees of high-risk settings: healthcare facilities, prisons and jails, long-term care facilities, homeless shelters, mycobacteriology labs	Persons with no risk factors for TB
Recent contacts of TB case patients	Recent immigrants (within 5 years) from high prevalence countries	
Fibrotic changes on chest radiograph consistent with prior TB	Injection-drug users	
Immunosuppression, including organ transplantation, ≥15 mg/day prednisone ≥30 days	Other conditions associated with increased risk of disease, including silicosis, diabetes mellitus, chronic renal failure, leukemias and lymphomas, lung cancer, head and neck cancer, weight loss ≥10% of ideal body weight, gastrectomy, jejunoileal bypass	

Adapted from CDC. Targeted tuberculin testing and treatment of latent tuberculosis infection. *MMWR Morb Mortal Wkly Rep* 2000; 49 (RR-6):1–51.

Table 63-2	Ability of TST and IGRAs to Predict Risk of Progression to Active TB			
	Sensitivity	**Specificity**	**Positive Predictive Value**	**Negative Predictive Value**
TST	90%–100%	29%–39%	2.7%–3.1%	99%–100%
IGRA	80%–90%	56%–83%	4%–8%	99%–100%

Pooled results from four published studies examining household contacts of an active TB case. Positive TST defined as a reaction >5 mm induration.

- TST sensitivity is reduced in immunosuppressed individuals, those with active infection, and in the first 8 to 12 weeks after primary infection; in the latter two situations, a negative TST is never sufficient to exclude infection.
- False positive TST results may occur from cross-reactions due to exposure to environmental mycobacteria including *M. avium-intracellulare* complex and *M. marinum*.
- BCG in infancy (established benefit) should not contribute to a positive TST after 4 to 5 years postvaccination. The effect of BCG vaccine later in life or due to boosting is more difficult to assess but may result in a positive TST up to 10 years later in 25% of recipients.
- Whole-blood interferon gamma release assays (IGRAs) based on quantification of IFN-γ released by sensitized lymphocytes in response to early secretory antigenic target-6 (ESAT-6) and culture filtrate protein-10 (CFP-10) are an alternative to TST. These antigens are common to all mycobacterium tuberculosis (MTB) isolates and pathogenic *M. bovis* strains but not BCG strains of *M. bovis*.
- Even though some mycobacteria (*M. szulgai, M. kansasii, M. marinum*) may produce false positive results, the specificity of IGRAs is superior to that of the TST. The sensitivity may be slightly less than the TST; however, the ability to identify individuals at risk for progression to active TB is similar (Table 63-2).
- Guidelines have been published for the use of IGRAs. Cost-effectiveness and managing discordant IGRAs and TST results remain unresolved issues.

Treatment for Latent Tuberculosis

- Risk of reactivation among those with LTBI is greatest in the first 2 years after infection.
- All newly TST positive individuals should be encouraged to take treatment for LTBI as recommended by regularly updated CDC guidelines (Table 63-3).
- Those who decline therapy for LTBI should be regularly evaluated for signs and symptoms of active TB.
- Baseline laboratory testing of liver function is not routinely indicated at the start of treatment for LTBI but should be performed for patients with known liver disorders or those at risk for chronic liver disease, HIV, pregnant women, women in the immediate postpartum period, and persons who use alcohol regularly.
- Active hepatitis and end-stage liver disease are relative contraindications to the use of isoniazid or pyrazinamide.
- Persons whose baseline liver function tests are abnormal and those at risk for liver disease should have routine laboratory testing throughout treatment. Additionally, laboratory testing is indicated for patients who develop symptoms of hepatotoxicity.

Table 63-3	Recommended Drug Regimens for Adults with Latent Tuberculosis Infection	
Drug	**Interval and Duration**	**Comments**
Isoniazid (INH)	Daily for 9 months	In HIV-infected patients, isoniazid may be administered concurrently with nucleoside reverse transcriptase inhibitors (NRTIs), protease inhibitors (PIs), or non-nucleoside reverse transcriptase inhibitors (NNRTIs).
	Twice weekly for 6–9 months	DOT must be used with this regimen.
	Daily for 6 months	Not indicated for HIV-infected patients, those with fibrotic lesions on chest radiographs or children.
Isoniazid and rifapentine	Weekly for 3 months	DOT must be used with this regimen. Not recommended for HIV-infected patients on antiretroviral agents (drug interactions not known). Not recommended for pregnant women (drug interactions not known).
Rifampin	Daily for 4 months	This regimen may be used for those who cannot tolerate isoniazid or for those who are contacts of patients with isoniazid-resistant, rifampin-susceptible TB.

Adapted from CDC. Targeted tuberculin testing and treatment of latent tuberculosis infection. *MMWR Morb Mortal Wkly Rep* 2000;49 (RR-6):1–51 and CDC. Recommendations for use of an Isoniazide and Rifapentine regimen with directly observed therapy to treat latent tuberculosis infection. *MMWR Morb Mortal Wkly Rep* 2011;60:1650–1653.

- Some experts recommend that isoniazid be discontinued if transaminase levels exceed three times the upper limit of normal in symptomatic patients and five times the upper limit of normal in asymptomatic patients.

ACTIVE PULMONARY TUBERCULOSIS

- Individuals who do not successfully halt replication of TB develop active disease. As mentioned above, disease may develop in any number of sites distant from the lungs.
- Patients with immunosuppression, HIV infection or born outside of the US have a higher reported incidence of extrapulmonary disease. Moreover, extrapulmonary involvement tends to increase in frequency with worsening immune compromise.
- Discussion of extrapulmonary TB is beyond the scope of this brief chapter.

Diagnosis of Active Pulmonary Tuberculosis

- Clinical manifestations of TB may include fever (the most easily quantified), malaise, poor appetite, weight loss, and night sweats.
- Hematologic manifestations of TB include an increased or decreased leukocyte count and anemia. Leukemoid reactions may occur. Monocytosis and eosinophilia have been reported.

- Cough is the most common symptom of pulmonary TB and ranges from being nonproductive early in disease to productive of sputum as disease progresses. Hemoptysis may rarely be a presenting symptom but usually is the result of previous disease.
- Rasmussen aneurysm (rupture of a dilated vessel in the wall of a cavity), bacterial or fungal infection in a residual cavity (mycetoma), or erosion of a lesion into an airway (broncholithiasis) should be suspected with hemoptysis.
- Pulmonary TB almost always causes abnormalities on plain chest radiographs. In HIV patients with pulmonary TB, a normal chest film is more common. In primary TB after recent infection, abnormalities are generally in the middle or lower lung zones, often associated with ipsilateral hilar adenopathy. Over time, after cell-mediated immunity develops, cavitation may occur.
- Active disease that develops as a result of reactivation of LTBI usually presents with imaging abnormalities in the apical segment of the upper lobes or the superior segment of the lower lobes of one or both lungs. Cavitation is also common.
- As disease progresses, scar formation with loss of lung volume and calcification may occur, and infection may be spread to other parts of the lungs, causing patchy infiltrates.
- Erosion of a parenchymal focus of TB into a blood or lymph vessel may lead to dissemination of the organism and a "miliary" (evenly distributed small nodules) pattern.
- Diagnosis and management of TB involves detection of mycobacteria, identification of the mycobacterial species, and determination of susceptibilities to antimycobacterial drugs.
- A series of at least three properly collected sputum specimens (material recovered from the lungs after a productive cough or sputum induced by nebulizer) should be obtained.
- For patients unable to produce sputum, three gastric aspirations performed early in the morning prior to eating or ambulating or specimens (washings, bronchoalveolar lavage, or transbronchial biopsy) from bronchoscopy may be substituted.
- Detection of acid-fast bacilli (AFB) in stained smears of a clinical specimen provides evidence of the presence of mycobacteria. Additionally, a quantitative estimation of the number of bacilli may be obtained, a useful piece of information when following response to therapy. 50% to 80% of patients with pulmonary TB will have positive sputum smears.
- Hospitalized patients should be placed in respiratory isolation until active pulmonary TB has been ruled out or until the patient has been treated and is no longer thought to be infectious.
- Outpatients should be instructed to remain at home and avoid contact with those at increased risk for acquiring TB until they are no longer thought to be infectious.
- Newer technologies of nucleic acid amplification have improved diagnostic speed and ability to confirm MTB species.
- All clinical specimens suspected of containing mycobacteria should be inoculated onto culture media for identification and drug susceptibility testing. In general, the sensitivity of culture is 80% to 85% with a specificity of approximately 98%.
- Any case of active TB that occurs in the United States must be reported to the local health department. Reporting is essential for contact investigation and control programs at local, state, and national levels.

Treatment of Active Pulmonary Tuberculosis

• Treatment decisions are based on several factors including drug susceptibility testing, burden of disease, and HIV status.

• Drug susceptibility tests should be performed on all initial isolates to identify an effective treatment regimen. These tests should be repeated if the patient continues to produce culture-positive sputum after 3 months of treatment or develops positive cultures after a period of negative cultures.

• Ten drugs are currently approved by the U.S. Food and Drug Administration for treating TB. Of these, first-line agents include isoniazid, rifampin, ethambutol, and pyrazinamide.

Drug-susceptible TB

• TB treatment regimens have an initial or "induction" phase of 2 months duration, followed by a continuation phase of either 4 or 7 months (6 to 9 months total). Table 63-4 lists CDC-recommended basic treatment regimens for drug-susceptible TB.

• Most patients should receive the 4-month continuation phase with the longer 7-month regimen reserved for patients with cavitary disease whose sputum culture after completion of 2 months of treatment is positive, patients whose initial phase of treatment did not include pyrazinamide, and those receiving once-weekly isoniazid and rifapentine whose sputum culture after the initial phase of treatment is positive.

• HIV-negative patients without cavitary disease and who have negative AFB smears after the initial phase of treatment may receive once-weekly isoniazid and rifapentine.

• The importance of compliance (completing therapy as prescribed) cannot be stressed enough. Poor compliance may lead to reemergence of symptomatic disease or TB bacteria that have become resistant to the drugs typically used for treatment.

Drug-susceptible TB in HIV

• Treatment of TB disease in the HIV-infected individual should involve an expert in the management of such patients whenever possible. Special issues among this group include the possibility of TB treatment failure, antiretroviral treatment

Table 63-4	Basic TB Disease Treatment Regimens	
Preferred Regimen	**Alternative Regimen**	**Alternative Regimen**
Initial Phase	*Initial Phase*	*Initial Phase*
Daily INH, RIF, PZA, and EMB for 56 doses (8 weeks)	Daily INH, RIF, PZA, and EMB for 14 doses (2 weeks), then twice weekly for 12 doses (6 weeks)	Thrice-weekly INH, RIF, PZA, and EMB for 24 doses (8 weeks)
Continuation Phase	*Continuation Phase*	*Continuation Phase*
Daily INH and RIF for 126 doses (18 weeks) or twice-weekly INH and RIF for 36 doses (18 weeks)	Twice-weekly INH and RIF for 36 doses (18 weeks)	Three times-weekly INH and RIF for 54 doses (18 weeks)

INH, isoniazid; RIF, rifampin; PZA, pyrazinamide; EMB, ethambutol.

failure, paradoxical temporary worsening of signs or symptoms of TB, and drug interactions and side effects.

- Drug interactions with rifampin and some protease inhibitors and nonnucleoside reverse transcriptase inhibitors are particularly problematic. Rifabutin has fewer interactions and may be used as an alternative to rifampin.
- The recommended treatment of TB in HIV patients is a 6-month regimen consisting of an initial phase of isoniazid, a rifamycin, pyrazinamide, and ethambutol for 2 months followed by a 4-month continuation phase of isoniazid and a rifamycin.
- Twice-weekly therapy may be considered in patients with less-advanced immunosuppression (CD4 counts ≥ 100/mcL). Once-weekly isoniazid and rifapentine for the continuation phase is not recommended for HIV patients.
- Prolonging treatment to 9 months by extending the continuation phase to 7 months is recommended in HIV patients with positive sputum cultures after 2 months of initial treatment.
- Directly observed therapy (DOT) should be used in all patients with HIV-related TB.

Drug-resistant TB

- Drug-resistant TB is resistant to at least one first-line antituberculous drug. Multidrug-resistant TB (MDR TB) is resistant to more than one antituberculous drug and at least isoniazid and rifampin.
- Treating and curing drug-resistant TB is difficult and must be individualized. Inappropriate management can have life-threatening consequences. Drug-resistant TB should be managed by or in close consultation with an expert in the disease.
- DOT always should be used in the treatment of drug-resistant TB to ensure adherence.

SUGGESTED READINGS

American Thoracic Society. Diagnostic standards and classification of tuberculosis in adults and children. *Am J Respir Crit Care Med* 2000;161:1376–1395.

American Thoracic Society, Centers for Disease Control and Prevention, and Infectious Diseases Society of America. Treatment of Tuberculosis. *MMWR Morb Mortal Wkly Rep* 2003;52(RR-11):1–77.

Centers for Disease Control and Prevention. Targeted Tuberculin Testing and Treatment of Latent Tuberculosis Infection. *MMWR Morb Mortal Wkly Rep* 2000;49 (RR-6):1–51.

Centers for Disease Control and Prevention. Updated guidelines for using interferon gamma release assays to detect *Mycobacterium tuberculosis* infection-United States, 2010. *MMWR Morb Mortal Wkly Rep* 2010;59(RR-5):1–25.

Centers for Disease Control and Prevention. Recommendations for use of an isoniazid and rifapentine regimen with directly observed therapy to treat latent tuberculosis infection. *MMWR Morb Mortal Wkly Rep* 2011;60:1650–1653.

Centers for Disease Control and Prevention. Trends in tuberculosis-United States 2011. *MMWR Morb Mortal Wkly Rep* 2012;61(11):181–185.

Dannenberg AM. Immune mechanisms in the pathogenesis of pulmonary tuberculosis. *Rev Infect Dis* 1989;11:S369–S378.

Dannenberg AM. Pathogenesis of pulmonary tuberculosis: host–parasite interactions, cell-mediated immunity, and delayed type hypersensitivity. In: Schlossberg D, ed. *Basic Principles in Tuberculosis*. 3rd ed. New York: Springer-Verlag; 1992.

Edwards D, Kirkpatrick CH. The immunology of mycobacterial diseases. *Am Rev Respir Dis* 1986;134:1062–1071.

Horsburgh CR, Rubin EJ. Clinical practice. Latent tuberculosis infection in the United States. *N Engl J Med* 2011;364(15):1441–1448.

Ichiyama S, Shimokata K, Takeuchi J, et al. Comparative study of a biphasic culture system (Roche MB check system) with a conventional egg medium for recovery of mycobacteria. *Tuber Lung Dis* 1993;74:338–341.

Jones B, Young S, Antoniskis D, et al. Relationship of the manifestations of tuberculosis to CD4 cell counts in patients with human immunodeficiency virus infection. *Am Rev Respir Dis* 1993;148:1292–1297.

Mazurek GH, Zajdowicz MJ, Hankinson AL, et al. Detection of *Mycobacterium tuberculosis* infection in United States Navy recruits using the tuberculin skin test or whole-blood interferon-γ release assays. *Clin Infect Dis* 2007;45:826–836.

Morgan MA, Horstmeier CD, DeYoung DR, et al. Comparison of a radiometric method (BACTEC) and conventional culture media for recovery of mycobacteria from smear-negative specimens. *J Clin Microbiol* 1983;18:384–388.

Small PM, Schecter GF, Goodman PC, et al. Treatment of tuberculosis in patients with advanced human immunodeficiency virus infection. *N Engl J Med* 1991;324:289–294.

Smith D, Wiengeshaus E. What animal models can teach us about the pathogenesis of tuberculosis in humans. *Rev Infect Dis* 1989;11:S385–S393.

www.cdc.gov/tb/

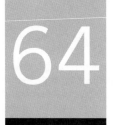

64 Mycobacterium avium Complex in the Immunocompetent Host

Cassandra D. Salgado

BACKGROUND

Nontuberculous mycobacterium (NTM) disease has been reported in most developed countries with incidence rates ranging from 1.0 to 1.8 cases per 100,000 persons. *Mycobacterium avium* complex (MAC) organisms are the most common cause of NTM disease worldwide. These organisms are commonly found in soil and water, including both natural and treated water, as well as wild and domesticated animals. Humans are thought to acquire disease via exposure (e.g., aerosolization) to these sources. There is no evidence that NTM (MAC) is able to be transmitted from animal to human or from human to human. Lung disease is the most common clinical manifestation of NTM (MAC); however lymphatic, skin, and soft tissue, as well as disseminated disease occur. This chapter focuses on pulmonary disease in the non-HIV host.

M. *avium* complex includes the species M. *avium* and M. *intracellulare*. Traditional laboratory characteristics such as physical appearance and biochemical testing cannot distinguish between these species and generally speciation is not clinically relevant; however, DNA probes have been developed for identification and may be useful for epidemiologic study. M. *avium* is the species more often encountered among patients with disseminated disease, whereas M. *intracellulare* is more common in respiratory infections.

Patient-specific risk factors for NTM disease include those that predispose to disseminated disease and those that predispose to lung disease. The interactions between the organism, macrophages, and lymphocytes (particularly T helper cells and natural killer cells) are important to protect the host from mycobacterial disease. Detailed discussion of the immunologic response is beyond the scope of this brief chapter; however, interleukin (IL)-12, interferon-gamma (INF-γ), and tumor necrosis factor-alpha (TNF-α) are all important. An immunologic defect, either acquired through disease (HIV or genetic) or through receipt of immunosuppressing medications, which disrupts these pathways, may predispose to disseminated disease. Underlying structural disease predisposes to respiratory infection. This includes chronic obstructive pulmonary disease (COPD), bronchiectasis, cystic fibrosis, pneumoconiosis, and previous cavitary lung infection from tuberculosis. Additionally, it has been described that women with pulmonary MAC infections with bronchiectasis have a similar body type, sometimes including a thin build, scoliosis, pectus excavatum, and mitral valve prolapse.

IFN-γ and IL-12 protect the host from mycobacteria largely through upregulation of TNF-α and a relationship between the use of TNF-α blocking agents (such as infliximab, adalimumab, and etanercept) and development of active *Mycobacterium tuberculosis* has been realized among patients with a history of latent tuberculosis; however, the risk associated with receipt of these agents and NTM (MAC) infection is not known. Expert opinion suggests that patients with active NTM disease should receive TNF-α blocking agents only if they are also receiving adequate therapy for NTM.

CLINICAL DISEASE

Pulmonary Disease

Almost all patients with pulmonary MAC have a chronic or recurring cough. Some have fever, fatigue, and malaise, some have dyspnea, sputum production, and hemoptysis. The range and severity of symptoms often correlates with stage of illness (mild in early disease and more severe in advanced disease). In patients with underlying lung disease, evaluation can be difficult. The clinician should take into account changes in the patient's baseline symptoms that cannot be otherwise explained and have a high index of suspicion for NTM. Chest auscultation may reveal rhonchi, crackles, or wheezing. NTM lung disease may present similar to tuberculosis with fibrocavitary lesions or may be characterized by nodular infiltrates associated with bronchiectasis. Thus, radiographic appearance will vary.

Fibrocavitary NTM (MAC) lung disease has been described predominately among middle-aged males who have a smoking and alcohol history. This form of disease almost always progresses within 1 to 2 years resulting in lung tissue destruction and ultimately respiratory failure. Fibrocavitary lesions tend to be thin walled with minimal surrounding parenchymal disease often with evidence of involvement of the overlying pleura. These lesions are often visible on plain chest x-ray.

Noncavitary NTM (MAC) lung disease has been described predominately among postmenopausal, nonsmoking, white females, often with the body type described above. This form of lung disease has been associated with a slower progression compared to fibrocavitary disease and appears as nodular and interstitial nodular infiltrates frequently of the right middle lobe or lingula. High-resolution computed tomography (CT) scan is needed to visualize these findings and they are described as small peripheral pulmonary nodules centered on the bronchovascular tree with cylindrical bronchiectasis often termed "tree-in bud" (Fig. 64-1).

Isolation of MAC in respiratory culture is essential for the diagnosis of lung disease; however, because the organism is ubiquitous in the environment, contamination of specimens does occur. Thus, a single positive sputum culture is often regarded as indeterminate for diagnosis. To fully optimize the utility of sputum analysis, patients should have at least three specimens collected, preferably in the morning, on separate days sent for acid-fast bacilli (AFB) staining and culture. For patients unable to produce sputum, induced sputum may be attempted but the validity of this specimen has not been established for diagnosis of NTM (MAC) lung disease. Bronchial lavage may also be useful for diagnosing NTM (MAC) lung disease and is often regarded as a more sensitive test compared to expectorated sputum. Rarely, in more difficult cases, a lung biopsy (generally transbronchial) may be needed for histopathology. Consultation with an expert experienced in diagnosing and caring for these patients is suggested.

Diagnosis of NTM (MAC) lung disease requires that the patient meet both clinical and microbiologic criteria. *Clinical criteria* include pulmonary symptoms, nodular or cavitary opacities on chest imaging, *and* exclusion of other diagnoses such as active tuberculosis or malignancy. *Microbiologic criteria* include positive culture results from at least two separate expectorated sputum samples, *or* a positive culture result from at least one bronchial wash or lavage, *or* a transbronchial or other lung biopsy with mycobacterial histopathologic features (granulomatous inflammation) and positive culture for NTM, or biopsy showing mycobacterial histopathologic features (granulomatous inflammation) and one or more sputum or bronchial washing that are culture positive for NTM.

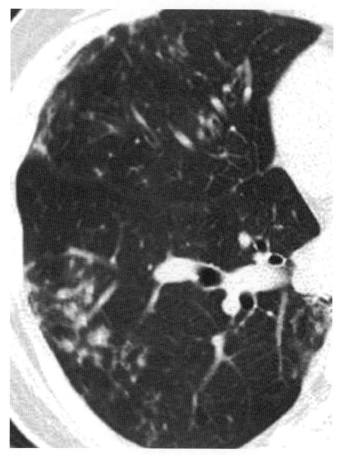

Figure 64-1 High-resolution CT Scan in a patient with MAC pulmonary disease. Bronchiectasis with centrilobular small nodules and tree-in-bud signs extending more than 2 cm from pleura, in superior segment of right lower lobe. (From Song JW, Koh WJ, Lee JY, et al. High-resolution CT findings of *Mycobacterium avium-intracellulare* complex pulmonary disease: correlation with pulmonary function tests. *AJR Am J Roentgenol* 2008;191:1010–1017, with permission.)

Routine antibiotic susceptibility testing for NTM (MAC) isolates remains an unresolved issue largely because in vitro susceptibility tests for antituberculosis drugs does not correlate with clinical response for MAC infections. In contrast, susceptibility testing for clarithromycin has correlated well with clinical response. MAC isolates from a patient's initial infection should undergo susceptibility testing to clarithromycin to establish baseline values. These isolates are usually susceptible (minimal inhibitory concentration [MIC] of 4 g/mL). Other clinical scenarios where susceptibility testing to clarithromycin is recommended is for patients who were previously treated with macrolide therapy to determine whether or not the isolate would still respond to a macrolide, or for patients currently receiving macrolide therapy for lung disease with suspected relapse or treatment failure. Relapse strains after treatment tend to have a higher MIC to clarithromycin (32 g/mL or greater) and will no longer respond to macrolide treatment. Extended in vitro susceptibility testing for macrolide-resistant MAC isolates (e.g., to the newer fluoroquinolones and linezolid) may be considered in consultation with an expert familiar with interpretation of the results.

TREATMENT

Drug Treatment of MAC Lung Disease

The use of traditional antituberculosis agents for the treatment of MAC lung disease has been associated with inconsistent results. Most of these agents have far less in vitro activity against MAC isolates than against *M. tuberculosis* and when used, relapse is common. The macrolide class of antibiotics, which have good in vitro activity against NTM and MAC, has emerged as a vital component of recommended therapy. Studies have reported that among patients who complete at least 6 months of a macrolide-containing regimen, 59% to 92% had conversion of sputum to AFB negative, with 12 months of consecutive negative sputum cultures on therapy. Additionally, intermittent therapy for MAC lung disease (three times weekly) may be considered for patients who meet certain criteria. This may be associated with lower medication side effects and cost. Patients who have severe nodular/bronchiectatic disease, cavitary disease, received previous treatment for MAC lung disease, or who have a history of underlying lung disease (COPD, bronchiectasis) would not be good candidates for intermittent therapy.

The optimal therapeutic regimen has yet to be established for MAC lung disease and treatment is often complicated by intolerance to the agents (Gastrointestinal [GI] intolerance primarily). It is also important to note that macrolides should never be used as monotherapy due to a low threshold for development of resistance among NTM (MAC) isolates. This is the result of a single point mutation that occurs on therapy in the macrolide-binding region (peptidyltransferase) of the 23S rRNA gene conferring resistance to all macrolides. Treatment regimen options for MAC lung disease are outlined in Table 64-1. The most widely used backbone of MAC therapy includes the macrolides, clarithromycin and azithromycin, and ethambutol. Companion drugs, usually a rifamycin or an aminoglycoside, are then considered based on the individual patient's disease state and desired aggressiveness of treatment.

Patients receiving rifabutin should be monitored for drug-related toxicity, particularly leukopenia and abnormal liver function tests. Patients receiving aminoglycoside therapy should be monitored for renal toxicity, ototoxicity, and vestibular toxicity. Ototoxicity and vestibular toxicity are generally not reversible, thus, careful instruction regarding signs and symptoms (vertigo, unbalanced gait, tinnitus, reduced hearing) and continued assessment are necessary. If signs or symptoms develop, the drug should be discontinued or the dosage decreased. Baseline audiometry testing with repeat testing at regularly scheduled intervals or with the onset of new symptoms is recommended.

The desired goals of therapy may vary from patient to patient but generally include symptomatic and microbiologic improvement. Patients should show signs of symptomatic improvement (decreased cough, dyspnea, and fatigue) within 3 to 6 months of therapy. The microbiologic treatment goal for MAC lung disease is the conversion of sputum cultures to negative. To document this response, sputum samples should be sent monthly during therapy for AFB smears and cultures. Three consecutive AFB-negative samples represent the desired endpoint. Patients should convert their sputum

Table 64-1	Therapy for MAC Lung Disease According to Disease Status and/or Severity

Initial therapy for nodular/bronchiectatic disease[a]
Macrolide (clarithromycin 1,000 mg or azithromycin 500–600 mg three times weekly) *plus* ethambutol 25 mg/kg three times weekly *plus* rifampin 600 mg three times weekly.

Initial therapy for cavitary disease
Macrolide (clarithromycin[b] 500–1,000 mg or azithromycin 250–300 mg daily) *plus* ethambutol 15 mg/kg daily *plus* rifampin 450–600 mg daily. Consider addition of aminoglycoside (streptomycin or amikacin) for the first 2–3 months of therapy at 10–15 mg/kg three times weekly.

Advanced (severe) or previously treated disease
Macrolide (clarithromycin[b] 500–1,000 mg or azithromycin 250–300 mg daily) *plus* ethambutol 15 mg/kg daily *plus* rifabutin 150–300 mg or rifampin 450–600 mg daily *plus* aminoglycoside (streptomycin or amikacin) at 10–15 mg/kg three times weekly.

[a]For some patients (mild nodular/bronchiectatic disease or drug intolerance) clarithromycin or azithromycin with ethambutol on a daily basis would be acceptable. No other two-drug regimen is recommended.
[b]For many patients, the dose of clarithromycin may need to be split (500 mg twice daily) or gradually increased because of gastrointestinal intolerance.
Adapted from Griffith DE, Aksamit T, Brown-Elliott BA, et al. An official ATS/IDSA statement: diagnosis, treatment, and prevention of nontuberculous mycobacterial diseases. *Am J Respir Crit Care Med* 2007;175:367–416.

to negative within 12 months on a macrolide-containing regimen. Failure to show clinical or microbiologic response to therapy should alert the clinician to the possibility of noncompliance, drug resistance (particularly macrolide resistance), or the presence of an anatomic abnormality (abscess, cyst, further cavitation). Optimal duration of therapy has not been established; however, most experts would recommend continuing treatment for 12 consecutive months of documented negative cultures. For patients who do not have the desired response to conventional macrolide-based therapy, an alternative drug regimen or surgery may be necessary.

Interpretation of sputum cultures that were initially negative but have converted to positive can be challenging. For patients who completed a full course of therapy and met clinical and microbiologic endpoints of successful therapy, new positive sputum cultures likely represent reinfection by a new MAC strain. For patients who met criteria but discontinued therapy after < 10 months of negative cultures, multiple positive cultures are likely to represent relapse of the original MAC strain.

The management of macrolide-resistant MAC lung infection is complex and should be done under the guidance of an expert. The treatment strategy associated with the most success includes both the use of an aminoglycoside combined with surgical resection. Additional agents that may have activity against MAC isolates include, clofazimine, cycloserine, ethionamide, capreomycin, and the newer fluoroquinolones.

Alternative and Adjunct Treatment of MAC Lung Disease

Patients whose disease is predominantly localized to one lung and who can tolerate surgery might also be considered for resection under some circumstances. These include poor response to conventional drug therapy, the development of macrolide-resistant MAC disease, or the presence of significant disease-related complications. Surgery has been associated with severe perioperative complications and thus patients should be referred to experienced surgeons at centers with extensive experience with mycobacterial surgery.

Consideration should also be given to the use of adjunctive therapies, in addition to antibiotics, for patients with MAC lung infection. These therapies are principally directed at the management of the structural changes that occur in the lungs (bronchiectasis). These include bronchodilators and smoking cessation as well as methods for increased mucus clearance (oscillating positive expiratory pressure devices, and high-frequency chest compression devices). Cardiovascular exercise and adequate nutrition may also be beneficial.

SUGGESTED READING

Ahn CH, McLarty JW, Ahn SS, et al. Diagnostic criteria for pulmonary disease caused by *Mycobacterium kansasii* and *Mycobacterium intracellulare*. *Am Rev Respir Dis* 1982;125:388.

Griffith DE, Aksamit T, Brown-Elliott BA, et al. An official ATS/IDSA statement: diagnosis, treatment, and prevention of nontuberculous mycobacterial diseases. *Am J Respir Crit Care Med* 2007;175:367–416.

Griffith DE, Brown-Elliott BA, Langsjoen B, et al. Clarithromycin-resistant *Mycobacterium avium* complex lung disease. *Am J Respir Crit Care Med* 2006;174:928–934.

Horsburgh CR. Epidemiology of disease caused by nontuberculous mycobacteria. *Semin Respir Infect* 1996;11:244.

Iseman MD, Buschman DL, Ackerson LM. Pectus excavatum and scoliosis: thoracic anomalies associated with pulmonary disease caused by *Mycobacterium avium* complex. *Am Rev Respir Dis* 1991;144:914.

Keane J. Tumor necrosis factor blockers and reactivation of latent tuberculosis. *Clin Infect Dis* 2004;39:300–302.

Lam PK, Griffith DE, Aksamit TR, et al. Factors related to response to intermittent treatment of *Mycobacterium avium* complex lung disease. *Am J Respir Crit Care Med* 2006;173: 1283–1289.

NCCLS (formerly National Committee for Clinical Laboratory Standards) Susceptibility testing of *Mycobacteria, Nocardiae,* and other Aerobic Actinomycetes; Approved Standard (M24-A) 2003.

Prince DS, Peterson DD, Steiner RM, et al. Infection with *Mycobacterium avium* complex in patients without predisposing conditions. *N Engl J Med* 1989;321:863.

Reich JM, Johnson RE. *Mycobacterium avium* complex pulmonary disease presenting as an isolated lingular or middle lobe pattern. The Lady Windemere syndrome. *Chest* 1992;101:1605.

Song JW, Koh WJ, Lee JY, et al. High-resolution CT findings of *Mycobacterium avium-intracellulare* complex pulmonary disease: correlation with pulmonary function tests. *AJR Am J Roentgenol* 2008;191:1070.

Teirstein AS, Damsker B, Kirschner PA, et al. Pulmonary infection with *Mycobacterium avium-intracellulare*: diagnosis, clinical patterns, treatment. *Mt Sinai J Med* 1990;57:209.

65 Atypical Mycobacteria Other than MAC

Abdel Kareem Abu Malouh and Jonathan P. Moorman

GENERAL FEATURES

The atypical or nontuberculous mycobacteria (NTM) are a group of organisms distributed widely in the environment, including in domestic and natural water supplies, soil, food, and animals. They possess an impermeable cell wall and can survive environments with high acidity or alkalinity. NTM are intrinsically resistant to chlorine and biocides and can escape the filtration process. This chapter focuses on atypical mycobacteria not including *Mycobacterium avium-intracellulare*, which is covered in an accompanying chapter.

CLINICALLY (SEE TABLE 65-1)

- Most species in this group are less virulent than TB and usually affect immunocompromised hosts.
- Risk factors for pulmonary disease include bronchiectasis, scoliosis, pectus excavatum, mitral valve prolapse, and cystic fibrosis.
- HIV and use of anti-TNF drugs are associated with disseminated disease.
- Nosocomial infections are associated with inoculation into the skin during surgical procedures such as cosmetic facial surgery, ophthalmic surgery (including LASIK), augmentation mammoplasty, median sternotomy, and liposuction.
- These mycobacteria do not cause latent infection, and there is no person-to-person transmission risk.
- Routes of infection include cutaneous, respiratory, GI, and parenteral.
- Isolation from clinical specimens may represent colonization, true infection, or contamination.
- *M. kansasii* and *M. szulgai* are almost always true pathogens when isolated from respiratory specimens.
- *M. simiae* and *M. fortuitum* are usually not respiratory pathogens (except in patients with chronic vomiting and aspiration) even if the nontuberculous mycobacterial diagnostic criteria are met.
- *M. gordonae* and *M. terrae* complex are almost always contaminants of respiratory specimens.
- Divided into slow growers and rapid growers depending on speed of growth on culture media
  - Rapid growers group include *M. abscessus*, *M. fortuitum*, and *M. chelonae* and usually grow within 7 days.
  - Slow growers group include *M. kansasii*, *M. marinum*, *M. ulcerans*, *M. szulgai*, and other rare mycobacteria. This group requires at least 2 to 3 weeks to grow.
- Some species may cause false-positive PPD and interferon release assays, such as *M. kansasii*, *M. marinum*, and *M. szulgai*.

Table 65-1	Atypical Mycobacteria: Presentation and Treatment		
Organism	**Presentation**	**Treatment**	**Comment**
Slow growing			
M. kansasii	Pulmonary disseminated	INH + rifampin + ethambutol	Clarithromycin, moxifloxacin, sulfamethoxazole, streptomycin also active and may be used for rifampin-resistant isolates
M. marinum	Skin lesions	Ethambutol + rifampin or clarithromycin	Minocycline-doxycycline and trimethoprim-sulfamethoxazole are also active, may need debridement
M. ulcerans	Skin disseminated	Mainly surgical debridement clarithromycin + rifampin to prevent relapse	Causes necrotic skin and soft tissue lesions ("Buruli" ulcer)
M. xenopi	Pulmonary disseminated	Clarithromycin + rifampin + ethambutol	Grows at higher temperatures (45°C); quinolones may be added for better response.
M. szulgai	Pulmonary, tenosynovitis, osteomyelitis	INH + ethambutol + rifampin	Always a potential pathogen favorable treatment outcomes
Rapid growing			
M. abscessus	Pulmonary Skin	Clarithromycin + amikacin + cefoxitin	Pulmonary disease difficult to treat Imipenem may be a substitute for cefoxitin.
M. chelonae	Skin disseminated, catheter-related	Clarithromycin ± imipenem or tobramycin	Resistant to cefoxitin, can lead to contact lens–associated keratitis
M. fortuitum	Skin, catheter-related, rarely pulmonary	Clarithromycin + doxycycline or trimethoprim-sulfamethoxazole or quinolone Start with IV agent (amikacin + imipenem or cefoxitin) for serious infections	Contains erm gene (inducible macrolide resistance); associated with gastroesophageal disorders such as achalasia; can lead to nail salon furunculosis

- Antibiotic susceptibility testing should be done for rapidly growing NTM species to guide therapy.
- Susceptibility testing is not needed for slowly growing NTM except for *M. kansasii* susceptibility to rifampin. In other species, there is no correlation between susceptibility tests and in vivo response to antimicrobials.

DIAGNOSIS OF ATYPICAL MYCOBACTERIAL DISEASES

The diagnosis of atypical mycobacteriosis can be complicated given that their presence may be representative of colonization, infection, or contamination. Guidelines for making a diagnosis of atypical mycobacterial infection can be found at http://www.idsociety.org/uploadedFiles/IDSA/Guidelines-Patient_Care/PDF_Library/NTM%20Disease.pdf.

M. kansasii
Clinical Features
- Considered the second most common cause of NTM disease in the United States and the most pathogenic
- Tap water is the major environmental reservoir.
- Divided into five to seven subspecies; serotype 1 is the major isolate responsible for human infections.
- Primarily affects middle-aged white men
- Risk factors include pneumoconiosis, COPD, previous mycobacterial disease, malignancy, and alcoholism.
- The combination of HIV infection and silicosis increases the susceptibility to *M. kansasii*.
- Pulmonary infections resemble the clinical course of MTB, with similar symptoms.
- Symptoms include cough and sputum production, hemoptysis, fever, night sweats, and weight loss.
- Chest x-ray changes are usually located in the lung apices and include cavitation (in 50% of cases), pleural scarring, and infiltrates.
- The same diagnostic criteria for MAC apply to infections with other NTM, including *M. kansasii*.
- Growth of *M. kansasii* in a single sputum culture should potentially represent true infection, especially in HIV-infected patients.
- Dissemination occurs in about 25% of HIV-infected patients, usually with a CD4 count of <50 cells/μL.

Treatment
- Susceptibility testing of *M. kansasii* for rifampin is recommended.
- Patients should receive a daily regimen including rifampin 10 mg/kg/day, ethambutol 15 mg/kg/day, INH 5 mg/kg/day, and pyridoxine 50 mg/day.
- An initial 2 months of ethambutol at 25 mg/kg/day is no longer recommended.
- For patients with rifampin-resistant *M. kansasii* disease, a three-drug regimen is recommended based on in vitro susceptibilities.
  - Active drugs include clarithromycin, azithromycin, moxifloxacin, ethambutol, sulfamethoxazole, and streptomycin.
- Patients should have close clinical monitoring with frequent sputum cultures for AFB organisms.
- Long-term relapse rates with rifampin-containing regimens are very low.

- Therapy is continued for 12 to 15 months after the first negative sputum culture.
- Surgery has no role in managing routine cases of pulmonary disease because of excellent outcomes with antimycobacterial therapy.
- Treatment for disseminated disease is the same as for pulmonary disease.
- An option for treating HIV-infected patients on HAART is to substitute a macrolide or moxifloxacin for the rifamycin.
- The isolation of *M. kansasii* from sputum of HIV-infected patient with advanced disease is an indication to obtain mycobacterial blood culture to rule out dissemination.
- There is no recommended prophylaxis or suppressive regimen for disseminated *M. kansasii* disease.

M. abscessus

Clinical Features

- Rapid growing mycobacteria that is endemic in the southeastern United States
- Considered the most virulent pulmonary pathogen among rapid growing mycobacteria
- Causes skin/soft tissue and bone disease following accidental trauma or surgery
- Usually causes localized cutaneous infections that can be cellulitic or nodular and may progress to ulceration with purulent drainage
  - Patients may develop a sporotrichoid appearance with ascending lymphadenitis.
  - Can cause cutaneous disseminated disease in patients with defects in cellular immunity or who are receiving glucocorticoids
- May also cause pulmonary disease in patients with underlying lung disease or in white, female nonsmokers without predisposing conditions
- Most patients with *M. abscessus* and no underlying lung disease have an indolent, slowly progressive course.
- More fulminant courses can occur in patients with gastroesophageal disorders and cystic fibrosis.

Treatment

- *M. abscessus* is uniformly resistant to the standard antituberculous agents.
  - Antibiotic susceptibility of all clinically significant isolates is recommended.
  - Usually susceptible to clarithromycin and amikacin
  - The macrolides are the only oral agents reliably active in vitro against *M. abscessus*.
- For serious skin and soft tissue and bone disease, clarithromycin 1 g daily or azithromycin 250 mg/day should be combined with a parenteral agent (amikacin, cefoxitin, or imipenem).
- Clarithromycin alone (500 mg twice daily) can be used for localized, less severe cases.
- Amikacin combined with high dose cefoxitin (up to 12 g/day) is recommended for initial therapy for severe soft tissue disease (minimum of 2 weeks) until clinical improvement is evident.
- Imipenem is an alternative to cefoxitin, with higher bioavailability.
- Duration of therapy is 4 months for serious soft tissue infections and 6 months for bone infections.
- Surgery is indicated for extensive disease, abscess formation, or where drug therapy is difficult.
- Removal of foreign bodies such as breast implants and catheters is important for recovery.
- No antibiotic regimen is curative for *M. abscessus* lung disease.

- The goal of therapy for pulmonary disease is symptomatic improvement, radiologic regression of infiltrates, or improvement in sputum culture positivity.
- Periodic administration of multidrug therapy, including a macrolide and one or more parenteral agents (amikacin, cefoxitin, or imipenem) or a combination of parenteral agents over several months, may help control symptoms and progression of *M. abscessus* lung disease.
- Moxifloxacin and linezolid and tigecycline have in vitro activity, but there is limited clinical experience with these agents.
- The only predictive curative therapy of limited (focal) *M. abscessus* lung disease is surgical resection of involved lung combined with multidrug chemotherapy.
- For patients with underlying esophageal or other swallowing disorders, treatment of the underlying condition can result in improvement of lung disease.

M. chelonae

Clinical Features
- Rapidly growing, ubiquitous NTM
- Causes skin/soft tissue and bone disease and disseminated disease in immunocompromised patients
- Reported to cause keratitis associated with contact lenses and ocular surgery, including LASIK
- Catheter-related infections and postsurgical wound infections have been reported.
- Rarely causes pulmonary disease
- Has led to pseudo-outbreaks due to contaminated bronchoscopes

Treatment
- Susceptibility testing should be performed to guide antibiotic selection.
- Usually susceptible to tobramycin, clarithromycin, and linezolid
  - Other possible active agents include imipenem, amikacin, clofazimine, doxycycline, and ciprofloxacin.
  - Cefoxitin is usually not active.
  - Localized skin infections can be treated with clarithromycin monotherapy (500 mg twice daily).
- For serious skin/soft tissue and bone infections, a minimum of 4 months of combination therapy is needed; for bone infections, 6 months of therapy is recommended.
- The addition of a second agent (tobramycin, imipenem, linezolid) to clarithromycin prevents acquired resistance to clarithromycin.
- For corneal infections, treatment involves topical and systemic agents.
  - Choices include amikacin, fluoroquinolones, clarithromycin, and azithromycin.
  - The outcome for corneal infections is usually poor, with many patients requiring corneal transplants.
- Effective treatment of lung infections is unclear, but treatment with clarithromycin and a second agent based on susceptibilities is likely to be successful.

M. fortuitum

Clinical Features
- Rapidly growing mycobacterium
- Causes pulmonary disease similar to *M. abscessus*, especially in patients with gastroesophageal disorders and chronic vomiting
- Also causes skin/soft tissue and bone infections

- Recent outbreaks in a nail salon with associated furunculosis reported secondary to *M. fortuitum*
- Can cause intravenous catheter-related infections
- Pseudo-outbreaks due to tap water—contaminated bronchoscopes also reported

Treatment
- Usually susceptible to the newer macrolides and quinolones, doxycycline, minocycline, sulfonamides, and amikacin
- Organism contains an inducible erythromycin methylase (erm) gene that confers resistance to macrolides, so macrolides should be used with caution (as 80% of isolates become resistant after treatment).
- For lung disease, treatment with at least two active agents based on susceptibility results should be given for at least 12 months of negative sputum cultures.
- For localized skin disease, may use monotherapy with clarithromycin, trimethoprim-sulfamethoxazole, or doxycycline for 3 to 4 months
- For serious skin and soft tissue infections, treatment with two active agents should be given for at least 4 months, with 6 months for bone infections.
- Initial IV regimens include amikacin with imipenem or cefoxitin, which can be switched to oral regimens after improvement.
- Surgery is indicated for extensive disease, abscess formation, or where drug therapy is difficult.
- Removal of foreign bodies and catheters is important for recovery.

M. marinum

Clinical Features
- Pigmented, slowly growing atypical mycobacteria
- Present in fish tanks and nonchlorinated swimming pools
- Grows optimally at 30°C, a lower temperature than is optimal for other mycobacteria
- Causes swimming pool granuloma or fish tank granuloma
  - Infection is usually acquired from a soft tissue injury to the hand in an aquatic environment.
  - Presents with chronic granulomatous soft tissue infection involving skin and bone in both healthy and immunocompromised hosts
  - The lesions appear as papules on an extremity, progressing to shallow ulceration and scar formation.
  - May be characterized by ascending lesions that resemble sporotrichosis

Treatment
- Usually susceptible to rifampin, rifabutin, ethambutol, clarithromycin, sulfonamides, and doxycycline
- Usually resistant to INH and pyrazinamide and quinolones
- Treatment is with two active agents for 1 to 2 months after resolution of symptoms, usually 3 to 4 months in total.
- Good outcomes obtained with combination of clarithromycin and ethambutol or ethambutol and rifampin
- Rifampin-containing regimens should be used for osteomyelitis.
- Susceptibility testing is not routinely recommended and should be reserved for cases of treatment failure.
- Surgical debridement may be needed, especially in cases of hand involvement and cases not responding to standard therapy.

M. ulcerans

Clinical Features and Treatment

- Causes indolent, progressive necrotic lesions of the skin and underlying tissue with scalloped edges, known as Buruli ulcers
- Endemic in Central and West Africa, Central and South America, and Southeast Asia
- Scarring and deforming contractures may result from extensive necrosis.
- Surgical debridement combined with skin grafting is the treatment of choice.
- Drug treatment with clarithromycin and rifampin may prevent relapse or metastasis of infections.
- Immunization with BCG reduces the risk of disease by 50%.

M. xenopi

Clinical Features and Treatment

- Obligate thermophile with an optimal growth temperature of 45°C
- Second to MAC as a cause of NTM lung disease in Canada, the United Kingdom, and other areas of Europe
- Causes pulmonary disease with apical cavitary lesions and skin and soft tissue infections
- Therapy is with a combination of clarithromycin, rifampin, and ethambutol.
- Therapeutic response may be enhanced with the addition of quinolones or clarithromycin to standard antituberculous therapy.

M. szulgai

Clinical Features and Treatment

- Slowly growing atypical mycobacteria, pigmented after exposure to light
- Causes lung disease similar to TB
- Almost always considered a pathogen in positive sputum cultures
- Can cause tenosynovitis of the hand, olecranon bursitis, osteomyelitis, keratitis, and renal and cutaneous infections
- Treatment is with three to four drugs for 12 months of negative sputum culture and for 4 to 6 months for extrapulmonary infections.

SUGGESTED READINGS

ATS/IDSA Statement. Diagnosis, treatment, and prevention of nontuberculous mycobacterial diseases. *Am J Respir Crit Care Med* 2007;175:367–416.
http://www.idsociety.org/uploadedFiles/IDSA/Guidelines-Patient_Care/PDF_Library/NTM%20Disease.pdf
  This excellent and comprehensive guideline provides a reasonable approach to diagnosing atypical mycobacteriosis and discusses the treatment options currently available based on the data for these often challenging clinical diseases.
Benator DA, Khan V, Gordin FM. *Mycobacterium szulgai* infection of the lung: case report and review of an unusual pathogen. *Am J Med Sci* 1997;313:346–351.
Cook J. Nontuberculous mycobacteria: opportunistic environmental pathogens for predisposed hosts. *Br Med Bull* 2010;96:45–59.
Faress JA, McKinney LA, Semaan MT, et al. *Mycobacterium xenopi* pneumonia in the southeastern United States. *South Med J* 2003;96:596–599.
Griffith D. Nontuberculous mycobacterial lung disease. *Curr Opin Infect Dis* 2010;23:185–190.
Griffith DE, Brown-Elliott BA, Wallace RJ Jr. Thrice-weekly clarithromycin-containing regimen for treatment of *Mycobacterium kansasii* lung disease: results of a preliminary study. *Clin Infect Dis* 2003;37:1178–1182.

Hadjiliadis D, Adlakha A, Prakash UB. Rapidly growing mycobacterial lung infection in association with esophageal disorders. *Mayo Clin Proc* 1999;74:45.

Kuritsky JN, Bullen M, Broome CV, et al. Sternal wound infections and endocarditis due to organisms of the *Mycobacterium fortuitum* complex: a potential environmental source. *Ann Intern Med* 1983;9:938–939.

Lewis FM, Marsh BJ, von Reyn CF. Fish tank exposure and cutaneous infections due to *Mycobacterium marinum*: tuberculin skin testing, treatment, and prevention. *Clin Infect Dis* 2003;37:390–397.

Taiwo B, Glassroth J. Nontuberculous mycobacterial lung diseases. *Infect Dis Clin North Am* 2010;24:769–789.

This recent review outlines the nontuberculous mycobacterial diseases and is an excellent general resource.

van Ingen J, Boeree MJ, van Soolingen D, et al. Resistance mechanism and drug susceptibility testing of nontuberculous mycobacteria. *Drug Resist Updat* 2012 Jun;15(3):149–161.

A very current review focusing on drug susceptibility testing for the various NTM. This contains an extremely thorough review of mechanisms of resistance in these organisms.

XIX Common Problems in Infectious Disease

Skin and Soft Tissue Infections

Mark B. Carr and Kelsey Burr

Infection of the skin and soft tissues varies depending on the depth and severity of tissue involvement. These factors are largely determined by microorganism and host factors.

Erysipelas is infection involving only the upper dermis and superficial lymphatics and is most often caused by *Streptococcus pyogenes* in a normal host.

Cellulitis involves the deeper dermis and subcutaneous fat along with deeper lymphatics. It is typically caused by *S. pyogenes* or *Staphylococcus aureus* and complicates chronic venous insufficiency edema of the lower extremities.

Necrotizing fasciitis is an acute life-threatening infection involving the subcutaneous fat and upper fascia and extending up to the dermal layer. Unlike erysipelas and cellulitis, it often does not present with erythematous changes in the skin.

MICROBIOLOGY

Erysipelas and cellulitis are mostly caused by beta-hemolytic streptococci and *S. aureus*. An increasing number of cases are now caused by methicillin-resistant strains of *S. aureus* (MRSA), which are acquired outside of the healthcare setting.

Haemophilus influenzae and other respiratory pathogens may cause infection involving the face as a complication of upper respiratory tract infection.

Other pathogens are usually associated with certain specific exposures, such as *Pasteurella* following a cat bite, *Erysipelothrix* following a fish scale–induced injury, or *Aeromonas* following a fresh water traumatic injury.

Necrotizing fasciitis involving the extremities is usually secondary to *S. pyogenes* but may also be caused by group C or G streptococci, primarily in the elderly.

Cases of necrotizing fasciitis due to *Vibrio vulnificus* are reported in mostly patients with chronic liver disease with acquisition through salt water exposure.

Increasingly cases of necrotizing fasciitis have been seen due to the USA 300 strain of MRSA.

Necrotizing fasciitis due to synergy between multiple pathogens and involving either a foot ulcer or the perineum, so-called Fournier gangrene, is most commonly seen in patients with poorly controlled diabetes mellitus.

Clostridium perfringens is associated with necrotizing cellulitis or myonecrosis in patients who have had wounds contaminated by soil or compromised by the presence of devitalized tissue.

EPIDEMIOLOGY

Erysipelas and cellulitis risks include being overweight, having chronic edema or chronic skin breakdown, and having a prior history of erysipelas or cellulitis.

Necrotizing fasciitis risks include diabetes mellitus and alcoholic liver disease but also may occur in a normal host.

CLINICAL

Erysipelas and cellulitis present with erythema, warmth, tenderness, and varying degrees of edema of the skin and soft tissues. Both are typically associated with fever and chills. Erysipelas produces raised skin with a well-demarcated edge and typically begins with sudden onset and progresses rapidly over hours. Cellulitis begins more gradually, progresses more slowly often over days, and usually has less distinct skin margins. Both have a predilection for the lower legs but may be seen elsewhere depending on the circumstances. Women with chronic arm lymphedema following lymph node dissection for breast cancer may develop cellulitis in the involved arm. Patients who sustain a puncture wound to the hand due to a cat bite or to the antecubital fossa due to intravenous drug use may also develop cellulitis of the involved arm. Cellulitis may involve the abdominal wall in morbidly obese patients without any obvious trauma. Cellulitis may involve the head and neck region as a complication of upper respiratory tract or oral cavity infections.

Patients with necrotizing fasciitis present with severe localizing pain along with fever and tachycardia. The involved area is often initially ecchymotic or faintly erythematous but typically progresses very rapidly over hours to include worsening edema, bullae formation, erythema, and sometimes crepitus.

DIAGNOSIS

The diagnosis of skin and soft tissue infections is largely clinical. All may be associated with signs of increased inflammation such as an elevated C-reactive protein or leukocytosis. Patients with uncomplicated cellulitis may be febrile but rarely have positive blood cultures, whereas these are positive in 60% to 70% of patients with necrotizing fasciitis. Superficial cultures are rarely diagnostic, but surgical specimens obtained in patients with necrotizing fasciitis are helpful in directing antimicrobial therapy.

CT or MRI may be useful in the diagnosis and management of patients with complicated cellulitis where patients have atypical features or are not responding to standard therapy. MRI is useful in the initial diagnosis of necrotizing fasciitis where the diagnosis is not obvious on clinical findings alone.

The primary differential diagnosis of cellulitis includes thrombophlebitis, contact dermatitis, and insect bite reactions.

TREATMENT

Intravenous empiric antibiotic therapy is indicated for hospitalized patients with skin and soft tissue infections. Patients with erysipelas and cellulitis should receive treatment directed against streptococci and staphylococci, including MRSA. Nafcillin and cefazolin are first-line agents with vancomycin or daptomycin given to cover MRSA. Treatment is continued until all signs of active infection have resolved which usually is 10 days but may vary depending on the patient's response to treatment. Patients routinely are transitioned to oral therapy as their situation allows or are discharged on intravenous antibiotics when a prolonged course of parenteral therapy is required.

Patients with necrotizing fasciitis require broad-spectrum empiric antibiotics directed against streptococci and staphylococci as well as gram-negative bacilli and anaerobes. Piperacillin-tazobactam or a carbapenem is typically given initially often along with antistaphylococcal agents. These patients require urgent surgical debridement along with supportive care. Multiple surgical debridements usually are required.

Clindamycin is advocated in the treatment of necrotizing fasciitis to decrease *S. pyogenes* toxin production. As well, clindamycin has been shown to overcome the "Eagle effect" where beta-lactams lose effectiveness due to the large inoculum of organisms in the stationary phase of growth.

Intravenous immunoglobulin infusions have been used in patients with necrotizing fasciitis in an effort to neutralize streptococcal toxins. However, to date, no conclusive benefit has been shown from this therapy.

Hyperbaric oxygen has also been shown in a limited number of observational studies to be additive to standard surgical debridement and antimicrobial therapy in patients with necrotizing fasciitis but is not considered part of routine treatment presently.

PREVENTION

Erysipelas and cellulitis prevention primarily depends on control of risk factors such as chronic venous stasis edema and tinea pedis. Where these persist despite aggressive measures, chronic suppression with penicillin has proven effective.

Necrotizing fasciitis prevention centers around control of risk factors such as optimal control of diabetes and wound care.

SUGGESTED READINGS

Bisno AL, Stevens DL. Streptococcal infections of skin and soft tissues. *N Engl J Med* 1996;334(4):240–245.

Chira S, Miller LG. *Staphylococcus aureus* is the most common identified cause of cellulitis: a systematic review. *Epidemiol Infect* 2010;138(3):313–317.

Corwin P, Toop L, McGeoch G, et al. Randomised controlled trial of intravenous antibiotic treatment for cellulitis at home compared with hospital. *BMJ* 2005;330(7483):129.

Daum RS. Clinical practice. Skin and soft-tissue infections caused by methicillin-resistant *Staphylococcus aureus*. *N Engl J Med* 2007;357(4):380–390.
   This review article provides a summary of current approaches to diagnosis and treatment of MRSA infections involving the skin.

Falagas ME, Vergidis PI. Narrative review: diseases that masquerade as infectious cellulitis. *Ann Intern Med* 2005;142(1):47–55.
   This article discusses the differential diagnosis of skin and soft infections and provides a detail differential.

Gabillot-Carre M, Roujeau JC. Acute bacterial skin infections and cellulitis. *Curr Opin Infect Dis* 2007;20(2):118–123.

Gonzalez MH. Necrotizing fasciitis and gangrene of the upper extremity. *Hand Clin* 1998;14(4):635–645, ix.

Gorwitz RJ, Jernigan DB, Powers JH, et al. Strategies for clinical management of MRSA in the community: summary of an experts' meeting convened by the Centers for Disease Control and Prevention. March 2006. Accessed July 2, 2007, at http://www.cdc.gov/ncidod/dhqp/pdf/ar/CAMRSA_ExpMtgStrategies.pdf
   This consensus document discusses strategies for managing MRSA based on published studies and expert opinion.

Hepburn MJ, Dooley DP, Skidmore PJ, et al. Comparison of short-course (5 days) and standard (10 days) treatment for uncomplicated cellulitis. *Arch Intern Med* 2004;164(15):1669–1674.

Miller LG, Perdreau-Remington F, Rieg G, et al. Necrotizing fasciitis caused by community-associated methicillin-resistant Staphylococcus aureus in Los Angeles. *N Engl J Med* 2005;352(14):1445–1453.

This study described an outbreak of community-acquired MRSA presenting as necrotizing fasciitis. The authors conclude that MRSA should be considered in individuals presenting with fasciitis, especially in areas endemic for community-acquired MRSA infections.

Pertel PE, Eisenstein BI, Link AS, et al. The efficacy and safety of daptomycin vs. vancomycin for the treatment of cellulitis and erysipelas. *Int J Clin Pract* 2009;63(3):368–375.

Seal DV. Necrotizing fasciitis. *Curr Opin Infect Dis* 2001;14(2):127–132.

Wong CH, Wang YS. The diagnosis of necrotizing fasciitis. *Curr Opin Infect Dis* 2005;18(2):101–106.

67 Community-Acquired Pneumonia
Wael E. Shams

I. DEFINITION

Community-acquired pneumonia is an acute infection of the pulmonary parenchyma that is associated with at least some symptoms of acute infection (such as fever, cough, expectoration, or pleuritic chest pain), accompanied by the presence of an acute infiltrate on a chest radiograph or auscultatory findings consistent with pneumonia (such as altered breath sounds or localized rales), in a patient not hospitalized or residing in a long-term care facility for ≥14 days before onset of symptoms.

II. EPIDEMIOLOGY

- Pneumonia ranks first as the cause of death from infection and ninth as the leading cause of death in general in the United States.
- More than 2 million cases of community-acquired pneumonia (CAP) occur each year in the United States, resulting in approximately 10 million physician visits, more than 50,000 deaths, and more than 500,000 hospitalizations, especially among elderly and those with underlying lung disease such as emphysema.

III. ETIOLOGY OF CAP

- CAP may be viral, bacterial, or fungal in etiology; however, a causative pathogen may not be identified in up to 50% to 60% of patients in spite of extensive laboratory testing.
- Etiologic viruses include the influenza viruses, respiratory syncytial virus, adenovirus, parainfluenza virus, herpes simplex virus, human metapneumovirus, and Hantavirus.
- The most commonly encountered bacteria include *Streptococcus pneumoniae* (20% to 60%), *Haemophilus influenzae* (2% to 31%), *Moraxella catarrhalis* (2% to 13%), and "atypical bacteria" such as *Mycoplasma pneumoniae* (13% to 37%), *Chlamydia pneumoniae* (6% to 17%), and the *Legionella* species (1% to 16%).
- Coinfection with atypical bacterial pathogens is estimated to occur in up to 48% of all patients with CAP.
- Enteric gram-negative bacteria are not common etiologies in CAP, yet they may be encountered in particular settings, such as use of alcohol associated with klebsiella pneumoniae, and diabetes mellitus, chronic steroid use, or structural lung disease association with *Pseudomonas aeruginosa*.
- *Pneumocystis jiroveci* (formerly *carinii*) and endemic fungi (*Cryptococcus neoformans, Histoplasma capsulatum, Blastomyces dermatitiditis, Coccidioides immitis*) constitute other etiologic agents that are often dependent on epidemiologic and host factors. The frequency of these pathogens varies with the setting in which the infection was acquired. Variables include the season of the year, geographic location, environmental exposure, and host factors such as age, smoking, alcohol use, and underlying illnesses.

- Similarly, atypical zoonotic pathogens such as *Chlamydia psittaci, Francisella tularensis,* and *Coxiella burnetii* may cause CAP in specific exposure scenarios, particularly, close contact with psittacine birds (psittacosis), deer or rabbits that are infested with ticks (tularemia), and parturient cat or sheep (Q fever), respectively. These zoonoses will be discussed separately in relevant sections, yet their initial presentation may mimic CAP.

IV. CLINICAL FEATURES

- Patients with CAP may present with systemic, nonspecific, pulmonary, or extrapulmonary symptoms.
- Systemic and nonspecific symptoms include fever or hypothermia, rigors, sweats, fatigue, and anorexia. Pulmonary symptoms include new cough with or without sputum production or change in color of respiratory secretions in a patient with chronic cough, chest discomfort, or the onset of dyspnea.
- Extrapulmonary symptoms may include headache, myalgias, earache, abdominal pain, and diarrhea. Atypical pathogens have been classically linked to extrapulmonary symptoms, for example, diarrhea, abdominal pain, and myalgia with *Legionella pneumophila*, headache and myalgia with *C. pneumoniae*, and earache with *M. pneumoniae*.
- Findings on exam include documentation of fever or hypothermia, tachypnea, tachycardia, hypotension, cyanosis, or even septic shock in severe cases with overwhelming infection. Local findings include diminished intensity of breath sounds over affected lung areas with bronchial quality of breath sounds, and crackles may be heard.

V. DIAGNOSIS

- Diagnosis is suggested by the clinical features and documented by the presence of new infiltrates on routine chest x-ray.
- Determination of the severity of pneumonia is important in order to plan the site of care, further laboratory workup, and treatment. The pneumonia PORT (pneumonia outcomes research team) severity index (PSI), or the modified British Thoracic Society (BTS) criteria are best used for this purpose. The PSI classifies patients in five mortality risk classes and advises outpatient therapy for classes I and II, management in an observational unit or short hospital stay for class III, and inpatient treatment for classes IV and V, respectively (Table 67-1).
- The modified BTS criteria identified five indicators of increased mortality including confusion (based on a specific mental test or disorientation to person, place, or time), BUN level >20 mg/dL, respiratory rate ≥30 breaths/minute, low blood pressure (systolic, <90 mm Hg; or diastolic, ≤60 mm Hg), and age ≥65 years with the acronym CURB-65. Patients with CURB-65 score of ≥2 should be admitted to hospital, and those with ≥3 should be managed in ICU setting.
- While a chest x-ray or other imaging technique is usually required to confirm the diagnosis of CAP, the low yield and infrequent positive impact on clinical care argue against the use of further tests for patients who will be treated on outpatient basis.
- Patients who will be treated in the hospital, especially those with severe pneumonia or comorbidities such as asplenia, chronic liver disease, active alcohol use, leukopenia, lung cavitation, pleural effusion, and patients who had recent travel, would benefit from further testing. Determination of the specific pathogen causing pneumonia in these settings will guide and may alter empiric therapy.

Table 67-1	Point Scoring System for Step 2 of the Prediction

Rule for Assignment to Risk Classes II, III, IV, and V.

Characteristic	Points Assigned[a]
Demographic factor	
Age	
Men	Age (year)
Women	Age (year) −10
Nursing home resident	+10
Coexisting illnesses[b]	
Neoplastic disease	+30
Liver disease	+20
Congestive heart failure	+10
Cerebrovascular disease	+10
Renal disease	+10
Physical examination findings	
Altered mental status[c]	+20
Respiratory rate ≥30/minute	+20
Systolic blood pressure ≤90 mm Hg	+20
Temperature <35°C or ≥40°C	+15
Pulse ≥125/minute	+10
Laboratory and radiographic findings	
Arterial pH <7.35	+30
Blood urea nitrogen ≥30 mg/dL	+20
Sodium <130 mmol/L	+20
Glucose ≥250 mg/dl (14 mmol/L)	+10
Hematocrit <30%	+10
Partial pressure of arterial oxygen <60 mm Hg[d]	+10
Pleural effusion	+10

[a]A total point score for a given patient is obtained by summing the patient's age in years (age—10 for women) and the points for each applicable characteristic. The points assigned to each predictor variable were based on coefficients obtained from the logistic regression model used in step 2 of the prediction rule (see the Methods section).

[b]Neoplastic disease is defined as any cancer except basal or squamous cell cancer of the skin that was active at the time of presentation or diagnosed within 1 year of presentation. Liver disease is defined as a clinical or histologic diagnosis of cirrhosis or another form of chronic liver disease, such as chronic active hepatitis. Congestive heart failure is defined as systolic or diastolic ventricular dysfunction documented by history, physical examination, and chest radiograph, echocardiogram, multiple-gated acquisition scan, or left ventriculogram. Cerebrovascular disease is defined as a clinical diagnosis of stroke or transient ischemic attack or stroke documented by magnetic resonance imaging or computed tomography. Renal disease is defined as a history of chronic renal disease or abnormal blood urea nitrogen and creatinine concentrations documented in the medical record.

[c]Altered mental status is defined as disorientation with respect to person, place, or time that is not known to be chronic, stupor, or coma.

[d]In the pneumonia PORT cohort study, an oxygen saturation of <90% percent on pulse oximetry or intubation before admission was also considered abnormal.

- Laboratory tests include pretreatment blood cultures, expectorated sputum for gram stain and culture, urine testing for *S. pneumoniae* and *L. pneumophila* antigens, and influenza A and B antigen screen during applicable season.
- Patients not responding to conventional therapy or presenting with complicated CAP may be considered for bronchoscopy, where bronchoalveolar lavage (BAL) specimens can be obtained. Various cultures for viral, bacterial, and fungal etiologies as well as PCR and DFA (direct fluorescent antibody) testing for specific pathogens can be set up from BAL samples.
- A direct transthoracic fine needle aspiration (FNA) may also be considered for patients with upper lobe pathology that may not be readily accessible by bronchoscopy.

VI. TREATMENT

- In addition to the severity of illness as determined the PSI or the CURB-65, the decision to hospitalize the patient should be based on assessment of preexisting conditions that may compromise the safety of homecare and clinical judgment.
- Direct admission to the ICU is also required for patients with septic shock requiring vasopressors or with acute respiratory failure requiring intubation and mechanical ventilation.
- The Infectious Disease Society of America (IDSA) and the American Thoracic Society (ATS) strongly recommend locally adapted guidelines to be developed and implemented in the management of CAP. These should take into account local care variables, relevant clinical outcomes, and local trends in antimicrobial resistance. Table 67-2 provides an example of locally adapted guidelines for the management of CAP among outpatients and inpatients.

VII. PROGNOSIS

- Most patients with CAP will recover well. Mortality among cases treated as outpatient are <1%, while inpatients have mortality rate that varies and may reach as high as 40% among elderly patients with comorbidities.

VIII. COMPLICATIONS

- Complications of pneumonia include respiratory failure, sepsis, lung abscess, and empyema.
- Comorbidities such as intrinsic lung disease, for example, COPD and lung tumor, immune deficiency status, diabetes mellitus, renal failure, liver cirrhosis, and poor dentition with witnessed aspiration may all contribute to these complications and select for certain pathogens.

IX. PREVENTION

- Prevention of CAP should be focused on smoking cessation and vaccination.
- Pneumococcal polyvalent polysaccharide vaccine is indicated for prophylaxis in patients ≥65 years of age and younger adults if they have risk factors such as heart disease, lung disease, kidney disease, alcoholism, diabetes, cirrhosis, sickle cell disease, splenectomized patients, and immune deficiency status, for example, HIV, and chronic steroid therapy. A conjugated, polyvalent pneumococcal vaccine has

Table 67-2 Model Antibiotic Selection Guide for Community-Acquired Pneumonia

Treatment Setting	Patient Type	First Line	Second Line	Alternative/ 3rd Line	Penicillin Allergic[a]	History of MRSA
Outpatient treatment	Previously healthy/*no* use of antimicrobials[b] in previous 3 months	Azithromycin	Doxycycline		Same as 1st or 2nd line	Doxycycline
	Presence of comorbidities[b] or use of antimicrobials in previous 3 months[c]	Amox-clav **or** cefuroxime **plus** azithromycin	Levofloxacin	Amox-clav **or** cefuroxime **plus** doxycycline	Same as 2nd line	Amox-clav **or** cefuroxime **or** levofloxacin **plus** doxycycline or SMZ/TMP
Inpatient, non-ICU[d]		Ceftriaxone **plus** azithromycin	Levofloxacin	Amp-sulb **plus** azithromycin	Same as 2nd line **or** vancomycin **plus** aztreonam **plus** azithromycin	Vancomycin **plus** 1st, 2nd, **or** 3rd line, **or** vancomycin **plus** aztreonam **plus** azithromycin
Inpatient, ICU[d]		Ceftriaxone **plus** azithromycin	Ceftriaxone **plus** levofloxacin	Pip-tazo **plus** azithromycin	levofloxacin **plus** aztreonam	Vancomycin **plus** 1st, 2nd, **or** 3rd line, **or** vancomycin **plus** aztreonam **plus** azithromycin
Special considerations	*P. aeruginosa* suspected[e]	Pip-tazo **plus** levofloxacin	Cefepime[f] **plus** levofloxacin	Pip-tazo **or** cefepime **plus** tobra[g] **plus** azithromycin	aztreonam **plus** tobra[g] **plus** levofloxacin	
	ESBL+ organism flagged, colonized, or infected	Ertapenem[f] **plus** azithromycin	Ertapenem[f] **plus** levofloxacin		Tigecycline[f] **plus** tobra[g]	
	Polymicrobial pneumonia complicating influenza	**Add** oseltamivir to selected antibacterial regimen				Vancomycin plus 1st or 2nd line

[a]Patients with a remote history of mild adverse reaction due to penicillin (e.g., skin rash) may receive cephalosporins or carbapenems; patients with history of serious allergic reaction to penicillin (e.g., breathing difficulties, swollen mucous membranes, SJS) should not receive penicillins, cephalosporins, or carbapenems but may receive aztreonam.

[b]Comorbidities include chronic heart, lung, liver, or renal disease; diabetes mellitus; alcoholism; malignancies; asplenia; immunosuppressing conditions; or drug therapy.

[c]Use a different class of antibiotic than the one the patient was previously treated with.

[d]For a witnessed aspiration, substitute amp-sulb or pip-tazo for ceftriaxone in non-ICU and ICU patients, respectively.

[e]Risk factors for *P. aeruginosa* include severe structural lung disease (e.g., advanced COPD/bronchiectasis), exposure to quinolones within the previous 3 months, chronic steroid therapy, and diabetes mellitus.

[f]Requires nonformulary consult

[g]If tobramycin is used, give one dose at 5mg/kg and then ask clinical pharmacist to adjust and redose according to patient-specific parameters.

- Amoxicillin-clavulanate 875 mg PO BID
- Ampicillin-sulbactam 3 gm IV q6hours
- Aztreonam 1 to 2 gm IV q8hours
- Azithromycin 500 mg IV qday
- Cefepime 1 to 2 gm IV q12hours
- Ceftriaxone 1 gm qday
- Cefuroxime 500 mg PO BID
- Doxycycline 100 mg PO/IV q12hours
- Ertapenem 1 gm IV qday
- Levofloxacin 750 mg IV qday
- Oseltamivir 75 mg PO BID
- Piperacillin-tazobactam 3.375 gm IV q6hours
- Sulfamethoxazole-trimethoprim (SMZ/TMP) 1 DS tab PO BID
- Tigecycline 50 mg IV q12hrs
- Tobramycin 5 mg/kg IV once[g]
- Vancomycin 15 mg/kg IV q12 to 24 hours

been recently approved for individuals >50 years of age as well. The CDC also recommends that smokers age 19 to 64 also receive the vaccine. Influenza vaccination during the influenza season also help to prevent CAP.

SUGGESTED READINGS

Bartlett JG, Dowell SF, Mandell LA, et al. Practice guidelines for the management of community-acquired pneumonia in adults. Infectious Diseases Society of America. *Clin Infect Dis* 2000;31:347–382.

Centers for Disease Control. http://www.cdc.gov/nchs/fastats/pneumonia.htm

Fine MJ, Auble TE, Yealy DM, et al. A prediction rule to identify low-risk patients with community-acquired pneumonia. *N Engl J Med* 1997;336:243–250.

This publication describes a prediction rule that effectively identifies individuals with CAP with low risk for complications.

Fry AM, Shay DK, Holman RC, et al. Trends in hospitalizations for pneumonia among persons aged 65 years or older in the United States, 1988–2002. *JAMA* 2005;294:2712–2719.

Gotfried MH. Epidemiology of clinically diagnosed community-acquired pneumonia in the primary care setting: results from the 1999-2000 respiratory surveillance program. *Am J Med* 2001;111:25S–29S; discussion 36S–38S.

Lim WS, van der Eerden MM, Laing R, et al. Defining community acquired pneumonia severity on presentation to hospital: an international derivation and validation study. *Thorax* 2003;58:377–382.

Mandell L, Bartlett J, Dowell S, et al. Update of practice guidelines for the management of community-acquired pneumonia in immunocompetent adults. *Clin Infect Dis* 2003;37:1405–1433.

Mandell LA, Wunderink RG, Anzueto A, et al. Infectious Diseases Society of America/American Thoracic Society consensus guidelines on the management of community-acquired pneumonia in adults. *Clin Infect Dis* 2007;44(suppl 2):S27–S72.

These consensus guidelines outline the management of CAP in adults and provide a reasonable framework for clinical care. Risk stratification is discussed.

Nair GB, Niederman MS. Community-acquired pneumonia: an unfinished battle. *Med Clin North Am* 2011;95(6):1143–1161.

Neill AM, Martin IR, Weir R, et al. Community acquired pneumonia: aetiology and usefulness of severity criteria on admission. *Thorax* 1996;51:1010–1016.

Ruiz M, Ewig S, Marcos MA, et al. Etiology of community-acquired pneumonia: impact of age, comorbidity, and severity. *Am J Respir Crit Care Med* 1999;397–405.

Shams W, Evans ME. Guide to selection of fluoroquinolones in patients with lower respiratory tract infections. *Drugs* 2005;65(7):949–991.

Watkins RR, Lemonovich TL. Diagnosis and management of community-acquired pneumonia in adults. *Am Fam Physician* 2011;83(11):1299–1306.

Woodhead MA, Macfarlane JT, McCracken JS, et al. Prospective study of the aetiology and outcome of pneumonia in the community. *Lancet* 1987;1(8534):671–674.

Antimicrobial dosing regimen considering normal renal function (call clinical pharmacist for dosing assistance in patients with renal dysfunction)

68 Prosthetic Joint Infections

Evgenia Kagan, Cassandra D. Salgado, and Camelia E. Marculescu

BACKGROUND

- The number of patients who undergo joint replacement surgery continues to increase. It has been projected that almost 3.5 million total knee arthroplasties will have been performed by 2030.
- Prosthetic joint infections (PJIs) have been associated with significant morbidity and may lead to poor functional outcomes. For primary joint replacement surgeries, infection rates are <1% for hip and shoulder prostheses, <2% for knee prostheses, and <9% for elbow prostheses; however, infection rates associated with revision procedures are as high as 20%.
- Risk factors for PJI include a history of rheumatoid arthritis, psoriasis, immunosuppression (either through medication or illness), poor nutritional status, obesity, diabetes mellitus, age of 70 years or older, presence of a malignancy and history of previous joint arthroplasty.
- Inoculation of microorganisms into the surgical wound most commonly occurs during the perioperative period (during surgery or immediately thereafter); however, hematogenous spread from a distant site of infection or contiguous spread from an adjacent site of infection may occur.

CLINICAL PRESENTATION AND DIAGNOSIS

- Infections may present as a superficial cellulitis, an abscess, or more deep seated involving the joint space. PJI are classified as early (<3 months after surgery), usually caused by highly virulent organisms (*Staphylococcus aureus* or gram-negative bacilli); delayed (3 to 24 months after surgery), usually caused by less virulent organisms (coagulase-negative staphylococci or *Propionibacterium acnes*); and late (more than 24 months after surgery), predominantly caused by hematogenous seeding.
- Early infection may present with acute onset of fever, joint pain, effusion, erythema, and warmth at the implant site. Clinically significant cellulitis and formation of a sinus tract with purulent discharge may also occur.
- Delayed infection usually presents with more subtle signs and symptoms such as implant loosening and persistent joint pain. Infection is often difficult to distinguish from aseptic failure and often a combination of preoperative and intraoperative tests are necessary for accurate diagnosis.
- Peripheral leukocyte count with differential may be normal or slightly elevated in the presence of infection.
- Low sensitivity C-reactive protein is almost always elevated surrounding surgery and typically returns to normal within weeks. Repetitive measurements establishing a pattern with clinical correlation are often more informative than a single value.

- Synovial fluid analysis is encouraged as a rapid, accurate test for differentiating infection from aseptic failure. Leukocyte count and differential values for diagnosing PJI are considerably lower than those for septic arthritis in native joints. In patients without underlying inflammatory joint conditions, a synovial fluid leukocyte count of >1,700 per cubic millimeter or >65% neutrophils is 94% to 97% sensitive and 88% to 98% specific for diagnosing PJI.

- Histopathologic diagnosis requires the presence of 1 to 10 or more neutrophils per high-power field (magnification of 400) and has a sensitivity of more than 80% and a specificity of more than 90% for diagnosis of PJI.

- Gram staining of synovial fluid and periprosthetic tissue for microbiologic diagnosis when positive has a specificity of >97%; however, if negative, a sensitivity of only 25%. Periprosthetic tissue cultures remain the most reliable means of diagnosing PJI and identifying the associated organism(s). At least three intraoperative tissue specimens should be sampled for culture. Superficial wound or sinus tract cultures should be avoided as they are often positive for colonization of surrounding skin. Periprosthetic cultures may be negative due to a low number of microorganisms, fastidious organisms, improper culturing technique or laboratory methods, or because of prior antimicrobial exposure. When possible, antimicrobial therapy should be discontinued for 2 weeks before tissue culturing to better detect low-grade infection (typically presents only with early loosening of the prosthesis and persistent pain, often without systemic or local clinical signs of infection).

- Plain radiographs may help diagnose infection, especially when done serially over time after implantation. Prosthesis loosening will appear as new subperiosteal bone growth. Transcortical sinus tracts are specific for infection. Implant migration and periprosthetic osteolysis can also occur without infection and thus expert opinion is often necessary for diagnosis. Arthrography is useful for detecting implant loosening, pseudobursae, and abscesses.

- Criteria for diagnosis of PJI include (1) isolation of the same organism in at least two cultures of synovial fluid or periprosthetic tissue, (2) purulence of synovial fluid at the implant site, (3) acute inflammation on histopathologic examination of periprosthetic tissue, or (4) presence of a sinus tract communicating with the prosthesis.

SURGICAL MANAGEMENT

- Management of PJI requires a multidisciplinary approach that includes adequate surgical debridement combined with long-term antimicrobial therapy. Eradicating the infection and improving the functional status of the joint is the ultimate goal of therapy. Often, a patient's comorbidities prohibit surgical intervention and thus medical treatment alone may be justified. Often in this clinical scenario, lifelong antibiotic suppression is utilized.

- Several surgical modalities exist for management of PJI and include debridement with retention of the prosthesis; a one-stage exchange where the infected prosthesis is removed and a new one implanted during the same surgery; a two-stage exchange where a resection arthroplasty is performed with delayed reimplantation during a second surgery; resection arthroplasty with or without arthrodesis; and amputation.

- Zimmerli and colleagues developed a validated treatment algorithm that has been associated with an overall success rate of more than 80%.

- Debridement with retention is a reasonable option for patients with early or acute hematogenous infection and the duration of symptoms is <3 weeks, the implant is stable, the soft tissue is in good condition, and an agent with activity against the organisms in the biofilm is available.

- If the duration of symptoms exceeds 3 weeks, retention of the implant is not advisable. A one-stage exchange is possible if the soft tissues are in good condition, there are no severe coexisting medical illnesses, and the organism(s) is readily treatable. In patients with compromised soft tissue, a two-stage exchange is preferred. After removal of the hardware, a spacer or external-fixation device is inserted to maintain the length of the extremity. Antibiotics are then administered until the new hardware is inserted. If possible, it is preferable to discontinue antibiotics 2 weeks prior to reinsertion so that reliable cultures may be obtained for determining duration of therapy.
- Permanent explantation or joint arthrodesis is usually performed in severely immunocompromised patients and in patients who would not have any functional benefit from arthroplasty.

MEDICAL MANAGEMENT

- Empiric antibiotic therapy is necessary when a patient with PJI presents with sepsis or complicated soft tissue infection and is thus not clinically stable enough to await the culture and sensitivity results. In this situation, the timing of infection (early, delayed, or late) may help with choosing an antibiotic regimen. In general, broader spectrum regimens are initially required to empirically cover for resistant gram-positive as well as gram-negative organisms.
- Definitive antimicrobial therapy should be directed toward the susceptibility pattern of the pathogen or pathogens isolated from appropriately obtained cultures. Table 68.1 offers recommended agents for specific organisms in the treatment of PJI.
- In staphylococcal PJI, rifampin is often used in combination with another active antibiotic as it has demonstrated activity for surface-adhering, slow-growing, and biofilm-producing microorganisms. It is important to note however that staphylococci may develop resistance to rifampin in rapid fashion and thus should never be used as monotherapy.

Table 68-1	Antimicrobial Therapy Options for Select Microorganisms in Adults with PJI[a]	
Microorganism	**Recommended**	**Alternative**
Methicillin-susceptible *Staphylococcus spp.*	IV Nafcillin 1.5–2 g every 4 hours or IV Cefazolin 1–2 g every 8 hours	IV Vancomycin 15 mg/kg every 12 hours or Oral or IV Levofloxacin 500–750 mg every 24 hours plus oral rifampin 300–400 mg every 12 hours[b]
Methicillin-resistant *Staphylococcus spp.*	IV Vancomycin 15 mg/kg every 12 hours	Oral or IV Linezolid 600 mg every 12 hours or Oral or IV Levofloxacin 500–750 mg every 24 hours plus oral rifampin 300–400 mg every 12 hours[b]

(Continued)

Table 68-1	Antimicrobial Therapy Options for Select Microorganisms in Adults with PJI[a] (Continued)	

Microorganism	Recommended	Alternative
Penicillin-susceptible *Enterococcus* spp[c]	IV penicillin G 20–24 million units over 24 hours continuous infusion or in six divided doses or IV Ampicillin 12 g over 24 hours continuous infusion or in six divided doses	IV Vancomycin 15 mg/kg every 12 hours
Penicillin-resistant *Enterococcus* spp[c]	IV Vancomycin 15 mg/kg every 12 hours	Oral or IV Linezolid 600 mg every 12 hours
Pseudomonas aeruginosa[d]	IV Cefepime 1–2 g every 12 hours or IV Meropenem 1 g every 8 hours or IV Imipenem 500 mg every 6–8 hours	Ciprofloxacin 750 mg oral or 400 mg IV every 12 hours or IV Ceftazidime 2 g every 8 hours
Enterobacter spp.	IV Meropenem 1 g every 8 hours or IV Imipenem 500 mg every 6–8 hours	IV Cefepime 1–2 g every 12 hours or Ciprofloxacin 750 mg oral or 400 mg IV every 12 hours
beta-hemolytic streptococci	IV penicillin G 20–24 million units over 24 hours continuous infusion or in six divided doses or IV Ceftriaxone 1–2 g every 24 hours	IV Vancomycin 15 mg/kg every 12 hours
Propionibacterium acnes and *Corynebacterium* spp.	IV penicillin G 20–24 million units over 24 hours continuous infusion or in six divided doses or IV Ceftriaxone 1–2 g every 24 hours or IV Vancomycin 15 mg/kg every 12 hours	IV Clindamycin 600–900 mg every 8 hours

[a]Dose based on normal renal and hepatic function.
[b]Levofloxacin–rifampin combination therapy for patients managed by debridement with retention. If organism is susceptible, co-trimoxazole or minocycline may be substituted.
[c]Addition of aminoglycoside for bactericidal synergy is optional.
[d]Addition of an aminoglycoside is optional.
Modified from Sia IG, Berbari EF, Karchmer AW. Prosthetic joint infections. *Infect Dis Clin North Am* 2005;19:885–914, with permission from Elsevier.

- Use of vancomycin, typically reserved for treatment of resistant gram-positive organisms or for patients with beta-lactam allergies, requires knowledge of dosing parameters to achieve appropriate trough levels. Serum vancomycin trough concentrations should be >10 mg/L to prevent the development of resistance, and generally levels of 15 to 20 mg/L are recommended if the minimum inhibitory concentration (MIC) of the organisms is 1 mg/L or higher.
- The implications of an increased vancomycin MIC for treatment of musculoskeletal infections is not well described but successful outcomes of therapy with vancomycin for methicillin-resistant staphylococcus aureus (MRSA) PJI have been inversely correlated to the vancomycin MIC. Alternative agents with activity against MRSA include linezolid, daptomycin, telavancin, trimethoprim–sulfamethoxazole, clindamycin, ceftaroline, and tigecycline.
- Duration of therapy has not been standardized; however, most clinicians familiar with the treatment of PJI generally recommend a several week course of intravenous antibiotics followed by oral suppression for 3 to 6 months. Zimmerli and colleagues suggest treatment duration for 3 months for infected hip prostheses and 6 months for infected knee prostheses.
- Long-term suppressive antimicrobial therapy (usually oral agents) is an option for patients in whom surgery is contraindicated or not desired. The goal of suppressive antibiotic therapy is to control symptoms and not to cure the infection.
- In summary, treatment of PJI requires consideration of the timing, virulence, and antimicrobial susceptibilities of the microorganism(s) involved, side effects of antimicrobial therapy, and condition of the host. When possible, treatment of these patients should be done under the guidance of an infectious disease specialist in close collaboration with the orthopedic surgeon.

PREVENTION

- Recommendations for prevention of surgical site infections have been published. Perioperative antimicrobial prophylaxis, directed toward organisms that may be introduced into the surgical site in the operating room, is recommended. Cefazolin has specifically been shown to reduce the risk of PJI. For obese patients, appropriate dosing of perioperative systemic antimicrobials is very important. For patients with beta-lactam or cephalosporin allergies, prophylaxis with vancomycin or clindamycin is recommended. Vancomycin prophylaxis should also be considered when known outbreaks of infection due to MRSA are occurring in an institution, when there are high endemic rates of MRSA surgical site infection, or in patient populations at high risk for MRSA colonization and infection.
- Other infection control measures have been designed to specifically address prevention of MRSA. These include transmission-based approaches such as (1) system-wide behavioral change strategies to promote adherence to hand hygiene, (2) enhanced environmental and equipment disinfection, and (3) active surveillance to identify patients harboring MRSA in order to utilize barrier precautions. Additionally, patient-centered approaches designed to prevent infection in the known colonized individual include MRSA decolonization regimens. The optimal regimen has yet to be described; however, most experts would recommend the use of topical agents such as intranasal mupirocin and chlorhexidine bathing. In certain circumstances, systemic antibiotics known to be active against the patient's MRSA isolate are used in combination with topical agents.

- Prevention strategies targeting procedure-related issues include the use of antimicrobial impregnated bone cements and placement of antimicrobial beads into the infected joint space. Additionally, modifiable patient-related risk factors for prevention of surgical site infection include perioperative blood glucose control (particularly for patients with diabetes), and minimizing immunosuppressive medications whenever possible.

SUGGESTED READINGS

Atkins BL, Athanasou N, Deeks JJ, et al. Prospective evaluation of criteria for microbiological diagnosis of prosthetic-joint infection at revision arthroplasty. *J Clin Microbiol* 1998;36:2932–2939.

Berbari EF, Hanssen AD, Duffy MC, et al. Risk factors for prosthetic joint infections: case control study. *Clin Infect Dis* 1998;27:1247–1254.

Goyal N, Aggarwal V, Parvizi J. Methicillin-resistant Staphylococcus aureus screening in total joint arthroplasty: a worthwhile endeavor. *J Knee Surg* 2012;25:37–43.

Herbert C, Robicsek A. Decolonization therapy in infection control. *Curr Opin Infect Dis* 2010;23:340–345.

Lentino JR. Prosthetic joint infections: bane of orthopedists, challenge for infectious disease specialists. *Clin Infect Dis* 2003;36:1157e61.

Mangram AJ, Horan TC, Pearson ML, et al. The Hospital Infection Control Practices Advisory Committee. Guideline for prevention of surgical site infection, 1999. *Infect Control Hosp Epidemiol* 1999;20:247–280.

Marculescu CE, Berbari EF, Hanssen AD, et al. Outcome of prosthetic joint infections treated with debridement and retention of components. *Clin Infect Dis* 2006;42:471–478.

Osmon DR, Hanssen AD, Patel R. Prosthetic joint infection: criteria for future definitions. *Clin Orthop Relat Res* 2005;437:89–90.

Sakoulas G, Moise-Broder PA, Schentag J, et al. Relationship of MIC and bactericidal activity to efficacy of vancomycin for treatment of methicillin-resistant Staphylococcus aureus. *J Clin Microbiol* 2004;42:2398–2402.

Sia IG, Berbari EF, Karchmer AW. Prosthetic joint infections. *Infect Dis Clin North Am* 2005;19:885–914.

Steckelberg JM, Osmon DR. Prosthetic joint infection. In: Bisno AL, Waldvogel FA, eds. 3rd ed. Washington, DC: *Am Soc Microbiol* 2000:173–209.

Trampuz A, Hanssen AD, Osmon DR, et al. Synovial fluid leukocyte count and differential for the diagnosis of prosthetic knee infection. *Am J Med* 2004;117:556–562.

Trampuz A, Steckelberg JM, Osmon DR, et al. Advances in the laboratory diagnosis of prosthetic joint infection. *Rev Med Microbiol* 2003;14:1–14.

Trampuz A, Zimmerli W. Prosthetic joint infections: update in diagnosis and treatment. *Swiss Med Wkly* 2005;135(17–18):243–251

Zimmerli W, Trampuz A, Ochsner PE. Prosthetic-joint infections. *N Engl J Med* 2004;351: 1645–1654.

69 Neutropenic Fever

Susan Harwell, Ashley Tyler, and Christopher Trabue

INTRODUCTION

With the advent of cytotoxic chemotherapy for both acute leukemia and solid organ tumors over the past half century, the landscape on oncologic medicine has dramatically changed. However, with improved survival rates and the prospect of cure also came the potential for overwhelming and sometimes fatal infection in the context of neutropenia. Guidelines for both the prevention and management of such infections have been developed and serve to provide a framework for the evaluation and treatment of these patients.

BACKGROUND/EPIDEMIOLOGY

I. DEFINITIONS

    a. Fever is defined as temperature ≥100.5°F.

    b. Neutropenia is defined as an absolute neutrophil count (ANC) ≤500 cells/mL or trend toward neutropenia.

II. MICROBIOLOGY

    a. Bacteriology has fluctuated wildly over the past five decades.

    b. Although gram-positive bacteria, including *Staphylococcus aureus* and coagulase-negative staphylococci, historically caused the majority of bloodstream infections in the 1980s and 1990s, gram-negative pathogens including multidrug-resistant gram-negative bacilli/extended spectrum beta-lactamase (ESBL)-producing gram-negative bacilli have emerged over the last decade.

    c. Common gram-positive pathogens in neutropenic patients

        i. Coagulase-negative staphylococci, including *Staphylococcus lugdunensis*

        ii. *S. aureus*, including methicillin-resistant *Staphylococcus aureus* (MRSA)

        iii. *Enterococcus* species, including vancomycin-resistant *Enterococcus* (VRE)

        iv. Viridans group streptococci

        v. *Streptococcus pneumoniae*

        vi. *Streptococcus pyogenes*

    d. Common gram-negative pathogens in neutropenic patients

        i. *Escherichia coli*

        ii. *Klebsiella pneumoniae*

        iii. *Enterobacter cloacae*

        iv. *Pseudomonas aeruginosa*

        v. *Acinetobacter* species

        vi. *Stenotrophomonas maltophilia*

e. Fungal pathogens

   i. *Aspergillus* species remain the most common cause of invasive fungal infection in neutropenic cancer patients.

   ii. Other common fungal pathogens in neutropenic cancer patients

      1. *Candida* species (including *Candida albicans* and non-*albicans* species such as *Candida krusei, Candida glabrata*, and *Candida tropicalis*)

      2. *Fusarium* species

      3. Agents of mucormycosis

PRINCIPLES OF THERAPY

I. FEVER DURING NEUTROPENIA IS ALWAYS CONSIDERED A MEDICAL EMERGENCY.

II. FEVER DURING NEUTROPENIA IS ALWAYS CONSIDERED AS DUE TO INFECTION, UNTIL PROVEN OTHERWISE.

III. NEUTROPENIC HOSTS OFTEN DO NOT DISPLAY SIGNS OR SYMPTOMS OF INFECTION.

IV. NEUTROPENIC HOSTS ARE UNIQUELY SUSCEPTIBLE TO ORDINARILY MUNDANE OR TRIVIAL INFECTIONS.

ASSESSMENT OF RISK

I. ALL CANCER PATIENTS WITH NEUTROPENIC FEVER SHOULD UNDERGO RISK ASSESSMENT TO DETERMINE LEVEL OF CARE, VENUE OF TREATMENT, EXTENT OF DIAGNOSTIC EVALUATION, AND SELECTION AND ROUTE OF EMPIRICAL ANTIBIOTIC THERAPY.

II. THE MULTINATIONAL ASSOCIATION FOR SUPPORTIVE CARE IN CANCER (MASCC) SCORING SYSTEM IS A USEFUL TOOL FOR DEFINING RISK IN SUCH PATIENTS (TABLE 69-1).

   a. MASCC score of <21 → High risk

   b. MASCC score of ≥21 → Low risk

III. HIGH-RISK PATIENTS (MASCC SCORE <21) INCLUDE THOSE WITH:

   a. Anticipated prolonged (>7 days duration) neutropenia

   b. Profound neutropenia (ANC ≤100 cells/mm^3) following cytotoxic chemotherapy

   c. Significant medical comorbid conditions, including

      i. Hypotension

      ii. Pneumonia

      iii. New-onset abdominal pain

      iv. Neurologic changes

Table 69-1	Multinational Association for Supportive Care in Cancer (MASCC)

Criteria	Score
Burden of disease: asymptomatic or mild illness	5
Normotensive: systolic blood pressure >90 mm Hg	5
No history of chronic obstructive pulmonary disease (COPD)	4
No history of previous invasive fungal infection	4
Normovolemic	3
Burden of disease: moderate illness	3
Outpatient	3
Age <60 years	2

Adapted from Klastersky, Paesmans M, Rubenstein EB, et al. The Multinational Association for Supportive Care in Cancer risk index: a multinational scoring system for identifying low-risk febrile neutropenic cancer patients. *J Clin Oncol* 2000;18(16):3038–3051.

      v. Oral or gastrointestinal mucositis that interferes with swallowing or causes severe diarrhea

      vi. Hepatic impairment

  IV. Low-risk patients (MASCC score ≥21) include those with

      a. Anticipated brief (≤7 days) duration of neutropenia

      b. No or few comorbidities

DIAGNOSTIC EVALUATION

I. THE DIAGNOSTIC EVALUATION SHOULD BEGIN WITH A THOROUGH HISTORY AND PHYSICAL EXAMINATION, WITH SPECIAL ATTENTION TO

  a. Skin, mucous membranes, and wounds if surgery has recently been performed

  b. Intravascular devices and catheters

  c. Gastrointestinal tract and intra-abdominal sources

  d. Genitourinary tract

  e. Lungs

II. INITIAL TESTS SHOULD INCLUDE

  a. Complete blood count with differential leukocyte count

  b. Serum electrolytes, blood urea nitrogen, and creatinine

  c. Hepatic function panel

  d. Two sets of blood cultures; if a central venous catheter is present, blood should also be collected from each lumen.

  e. Chest radiograph

III. MORE FOCUSED TESTING MAY ENSUE BASED ON THE INITIAL CLINICAL EVALUATION

MANAGEMENT

I. HIGH-RISK PATIENTS WITH MASCC SCORE OF <21, ANTICIPATED DURATION OF NEUTROPENIA OF <7 DAYS, SIGNIFICANT COMORBIDITIES, OR CLINICAL INSTABILITY SHOULD BE HOSPITALIZED.

II. GENERAL MEASURES

a. Hand hygiene should be maintained for all patients hospitalized with neutropenic fever and remains the most effective means of preventing infection.

b. There are no specific policies for isolation of neutropenic patients; isolation of such patients should be in line with institutional policies and guidelines.

c. Although standard protocol for neutropenic patients, the "neutropenic diet" with avoidance of luncheon meats and raw vegetables has not been shown to reduce rates of infection or mortality.

d. Careful attention to skin care and oral care with daily showers, dental hygiene, and routine examination of mucous membranes, IV catheter sites, and perineum should be undertaken.

e. Plants and flowers should not be allowed in neutropenic patients' rooms due to potential harboring of invasive molds.

III. ANTIBIOTIC THERAPY FOR NEUTROPENIC FEVER

a. For most high-risk patients, monotherapy with an antipseudomonal beta-lactam agent will suffice for initial therapy (Table 69-2).

b. Indications for initial empiric coverage of gram-positive organisms

   i. Hemodynamic instability or severe sepsis

   ii. Pneumonia

   iii. Positive blood culture for gram (+) bacteria with pending susceptibility

   iv. Suspected central venous catheter–related infection

   v. Skin or soft tissue infection

   vi. Colonization with MRSA, VRE, or penicillin-resistant *S. pneumoniae*

   vii. Severe mucositis if receiving fluoroquinolone prophylaxis or recent ceftazidime therapy

c. For low-risk patients able to take and absorb oral antibiotics, oral ciprofloxacin plus amoxicillin-clavulanate is recommended; the patient should also be observed in clinic 4 to 24 hours to ensure tolerability of antibiotics and clinical stability.

IV. MODIFICATION OF ANTIMICROBIAL THERAPY

a. Changes to antibiotic therapy should be based primarily on clinical data, response to therapy, and microbiology.

b. Unexplained fever alone should not alone prompt changes to empiric therapy if the patient remains clinically stable.

c. Gram-positive coverage may be stopped after 2 days if there is no clinical or microbiologic indication to continue treatment.

Table 69-2	Antimicrobial Therapy for Febrile Neutropenia—High Risk	

	Antimicrobial Treatment	Comments
Broad-spectrum monotherapy. (Includes coverage of *Pseudomonas aeruginosa*)	Piperacillin-tazobactam Cefepime	Ceftazidime no longer recommended due to decreased activity vs. gram (−) bacteria and lack of coverage of gram (+) bacteria, including *Streptococcus species*
	Meropenem, imipenem, or doripenem	Consider if previous infection with ESBL-producing gram (−) bacteria

Consider adding coverage of the following pathogens if at increased risk or if grown from cultures:

Methicillin-Resistant *Staphylococcus aureus* (MRSA)	Vancomycin, linezolid, or daptomycin	Consider adding based on clinical indications
Vancomycin-resistant *Enterococcus faecium* (VRE)	Linezolid or daptomycin	Consider if previous infection or colonization with VRE, especially in the setting of leukemia and/or hematopoiefic stem cell transplant (HSCT) recipients

Consider adding empiric antifungal therapy for prolonged fever 4–7 days, if no source identified:

Antifungal therapy	Triazole antifungal agents: voriconazole, posaconazole, itraconazole	Note that fluconazole is not recommended as empiric therapy due to poor activity against *Aspergillus* species.
	Echinocandin antifungal agents (caspofungin, anidulafungin, micafungin)	Preferred therapy if fluconazole prophylaxis given previously
	Amphotericin B preparations	Higher toxicity profile

Adapted from Freifeld AG, Bow EJ, Sepkowitz A, et al; Infectious Diseases Society of America. Clinical practice guideline for the use of antimicrobial agents in neutropenic patients with cancer: 2010 update by the infectious diseases society of America. *Clin Infect Dis* 2011;52(4):e56–e93.

    d. Patients who worsen clinically with sepsis, hemodynamic instability, or organ failure should have their diagnostic evaluation intensified and empiric therapy broadened to include resistant gram-positive and gram-negative bacteria, anaerobic bacteria, and fungi.

    e. Empirical antifungal therapy should be considered in patients with persistent fever after 4 to 7 days of empirical antibiotics.

V. DURATION OF TREATMENT

a. Both antibiotic selection and duration of therapy should be tailored toward the pathogen and site of infection whenever possible.

b. In patients in whom a source of infection or fever is not found, antibiotics should be continued until the ANC is ≥500 cells/mL.

VI. ANTIFUNGAL THERAPY

a. In high-risk patients with prolonged fever of 4 to 7 days, antifungal therapy targeting invasive fungal pathogens is recommended.

b. Antifungal agents for empiric treatment of neutropenic fever

   i. Voriconazole

   ii. Echinocandin antifungal agents (caspofungin, anidulafungin, micafungin)

   iii. Posaconazole

   iv. Liposomal amphotericin B

c. A targeted approach to identify invasive fungal infection should also accompany empiric antifungal therapy and may include

   i. Serum galactomannan assay (to identify invasive aspergillosis)

   ii. High-resolution CT scans of the chest and sinuses

VII. ANTIVIRAL THERAPY

a. It is not recommended to administer antiviral agent as empiric therapy, unless there is suspicion for underlying viral infection.

VIII. PROPHYLAXIS (TABLE 69-3)

Table 69-3	Prophylactic Antimicrobial Therapy for Febrile Neutropenia	
Prophylaxis	**Indication**	**Recommendation**
Antibiotic	High risk with anticipated ANC ≤100 for >7 days	Levofloxacin, ciprofloxacin
Antifungal	Induction chemotherapy for acute myelogenous leukemia (AML) or intensive therapy for advanced myelodysplastic syndrome (MDS)	Posaconazole
	Allogeneic HSCT recipients or intensive remission-induction or salvage induction chemotherapy for acute leukemia	Fluconazole Alternatives: voriconazole, itraconazole, posaconazole, echinocandins
	HSCT recipients with prior invasive *Aspergillus* sp., anticipated neutropenia ≥2 weeks, or prolonged neutropenia immediately prior to HSCT	Voriconazole Posaconazole Echinocandins

Table 69-3	Prophylactic Antimicrobial Therapy for Febrile Neutropenia (*Continued*)	
Prophylaxis	**Indication**	**Recommendation**
Antiviral	Herpes simplex virus (HSV)-seropositive autologous or allogeneic HSCT recipients, patients undergoing induction therapy for acute leukemia	Acyclovir
Hematopoietic growth factors (G-CSF)	Patients in whom the risk of fever and neutropenia is significant (≥20%)	Filgrastim, pegfilgrastim

Adapted from Freifeld AG, Bow EJ, Sepkowitz A, et al; Infectious Diseases Society of America. Clinical practice guideline for the use of antimicrobial agents in neutropenic patients with cancer: 2010 update by the infectious diseases society of America. *Clin Infect Dis* 2011;52(4):e56–e93.

SUGGESTED READINGS

de Naurois J, Novitzky-Basso I, Gill MJ, et al; ESMO Guidelines Working Group. Management of febrile neutropenia: ESMO Clinical Practice Guidelines. *Ann Oncol* 2010;21(suppl):v252–v256.

The European Society for Medical Oncology published this guideline on the management of neutropenic fever in 2010, which provides a concise, evidence-based summary of risk assessment, evaluation, and treatment.

Ellis M. Febrile neutropenia. *Ann N Y Acad Sci* 2008;1138:329–350.

This publication is a comprehensive review of febrile neutropenia and details the history of febrile neutropenia in cancer patients, epidemiology, shifts in bacteriology, evaluation, and treatment.

Freifeld AG, Bow EJ, Sepkowitz KA, et al; Infectious Diseases Society of America. Clinical practice guideline for the use of antimicrobial agents in neutropenic patients with cancer: 2010 update by the infectious diseases society of America. *Clin Infect Dis* 2011;52(4):e56–e93.

The Infectious Diseases Society of Amercia (IDSA) published this latest guideline in 2010, which provides an in-depth perspective on evaluation and management of cancer patients with neutropenic fever.

Klastersky J, Paesmans M, Rubenstein EB, et al. The Multinational Association for Supportive Care in Cancer risk index: a multinational scoring system for identifying low-risk febrile neutropenic cancer patients. *J Clin Oncol* 2000;18(16):3038–3051.

70 Influenza

Santosh Dhungana and Paul C. McNabb

INTRODUCTION

- Historically and clinically, influenza is the most important viral respiratory disease of mankind, killing up to 500,000 people every year on a global basis.
- RNA virus of the *Orthomyxoviridae* family
- Three types: Influenza A/B/C; A and B are the most important pathogens in humans.
- Virus consists of eight single strands of RNA contained in a lipoprotein envelope studded with two antigenic proteins:
  - Hemagglutinin (HA), with 16 known antigenic types, allows attachment and entry to host respiratory mucosa.
  - Neuraminidase (N), with nine known antigenic types, allows the budding of newly replicated virus from cells.
- Influenza A has an error-prone RNA polymerase, creating subtle changes in the nature of HA and N, resulting in *antigenic drift*. This is the main factor necessitating annual vaccination with the most current strains of virus.
- Influenza A can also undergo reassortment of the RNA genome. This occurs when two different viruses simultaneously coinfect a host cell, creating a novel combination of HA and N. This is called *antigenic shift* and is the cause of pandemic spread of influenza.
- There were three pandemics in the 20th century and thus far one in the 21st century. The 1918 pandemic resulted in 50 million deaths, most occurring disproportionately in healthy young adults.
- Influenza virus can at times cause zoonotic infection. This was shown to occur recently when avian influenza (H5N1), also known as bird flu, crossed species boundaries and caused human infection. Only rarely was the virus subsequently able to be transmitted person to person.
- The 2009 pandemic flu was a variant of seasonal H1N1. It was a quadruple reassortment of two swine strains, one human strain, and one avian strain.
- Influenza B has far lesser propensity for antigenic changes, and only antigenic drifts in the HA have been described.
- H3N2 and seasonal H1N1 are the two most common influenza A subtypes in circulation, in addition to influenza B.

EPIDEMIOLOGY

- Influenza causes an average of 200,000 hospitalizations and 41,000 deaths in a typical endemic year in the United States.[1,2]
- Elderly populations have the highest rate of hospitalization following influenza.[1]
- CDC in collaboration with WHO publishes weekly updates on the activity of influenza virus throughout the world, which is accessible at www.cdc.gov/flu/weekly.

- The peak influenza activity in northern latitudes is in late fall and winter, with late January and early February being the peak season in the United States.
- Infected individuals shed virus from 1 day prior and 5 to 6 days after the onset of symptoms[3] with peak at day 2 to 3. Prolonged shedding occurs in hospitalized patients with severe disease and immunocompromised patients.[4,5]
- Influenza virus is transmitted both by aerosols induced by cough/sneeze and by contact with contaminated surfaces.
- The virus is inactivated by sunlight, disinfectants, and detergents.

CLINICAL FEATURES

- During an epidemic period, the presence of fever, cough, and illness duration <7 days has a sensitivity of 78% and specificity of 73% of being influenza.[6] Other symptoms include sore throat, hoarseness, and myalgias.
- Most cases of influenza are self-limited, though complications occur with increased frequency in high-risk populations.
- High-risk populations include:
  - Unvaccinated infants 12 to 24 months of age
  - Patients 65 years and older
  - Patients with chronic pulmonary diseases like asthma, COPD, or cystic fibrosis
  - Patients with hemodynamically significant cardiac disease
  - Patients with hemoglobinopathies, chronic renal failure, cancer, and diabetes mellitus
  - Patients with neuromuscular, cognitive, or seizure disorders that impair handling of respiratory secretions
  - Residents of long-term care institutions
  - Patients on immunosuppressive medications or with immunosuppressive conditions including HIV.[7]
- Some influenza strains have the capacity to induce an uncontrolled and highly destructive immune response, largely mediated by proinflammatory cytokines, resulting in ARDS and multisystem organ failure. This response to infection is capable of inducing high case fatality rates in healthy individuals aged 18 to 40.[8]
- Complications include:
  - Secondary bacterial pneumonia:
    ○ Viral neuraminidase contributes to the adherence of *Streptococcus pneumoniae* and increases the chance of bacterial pneumonia.[9]
    ○ Pneumococcus is the most common bacterial pathogen, followed by *Staphylococcus aureus*, with increasing incidence of community-acquired MRSA.[10]
  - Viral pneumonia:
    ○ Radiographic manifestations include bilateral reticulonodular opacities with or without consolidation.
    ○ Patients with primary influenza pneumonia present more acutely than patients with uncomplicated disease and often develop respiratory failure.
  - Rare complications include:
    ○ Guillain-Barre syndrome[11]
    ○ Rhabdomyolysis and acute renal failure[12]
    ○ Aseptic meningitis and encephalitis
    ○ Transverse myelitis
    ○ Myocarditis and pericarditis
    ○ Reye syndrome with the use of salicylates in children[13,14]

DIAGNOSIS

- Diagnostic testing is recommended for patients presenting with ILI (influenza like illness) of <5 days duration:
  - Who are at high risk as described above
  - Who are hospitalized or develop symptoms during hospitalization
  - Elderly patients and infants with sepsis or fever of unknown origin
  - Healthcare workers in an institution that is experiencing an influenza outbreak
  - Returning travelers from a country epidemiologically linked to an influenza outbreak[7]
- Diagnostic tests include:
  - Rapid tests utilizing EIA (enzyme linked immunosorbent assay) for antigen detection. These results are available in 20 minutes, but false negatives are common. The test may not be able to distinguish between influenza A and B and the subtype of influenza A.
  - Direct or indirect immunofluorescence detection of antigen in respiratory epithelial cells. These tests have high sensitivity[15] but require fluorescence microscopy.
  - Reverse transcriptase polymerase chain reaction (RT-PCR). This is the most sensitive and specific method, and results are available in 2 hours. RT-PCR can differentiate between different subtypes of influenza A, including avian flu (H5N1) and pandemic H1N1.
  - Viral cultures. These are useful only for public health purposes, as they require careful transport and 3 to 10 days before results are known.
  - Serologic tests using EIA, complement fixation, or hemagglutination inhibition. These are not useful for timely clinical management and require paired serum samples.
- When influenza is circulating within the community, antiviral therapy may be appropriate based on clinical symptoms alone.[16]
- By contrast, patients who present outside the context of an influenza outbreak and are at low risk for complications should be tested before antiviral treatment.[17]
- Nasopharyngeal aspirates and swabs are the preferred specimens and have significantly higher yield than oropharyngeal specimens or sputum.[18]

TREATMENT

- Treatment with antiviral chemotherapy is recommended for patients with laboratory-confirmed or highly suspected influenza infection who present within 48 hours of symptom onset and are:
  - Desirous of shortening the duration of the illness
  - Hospitalized
  - At high risk of complications
  - In contact with persons at high risk of complications
  - Pregnant
  - Residents of a long-term care facility
  - Above 65 years of age
  - Manifesting signs of progressive disease[7]
- Treating high-risk patients even after the 48-hour window has passed has been shown to reduce complications.
- Neurominidase inhibitors are the most active antiviral agents:
  - Oseltamivir, 75 mg PO twice daily for 5 days
  - Zanamivir, 10 mg (two inhalations) twice daily for 5 days
  - Double dose in severely ill or immunocompromised patients or in avian influenza.[19]

- Zanamivir is contraindicated in those with reactive airway disease as it can cause severe bronchospasm.[20]
- Adamantanes (M2 protein inhibitors) including amantadine and rimantadine should not be used due to high level of resistance in both H3N2 and influenza B.[19,21]
- Early treatment reduces:
  - Symptomatology by approximately 1 day[22]
  - Lower respiratory tract complications[23]
  - Systemic complications[24]
  - Rate of hospitalizations[25]
  - Mortality
  - Viral shedding[26,27]
- Emerging resistance to oseltamivir has been reported in areas with widespread use of the drug secondary to a H275Y mutation.[21] The virus still remains sensitive to zanamivir, however.
- Newer agents undergoing trial include:
  - Single-dose inhaled laninamivir[28]
  - Single intravenous dose of peramivir[29]
  - Sialidase inhibitor
  - Polymerase inhibitor
  - Monoclonal antibodies[30]
  - Sphingosine analog[31]
- Patients with secondary bacterial pneumonia require treatment with third-generation cephalosporins or respiratory quinolones (levofloxacin or moxifloxacin) plus vancomycin if the suspicion for *S. aureus* is high.
- Salicylates should be avoided for symptom management in children and those <18 years of age due to risk of Reye syndrome.

PREVENTION

Avoidance:
- Includes:
  - Contact isolation of patients
  - Droplet precautions with facemasks[32]
  - Cough etiquette
  - Hand washing after caring for the patient
  - Ill healthcare workers refraining from work
  - Continued isolation for seven days after symptom onset or 24 hours after resolution of symptoms, whichever is longer
  - Prolonged isolation in children and the immunosuppressed due to long periods of viral shedding
- Airborne isolation utilizing N95 respirators appears unnecessary,[33] though it is recommended in the clinical setting where there is aerosol generation such as intubation, CPR, bronchoscopy, etc.

Immunization:

- Available types of vaccines include:
  - Intramuscular trivalent inactivated influenza vaccine (trade names: *Fluvirin, Fluzone, Fluarix*) containing the three seasonal strains (two influenza A and one influenza B) predicted by the WHO to be the dominant strains for the next flu season
  - Intranasal live attenuated influenza vaccine (LAIV) (trade name: *FluMist*)

- Higher dose inactivated influenza vaccine approved for use in patients above the age of 65.[34]
- Monovalent vaccines available for use during pandemics (2009 H1N1)
- Immunization is exceedingly important and is effective in reducing:
  - The incidence of pneumonia
  - Hospital admission for influenza as well as for respiratory/cardiac diseases and stroke[35]
  - All-cause mortality[36,37]
  - Influenza-associated antibiotic prescription[38]
  - Work absence and febrile respiratory illness in healthcare workers[39]
  - Mortality in healthcare institutions[40]
- Trivalent inactivated vaccine is recommended for the entire population before the start of influenza season.
- The degree of protection may vary widely (10% to 90%) depending on the antigenic match between the vaccine and the actual influenza virus circulating in the population.[41,42]
- Children under the age of 9 years require two doses separated by at least 4 weeks.
- Intranasal LAIV is approved by FDA for use in people up to the age of 49. LAIV seems to be more efficacious than the inactivated vaccine in children <6 years of age, while the reverse is true in the adult population.[43]
- LAIV is contraindicated in:
  - Immunosuppressed patients
  - Those at high risk of influenza complications
  - Pregnant women
  - Those with h/o Guillain-Barre syndrome[44]
- Adverse reactions to influenza immunization include local soreness at the injection site and nasal stuffiness/sore throat in the case of intranasal vaccine. Both vaccines are contraindicated in those with egg allergy.
- Dual pneumococcal and influenza vaccination is superior to either vaccine alone in reducing complications in the elderly.[45]
- Newer advances include:
  - Cell culture–derived vaccines[46]
  - Utilization of adjuvants to amplify the immune response, including oil-in-water emulsions
  - "Universal vaccines" utilizing highly preserved epitopes like the matrix 2 protein, which may provide long-lasting immunity[47]
  - Intradermal delivery allowing conservation of the vaccine during epidemics[48]

Chemoprophylaxis:

- Postexposure chemoprophylaxis is useful in a number of settings, including:
  - High-risk patients who did not get vaccinated
  - Allergy to egg
  - Other contraindications to vaccine
  - Immunosuppressed patients who are expected to have decreased efficacy to the vaccine
  - Those vaccinated within 2 weeks of exposure, as antibody response takes 2 weeks to develop [7]
  - Unvaccinated healthcare workers
  - Close contacts of person at high risk of developing influenza complications
  - All residents of long-term care facilities that are experiencing influenza outbreak, regardless of their vaccination status[7]

- Documented low level of antigenic match between the vaccine and the virus in circulation
- Vaccine shortage
- Recommended regimens include once daily dose of either oseltamivir (75 mg daily) or zanamivir (10 mg inhalation daily).[49,50]
- Chemoprophylaxis should be continued for at least 10 days following exposure in household setting and in high-risk populations, for as long as the virus is circulating in the community.[7]
- Adamantanes should be avoided as chemoprophylaxis.[51]

REFERENCES

1. Thompson WW, Shay DK, et al. Influenza-associated hospitalizations in the United States. *JAMA* 2004;292(11):1333–1340.
   National Hospital Discharge Survey (NHDS) data and WHO surveillance data were used and showed that significant numbers of influenza-associated hospitalizations in the United States occur among the elderly, and the numbers have increased substantially over the last 2 decades due in part to the aging of the population.
2. Dushoff J, Plotkin JB, et al. Mortality due to influenza in the United States–an annualized regression approach using multiple-cause mortality data. *Am J Epidemiol* 2006;163(2):181–187.
   This study estimates annual mortality from influenza via regression analysis.
3. Carrat F, Vergu E, et al. Time lines of infection and disease in human influenza: a review of volunteer challenge studies. *Am J Epidemiol* 2008;167(7):775–785.
   Volunteers are challenged with influenza virus to establish the time line of infection, viral shedding, and other characteristics of the disease.
4. Gooskens J, Jonges M, et al. Prolonged influenza virus infection during lymphocytopenia and frequent detection of drug-resistant viruses. *J Infect Dis* 2009;199(10):1435–1441.
   Prolonged influenza virus infection was associated with lymphocytopenia, lower respiratory tract infection, and development of drug resistance during antiviral therapy.
5. Lee N, Chan PK, et al. Viral loads and duration of viral shedding in adult patients hospitalized with influenza. *J Infect Dis* 2009;200(4):492–500.
   This 1-year prospective, observational study involving adults hospitalized with influenza showed that patients hospitalized with severe influenza have more active and prolonged viral replication.
6. Walsh EE, Cox C, et al. Clinical features of influenza A virus infection in older hospitalized persons. *J Am Geriatr Soc* 2002;50(9):1498–1503.
   Prospective study showing that older persons with fever, cough, and brief illness likely have diagnosis of influenza.
7. Harper SA, Bradley, JS. et al. Seasonal influenza in adults and children—diagnosis, treatment, chemoprophylaxis, and institutional outbreak management: clinical practice guidelines of the Infectious Diseases Society of America. *Clin Infect Dis* 2009;48(8): 1003–1032.
   Guidelines for the treatment of persons with influenza virus infection were prepared by an Expert Panel of the Infectious Diseases Society of America.
8. Osterholm MT. Preparing for the next pandemic. *N Engl J Med* 2005;352:1839–1842.
   Succinct review of pandemic influenza and its proposed mechanism to evoke a highly destructive immune response
9. Peltola VT, Murti KG, et al. Influenza virus neuraminidase contributes to secondary bacterial pneumonia. *J Infect Dis* 2005;192(2):249–257.
   Mouse model showing the causative role of neuraminidase in bacterial pneumonia.
10. Kallen AJ, Brunkard J, et al. *Staphylococcus aureus* community-acquired pneumonia during the 2006 to 2007 influenza season. *Ann Emerg Med* 2009;53(3):358–365.

S. aureus community-acquired pneumonia occurs with or after influenza. In this series, patients were often otherwise healthy young people and mortality rates were high.

11. Sivadon-Tardy V, Orlikowski D, et al. Guillain-Barre syndrome and influenza virus infection. *Clin Infect Dis* 2009;48(1):48–56.
    Case series on influenza virus infection as the cause of GBS.

12. Naderi AS, Palmer, BF. Rhabdomyolysis and acute renal failure associated with influenza virus type B infection. *Am J Med Sci* 2006;332(2):88–89.
    Case report on influenza causing rhadomyolysis.

13. Glasgow JF. Reye s syndrome: the case for a causal link with aspirin. *Drug Saf* 2006;29(12):1111–1121.
    Review article on Reye syndrome

14. Ninove L, Daniel L, et al. Fatal case of Reye's syndrome associated with H3N2 influenza virus infection and salicylate intake in a 12-year-old patient. *Clin Microbiol Infect* 2011;17(1):95–97.
    Case report of Reye syndrome in a 12-year-old male patient during an influenza A (H3N2) infection for which he received salicylates

15. Landry ML, Cohen S, et al. Real-time PCR compared to Binax NOW and cytospin-immunofluorescence for detection of influenza in hospitalized patients. *J Clin Virol* 2008;43(2):148–151.
    The accuracy of real-time RT-PCR should greatly improve the diagnosis of influenza in hospitals using simple rapid flu tests.

16. Monto AS, Gravenstein S, et al. Clinical signs and symptoms predicting influenza infection. *Arch Intern Med* 2000;160(21):3243–3247.
    Retrospective, pooled analysis of baseline signs and symptoms from phase 2 and 3 clinical trial participants reveals that when influenza is circulating within the community, patients with cough and fever are likely to have influenza.

17. Sintchenko V, Gilbert, GL. et al. Treat or test first? Decision analysis of empirical antiviral treatment of influenza virus infection versus treatment based on rapid test results. *J Clin Virol* 2002;25(1):15–21.
    Patients with flu-like illness, who present outside the influenza outbreak and are considered to be at low risk, should be tested to confirm the diagnosis before starting antiviral treatment.

18. Lieberman D, Shimoni A, et al. Identification of respiratory viruses in adults: nasopharyngeal versus oropharyngeal sampling. *J Clin Microbiol* 2009;47(11):3439–3443.
    This comparison of different methods of virus sampling showed that nasopharyngeal sampling has a higher rate of sensitivity than oropharyngeal sampling.

19. Fiore AE, Fry A, et al. Antiviral agents for the treatment and chemoprophylaxis of influenza—recommendations of the Advisory Committee on Immunization Practices (ACIP). *MMWR Recomm Rep* 2011;60(1):1–24.
    This report updates previous recommendations by CDC's Advisory Committee on Immunization Practices (ACIP) regarding the use of antiviral agents for the prevention and treatment of influenza.

20. Kiatboonsri S, Kiatboonsri C, et al. Fatal respiratory events caused by zanamivir nebulization. *Clin Infect Dis* 2010;50(4):620.
    Case series reporting fatal respiratory complications during zanamivir inhalational use.

21. Weinstock DM, Zuccotti, G. Adamantane resistance in influenza A. *JAMA* 2006;295(8):934–936.
    Review article on adamantane resistance.

22. Jefferson TO, Demicheli V, et al. Neuraminidase inhibitors for preventing and treating influenza in healthy adults. *Cochrane Database Syst Rev* 2006;3:CD001265.
    Cochrane database review that concluded that NIs have low effectiveness and should not be used in routine seasonal influenza but should be used in a serious epidemic or pandemic influenza.

23. Hernan MA, Lipsitch M.. Oseltamivir and risk of lower respiratory tract complications in patients with flu symptoms: a meta-analysis of eleven randomized clinical trials. *Clin Infect Dis* 2011;53(3):277–279.
   This independent reanalysis of 11 randomized clinical trials shows that oseltamivir treatment reduces the risk of lower respiratory tract disease.

24. Silagy CA, Campion, K. Effectiveness and role of zanamivir in the treatment of influenza infection. *Ann Med* 1999;31(5):313–317.
   Review article on the efficacy of Zanamivir

25. McGeer A, Green KA, et al. Antiviral therapy and outcomes of influenza requiring hospitalization in Ontario, Canada. *Clin Infect Dis* 2007;45(12):1568–1575.
   This prospective cohort study in Canada showed that treatment with antiviral drugs was associated with a significant reduction in mortality among patients hospitalized with influenza.

26. Nicholson KG, Aoki FY, et al. Efficacy and safety of oseltamivir in treatment of acute influenza: a randomised controlled trial. Neuraminidase Inhibitor Flu Treatment Investigator Group. *Lancet* 2000;355(9218):1845–1850.
   Oseltamivir is effective and well tolerated in the treatment of natural influenza infection in adults.

27. Ng S, Cowling BJ, et al. Effects of oseltamivir treatment on duration of clinical illness and viral shedding and household transmission of influenza virus. *Clin Infect Dis* 2010;50(5):707–714.
   Prospective study showing the efficacy of oseltamivir treatment.

28. Watanabe A, Chang SC, et al. Long-acting neuraminidase inhibitor laninamivir octanoate versus oseltamivir for treatment of influenza: A double-blind, randomized, noninferiority clinical trial. *Clin Infect Dis* 2010;51(10):1167–1175.
   Single inhalation laninamivir is effective for the treatment of seasonal influenza, including that caused by oseltamivir-resistant virus.

29. Kohno S, Kida H, et al. Efficacy and safety of intravenous peramivir for treatment of seasonal influenza virus infection. *Antimicrob Agents Chemother* 2010;54(11):4568–4574.
   Randomized trial showing the efficacy of single intravenous dose peramivir in subjects with uncomplicated seasonal influenza virus infection.

30. Koudstaal W, Koldijk MH, et al. Pre- and postexposure use of human monoclonal antibody against H5N1 and H1N1 influenza virus in mice: viable alternative to oseltamivir. *J Infect Dis* 2009;200(12):1870–1873.
   This murine study reveals that a single injection of monoclonal antibody against influenza outperforms a 5-day course of treatment with oseltamivir with respect to both prophylaxis and treatment of lethal H5N1 and H1N1 infections.

31. Marsolais D, Hahm B, et al. A critical role for the sphingosine analog AAL-R in dampening the cytokine response during influenza virus infection. *Proc Natl Acad Sci U S A* 2009;106(5):1560–1565.
   Sphingosine analogs display useful potential for controlling the immunopathology caused by influenza virus.

32. Cowling BJ, Chan KH, et al. Facemasks and hand hygiene to prevent influenza transmission in households: a cluster randomized trial. *Ann Intern Med* 2009;151(7):437–446.
   Face masks and hand hygiene are crucial in preventing influenza transmission.

33. Radonovich LJ, Bender BS. ACP Journal Club. Surgical masks were noninferior to N95 respirators for preventing influenza in health care providers. *Ann Intern Med* 2010;152(6):JC3–2.
   Simple surgical masks are as effective as N95 in the prevention of influenza in hospital setting.

34. Falsey AR, Treanor JJ, et al. Randomized, double-blind controlled phase 3 trial comparing the immunogenicity of high-dose and standard-dose influenza vaccine in adults 65 years of age and older. *J Infect Dis* 2009;200(2):172–180.

Use of high-dose influenza vaccine in elderly populations improves efficacy of immunization.

35. Nichol KL, Nordin J, et al. Influenza vaccination and reduction in hospitalizations for cardiac disease and stroke among the elderly. *N Engl J Med* 2003;348(14):1322–1332.
    In the elderly, vaccination against influenza is associated with reductions in hospitalization for heart disease, cerebrovascular disease, and pneumonia, as well as the risk of death from all causes during influenza seasons.

36. Jefferson TD, Rivetti D, et al. Efficacy and effectiveness of influenza vaccines in elderly people: a systematic review. *Lancet* 2005;366(9492):1165–1174.
    In long-term care facilities, where vaccination is most effective against complications, the aims of a vaccination campaign are fulfilled.

37. Talbot HK, Griffin MR, et al. Effectiveness of seasonal vaccine in preventing confirmed influenza-associated hospitalizations in community dwelling older adults. *J Infect Dis* 2011;203(4):500–508.
    Prospective study on the efficacy of seasonal vaccines.

38. Kwong JC, Maaten S, et al. The effect of universal influenza immunization on antibiotic prescriptions: an ecological study. *Clin Infect Dis* 2009;49(5):750–756.
    The Canadian province of Ontario introduced universal influenza immunization in 2000, offering free vaccines to the entire population. Universal immunization was associated with reduced influenza-associated antibiotic prescriptions.

39. Wilde JA, McMillan JA, et al. Effectiveness of influenza vaccine in health care professionals: a randomized trial. *JAMA* 1999;281(10):908–913.
    Influenza vaccine is effective in preventing infection by influenza A and B in health care professionals and may reduce reported days of work absence and febrile respiratory illness.

40. Carman WF, Elder AG, et al. Effects of influenza vaccination of health-care workers on mortality of elderly people in long-term care: a randomised controlled trial. *Lancet* 2000;355(9198):93–97.
    Vaccination of health care workers can reduce mortality in elderly patients.

41. Belongia EA, Kieke BA, et al. Effectiveness of inactivated influenza vaccines varied substantially with antigenic match from the 2004-2005 season to the 2006-2007 season. *J Infect Dis* 2009;199(2):159–167.
    This study illustrates how the antigenic match between the vaccine and the circulating strain of virus affects the efficacy of the vaccine.

42. Beran J, Vesikari T, et al. Efficacy of inactivated split-virus influenza vaccine against culture-confirmed influenza in healthy adults: a prospective, randomized, placebo-controlled trial. *J Infect Dis* 2009;200(12):1861–1869.
    Excellent study on efficacy of the inactivated split virus vaccine

43. Monto AS, Ohmit SE, et al. Comparative efficacy of inactivated and live attenuated influenza vaccines. *N Engl J Med* 2009;361(13):1260–1267.
    Randomized trial comparing the efficacy of inactivated and live attenuated vaccines during the influenza season.

44. Fiore AE, Uyeki TM, et al. Prevention and control of influenza with vaccines: recommendations of the Advisory Committee on Immunization Practices (ACIP), 2010. *MMWR Recomm Rep* 2010;59(RR-8):1–62.
    This report updates the 2009 recommendations by CDC's Advisory Committee on Immunization Practices (ACIP) regarding the use of influenza vaccine for the prevention and control of influenza.

45. Hung IF, Leung AY. Prevention of acute myocardial infarction and stroke among elderly persons by dual pneumococcal and influenza vaccination: a prospective cohort study. *Clin Infect Dis* 2010;51(9):1007–1016.
    In this important trial, dual vaccination with pneumococcal vaccine and trivalent influenza vaccine was effective in protecting elderly persons with chronic illness from developing complications from respiratory, cardiovascular, cerebrovascular diseases, and death.

46. Frey S, Vesikari T, et al. Clinical efficacy of cell culture-derived and egg-derived inactivated subunit influenza vaccines in healthy adults. *Clin Infect Dis* 2010;51(9):997–1004.
This trial compared the efficacy of cell culture–derived influenza vaccine (CCIV) and egg-derived trivalent inactivated vaccine (TIV) with placebo against laboratory-confirmed influenza illness in healthy adults. Both CCIV and TIV were effective in preventing influenza.

47. Lambert LC, Fauci, AS. Influenza vaccines for the future. *N Engl J Med* 2010;363(21): 2036–2044.
Future technologies in the pipeline for producing influenza vaccines.

48. Belshe RB, Newman FK, et al. Serum antibody responses after intradermal vaccination against influenza. *N Engl J Med* 2004;351(22):2286–2294.
Reduced dose intradermal vaccine is effective in certain age groups.

49. Welliver R, Monto AS, et al. Effectiveness of oseltamivir in preventing influenza in household contacts: a randomized controlled trial. *JAMA* 2001;285(6):748–754.
Excellent study showing the efficacy of postexposure prophylaxis with oseltamivir.

50. LaForce C, Man CY, et al. Efficacy and safety of inhaled zanamivir in the prevention of influenza in community-dwelling, high-risk adult and adolescent subjects: a 28-day, multicenter, randomized, double-blind, placebo-controlled trial. *Clin Ther* 2007;29(8): 1579–1590; discussion 1577–1578.
This study investigated the efficacy and safety of zanamivir in preventing influenza in community-dwelling adult and adolescent subjects at high risk for complications of influenza.

51. Hayden FG, de Jong MD. Emerging influenza antiviral resistance threats. *J Infect Dis* 2011;203(1):6–10.
Review article on emerging antiviral resistance amongst influenza viruses.

Lymphadenopathy and Fever

Jonathan P. Moorman

Generalized lymphadenopathy with associated fever is a symptom complex common to many different disease entities. Persistent generalized lymphadenopathy is defined as two or more extrainguinal sites lasting for 3 to 6 months with no other cause. Illnesses such as infection, autoimmune disorders, malignancy, and drug hypersensitivity may all present with fever and lymph node enlargement.

INFECTIOUS DISEASES

- The range of **infectious diseases** that can cause generalized lymphadenopathy is extensive, and initial evaluation of the patient will require a detailed history. Clinical clues may be found in the symptoms, a system review to include epidemiology, and the social/occupational history.
  - **Fungal diseases** such as histoplasmosis and coccidioidomycosis may be suggested by exposure history and geographic setting. A history of contact with sheep or employment in a slaughterhouse or drinking unpasteurized milk suggests **brucellosis** should be considered. Contact with ticks or rodents suggests the possibility of **tularemia**. Contact with cats might be a clue to **cat scratch disease** or **toxoplasmosis**. The patient should be asked about exposure to **tuberculosis** or travel to areas where **trypanosomal** or **leishmanial** organisms are endemic. Table 71-1 lists infectious diseases that have been associated with generalized lymphadenopathy.
  - A detailed history of sexual activities and risk factors for **AIDS** needs to be obtained. HIV disease may present with lymphadenopathy in association with **acute retroviral syndrome**. Generalized lymphadenopathy may occur in HIV disease in association with **non-Hodgkin lymphoma**. **Secondary syphilis** and **lymphogranuloma venereum** can also cause fever and diffuse lymphadenopathy with or without HIV disease.

AUTOIMMUNE DISORDERS

- In the evaluation of the patient with fever and lymphadenopathy, a history of joint pain, rash, other lupus clinical signs and symptoms, dry mouth, and dry eyes should be obtained.
- Rheumatoid arthritis, systemic lupus erythematosus (SLE), and Sjögren syndrome are the most common autoimmune disorders to cause lymphadenopathy.
- Lymphadenopathy is present in 75% of rheumatoid arthritis patients at some point in the illness. Enlarged nodes may or may not occur in association with inflamed joints, and fever is also common. Pathology will show reactive lymphoid hyperplasia.
- Lymphadenopathy occurs in 25% to 70% of patients with SLE. Fever and lymphadenopathy can be the initial symptoms.
- Sjögren syndrome will cause dry eyes and dry mouth with lymphocytic infiltration of salivary and lacrimal glands. Fever is less commonly associated with this syndrome.

Table 71-1	Infectious Causes of Generalized Lymphadenopathy

Streptococcal and Staphylococcal Infection
Bartonella spp. (cat scratch fever and bacillary angiomatosis)
Secondary syphilis
Tuberculosis/atypical mycobacteria
Brucellosis
Tularemia
T. whippeli (Whipple disease)
HIV disease—acute retroviral syndrome
CMV
Infectious mononucleosis

DRUG HYPERSENSITIVITY AND UNUSUAL SYSTEMIC DISEASES

- Hypersensitivity reactions to drugs are an increasingly common cause of diffuse lymphadenopathy. Fever, rash, or eosinophilia may be part of the syndrome.
- **Phenytoin, carbamazepine, sulfa drugs, and other antibiotics** are most commonly implicated, but many different drugs can produce this syndrome. Reactions occur within weeks to months of initiation of the medication. A wide range of pathology, from reactive hyperplasia to malignancy, may be seen.
- **Sarcoidosis** is a systemic disease of unknown cause that usually affects middle-aged adults. The disease usually presents with bilateral hilar adenopathy, skin lesions, pulmonary infiltrates, and ocular symptoms. The liver, spleen, salivary glands, kidneys, and central nervous system also may be involved. Histology shows noncaseating epithelioid granulomas. Fever and generalized lymphadenopathy would be an unusual presentation.
- **Whipple disease** is a systemic infectious disease presenting with fever, weight loss, arthralgia, and gastrointestinal symptoms of diarrhea and abdominal pain. The disease is caused by *Tropheryma whippeli*, an actinomycete, which can be seen on small bowel biopsy with periodic acid Schiff stain and can now be propagated in vitro. Peripheral lymphadenopathy as the sole clinical manifestation is rare but has been reported. The disease can mimic sarcoidosis or tuberculosis.

LYMPHOPROLIFERATIVE DISORDERS

- Benign and malignant lymphoproliferative disorders may present with fever and lymphadenopathy. Lymphoproliferative disorders that are benign, clonal, and malignant must be included in the differential diagnosis.
- **Kikuchi disease** is a benign reactive lymphoproliferative disorder with a histiocytic lymphadenitis; it is characterized by fever, leukopenia, and lymphadenopathy, which can be cervical or generalized, and resolves spontaneously after several months.
- **Castleman disease** is a rare atypical lymphoproliferative disorder that may present as benign lymphadenopathy; it has been associated with human herpesvirus-8 (HHV-8) and HIV.
- Atypical lymphoproliferative disorders have potential for developing a malignant phenotype. These include diseases such as angioimmunoblastic lymphadenopathy with dysproteinemia (AILD).

- **AILD** presents with a several-week history of fever, night sweats, weight loss, and generalized lymphadenopathy. Coombs-positive hemolytic anemia and polyclonal hypergammaglobulinemia are usually present. Lymph nodes are characterized by destruction of nodal architecture and a pleomorphic cellular infiltrate.
- The most likely lymphoproliferative disorders to present with fever and lymphadenopathy are **non-Hodgkin** and **Hodgkin lymphoma**.
- On physical examination, it must be determined whether lymph node enlargement is localized or generalized.
  - Localized adenopathy in the neck suggests pharyngitis or intraoral infection. Careful examination of the face, ears, throat, and mouth will follow.
  - Hodgkin disease may present as cervical adenopathy.
  - Enlarged posterior cervical nodes may be caused by scalp infection or systemic disease, such as toxoplasmosis.
  - If axillary adenopathy is the finding, examination of the breast and arms is most important. Cat scratch fever, staphylococcal and streptococcal infection, sporotrichosis, and lymphoma can cause isolated axillary adenopathy.
  - Isolated inguinal adenopathy is not uncommon in the general population but may be caused by infections of the genitalia or perineum.
- Generalized adenopathy, particularly when accompanied by night sweats and weight loss, should suggest the diagnosis of AIDS in any high-risk patient.
  - Lymphoma may present as generalized adenopathy but typically at advanced stages. Many infectious processes, as described in Table 71-1 and including infectious mononucleosis, toxoplasmosis, and cat scratch fever, present with generalized lymphadenopathy.

DIAGNOSIS

- The laboratory evaluation of fever and generalized adenopathy proceeds according to clinical clues. All patients should have a **complete blood count** (CBC), with review of a blood smear for atypical lymphocytes and other abnormal cells. If the patient appears toxic, **blood cultures** should be obtained to rule out subacute endocarditis, tularemia, or brucellosis.
  - A serologic test for Epstein-Barr virus (EBV), VDRL test for syphilis, IgM determination for toxoplasmosis, and HIV serology and HIV viral load testing for AIDS are indicated. A cytomegalovirus (CMV) IgM and PCR testing for CMV should be obtained.
  - Some authors have recommended that EBV, HIV, and CMV infection and toxoplasmosis be ruled out first, with the investigation then proceeding to diseases caused by other agents.
  - Agglutinin tests for brucellosis and tularemia and serology for histoplasmosis along with urine histoplasma antigen and serology for coccidioidomycosis may be obtained based on the index of suspicion for these processes.
  - Antinuclear antibody and rheumatoid factors may be supportive of a diagnosis of SLE or Still disease. A chest radiograph showing hilar adenopathy will require evaluation for tuberculosis, sarcoidosis, or lymphoma.
- Definitive diagnosis may require lymph node biopsy.
  - Slap et al. studied 123 young patients who had undergone biopsy of enlarged peripheral lymph nodes. In 42% of the cases, biopsy results led to specific treatment.

- Patients found to have granuloma or tumor were more likely to have abnormal findings on chest radiograph, lymph nodes >2 cm in diameter, a history of night sweats or weight loss, and a hemoglobin level of <10 g/dL.
- Patients with a recent history of ear, nose, and throat symptoms were less likely to have a biopsy result that led to specific therapy.
- Excisional biopsy is generally preferred.
  - Fluctuant nodes and needle aspiration may be sufficient for diagnosis.
  - Inguinal nodes should be avoided for biopsy because they frequently show non-specific reactive hyperplasia.
  - Supraclavicular nodes and scalene nodes have the highest yield.
  - The node itself should be divided between the pathology and microbiology laboratories.
- When a definitive diagnosis cannot be made by biopsy, careful follow-up is required.
  - If anemic, bone marrow biopsy may be considered.
  - If the patient has an associated hepatitis, liver biopsy may be considered.

SUGGESTED READINGS

Alkan S, Beals TF, Schnitzer B. Primary diagnosis of Whipple disease manifesting as lymphadenopathy: use of polymerase chain reaction for detection of Tropheryma whippelii. *Am J Clin Pathol* 2001;116:898.

Bonekamp D, et al. Castleman's Disease: the Great Mimic. *Radiographics* 2011;31(6):1793–1807.

Brown JR, Skarin AT. Clinical mimics of lymphoma. *Oncologist* 2004;9:406.
  Comprehensive review of conditions that must be differentiated from lymphoma, including differential for lymphadenopathy and fever

Bujak JS, et al. Juvenile rheumatoid arthritis presenting in the adult as fever of unknown origin. *Medicine (Baltimore)* 1973;52:431.

Case records of the Massachusetts General Hospital. Weekly clinicopathological exercises. Case 30-1977. *N Engl J Med* 1977;297:206–211.
  A discussion of the pathology of Hodgkin disease, toxoplasmosis, angioimmunoblastic lymphadenopathy, and Lennert lesion

Chau I, et al. Rapid access multidisciplinary lymph node diagnostic clinic: analysis of 550 patients. *Br J Cancer* 2003;88:354.
  Most patients with diffuse lymphadenopathy had toxoplasmosis, tuberculosis, HIV disease, or EBV infection.

De Vriese AS, et al. Carbamazepine hypersensitivity syndrome: report of four cases and review of the literature. *Medicine* 1995;74:144.

Greenfield S, Jordan MC. The clinical investigation of lymphadenopathy in primary care practice. *JAMA* 1978;240:1388.
  This review provides an algorithm for the investigation of lymphadenopathy. Newer technologies such as PCR are not addressed.

Hjalgrim H, et. al. Characteristics of Hodgkin's lymphoma after infectious mononucleosis. *N Engl J Med* 2003;349:1324.

Lamp LW, Scott MA. Cat scratch disease: historical, clinical, and pathologic perspective. *Am J Clin Path* 2004;121:S71.

Melikoglu MA, Melikoglu M. The clinical importance of lymphadenopathy in systemic lupus erythematosus. *Acta Reumatol Port* 2008;33(4):402–406.

Montoya JG, Remington JS. Studies on the serodiagnosis of toxoplasmic lymphadenitis. *Clin Infect Dis* 1995;20:781.

Saltzstein SL, Ackerman IV. Lymphadenopathy induced by anticonvulsant drugs and mimicking clinically and pathologically malignant lymphomas. *Cancer* 1959;12:164.

Sinclair S, Beckman E, Ellman L. Biopsy of enlarged superficial lymph nodes. *JAMA* 1974;228:602.

Slap GB, Brooks JSJ, Schwartz JS. When to perform biopsies of enlarged peripheral lymph nodes in young patients. *JAMA* 1984;252:1321.

This study reviews the records of 123 young patients to determine which had biopsy results that led to a specific therapy. Those with abnormal findings on chest x-ray films, a node >2 cm, night sweats, or weight loss benefited from biopsy diagnosis.

72 Fever of Unknown Origin

Amit Kalra and Jonathan P. Moorman

DEFINITION

Fever of unknown origin (FUO) was defined by Petersdorf and Beeson in 1962:

1. Temperature of >101°F (38.3°C) on several occasions
2. Duration of fever >3 weeks
3. Failure to reach diagnosis despite 1 week of inpatient investigations

Durack and Street recommended another revised system of classification of FUO:

1. Classic
2. Nosocomial
3. Neutropenic
4. HIV-associated FUO

Newer definition of FUO outlines describes three outpatient visits or 3 days in the hospital without finding the cause for fever, or 1 week of intensive investigations.

ETIOLOGIES

1. **Infections:** (most common cause)
   A. Bacterial: localized or systemic
      - Pyogenic infections: appendicitis, cholecystitis, diverticulitis, dental abscess, liver abscess, osteomyelitis, pelvic inflammatory disease, pancreatitis abscess, perirectal abscess, sinusitis, suppurative thrombophlebitis, recurrent aspiration
      - Systemic infections: subacute bacterial endocarditis, gonococcemia, Lyme disease, Legionnaires disease, leptospirosis, borreliosis, salmonellosis
   B. Mycobacterial: tuberculosis
   C. Fungal: cryptococcus, histoplasmosis
   D. Rickettsial
   E. Mycoplasma
   F. Chlamydia
   G. Viral: CMV, EBV, HIV, viral hepatitis
   H. Parasitic: malaria, toxoplasmosis, trypanosomiasis
2. **Neoplasms:** benign or malignant
   A. Lymphoma
   B. Leukemia
   C. Renal cell carcinoma
   D. Hepatocellular carcinoma
   E. Atrial myxoma

3. **Connective tissue disorders:** lupus, polymyalgia rheumatica, giant cell arteritis
4. **Granulomatous disease:** sarcoidosis, granulomatous hepatitis
5. **Metabolic and inherited diseases including endocrine causes:** thyroiditis, pheochromocytoma
6. **Thermoregulatory disorder**
7. **Miscellaneous causes:**
    - **A.** Drugs, including allopurinol, antihistamine, aspirin, clofibrate, erythromycin, captopril, quinidine, nitrofurantoin, penicillins
    - **B.** Deep vein thrombosis
    - **C.** Pulmonary embolism
    - **D.** Superficial thrombophlebitis
    - **E.** Factitious fever
    - **F.** Postmyocardial infarction
    - **G.** Hematoma
    - **H.** Periodic fever
    - **I.** Gout/pseudogout
    - **J.** Familial Mediterranean fever

EVALUATION OF PATIENT WITH FUO: GENERAL APPROACH

FUO is a diagnostic challenge for the internists and infectious disease specialists. Initial workup starts with a detailed comprehensive history, including but not limited to country of origin of the patient, travel history, exposure to pets, occupational history, past medical history including history of exposures to drugs (immunosuppressive, immunomodulatory, monoclonal antibodies), and occupational history. Sometimes, repeat history from the patient and even the family members and friends is of worth in refining the diagnostic cues to find the underlying cause of the fever. A complete physical examination is key. This can be supplemented with basic laboratory studies to include complete blood count, blood chemistries with liver function tests, blood cultures, and urinalysis with cultures. Any expensive investigation must be weighed considering in mind the benefits versus cost and the concrete need for the requested investigation.

PHYSICAL EXAMINATION

- General appearance
- HEENT (head, eyes, with funduscopic examination, ears, nose, throat)
- Mucosa: oral or genital ulceration, mucous patches, vesiculations, urethral or genital discharge
- Cutaneous: complete cutaneous examination for any evidence of rash, any parasitic infestation, vesiculobullous disease, ulceration, palms and soles, pressure ulcer sites, interdigital web spaces, intravenous line sites, costochondral tenderness, temporal tenderness, any rash in a dermatomal pattern
- Nails: splinter hemorrhages, onycholysis, ingrown toenail
- Neck: lymphadenopathy, thyroid mass
- Heart: rub, murmur
- Lungs: rub, rales
- Abdomen: localized or diffuse tenderness, hepatosplenomegaly
- Pelvic examination: cervical motion tenderness, adnexal tenderness, masses

- Rectal: any ulceration or prostate tenderness
- Musculoskeletal: joint effusion

LABORATORY WORKUP

- Complete blood count with differential
- Blood chemistries with liver function test including the serum bilirubin
- Peripheral blood smear
- Urinalysis
- Urine culture
- Blood culture
- Sputum culture
- C-reactive protein
- Erythrocyte sedimentation rate
- VDRL
- HIV testing
- Fluid culture
- Lumbar puncture
- Bone marrow aspiration (with biopsy) for culture and histopathology
- PPD skin testing
- Connective tissue profile (ANA, rheumatoid factor)
- Fungal serology
- Viral serology or PCR

DIAGNOSTIC IMAGING

- Chest x-ray
- Echocardiogram (transthoracic echocardiogram/transesophageal echocardiogram to exclude any valvular vegetation)
- CT chest/abdomen/pelvis with oral and/or intravenous contrast
- Gallium or indium or FDG PET scans

TREATMENT

Any treatment of FUO that is infectious in origin should be targeted with specific antibiotics with suitable dose and duration. If the cause of the fever is unknown, empiric antibiotics or steroids should be withheld pending evaluation unless the patient is hemodynamically unstable or immunocompromised. Steroids and antipyretic agents can conceal the pattern of the fever, can mask important clinical clues, and can lead to partial treatments with relapse; antipyretics rarely make patients more comfortable. In cases of suspected drug fever, a trial of holding the suspected drug can be helpful. Any patient with undiagnosed weight loss or other constitutional signs and symptoms should be referred for the appropriate consultation(s).

PROGNOSIS

General prognosis for FUO depends upon the underlying etiology of the fever. About 5% to 15% of patients remain undiagnosed, but the majority of these recover. FUO lasting more than 6 months carries a good prognosis but requires repeat evaluations and testing as appropriate.

SUGGESTED READINGS

Cunha BA. Fever of unknown origin: focused diagnostic approach based on clinical clues from the history, physical examination, and laboratory tests. *Infect Dis Clin North Am* 2007;21:1137–1187.

This review provides an excellent compendium of the various causes of FUO based upon frequency of occurrence. The clinical summaries table also provides reasonable diagnostic measures.

Durack DT, Street AC. Fever of unknown origin—reexamined and redefined. In: Remington JS, Swartz MN, eds. *Current clinical topics in infectious diseases*, vol III. Boston, MA: Blackwell Science; 1991:35–51.

Knockaert DC, Vanneste LJ, Vannester SB, et al. Fever of unknown origin in the 1980s: an update of the diagnostic spectrum. *Arch Intern Med* 1992;152:51–55.

Knockaert DC, Dujardin KS, Bobbaers HJ. Long-term follow up of patients with undiagnosed fever of unknown origin. *Arch Intern Med* 1996;156(6):618–620.

This study followed 61 individuals with FUO for which a diagnosis could not be made despite evaluation in the hospital setting. They found that FUO was rarely the ultimate cause of death.

Mayo J, Collazos J, et al. Fever of unknown origin in the setting of HIV infection: guidelines for a rational approach. *AIDS Patient Care STDS* 1998;12:373–378.

This guideline provides a reasonable approach to FUO in the setting of HIV, with the most common etiologies (disseminated MAC, PCP, CMV, and lymphoma) being discussed.

Meller J, Sahlmann CO, Scheel AK. 18F-FDG PET and PET/CT in fever of unknown origin. *J Nucl Med* 2007;48:35–45.

Petersdorf RG, Beeson PB. Fever of unexplained origin: report on 100 cases. *Medicine* 1961;40:1–30.

This classic report details the underlying causes of FUO in a large cohort of patients, describing the three major etiologies: infections, malignancy, and connective tissue disorders.

Epstein-Barr Virus

Amit Kalra and Jonathan P. Moorman

INTRODUCTION

Epstein-Barr virus (EBV) belongs to the family of gamma herpesviridae. EBV is a double-stranded DNA lymphocytotropic virus that induces both latent and lytic infection in animals and humans. This virus can cause not only primary infection but also lymphoproliferative disorders including lymphoreticular malignancies and other systemic manifestations.

EPIDEMIOLOGY

EBV infection is ubiquitous throughout the world, and 95% of individuals generate antibodies to the virus by the time they reach adulthood. In the United States, the peak incidence is from ages 15 to 24, and the overall incidence is approximately 500 cases/100,000/year. In developing countries or lower socioeconomic populations, children contract the infection at an early age. Infection spreads primarily through salivary secretions or occasionally through sexual contact.

PATHOGENESIS AND MICROBIOLOGY OF EBV INFECTION

- EBV is a linear DNA virus with core DNA surrounded by capsid and glycoprotein.
- Primary target cells of EBV are human epithelial cells, human B cells, T cells, salivary gland cells, natural killer (NK) cells, macrophages/monocytes, and endothelial cells.
- Reservoir for infection is the latently infected B cell.
- Incubation period from infection to symptoms is 30 to 50 days.
- A robust CD4+ and CD8+ T-cell response may be responsible for the clinical syndrome of mononucleosis.

CLINICAL FEATURES OF EBV-INDUCED INFECTIOUS MONONUCLEOSIS

- Often subclinical in early childhood
- Classic EBV infection is characterized by the triad of pharyngitis, fever, and lymphadenopathy.
- Myalgia, headache, malaise, headache, anorexia, abdominal discomfort, chills, arthralgia, rash, hepatomegaly, splenomegaly, and jaundice may occur.
- Treatment with ampicillin will lead to a rash in the vast majority of patients.
- Complications include splenic rupture, neurologic involvement, airway obstruction, hepatitis, hemolytic anemia, and cytopenias.
- Differential diagnosis would include streptococcal pharyngitis, acute HIV infection, lymphoma, cytomegalovirus (CMV), Bartonella infection/cat scratch disease, drug reactions, viral hepatitis, measles, mumps, rubella, roseola, secondary syphilis, and toxoplasmosis.

Major Diseases Attributed to EBV

Primary Infections	Lymphoproliferative Disorders
Infectious mononucleosis	Burkitt lymphoma
Meningoencephalitis	Hodgkin lymphoma
Gianotti-Crosti syndrome	Nasopharyngeal carcinoma
Hemophagocytic syndrome	CNS lymphoma in AIDS
	HIV-associated oral hairy leukoplakia
	Leiomyosarcoma (immunosuppressed)
	Posttransplant lymphoproliferative disorders (PTLD)

Less Common Systemic Manifestations of EBV Infection

Cranial nerve palsies (VII most common)
Guillain-Barre syndrome
Acute transverse myelitis
Peripheral neuritis
Encephalitis
Laryngotonsillar obstruction
Autoimmune hemolytic anemia
Myocarditis
Pericarditis
Interstitial nephritis
Vasculitis
Hepatitis
Hypo-/hypergammaglobulinemia

LABORATORY EVALUATION

- Common findings include lymphocytosis (approximately 75% of patients will have elevations >60% to 70%); atypical lymphocytes of >10% are commonly noted.
- Leukemoid reactions
- Thrombocytopenia or neutropenia may be seen.
- Elevated hepatic transaminases, LDH, and/or alkaline phosphatase are often seen.

Interpretation of Serology

- **Heterophile antibodies**: These are nonspecific IgM antibodies, which rely on the polyclonal activation of the B cells. A heterophile antibody titer of more than 1:40 is usually diagnostic for infectious mononucleosis in patients with clinical features of infectious mononucleosis and atypical lymphocytes. It is not diagnostic of EBV infection per se because infectious mononucleosis can be caused by other infectious agents as well. These tests are not reliable in children under age 12.
- **Viral capsid antigen (VCA) antibodies**: IgM and IgG antibodies to VCA along with heterophile antibodies are the most commonly used antibodies tested in clinical practice for determination of EBV infection. IgM antibodies generally denote

acute infection, and IgG antibodies denote the evidence of prior infection, or the stage of convalescence. VCA IgG antibody titer develops in the initial 2 to 3 months postinfection and can be found in more than 90% of infected individuals.

- **Epstein-Bars Nuclear Antigen (EBNA) antibody**: EBNA IgG antibodies are produced late in the infection; their presence generally indicates prior infection.
- **EBV DNA**: Quantitative EBV DNA has been found to be useful in AIDS patients with lymphoma and has been used in the setting of organ transplantation, PTLD, and nasopharyngeal carcinoma. While preserved primarily for immunosuppressed individuals, EBV DNA is detectable at high levels in the setting of acute infectious mononucleosis but drops to low or undetectable levels after several weeks to months. A healthy carrier may have detectable EBV DNA in whole blood at steady state but at very low levels (1 to 50 copies EBV DNA/1×10^6 white blood cells).

Interpretation of EBV Serologies

	VCA IgG	VCA IgM	EBNA IgG
Acute EBV	Positive/negative	Positive	Negative
Chronic EBV	Positive	Negative	Positive

TREATMENT OPTIONS

Treatment of the EBV is usually supportive in nature, and the majority recover with no sequelae. Acyclovir has been used in the management of oral hairy leukoplakia due to the lytic nature of EBV in this disease; relapse upon cessation is common. Steroids have been generally reserved for the treatment of severe thrombocytopenia, autoimmune hemolytic anemia, myocarditis, pericarditis, neurologic complications, and for significant pharyngeal edema due to lymphadenopathy. There is still no definite therapeutic option for the management of the EBV infection.

SUGGESTED READINGS

Balfour HH Jr, et al. A virologic pilot study of valacyclovir in infectious mononucleosis. *J Clin Virol* 2007;39:16–21.
   This randomized study found that treatment with valacyclovir leads to decreased EBV shedding during therapy and reduced severity of symptoms, but no differences in EBV DNA viral loads between treatment and control populations.
Candy B, Hotopf M. Steroids for symptom control in infectious mononucleosis. *Cochrane Database Syst Rev* 2006;3:CD004402.
   This Cochrane review found insufficient evidence for a benefit from steroids for EBV infection based on the limited literature.
Gulley ML, Tang W. Laboratory assays for Epstein-Barr virus-related disease. *J Mol Diagnostics* 2008;10:279–292.
   This excellent review article discusses the current laboratory assessments for EBV infection, including the role of testing in the setting of EBV-related tumors developing following immunosuppression.
Iwatsuki K, Yamamoto T, Tsuji K, et al. A spectrum of clinical manifestations caused by host immune responses against Epstein-Barr virus infections. *Acta Med Okayama* 2004;58(4):169–180.

Klutts JS, Ford BA, Perez NR, et al. Evidence-based approach for interpretation of Epstein-Barr virus serological patterns. *J Clin Microbiol* 2009;47(10):3204–3210.

Luzuriaga K, Sullivan JL. Infectious Mononucleosis. *N Engl J Med* 2010;362:1993–2000.
   This review article provides an excellent resource for the general understanding of EBV infection leading to infectious mononucleosis. The author concisely discusses treatment modalities.

Miller, M. Epstein–Barr virus biology, pathogenesis, and medical aspects. In: Fields BN, Knipe DM, eds. *Virology*. 2nd ed. New York, NY: Raven Press; 1990:1921–1958.

Straus SE, Cohen JI, Tosato G, et al. *Ann Intern Med* 1993;118(1):45–58.

Index

Pages followed by f indicate figures; pages followed by t indicate tables.

A

Abacavir
 drug interactions in, 22t
 pregnancy and HIV infection, 44t
Acanthamoeba, encephalitis, 138t
Acid-fast negative protozoans, 187–188t
Acid-fast organisms, 189t
Acinetobacter baumannii, carbapenem-resistant, 304t
Acinetobacter spp.
 antimicrobial therapy, 430
 breakpoints for, 419t
Acquired immunodeficiency syndrome (AIDS). *See* Human immunodeficiency virus (HIV)
Acyclovir
 for genital herpes, 88–89, 88t, 89t
 for herpes zoster, 143t
 intermittent hemodialysis and continuous renal replacement therapy, 467t
 in pregnancy, 525
 varicella-zoster virus disease, 13t, 14t
Adefovir, hepatitis B infection, 56t
Adenoviruses, enteric, traveler's diarrhea, 192
Adjusted body weight (ABW), 457t, 458t
Adult immunizations, HIV infection, 40
Aeromonas, treatment of, 190t
African spotted fever, 198t
Albendazole, diarrhea, 385t
Amikacin, 439
 aminoglycosides, therapeutic drug monitoring, 447, 448t
 breakpoints, 418t, 419t
 health care-associated urinary tract infection, 263t
 intermittent hemodialysis and continuous renal replacement therapy, 467t
 peritoneal dialysis, 470t
Aminoglycosides
 Mycobacterium avium complex (MAC), 553t
 obesity effects on, 457t
 therapeutic drug monitoring
  high-dose extended interval method, 447, 447t, 449
  recommended therapeutic goals, dosing, and monitoring, 448t
  three-compartment model, 446–447
  traditional dosing method, 447
Amitriptyline, for postherpetic neuralgia, 144t

Amoxicillin
 anthrax, 519
 Chlamydia trachomatis, 83
Amoxycillin-clavulinic acid, for animal bites, 321t
Amphotericin, 485–486
 adverse reactions, 485t
 peritoneal dialysis, 470t
Amphotericin B
 candidiasis, 493t
 cryptococcal meningitis, 11t
 cryptococcosis, 494t
 dimorphic fungi, 496t
 endemic fungal infections, 405
 Histoplasma capsulatum infections, 12t
 for histoplasmosis, 408–409t
 lipid-associated formulations, 486
Ampicillin, 298
 breakpoints, 418t
 for endocarditis, infectious, 239t, 240t
 Enterobacteriaceae, innate resistance of, 427t
 intermittent hemodialysis and continuous renal replacement therapy, 467t
 for meningitis, acute bacterial, 127, 127t
 peritoneal dialysis, 470t
 for prosthetic joint infections, 578t
 renal impairment, antibiotic dosage adjustments, 463t
Ampicillin-sulbactam
 Bacteroides group organisms, percent resistance of, 433t
 breakpoints, 418t
 for endocarditis, infectious, 242t
 Enterobacteriaceae, innate resistance of, 427t
 intermittent hemodialysis and continuous renal replacement therapy, 467t
 non-*Bacteroides* group organisms, percent resistance of, 433t
 pelvic inflammatory disease, 76t
 peritoneal dialysis, 470t
 renal impairment, antibiotic dosage adjustments, 463t
Amprenavir, minimum trough concentrations, 452t
Anaerobes, 432
Anal warts, recommended regimens, 96
Anaplasma phagocytophilum. See Human granulocytic anaplasmosis
Anemia, hemolytic, 212